Essentials
for
Health
and
Wellness

Essentials for Health and Wellness

SECOND EDITION

Gordon Edlin

John A. Burns School of Medicine
University of Hawaii

Eric Golanty

Las Positas College

Kelli McCormack Brown

Department of Community and Family Health
University of South Florida

Jones and Bartlett Publishers

Sudbury, Massachusetts
Boston   Toronto   London   Singapore

World Headquarters
Jones and Bartlett Publishers
40 Tall Pine Drive
Sudbury, MA 01776
978-443-5000
info@jbpub.com
www.jbpub.com

Jones and Bartlett Publishers Canada
2100 Bloor Street West
Suite 6-272
Toronto, ON M6S 5A5
CANADA

Jones and Bartlett Publishers International
Barb House, Barb Mews
London W6 7PA
UK

All resource addresses, telephone numbers and web addresses found in Essentials for Health and Wellness, Second Edition have been checked and are correct at time of printing. Jones and Bartlett Publishers is not responsible for changes in resource addresses, telephone numbers or web addresses.

Library of Congress Cataloging-in-Publication Data
Edlin, Gordon, 1932–
    Essentials for health and wellness / Gordon Edlin, Eric Golanty, Kelli McCormack
Brown.—2nd ed.
        p. ; cm.
    Includes bibliographical references and index
    ISBN 0-7637-1154-3 (annotated instructor's ed. : pbk.) — ISBN 0-7637-0909-3 (student
ed. : pbk.)
        1. Health. 2. Holistic medicine. I. Golanty, Eric. II. Brown, Kelli McCormack. III.
Title.
    [DNLM: 1. Holistic Health. W 61 E23e 1999]
    RA776 .E239 1999
    613—dc21   99-044542

Student Edition ISBN 0-7637-0909-3

Chief Executive Officer: Clayton E. Jones
Chief Operating Officer: Donald W. Jones, Jr
President: Tom Walker
V.P., Sales and Marketing: Tom Manning
V.P., Senior Managing Editor: Judith H. Hauck
V.P., Director of Interactive Technology: Mike Campbell
Director of Production and Design: Anne Spencer
Manufacturing Director: Therese Bräuer
Senior Acquisitions Editor: Paul Shepardson
Associate Editor: Amy Austin
Senior Marketing Manager: Jennifer M. Jacobson

Developmental Editor: Ohlinger Publishing Services
Senior Production Editor: Lianne Ames
Production Editor: Linda S. DeBruyn
Design: Merce Wilczek
Editorial Production Services, Typesetting:
    The Clarinda Company
Anatomical Illustration: Imagineering Scientific and
    Technical Artworks
Cover Design: Stephanie Torta
Printing and Binding: Banta
Cover Printing: Banta

Unless otherwise acknowledged, all photographs are the property of Jones and Bartlett Publishers

Printed in the United States of America
03 02 01 00 99 10 9 8 7 6 5 4 3 2 1

Brief Contents

Contents

Part 2   Eating and Exercising Toward a Healthy Life-Style   59

Part 5   Explaining Drug Use and Abuse   251

Part **6** Making Healthy Choices 301

Feature Contents

Global Wellness

Preface for the Student

Our goal in writing this textbook is to provide you with the information you need to understand and implement the basic principles of physical, mental, and spiritual wellness. We have provided the most up-to-date tools, information, exercises, and humor to motivate you toward making healthy changes in your life and developing a life-style that will promote lifelong wellness. We believe that the key to health is self-responsibility for one's behaviors (both positive and negative)—for overeating or undereating, for drinking alcohol or smoking, for taking drugs or engaging in stressful activities, and for living in harmony with the environment. We also believe that health involves our entire being and is not a matter of repairing broken parts.

What does it mean to be healthy and well? Often, we equate health with being a certain ideal weight, exercising regularly, not smoking, or never catching a cold. But a holistic view of health encompasses many more of our behaviors. Answer the following questions and see if your opinion about your health changes:

- If you drink, do you drink responsibly (e.g., you do not get drunk or drink and then drive)?
- Do you get enough sleep (at least 8 hours a night)?
- Are you able to cope with stressful situations without getting angry, anxious, or depressed?
- Are your interpersonal relationships satisfying?
- If you are sexually active, do you use fertility control and practice safer sex?
- Does your diet consist of fast food, pizza, and ice cream?
- Do you exercise regularly?
- Do you take time to enjoy nature?
- Are you involved in your community?

Remember, we all engage in unhealthy behaviors from time to time, but you should know that these behaviors are things that you can change. Wellness is a process, not a place. We hope that, in your use of this textbook, you will become aware of your unhealthy behaviors, and we hope that we can motivate you to change and give you some strategies for making that change. We want you to achieve lifelong wellness through self-responsibility.

We have developed a number of features to help you in your study of the material.

Each chapter begins with a list of Learning Objectives to help you focus on the most important concepts in that chapter.

Learning Objectives

1. Explain Maslow's hierarchy of needs and the role it plays in emotional wellness.
2. Identify several strategies for coping with emotional distress.
3. Identify several defense mechanisms.
4. Identify and explain fear and phobia.
5. Explain the characteristics of depression.
6. Discuss the prevalence and several signs of suicide.
7. Discuss the importance of sleep for mental well-being.
8. Identify characteristics of schizophrenia.

Key Terms are defined on the page on which they are introduced. For review, terms are available in a flash card format on the text's website (www.jbpub.com/hwonline).

Epigrams enliven each chapter with both serious and humorous quotations about health.

Certain key topics in each chapter are highlighted with a **Web Icon**, 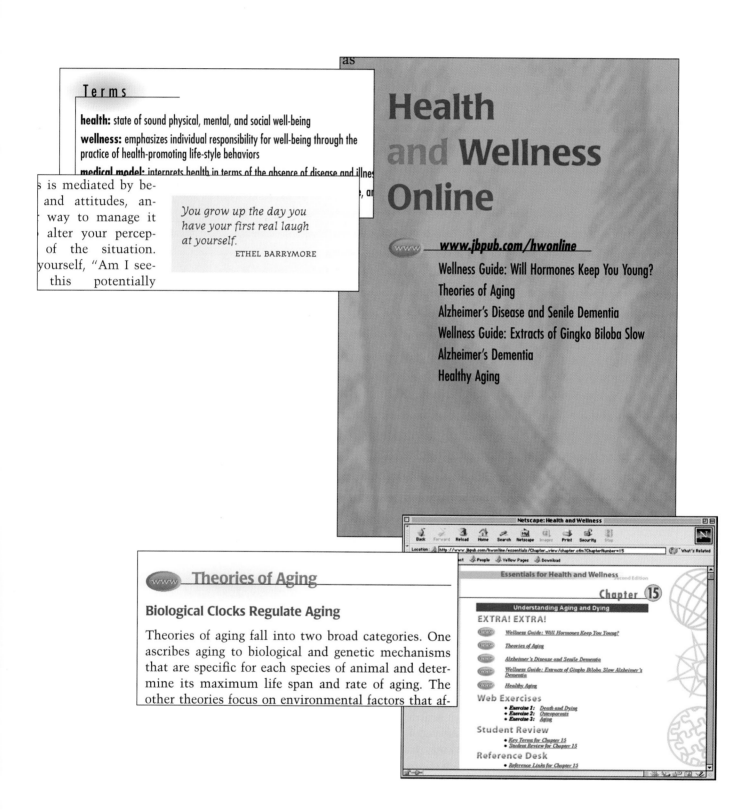 indicating that additional or up-to-date information is available on the website. **Health and Wellness Online** (www.jbpub.com/hwonline) is a valuable resource for you to use for research, to prepare for tests, or just to find out more about a topic.

Terms

health: state of sound physical, mental, and social well-being

wellness: emphasizes individual responsibility for well-being through the practice of health-promoting life-style behaviors

medical model: interprets health in terms of the absence of disease and illnes

s is mediated by be- and attitudes, an- way to manage it alter your percep- of the situation. yourself, "Am I see- this potentially

You grow up the day you have your first real laugh at yourself.
ETHEL BARRYMORE

Health and Wellness Online

www.jbpub.com/hwonline

Wellness Guide: Will Hormones Keep You Young?

Theories of Aging

Alzheimer's Disease and Senile Dementia

Wellness Guide: Extracts of Gingko Biloba Slow

Alzheimer's Dementia

Healthy Aging

Theories of Aging

Biological Clocks Regulate Aging

Theories of aging fall into two broad categories. One ascribes aging to biological and genetic mechanisms that are specific for each species of animal and determine its maximum life span and rate of aging. The other theories focus on environmental factors that af-

Netscape: Health and Wellness

Back Forward Reload Home Search Netscape Images Print Security Stop

Location: http://www.jbpub.com/hwonline/essentials/Chapter_view/chapter.cfm?ChapterNumber=15   What's Related

net   People   Yellow Pages   Download

Essentials for Health and Wellness   Second Edition

Chapter 15

Understanding Aging and Dying

EXTRA! EXTRA!

Wellness Guide: Will Hormones Keep You Young?

Theories of Aging

Alzheimer's Disease and Senile Dementia

Wellness Guide: Extracts of Gingko Biloba Slow Alzheimer's Dementia

Healthy Aging

Web Exercises
- *Exercise 1:* *Death and Dying*
- *Exercise 2:* *Osteoporosis*
- *Exercise 3:* *Aging*

Student Review
- *Key Terms for Chapter 15*
- *Student Review for Chapter 15*

Reference Desk
- *Reference Links for Chapter 15*

Current and interesting topics are highlighted in boxes to give a complete perspective in your study of health and wellness. **Managing Stress** boxes give you practical strategies for coping with stress; **Wellness Guides** offer tips, techniques, and steps toward a healthy life-style and self-responsibility; and **Global Wellness** boxes explore health and wellness topics as they affect different cultures.

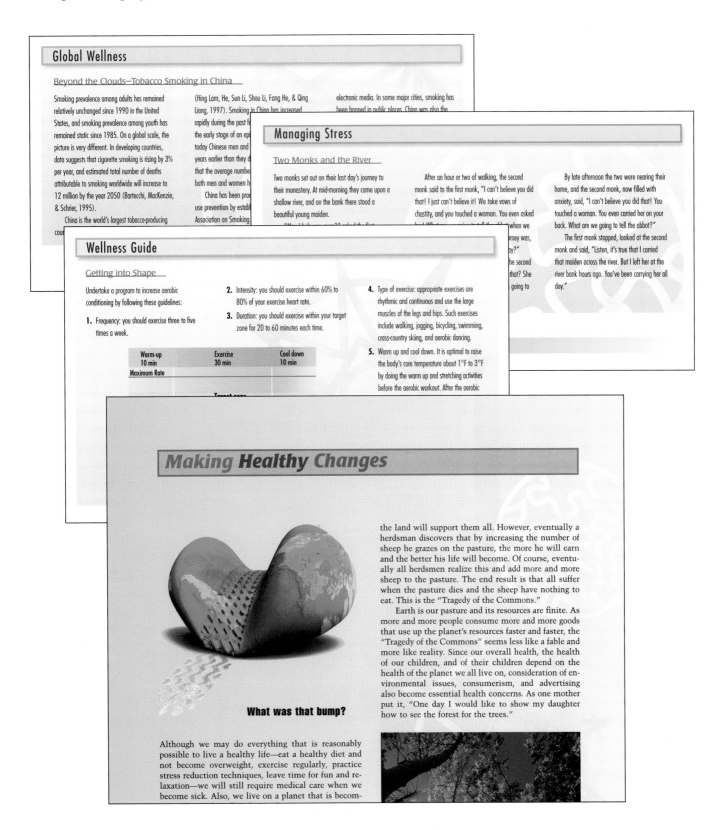

Global Wellness

Beyond the Clouds—Tobacco Smoking in China

Smoking prevalence among adults has remained relatively unchanged since 1990 in the United States, and smoking prevalence among youth has remained static since 1985. On a global scale, the picture is very different. In developing countries, data suggests that cigarette smoking is rising by 3% per year, and estimated total number of deaths attributable to smoking worldwide will increase to 12 million by the year 2050 (Bartecchi, MacKenzie, & Schrier, 1995).

China is the world's largest tobacco-producing cou

(Hing Lam, He, Sun Li, Shou Li, Fang He, & Qing Liang, 1997). Smoking in China has increased rapidly during the past f the early stage of an epi today Chinese men and years earlier than they d that the average number both men and women h

China has been pro use prevention by establ Association on Smoking

electronic media. In some major cities, smoking has been banned in public places. China was also the

Managing Stress

Two Monks and the River

Two monks set out on their last day's journey to their monastery. At mid-morning they came upon a shallow river, and on the bank there stood a beautiful young maiden.

After an hour or two of walking, the second monk said to the first monk, "I can't believe you did that! I just can't believe it! We take vows of chastity, and you touched a woman. You even asked

By late afternoon the two were nearing their home, and the second monk, now filled with anxiety, said, "I can't believe you did that! You touched a woman. You even carried her on your back. What are we going to tell the abbot?"

The first monk stopped, looked at the second monk and said, "Listen, it's true that I carried that maiden across the river. But I left her at the river bank hours ago. You've been carrying her all day."

Wellness Guide

Getting into Shape

Undertake a program to increase aerobic conditioning by following these guidelines:

1. Frequency: you should exercise three to five times a week.

2. Intensity: you should exercise within 60% to 80% of your exercise heart rate.

3. Duration: you should exercise within your target zone for 20 to 60 minutes each time.

Warm-up 10 min	Exercise 30 min	Cool down 10 min
Maximum Rate		

4. Type of exercise: appropriate exercises are rhythmic and continuous and use the large muscles of the legs and hips. Such exercises include walking, jogging, bicycling, swimming, cross-country skiing, and aerobic dancing.

5. Warm up and cool down. It is optimal to raise the body's core temperature about 1°F to 3°F by doing the warm up and stretching activities before the aerobic workout. After the aerobic

Making Healthy Changes

What was that bump?

Although we may do everything that is reasonably possible to live a healthy life—eat a healthy diet and not become overweight, exercise regularly, practice stress reduction techniques, leave time for fun and relaxation—we will still require medical care when we become sick. Also, we live on a planet that is becom-

the land will support them all. However, eventually a herdsman discovers that by increasing the number of sheep he grazes on the pasture, the more he will earn and the better his life will become. Of course, eventually all herdsmen realize this and add more and more sheep to the pasture. The end result is that all suffer when the pasture dies and the sheep have nothing to eat. This is the "Tragedy of the Commons."

Earth is our pasture and its resources are finite. As more and more people consume more and more goods that use up the planet's resources faster and faster, the "Tragedy of the Commons" seems less like a fable and more like reality. Since our overall health, the health of our children, and of their children depend on the health of the planet we all live on, consideration of environmental issues, consumerism, and advertising also become essential health concerns. As one mother put it, "One day I would like to show my daughter how to see the forest for the trees."

Chapters conclude with **Critical Thinking About Health**—a set of questions that present thought-provoking or controversial situations and ask you to examine your opinions and explore your biases.

End-of-chapter material includes **Health in Review,** a brief review of the chapter, **Health and Wellness Online,** a glimpse at the resources available on the Web; **References;** and **Annotated Suggested Readings.**

Making Healthy Changes sections appear at the end of each of the six parts of the text and give you the tools you need for making behvaioral and life-style changes that will improve your health and wellness. These Making Healthy Changes sections provide specific exercises and suggestions for improving emotional wellness, managing stress, increasing physical activity, improving diet, and becoming a wise consumer. This last

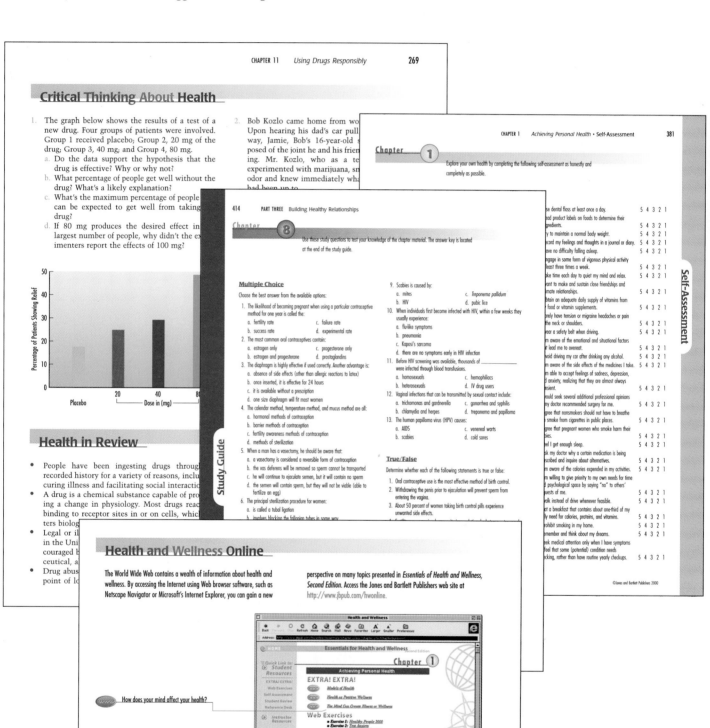

theme, becoming a wise consumer, is a topic that we think is increasingly important because the marketing of health-enhancing products directly to consumers has grown immensely in the past few years. Consumers are besieged with ads for new drugs, food supplements, herbs, and devices that claim to reduce weight, eliminate anxiety, prevent aging, renew sexual vigor, and improve health in every way imaginable. The unwise consumer can easily go bankrupt purchasing a dazzling array of health products. Self-responsibility is essential to avoid the perils of overconsuming "health products." We provide guidelines throughout Making Healthy Changes so you can make sensible, economic choices in the products you choose to purchase.

Finally, **self-assessments** and **activities** to explore your own health are provided at the end of the text. A **Built-in Study Guide** includes sample test questions for each chapter to assess your knowledge of the material.

A Note of Thanks

Throughout the two editions of *Essentials for Health and Wellness*, many people have contributed support and guidance. This book has benefited greatly from their comments, opinions, thoughtful critiques, expert knowledge, and constructive suggestions. We are most appreciative for their participation in this project.

Reviewers

Pat Alsader, Planned Parenthood of West Central Illinois
David Anspaugh, Memphis State University
Judy B. Baker, East Carolina University
N.K. Bhagavan, University of Hawaii Medical School
Nancy J. Binkin, Centers for Disease Control and Prevention, Atlanta
David Birch, Indiana University
Donald Calitri, Eastern Kentucky University
Barbara Coombs, San Francisco City College
Linda Chaput, W.H. Freeman, New York
Dorothy Coltrin, De Anza College
Geoffrey Cooper, Harvard Medical School
Judy Drolet, Southern Illinois University at Carbondale
Philip Duryea, University of New Mexico
JoAnna Nicholas Eidson, Spoon River College
Seymour Eiseman, California State University – Northridge
Carol Ellison, Berkeley, California
Tiffany Fennell, Mississippi State University
Marianne Frauenknecht, Western Michigan University
Nicole Gegel, Illinois State University
Brian F. Geiger, University of Alabama at Birmingham

Mal Goldsmith, Southern Illinois University at Edwardsville
Allan C. Henderson, California State University – Long Beach
Sherry Hineman, University of California – San Diego
Leo Hollister, Stanford Medical Center
Kathy E. Houston, State University of West Georgia
Stanley Inkelis, Harbor General Hospital
John Janowiak, Appalachian State University
William Kane, University of New Mexico
Mark Kittleson, Southern Illinois University at Carbondale
Dawn Larsen, Mankato State University
Will Lotter, University of California, Davis
Beverly Saxton Mahoney, The Pennsylvania State University
Mary Martin, University of California – San Francisco
Jennifer McLean, Corning Community College
Marion Micke, Illinois State University
Anne Nadakavukaren, Illinois State University
Marion Nestle, University of California – San Francisco
Roberta Ogletree, Southern Illinois University at Carbondale
Larry Olsen, The Pennsylvania State University
David Phelps, Oregon State University
Richard Plant, South Middlesex Community College
Lynn Poulson, Snow College
Bruce Ragon, Indiana University
Kerry J. Redican, Virginia Technical University
Dwayne Reed, Buck Center for Research in Aging
Janet Reis, University of Illinois at Urbana – Champaign
Tim Knickelbein, Normandale Community College
Brian Luke Seaward, University of Colorado – Boulder
Sam Singer, University of California – Santa Cruz
Susan Spreecher, Illinois State University
David R. Stronck, California State University – Hayward
John Struthers, Planned Parenthood of Sacramento County
Karen Vail-Smith, East Carolina University
Bryan Williams, University of Arkansas
Carol Wilson, University of Nevada at Las Vegas
Richard Wilson, Western Kentucky University

Acknowledgements

This book could not have been published without the efforts of the staff at Jones and Bartlett Publishers and the *Essentials for Health and Wellness* team: Judy Hauck, Vice President and Senior Managing Editor; Paul Shepardson, Senior Acquisitions Editor; Amy Austin, Associate Editor; Lianne Ames, Senior Production Editor; Linda DeBruyn, Production Editor; Jennifer Jacobson, Senior Marketing Manager; Michael Campbell, Director of Interactive Technology; Michael DeFronzo, Web

Designer; Dean Wetherbee, Web Designer; Scott Smith, Interactive Technology Product Manager; and Ohlinger Publishing Services. We would also like to thank Brian Luke Seaward, Ph.D., University of Colorado, Boulder; James Walsh; Esther M. Weekes; Martin Schulz; Shae Bearden; Rocky Young; Bharti Temkin; Laura Jones-Swann M.ED., LCDC, Texas Tech University; and Scott O. Roberts, Ph.D., FAACVPR, Texas Tech University. To all we express our appreciation.

I want to thank Gordon Edlin for being a magnificent co-author and fantastic friend throughout our 20 years of working on Health and Wellness *together.*
E.G.

What we do is not in isolation; therefore, I would like to thank my husband, Dennis, for his support of my professional life as a health educator, professor, teacher, and mentor.
K.M.B.

Gordon Edlin
John A. Burns School of Medicine
University of Hawaii
Honolulu, Hawaii 96822

Eric Golanty
Las Positas College
Livermore, California 94550

Kelli McCormack Brown
Department of Community and Family Health
University of South Florida
Tampa, Florida 33612-3805

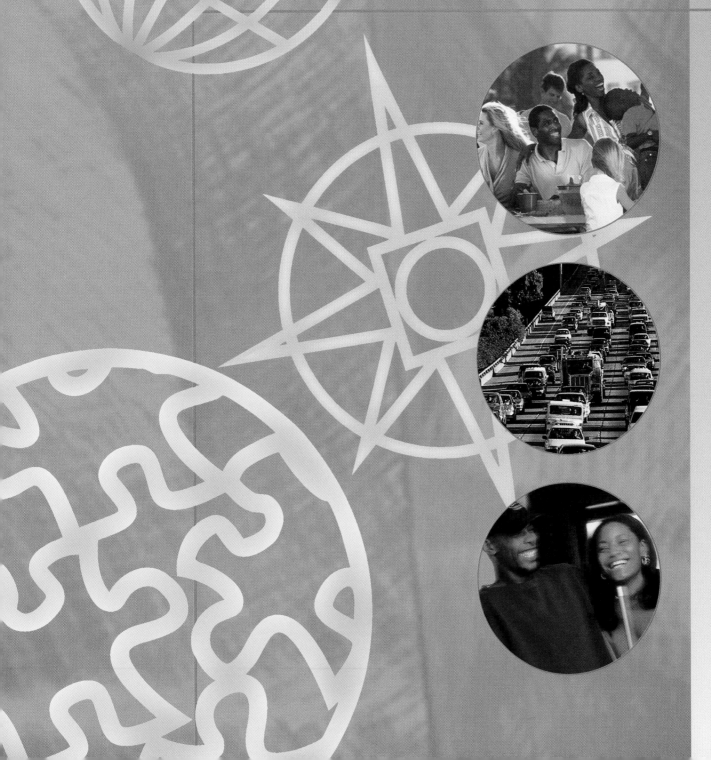

Part 1

Achieving Wellness

Learning Objectives

1. Describe what it means to be healthy.
2. Describe the medical, environmental, and holistic, or wellness, models of health.
3. Explain the wellness continuum and its impact on personal health.
4. Identify and describe the six dimensions of wellness.
5. Describe the personal qualities that are associated with the six dimensions of wellness.
6. Explain the philosophy of holistic health.
7. List the three most common actual causes of death and explain how life-styles and behaviors contribute to disease.
8. Describe how the mind contributes to illness.
9. Understand how spirituality enhances health.
10. Explain the importance of the national health objectives for the year 2000 and 2010.
11. Discuss the Health Belief Model and the Transtheoretical Model and how they relate to behavior change.

Exercises and Activities

WORKBOOK
How Well Are You?

Health and Wellness Online

 www.jbpub.com/hwonline

Models of Health

Health as Positive Wellness

The Mind Can Create Illness or Wellness

Chapter 1

Achieving Personal Health

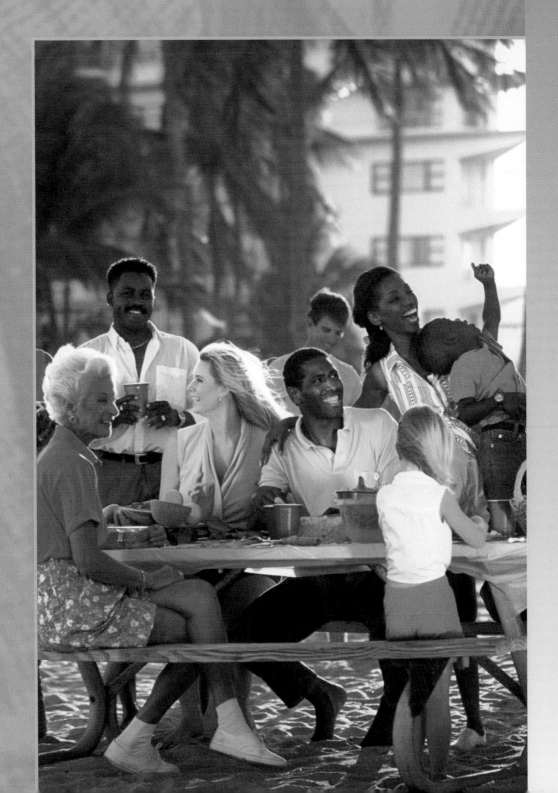

Ask people what they mean by "being healthy" or "feeling well" and you probably will get a variety of answers. Most people usually think of health as the absence of disease. But what about someone who has a relatively harmless genetic disorder, such as an extra toe? Is this individual less healthy than a person with the usual number of toes? Different perhaps, but not necessarily less healthy. Are you less well when you are struggling with a personal problem than when you are out having fun? Finding an acceptable, generally useful definition of health or wellness is not a simple task.

> The only way to keep your health
> is to eat what you don't want . . .
> Drink what you don't like . . .
> And do what you'd rather not.
> MARK TWAIN

It is true that not feeling sick is one important aspect of health. Just as important, however, is the idea that health is a sense of optimum well-being—a state of physical, mental, emotional, social, and spiritual wellness. Contained in this view is the idea that health can be obtained by living in harmony with yourself, with other people, and with the environment. Health is gained and maintained by exerting self-responsibility for reducing exposure to health risks and for maximizing good nutrition and exercise.

Throughout this book, we show you ways to maximize your health by understanding how your mind and body function, how to avoid harmful chemicals, how to make informed decisions about health and health care, and how to be responsible for your actions and behaviors. Learning to be responsible for the degree of health and energy you want while you are young helps to ensure life long wellness and the capacity to cope with sickness when it does occur.

Defining Health and Wellness

Health, like love or happiness, is a quality of life that is difficult to define and virtually impossible to measure. **Health** is defined differently among experts, but all definitions have a common theme: self-responsibility and adopting a healthy life-style.

> Health is a state of complete physical, mental, and social well-being and not merely the absence of disease or infirmity.
> —*World Health Organization, 1947*

Wellness has been defined as

> an approach to personal health that emphasizes individual responsibility for well-being through the practice of health-promoting lifestyle behaviors.
> —*Hurley and Schlaadt, 1992*

Wellness is many times referred to in a broader context than health, which sometimes means only physical health. For the purposes of this book, we consider health multidimensional, involving the whole person's relation to the total environment. We refer to wellness as a process of moving toward optimal health.

 ## Models of Health

Scientists and health educators have developed three main ways to define health: (a) the medical model, (b) the environmental model, and (c) the wellness, or holistic, model. How you approach being healthy and well in many ways depends on your personal definition of health.

The Medical Model

The **medical model's** main tenet is that health is the absence of one or more of the "five Ds"—death, disease, discomfort, disability, and dissatisfaction. In other words, if you are not sick or dying, you are considered to be in the best attainable state of health. Followers of the medical model rely almost exclusively on biological explanations of disease and illness and tend to interpret disease and illness in terms of malfunction of individual organs, cells, and other biological systems, e.g., liver disease, heart disease, or sickle cell anemia.

Within the medical model, the health of a population is measured in terms of **vital statistics,** which are data on the degree of illness (**morbidity**) and the numbers of deaths (**mortality**) in a given population. Vital statistics include **prevalence** (the predominance of a disease in a population) and **incidence** (the frequency

Terms

health: state of sound physical, mental, and social well-being

wellness: emphasizes individual responsibility for well-being through the practice of health-promoting life-style behaviors

medical model: interprets health in terms of the absence of disease and illness

vital statistics: numerical data relating to birth, death, disease, marriage, and health

morbidity: ratio of persons who are diseased to those who are well in a given community

mortality: death rate: number of deaths per unit of population (e.g., per 100; 10,000; or 1,000,000) in a specific region, age range, or other group

prevalence: predominance of a particular disease

incidence: frequency of occurrence of a particular disease

environmental model: modern analyses of ecosystems and environmental risks to health, such as socioeconomic status, education, and various environmental factors that affect health

at which certain diseases occur). These statistical measurements allow comparisons between populations and also within the same population over time.

The medical model tends not to deal with social problems that affect health and only with difficulty integrates mental and behavioral issues that do not derive from diseased organs. In the medical model, health is restored by curing a disease or by restoring function to a damaged body part. Because of its exclusive focus on biological processes, the medical model is of limited value. It does not help us understand psychological and social factors that affect health and contribute to disease.

The reliance on biological interpretations of illness has contributed greatly to the success of the medical model. Anyone who has been cured of a serious infection by taking antibiotics or undergone a lifesaving surgical procedure can attest to that. On the other hand, that same reliance on biological thinking has not furthered understanding of health and illness in terms of psychological and social factors, nor has it been very successful in fostering health by preventing disease caused by unhealthy life-styles and destructive behaviors.

The Environmental Model

The **environmental model** of health emerged with modern analyses of ecosystems and environmental risks to human health. In this model, health is defined in terms of the quality of a person's adaptation to the environment as conditions change. This model (Figure 1.1) includes the effects on personal health of socioeconomic status, education, and multiple environmental factors.

> *I may have faults, but being wrong ain't one of them.*
>
> JIMMY HOFFA

Unlike the medical model, which focuses on diseased organs and biological abnormalities, the environmental model focuses on conditions outside the individual that affect his or her health. These conditions include the quality of air and water, living conditions, exposure to harmful substances, socioeconomic conditions, social relationships, and the health-care system.

In many respects the environmental model of health is similar to ancient Asian and Native American philosophies that associate health with harmonious interactions with fellow creatures and the envi-

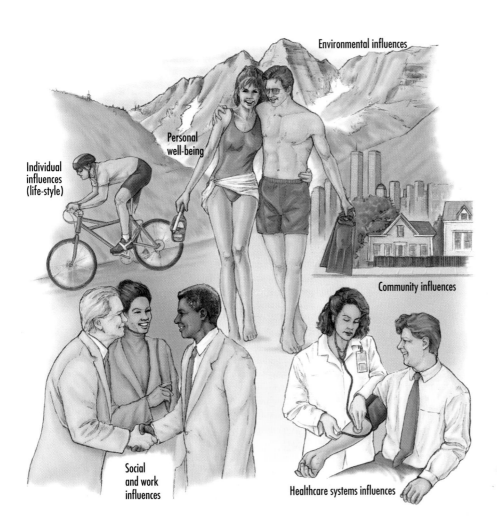

Environmental influences

Personal well-being

Individual influences (life-style)

Community influences

Social and work influences

Healthcare systems influences

FIGURE 1.1   Environmental Health Model This model takes into account all factors that interact with one another to affect one's health.

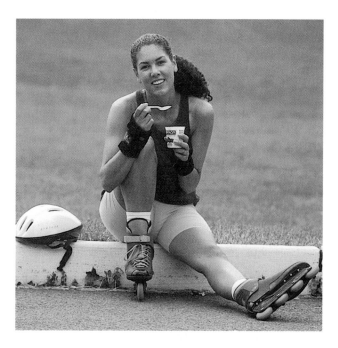

A healthy life-style depends on exercise and good nutrition.

ronment. In particular, as the environment changes, one's interaction with it must change to remain in harmony. Illness is interpreted as disharmony of human and environmental interactions.

The Holistic Model

The holistic, or wellness, model defines health in terms of the whole person, not in terms of diseased parts of the body. The **holistic model** encompasses the physiological, mental, emotional, social, spiritual, and environmental aspects of individuals and communities. It focuses on optimal health, prevention of disease, and positive mental and emotional states.

The holistic model incorporates the idea of spiritual health, which is not considered in the medical model. Unlike the medical model, which assumes that a person who is not sick or not suffering from a disease is as healthy as possible, the holistic model proposes that health is a state of optimum or positive wellness.

Wellness is much more than physical health; it addresses mental, emotional, and spiritual aspects of a person, as well as the relationships among these di-

mensions. The wellness continuum helps delineate between the medical concept of health and the wellness concept (Figure 1.2). Most people find themselves in the neutral area of the continuum. Most of us, however, can remember moving toward disability and also moving toward optimal health or high-level wellness.

One may move from a state of illness or disease back to the neutral point many times with the help of medical care. The wellness continuum also includes prevention, which means taking positive actions to prevent acute and chronic illnesses.

Wellness is not static; it is a dynamic process that takes into account all the decisions we make daily, such as which foods we eat, the amount of exercise we get, and whether we drink alcohol before driving, wear safety belts, or smoke cigarettes. Every choice we make potentially affects health and wellness.

In this book we discuss aspects of all of the different models of health wherever appropriate. The models themselves are abstractions of ideas, but in real life one needs to use whatever is practical to optimize health and well-being. Health depends very much on each person's perception. People with a disease may live joyful, positive, healthy lives; people without a disease may be despondent, unhappy, and feel sick. People need attainable goals to promote wellness and to live harmoniously with family, friends, and the environment.

Dimensions of Health and Wellness

Because wellness is dynamic and continuous, no dimension of wellness functions in isolation. When you have a high level of wellness or optimal health, all dimensions are integrated and functioning together. The person's environment (including work, school, family, community), and his or her physical, emotional, intellectual, occupational, spiritual, and social dimensions of wellness are in tune with one another to produce harmony. Health educators commonly refer to six dimensions of health and wellness: emotional, intellectual, spiritual, occupational, social, and physical:

- **Emotional wellness** requires understanding emotions and coping with problems that arise in everyday life.

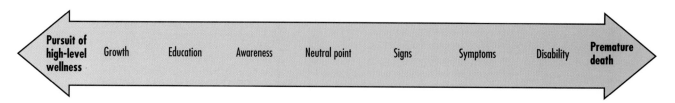

| Pursuit of high-level wellness | Growth | Education | Awareness | Neutral point | Signs | Symptoms | Disability | Premature death |

FIGURE 1.2 **The Wellness Continuum** The wellness continuum allows you to visualize the difference between wellness and the medical approaches to health.

Managing Stress

Harmony and Peace

Many Native American cultures and tribes incorporate the idea of harmonious interactions with nature, animals, and other people in their religions.

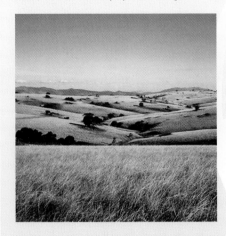

The first peace,
which is the most important,
is that which comes from
within the souls of men when they
realize their relationship,
their oneness, with the universe
and all its powers,
and when they realize that
at the center of the universe dwells
Wakan-Tanka, and that
this center is really everywhere,
it is within each of us.
This is the real peace, and the others are
but reflections of this.
The second peace is that which is

made between two individuals,
and the third is that
which is made between two nations.
But above all you should
understand that there can never be peace
between nations until there is
first known that true peace which . . .
is within the souls of men.

Black Elk
The Sacred Pipe

Source: From *The Sacred Pipe: Black Elk's Account of the Seven Rites of the Oglala Sioux,* by Joseph Epes Brown. Copyright © 1953, 1989 by the University of Oklahoma Press.

- **Intellectual wellness** involves having a mind open to new ideas and concepts. If you are intellectually healthy, you seek new experiences and challenges.
- **Spiritual wellness** is the state of harmony with yourself and others. It is the ability to balance inner needs with the demands of the rest of the world.
- **Occupational wellness** is being able to enjoy what you are doing to earn a living and contribute to society, whether it be going to college, working as a secretary, doctor, construction manager, or accountant. In a job, it means having skills such as critical thinking, problem solving, and communicating well.
- **Social wellness** refers to the ability to perform social roles effectively, comfortably, and without harming others.
- **Physical wellness** is a healthy body maintained by eating right, exercising regularly, avoiding harmful habits, making informed and responsible decisions about health, seeking medical care when needed, and participating in activities that help prevent illness.

Health as Positive Wellness

If freedom from sickness isn't all there is to health, then what else is involved? The World Health Organization (WHO) defines health as "a state of complete physical, mental, and social well-being and not merely the ab-

sence of disease and infirmity." This definition is so broad and covers so much that some people find it meaningless. Its universality, however, is exactly right. Peoples' lives, and therefore their health, are affected by every aspect of life: environmental influences such as climate; the availability of nutritious food, comfortable shelter, clean air to breathe, and pure water to drink; and other people, including family, lovers, employers, coworkers, friends, and associates of various kinds.

The WHO definition of health takes into account not only the condition of your body but also the state of your mind. Your mental processes are perhaps the most important influences on your health, because

Terms

holistic model: encompasses the physiological, mental, emotional, social, spiritual, and environmental aspects of health

emotional wellness: understanding emotions and knowing how to cope with problems that arise in everyday life, and how to endure stress

intellectual wellness: having a mind open to new ideas and concepts

spiritual wellness: state of balance and harmony with yourself and others

occupational wellness: enjoyment of what you are doing to earn a living and contribute to society

social wellness: ability to perform the expectations of social roles effectively, comfortably, and without harming others

physical wellness: maintenance of your body in good condition by eating right, exercising regularly, avoiding harmful habits, and making informed responsible decisions about your health

Managing Stress

The Rainbow of Human Energy

In truth, we know that we cannot separate the mind from the body, nor can we separate the mind from emotions, or the body from the soul. All aspects are integrated. Through the recent insights of quantum physics, we know that everything, including our thoughts and feelings, consists of energy. This is what the wisdom keepers and shamans have known for millennia. Renowned physicist David Bohm addressed the spiritual nature of health in terms of quantum physics. He used the term coherence to describe the harmony among the energies of body, mind, and spirit, which gives a sense of wholeness that can only be described as "inner peace." As we continue to explore the issues of health and illness, some interesting facts come to light which support the holistic concept that the whole is greater than the sum of the parts. Spontaneous remissions and healing through prayer are two of many phenomena that cannot be explained by the mechanistic model. In fact, the new paradigm suggests that we are not a mind in a body, but a body in a mind.

Try the following exercise: Keeping in mind the concept of coherence in this new paradigm, take a moment to reflect on your whole being — all that you are, not just your body. You can begin by thinking about your physical body — your senses, organs, bones, tissue, and fluids. Visualize all the organs, tissues, and fluids working in cooperation with each other (coherence). Imagine that every cell in your body, like the needle of a compass, is headed north. Next, imagine that a layer of energy surrounds and permeates your body. This layer of energy is aqua. This represents what is known as your emotional body. Imagine this layer of blue energy around your body like warm Caribbean water. Imagine what it would feel like to sense harmony between your emotions and physical body. Next, imagine that superimposed over this aqua-blue layer is a layer of energy deeper in color — indigo blue. This color represents your intellect and the powers of the mind. When all thoughts are focused in the same direction, you have coherence at this level of energy as well. Finally, visualize that superimposed on the layer of indigo blue is a layer of violet, a color that often represents the spiritual nature of humanity. As you envision these colors, think and sense coherence — the integration, balance, and harmony of your mind, body, spirit, and emotions. Know that there is no separation of body, mind, and spirit and the whole is truly greater than the sum of the parts.

they determine how you deal with your physical and social surroundings, what attitudes about life you have, and how you interact with others.

Health as the totality of a person's existence is the holistic view, which recognizes the interrelatedness of the physical, psychological, emotional, social, spiritual, and environmental factors that contribute to the overall quality of a person's life. No part of the mind, body, or environment is truly separate and independent.

The philosophy of holistic health is not incompatible with the practice of conventional medicine. Rather, it emphasizes a view that has gained wide acceptance among members of the medical community—that each person has the capacity and the responsibility for optimizing his or her sense of well-being, for self-healing, and for the creation of conditions and feelings that help prevent disease. Holistic health is hardly a revolutionary idea; the Old English root of our word *health* (*hal,* meaning sound or whole) implies that there is more to health than freedom from sickness.

Positive wellness involves (a) being free from symptoms of disease and pain as much as possible; (b) being active, able to do what you want and what you must at the appropriate time; and (c) being in good spirits and feeling emotionally healthy most of the time. These characteristics indicate that health is not something suddenly achieved at a specific time, like getting a college degree. Rather, health is a *process*— indeed, a way of life—through which you develop and encourage every aspect of your body, mind, and feelings to interrelate harmoniously as much of the time as possible.

The Philosophy of Holistic Health

The philosophy of holistic health emphasizes the unity of the mind, spirit, and body. Therefore, symptoms of illness and disease may be viewed as an imbalance in a person's total state of being and not simply as the malfunction of a particular part of the body. Consider, for example, a common minor illness: the headache. About 80% to 90% of American adults experience at least one headache each year. Although a headache can be the result of brain injury or the symptom of another illness, more often it is caused by emotional stress that produces a tightening of the muscles in the head and neck. These contracting muscles increase the blood pressure in the head, thereby causing the pain of headache.

Most people try to relieve a headache by taking aspirin or some other analgesic drug that can alter the physiological mechanisms that produce the pain. In contrast, someone using the holistic approach would first try to determine the *source* of the tensions— worry, anger, or frustration—and then work to reduce

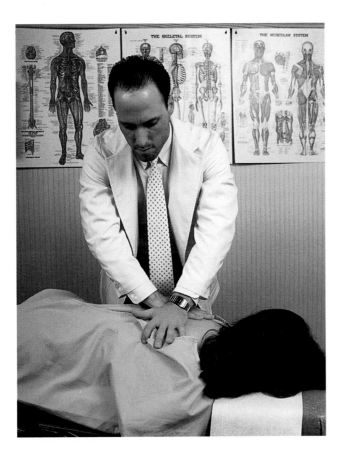

Many alternative medical practices, such as chiropractic, massage, and acupuncture, are now considered legitimate medical treatments and are often covered by insurance.

or eliminate the tensions. Similarly, an upset stomach cannot be regarded as simply the result of excessive secretion of stomach acid, requiring an antacid to bring relief. In many cases, the upset results from unexpressed hostility or fear. You are probably aware that such common events as taking an examination or having a dispute with someone can cause uncomfortable feelings in the stomach.

The holistic approach emphasizes self-healing, the maintenance of health, and the prevention of illness, rather than the treatment of symptoms and disease. A holistic approach integrates medical technology into a broader treatment that looks not only at a person's symptoms, but also at the sources of disharmony. From the holistic point of view, illness is the result of some imbalance in the harmonious interaction of the body, mind, and environment. Thus, to the extent that we can follow a program of positive wellness and create a healthy environment, we can be free of disease.

Some of the great advances in medicine have resulted from considering illness solely in terms of the affected bodily organ. Indeed, devoting medical attention to one specific ailing part of the body is sometimes the most efficient way to treat a medical problem, which is why we have specialists who are experts in treating diseases of different body parts, such as heart specialists, gastrointestinal specialists, podiatrists, gynecologists, and so on.

Some health professionals have criticized those who advocate holistic health practices and holistic medicine, arguing that the concepts and methods are

Wellness Guide

Whole-Person Wellness

A person with emotional wellness is able to:

- Maintain a sense of humor.
- Recognize feelings and appropriately express them.
- Strive to meet emotional needs.
- Take responsibility for his or her behavior.

A person with intellectual wellness is able to:

- Communicate effectively in speaking and in writing.
- See more than one side of an issue.
- Keep abreast of global issues.
- Exhibit good time-management skills.

A person with spiritual wellness is able to:

- Examine personal values and beliefs.
- Search for meanings that help explain the purpose of life.
- Have a clear understanding of right and wrong.
- Appreciate natural forces in the universe.

A person with occupational wellness is able to:

- Feel a sense of accomplishment in his or her work.
- Balance work and other aspects of life.
- Find satisfaction in being creative and innovative.
- Seek challenges at work.

A person with social wellness is able to:

- Develop positive relationships with loved ones.
- Develop relationships with friends.
- Enjoy being with others.
- Effectively communicate with others who may be different.

A person with physical wellness is able to:

- Exercise regularly and select a well-balanced diet.
- Participate in safe, responsible sexual behavior.
- Make informed choices about medicinal use and medical care.
- Maintain a positive, health-promoting life-style.

antiscientific and hence harmful. Holistic medicine is not antiscientific. By encouraging individuals to take personal command of their health, including how they use medical services, holistic health practices are likely to be less harmful than some modern medical practices, such as unnecessary surgery.

Taking Responsiblity for Your Health

Not so many years ago, people were subject to a variety of diseases over which they had little or no control. In the early part of the twentieth century, infectious diseases caused by organisms were the leading causes of death in the United States. Modern public health methods and modern drugs, such as antibiotics, were not available. In 1918, millions of people around the world died from influenza, the cause of which was unknown at that time (Table 1.1).

Today, the leading causes of illness and death are not due to infections, but to "life-style diseases." These diseases, such as heart disease and cancer, result from environmental factors, people's behaviors, and the ways in which they choose to live.

Heart disease results primarily from today's lifestyles, although recent evidence suggests that certain bacterial infections may also contribute to heart disease. Behaviors contributing to heart disease include overeating and overweight, which contribute to high cholesterol (see chapter 5); cigarette smoking (see chapter 12); lack of exercise (see chapter 6); and stress (see chapter 2), which can lead to high blood pressure (see chapter 10). Cancer is associated with both nutritional (see chapter 4) and environmental factors (see

TABLE 1.1   Ten Leading Causes of Death for All Ages, All Races, and Both Sexes, 1900, 1987, and 1997

1900	1987	1997
1. Tuberculosis	Heart disease	Heart disease
2. Pneumonia	Cancer	Cancer
3. Diarrhea and enteritis	Stroke	Stroke
4. Heart disease	Injuries	Chronic obstructive pulmonary disease (COPD)
5. Liver disease	Bronchitis and emphysema	Accidents, including motor vehicle accidents
6. Injuries	Pneumonia and influenza	Pneumonia and influenza
7. Stroke	Diabetes	Diabetes
8. Cancer	Suicide	HIV infection
9. Bronchitis	Chronic liver disease	Suicide
10. Diphtheria	Arteriosclerosis	Chronic liver disease and cirrhosis

chapter 10). Improper nutrition, smoking cigarettes, and exposure to hazardous substances in the environment initiate biological changes that can result in cancer. An unhealthy life-style is also at the root of suicide and homicide (alcohol, drugs, and stress), accidents (alcohol use and stress), and cirrhosis of the liver (alcohol abuse).

Life-style and Health

When a person dies, the cause of death is generally identified in terms of the organ system that failed

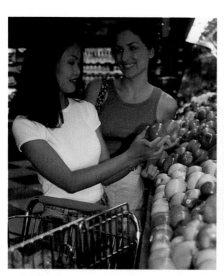
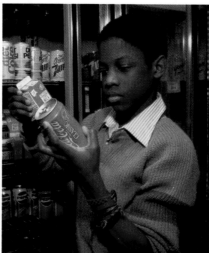
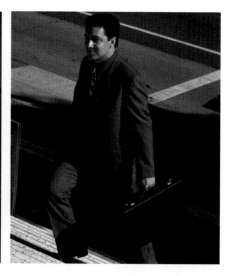

Simple behaviors in our everyday lives can postively affect health: eat 5 servings of fruits and vegetables every day, read food labels to make wise choices; and walk to work whenever possible.

Wellness Guide

Health Issues for College Students

What health issues face North America's 15 million college students as we approach the next century? Here's what college and university health educators and medical professionals think the answers are (Grace, 1997).

Sexual health. More than any others, sexual issues have the potential to affect the health of college students. These include sexually transmitted diseases (7% to 10% of college students carry an undiagnosed STI), unintended pregnancy, and sexual assault, especially acquaintance or date rape.

Sexuality is also related to issues of self-esteem, peer acceptance, loneliness, and relieving academic stress with superficial sexual relationships, all of which have the potential to produce psychological harm and establish negative attitudes and behavior that may impair future sexual and intimate relationships.

Substance abuse. The abuse of alcohol, drugs, tobacco, and food is related to trying to gain peer acceptance, unhealthy role modeling in families and in society-at-large, and trying to cope with psychological distress. Students whose parents abuse substances often have a tendency for substance abuse. Alcohol abuse is related to the majority of sexual assaults, unintended pregnancies (from not using contraceptives properly or at all), and the transmission of STIs (from not practicing safe sex).

Mental health. Failure to achieve, academic stress, lack of social support, difficulty adjusting to young adulthood, and pressures to fit in socially all contribute to emotional problems (especially anxiety and depression) that may impair a student's academic performance and sense of well-being. They can also lead to stress-related physical illnesses.

Competitive academic environments can create feelings of inferiority, insecurity, and emotional distress.

Food and weight. Many students are highly concerned about their body size and shape and may become malnourished to meet their perceptions of social ideality. Eating disorders, such as bulimia and anorexia nervosa, affect a large number of students (see chapter 5).

Health care. A large proportion of college students in the United States have limited access to health care because their colleges do not have comprehensive services for students or they do not have private health insurance.

Accidents and injuries. Many students are susceptible to automobile accidents (often alcohol-related) and sports injuries.

and resulted in the person's death, e.g., heart disease, cirrhosis of the liver, cancer of the lung. This may not, however, identify the root causes of that death. For example, saying someone died of lung cancer does not tell us that *actual* cause of death was smoking 2½ packs of cigarettes a day for 25 years. When deaths are examined for their actual causes and not simply what is reported on death certificates, the results show that approximately *half* of the 2.1 million deaths in the United States each year are due to life-style factors (Table 1.2), and by extension, that many, many deaths could be prevented if people lived more healthfully (McGuiness and Foege, 1993).

Leading the list of life-shortening behaviors is tobacco use, which is responsible for more than 400,000 American deaths per year. Smoking cigarettes and cigars, chewing tobacco, and being exposed to second hand smoke contribute substantially to deaths caused by cancer of all kinds, heart disease, high blood pressure, stroke, bronchitis, chronic obstructive pulmonary disease (COPD), pneumonia, low birth weight, and burns from fires. The enormous toll on life and health exacted by tobacco use is the reason that health agencies, doctors, and governments overwhelmingly recommend limiting tobacco use (see chapter 12).

TABLE 1.2   **Number of Preventable Deaths in the United States in 1990**
Estimates are from data including actual numbers (firearm deaths) and calculated risks (tobacco deaths). More than 1 million deaths are caused by life-styles and behaviors—all preventable deaths.

Cause	Deaths Estimated No.	Percentage of Total Deaths
Tobacco	400 000	19
Diet/activity patterns	300 000	14
Alcohol	100 000	5
Microbial agents	90 000	4
Toxic agents	60 000	3
Firearms	35 000	2
Sexual behavior	30 000	1
Motor vehicles	25 000	1
Illicit use of drugs	20 000	<1
Total	1 060 000	50

Source: McGuinnis and Foege (1993). Actual causes of death in the United States. *Journal of the American Medical Association, 270,* 2207–2212.

Next to tobacco use, unhealthy diet and activity patterns contribute the most to death in the U.S. Consumption of high levels of cholesterol and saturated fat in foods is associated with heart disease, several types of cancer, and stroke. High-calorie consumption coupled with low levels of physical activity predisposes people to overweight, diabetes, and high blood pressure. A sedentary life-style is responsible for 23% of deaths from the leading chronic diseases (heart disease, high blood pressure, stroke, and diabetes).

Americans will always do the right thing . . . after they have exhausted all the other possibilities.
WINSTON CHURCHILL

Drug use and abuse are responsible for 120,000 American deaths each year. Misuse of alcohol accounts for nearly 100,000 deaths each year directly from alcohol toxicity and medical complications therefrom (e.g., liver and pancreatic disease), motor vehicle and other types of accidents, and homicides. Another 20,000 deaths annually are attributable to the use of both legal and illegal drugs other than alcohol. These include deaths from deliberate overdose, accidental overdose, and fatal accidents caused by intoxication.

The transmission of infectious agents accounts for over 120,000 deaths. Unsafe sex and injection drug use contribute to thousands of new cases of AIDS each year. Transmission of hepatitis B virus by unsafe sex and injection drug use and of other strains of hepatitis virus via fecal contamination of food results in thousands of cases of fatal liver failure. Overuse of antibiotics has produced bacterial strains that are resistant to antibiotics, resulting in infections that are difficult (and occasionally impossible) to treat.

Social factors cause fatalities, also. For example, exposure to toxic agents in the workplace and elsewhere account for 60,000 deaths per year. Firearms used in homicides, suicides, and accidental shootings are responsible for 35,000 deaths. Motor vehicle accidents cause another 47,000 deaths. Lack of access to medical care—a condition that affects the one third of American families who have no health insurance—contributes to thousands of deaths each year as well.

The Mind Can Create Illness or Wellness

The power of the mind to affect the health of the body is illustrated by **psychosomatic illnesses.** When a person is subjected to stress or emotional upset, changes in the body may manifest as diseases (Figure 1.3). The terms *psycho* (mind) and *soma* (body) emphasize the connection between the mind and the body with respect to health.

Many people believe that if a person has a psychosomatic illness, he or she is imagining it, that it is "all in

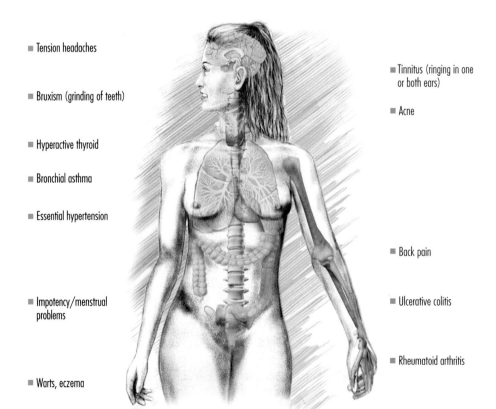

- Tension headaches
- Bruxism (grinding of teeth)
- Hyperactive thyroid
- Bronchial asthma
- Essential hypertension
- Impotency/menstrual problems
- Warts, eczema

- Tinnitus (ringing in one or both ears)
- Acne
- Back pain
- Ulcerative colitis
- Rheumatoid arthritis

FIGURE 1.3   Psychosomatic Illnesses
Many diseases and disorders of the body are partly caused by thoughts and feelings in the mind that produce psychosomatic illnesses.

Wellness Guide

Using Your Mind to Improve Health

- Become more aware of the power your mind has to improve health, hasten healing, and help you perform better in school and in other activities. Belief in yourself, in prayer, or in a particular treatment can facilitate healing and help prevent sickness.
- Use mental images that feel right to you to reduce exam anxiety and to improve performance in sports or other activities. Avoid negative mental images and thoughts such as "I feel lousy," or "I'm too tired to run," or "I just know I can't do that." Use your mind to create positive images and thoughts. You can reverse what seems to be a "bad" day by suggesting to yourself that things are going to change and improve.
- Practice a daily mental relaxation technique in a place that is comfortable and quiet. Use the time to "talk" to your body to promote healing or to change behaviors. Visualize scenes from the past or the future that you know are healthy and constructive. As you become more adept at using your mind, you will find new ways to use mental relaxation in all aspects of your life. *(Notice how we inserted a positive suggestion.)*

the mind." This is not true. The symptoms of a headache brought on by stress can be just as severe as one brought on by being hit over the head with a bat. In one case, stress has caused a change in the flow of blood through the head, and in the other case, blood vessels may have been damaged by the injury. Psychosomatic illnesses are as real as a cold brought on by a virus.

Western medicine is not well equipped to deal with psychosomatic illnesses. Although physicians can treat the symptoms, they are not well trained to help with the underlying mental states that cause the illness. On the other hand, Buddhist and Chinese medicine take the position that all sickness, to some degree, is brought on by a person's state of mind. In Western medicine, if a physician cannot find an organic cause for symptoms, the patient may be advised to see a psychologist or given a drug to mask symptoms.

This view should not be interpreted to mean that sickness is brought on just by a person's state of mind, but that our psychological state, at any time, may invite illness. In order for an emotional or mental state to change physiology, a process called **somatization** must occur. Somatization refers to the occurrence of physical symptoms in a person without the presence of disease or injury that can be detected medically.

Psychological and social problems may contribute to pain, fatigue, nausea, diarrhea, sexual dysfunction, and other symptoms that are classified as **somatization disorders** (McCahill, 1995). It is estimated that 25% to 75% of all patients who visit primary care physicians suffer from somatization disorders. These are difficult to treat, time-consuming for physicians to diagnose, and expensive for the health care system.

Image Visualization

One of the most effective ways to promote wellness and change undesirable behaviors is through the use of **image visualization.** Many mind-body healing tech-

niques employ some form of image visualization. For example, frightening scenes from the past, especially from early childhood, can be reexperienced while a person is in a state of mental relaxation brought on by hypnosis or some other technique. As the scenes and emotional upsets are visualized in the mind, they can be reinterpreted and reprogrammed to change their negative effects on health and behaviors. Mental imagery can also be used to reduce pain; hasten healing; improve performance in sports; change smoking, drinking, or eating behaviors; and help control compulsive urges to gamble. At one time or another in our lives, we all daydream or run an "internal movie," fantasizing our hopes and fears. During such fantasies we visualize experiences and create feelings. Image visualization can change body temperature, blood flow, heartbeat, breathing rate, production of hormones, and other body processes regulated by the brain.

> We are what we pretend to be, so we better be very careful what we pretend to be.
>
> KURT VONNEGUT, *MOTHER NIGHT*

Most psychologists who work with athletes to improve physical performance use image visualization. The so-called inner games of tennis, golf, skiing, and

Terms

psychosomatic illnesses: physical illnesses brought on by negative mental states such as stress or emotional upset

somatization: occurrence of physical symptoms without any bodily disease or injury being present

somatization disorder: prolonged pain and other symptoms that are not due to disease or injury

image visualization: use of mental images to promote healing and change behaviors

skating are based on image visualization. Baseball players in a batting slump use relaxation and visualization to "see" themselves getting hits. Basketball players use the technique to "see" their free throws going cleanly through the hoop.

Image visualization is also the secret to improved sexual responses and enjoyment. Sexual arousal begins in the mind and negative thoughts or fears can stifle the sexual responses. The sex organs are particularly sensitive to images generated in the mind. Most sex therapists use relaxation techniques and image visualization to help clients improve their sexual experiences. Tension related to sexual performance is usually the main reason for not experiencing the desired sexual sensations. In all areas of your life, begin to use your mental powers more to enhance health and improve performance in daily tasks.

 ## National Health Objectives

In 1979 the first *Surgeon General's Report on Health Promotion and Disease Prevention* was released. Its purpose was to create a public health revolution. The strategy was to emphasize prevention of disease. The focus was on personal responsibility for one's own health by reducing risky habits. The report indicated that, for the public health revolution to succeed, social changes must also take place to deal with poverty, lack of education, inadequate housing, hunger, drug use, and so on. The report identified five public health goals that were measurable and could be achieved by 1990 (Table 1.3).

In 1980 the United States Department of Health and Human Services (USDHHS) published *Promoting Health/Preventing Disease: Objectives for the Nation*,

which provides quantifiable objectives necessary to obtain the broad goals set in the *Surgeon General's Report* of 1979. A total of 226 specific objectives were established for 15 priority areas identified in the *Surgeon General's Report*. Within each priority, the nature and extent of problem, prevention and promotion measures, specific objectives, principal assumptions, and data sources were outlined and discussed.

Healthy People 2000

Efforts by local, state, and federal governments have led to *Healthy People 2000* (USDHHS, 1990), the nation's vision for a new century characterized by enhancing quality of life, reducing preventable death and disability, and reducing the disparity in the health status of people within American society. The framework of *Healthy People 2000* consists of three broad goals:

1. Increase the length of healthy life for Americans.
2. Reduce health disparities among Americans.
3. Achieve access to preventive health services for all Americans.

Grouped under the broad categories of health promotion, health protection, and preventive services, the more than 300 national objectives are organized into 22 priority areas. This framework provides direction for individuals to change personal behaviors and for organizations and communities to support good health through health promotion policies.

Healthy People 2000: Midcourse Review

In 1995, the mid-decade review of *Healthy People 2000* showed that the U.S. was moving in the right direction on more than two thirds of the national objectives for which data was available. The midcourse review shows that partnerships among all levels of government and the private sector can make a positive difference in an individual's health status. Trends during the first five years of the decade indicate that life expectancy continues to increase, heart disease and stroke deaths continue to decline, and Americans are changing their diets toward the goals of less fat and more fruits and vegetables. Although these are hopeful trends, America still faces many significant challenges. Americans who have disabilities, come from low-income families, or are members of minority groups continue to experience disproportionately worse health outcomes than other Americans (USDHHS, 1996).

Goals for 2010

Healthy People 2010 is being developed with a greater understanding of advances in preventive therapies, vaccines and other pharmaceuticals, assistive tech-

TABLE 1.3   1990 Health Status Goals for U.S. Population Set in 1979

Age group (years)	1990 goal*	Special focus
Healthy infants (birth to age 1)	35% fewer deaths	Low birth weight Birth defects
Healthy children (ages 1–14)	20% fewer deaths	Growth and development Injuries
Healthy adolescents and young adults (ages 15–24)	20% fewer deaths	Motor vehicle injuries Alcohol and drug use
Healthy adults (ages 25–64)	25% fewer deaths	Heart attacks Strokes, cancers
Healthy older adults (age 65+)	20% fewer sick days	Functional independence Influenza, pneumonia

*Relative to 1977

Source: U.S. Department of Health, Education, and Welfare, *Healthy People: The Surgeon General's Report on Health Promotion and Disease Prevention* (Washington, D.C.: U.S. Government Printing Office, 1979), pp. ix–x.

nologies, and computerized systems; a heightened awareness and demand for preventive health services and quality health care; and changes in demographics, science, technology, and disease spread that will affect public health into the twenty-first century. Global forces, including food supplies, emerging infectious diseases, and environmental interdependence, will present new public health challenges. While the federal government will take the lead in developing the initial draft objectives, this process is designed to be very participatory.

Healthy People 2010 is the contribution of the U.S. to the World Health Organization's (WHO) *Health for All* strategy. The U.S. effort will be characterized by intersectoral collaboration and community participation. Through national objectives, the U.S. can provide models for world policy and strategies for health improvement for the world's population.

Spirituality and Health

Much of our culture's traditional thinking about health tends to view states of wellness and illness as being affected only by physical processes that are amenable to objective, scientific study. Many people believe, however, that spiritual feelings and experiences—those that are not necessarily achieved by the application of logic and critical thought but that are more intuitive and subjective—can affect a person's health. Indeed, nearly all physicians endorse the idea that a spiritual dimension to life can aid healing (Harvard Health Letter, 1998), and research shows that people with higher levels of intrinsic spirituality tend to be healthier (McBride et al., 1998).

Spiritual experiences tend to engender feelings of compassion and empathy; peace of mind; relatedness and communion with a force, power, or set of values larger than oneself; and harmony with the environment (Dyson et al., 1997). These feelings are believed to be a cornerstone of health because they represent a balance between the inner and outer aspects of human experience. For some, the spiritual dimension of life is embodied in the practice of a specific religion. For others, the spiritual dimension is nonreligious and simply part of a personal philosophy. Many practices can help people experience the spiritual realms of existence—prayer, meditation, yoga, musical and artistic endeavors, and helping others are but a few common ones.

Becoming more spiritually aware, regardless of the chosen path, can lead to a healthier life. Being in touch with your spiritual feelings helps you handle life's ups and downs with understanding and compassion for yourself and others. You become open to love

in the highest sense of its meaning, which is acceptance and tolerance. You begin to love yourself despite your problems and hang-ups. You love your family and friends when relations are strained. You see beauty and harmony in more and more aspects of living. And occasionally—however fleetingly—you may experience the truly wondrous feeling of being completely and joyfully alive.

> *Heavy thoughts bring on physical maladies; when the soul is oppressed so is the body.*
>
> MARTIN LUTHER

Making Healthy Changes

> *One day while out walking, the Buddha and some of his students encountered a line of ants in their path. One of the students said, "Master, why are the ants crossing the road?" The Buddha replied, "Because they want to be happy."*

A major assumption of health education is that nearly everyone has a basic desire to be healthy and well, but that many people acquire habits of thought and behavior that may make them less well rather than more. One goal of health education, therefore, is to encourage people to give up less-healthy attitudes and behaviors and adopt ones that lead to greater health, wellness, and satisfaction in life.

It is said that knowledge is power, but with regard to living healthfully, that isn't always the case. Almost everyone knows that smoking cigarettes, driving after drinking alcohol, and eating junk food are unhealthy, but many people do those things anyway. Simply knowing what to do is no guarantee that a person will do it. One reason for this is that an unhealthy attitude or behavior is rewarding in some way, even if it is harmful in some other way (for example, smoking cigarettes to relieve stress). Also, a variety of biological, social, and psychological forces help maintain an attitude or behavior: A smoker may want to stop, but if many of his or her friends smoke, stopping may jeopardize the smoker's friendships. For a change to occur, the person has to believe that the benefits of change outweigh the costs. Rituals such as New Year's resolutions and slogans such as "just do it" offer unrealistic models of how habits are changed. Desire and will power alone are insufficient; research, planning, and enlisting social support are required as well.

Health behavior change models are classified as individual change models, interpersonal change models, and community models or interventions. We will look at two individual change models and how they apply to an ability to make positive, healthy changes or maintain a healthy lifestyle.

The Health Belief Model

The Health Belief Model (HBM) was originally developed as a systematic method to explain and predict preventive health behavior, but it has been revised to include general health motivation for the purpose of distinguishing illness and sick-role behavior from health behavior. Key aspects of the model are described as:

Perceived Susceptibility Each individual has his or her own perception of the likelihood of experiencing a condition that would adversely affect his or her health. Individuals vary widely in their perception of susceptibility to a disease or condition. Those at the low end of the extreme deny the possibility of contracting an adverse condition. Individuals in a moderate category admit to a statistical possibility of disease susceptibility. Individuals at the high extreme of susceptibility feel there is real danger that they will experience an adverse condition or contract a given disease.

Perceived Seriousness Perceived seriousness refers to the beliefs a person holds concerning the effects of a given disease or condition on his or her state of affairs. These effects can be considered from the point of view of the difficulties that a disease would create—for instance, pain and discomfort, loss of work time, financial burdens, difficulties with family, problems with relationships, and susceptibility to future conditions. It is important to include these emotional and financial burdens when considering the seriousness of a disease or condition.

Perceived Benefits of Taking Action Taking action toward the prevention of disease or toward dealing with an illness is the next step after an individual has accepted the susceptibility of a disease and recognized its seriousness. The direction of action that a person chooses will be influenced by his or her beliefs regarding the action.

Barriers to Taking Action Action may not take place even though an individual may believe that the benefits to taking action are significant. This may be because of barriers, which can include inconvenience, cost, unpleasantness, pain, or upset. These characteristics may lead a person away from taking the desired action.

Cues to Action An individual's perception of the levels of susceptibility and seriousness provide the force to act. Benefits, minus barriers, provide the path of action. However, "cues to action" may be required for the desired behavior to occur. These cues to action may be internal or external.

The Transtheoretical Model

One of the most influential models of health behavior change is the Transtheoretical Model, or Process of Change Model (Prochaska, DiClemente, & Norcross, 1992). This model recognizes that change occurs through the following stages:

Precontemplation The person is not considering changing a particular behavior any time in the foreseeable future. Many individuals in this stage are unaware or underaware of their problems. Information is important during this stage.

Contemplation The person becomes aware that change is desirable but has not committed to act. The person often focuses on why it would be difficult to change. Information on options on how to change the behavior can be helpful during this stage.

Preparation The person desires change and commits to making that change in the near future, usually within the next 30 days. Instead of thinking why he or she can't take action, the focus is on what can be done to begin. The person creates a realistic plan for making a change, including overcoming obstacles. This stage may include announcing the change to friends and family, researching how to make the change, making a calendar, or setting up a diary or journal to record progress and obstacles to progress.

Action The person implements the plan. The old behavior and the environmental situations that reinforced that behavior are stopped and new behaviors and environmental supports are adopted. Obstacles are expected and noted, and strategies for overcoming them are implemented. Progress through this stage may take 6 months or more.

Maintenance The person strengthens the change, recognizing that lapses and even temptations to give up will occur. "Ebb and flow" are to be expected and not to be seen as failures. The person can remind himself or herself of the many benefits of and gains from the behavior change to help combat relapse.

Termination The person is not tempted to return to the previous behavior.

At the end of each major section of this book, you will find an activity section called *Making Healthy Changes*. This program is intended to give you specific suggestions for healthier living. It is designed to make you question common unhealthy behaviors and work toward slowly changing them. These changes will require motivation on your part to try all or some of the activities, so be aware of the steps toward behavior change described above.

Critical Thinking About Health

1. As pointed out in this chapter, the major health issues of college students are sexual health, mental health, substance abuse, weight, accidents and injuries, and health care. Discuss which of these issues is of most concern to you personally. Explain your reasons and worries. How can you deal with your concerns in a way that will improve your health?

2. Describe one lifestyle or behavior that you routinely engage in that you regard as destructive to your health (smoking, for example). Discuss your reasons for continuing to engage in this unhealthy behavior. Consider what you might do to change this behavior and list the steps you would take to accomplish the healthy change. Do you believe that you can make the healthy change?

3. Suppose that someone you know is suffering from frequent, severe headaches (several times a week) and does not know what to do about the problem

other than to take acetaminophen or aspirin. Based on your own health experiences, explain the advice that you would give such a friend. Consider all the alternatives discussed in this chapter and any others that you think might be helpful. Develop an approach to ending this person's headaches that you think is both appropriate and likely to solve the problem. Give reasons for the approach that you recommend.

4. Imagine that you are the Surgeon General of the United States, who formulates national health policy. (A former Surgeon General, C. Everett Koop, formulated the crusade against tobacco smoking a generation ago). Describe what you believe is the primary health problem in the U.S. today. Justify your choice with as many facts as you can find. Describe the steps you believe should be taken by government, private companies, organizations, and individuals to eradicate this health problem.

Health in Review

- Health is not only the absence of disease but also is living in harmony with oneself, friends and relatives, and the environment.
- Health means being responsible for preventing personal illness and injuries as well as knowing when to seek medical help.
- The three models used to describe health are medical, environmental, and holistic, or wellness.
- The wellness continuum ranges from high-level wellness to premature death.
- A holistic approach to health emphasizes prevention of disease and injury and self-responsibility for nutrition, exercise, and other aspects of lifestyle that promote wellness.
- The dimensions of wellness are emotional, intellectual, spiritual, occupational, social, and physical.
- Many chronic diseases (e.g., diabetes, heart disease, cancer) are primarily attributable to un-

healthy living habits. Taking responsibility for your health while you are young is the best way to reduce the risk of chronic disease later in life.
- Unhealthy lifestyles and behaviors are responsible for half of all deaths in the United States each year.
- Psychosomatic illnesses are physical symptoms caused by stress, anxiety, and emotional upset in the absence of any organic disease.
- Image visualization is effective in reducing anxiety and stress, in modifying behaviors, and in enhancing performance on exams and in sports.
- Spiritual awareness is an essential part of maintaining wellness and preventing illness.
- *Healthy People 2000* is the nation's vision for the new century, characterized by enhancing quality of life, reducing the incidence of preventable diseases and premature deaths, and reducing disparity in health status among different demographic groups.

Health and Wellness Online

The World Wide Web contains a wealth of information about health and wellness. By accessing the Internet using Web browser software, such as Netscape Navigator or Microsoft's Internet Explorer, you can gain a new perspective on many topics presented in *Essentials of Health and Wellness, Second Edition.* Access the Jones and Bartlett Publishers web site at http://www.jbpub.com/hwonline.

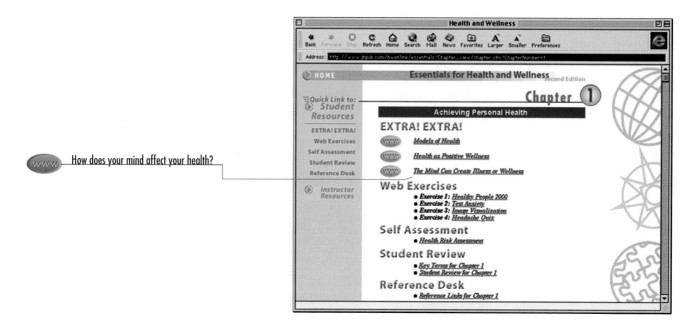

References

Douglas, K. A., Collins, J. L., Warren, C., Kann, L., Gold, R., Clayton, S., Ross, J. G., & Kolbe, L. J. (1997). Results from the 1995 national college health survey. *Journal of American College Health, 46,* 55–61.

Dyson, J., Cobb, M., & Forman, D. (1997). The meaning of spirituality: A literature review. *Journal of Advances in Nursing, 26,* 1183–1188.

Grace, T. W. (1997). Health problems of college students. *Journal of American College Health, 45,* 243–250.

Making a place for spirituality. (1998). *Harvard Health Letter 23(4),* 1–3.

McBride, J. L., Borrks, A. G., & Pilkington, L. (1998). The relationship between a patient's spirituality and health experiences. *Family Medicine, 30,* 122–126.

McCahill, M. E. (1995, February 15). Focus on the somatoform disorders. *Hospital Practice,* 59–66.

Prochaska, J. O., DiClemente, C. C., & Norcross, J. (1992). In search of how people change: Applications to addictive behaviors. *American Psychologist, 47,* 1102–1114.

United States Department of Health and Human Services. (1979). *Healthy people: The Surgeon General's report on health promotion and disease prevention.* (PHS 79-55071). Washington, DC: U.S. Government Printing Office.

United States Department of Health and Human Services. (1996). *Healthy people 2000: Midcourse review and 1995 revisions.* Washington, DC: U.S. Government Printing Office.

Suggested Readings

Anders, G. (1996). *Health against wealth.* New York: Houghton Mifflin. A journalist's examination of the health care industry and the need for people to take responsibility for their own health.

Hurley, J. S., & Schlaadt, R. G. (1992). *The Wellness life-style.* Guilford, CT: Dushkin Publishing Group. A book that helps you think critically about your life-style and offers suggestions for change.

McGinnis, J. M., & Foege, W. H. (1993). Actual causes of death in the United States. *Journal of the American Medical Society, 270,* 2207–2212. Shows that half of all deaths in the United States are caused by unhealthy lifestyle choices and behaviors.

Miller, E. (1997). *Deep healing: The essence of mind/body medicine.* New York: Hay House. Stories, reflections, and case studies that illustrate how mental imagery, positive thinking, and other basics of mind-body medicine contribute to health and longevity.

Ornish, D. (1998). *Love and survival: The scientific basis for the healing power of intimacy* New York: HarperCollins. Discusses how personal intimacy and other aspects of emotional well-being contribute to better health, including stronger immune systems, better cardiovascular functioning, and longer life expectancies.

Taylor, E., Lee, C. T. & Young, J. D. (1997, May 15). Bringing mind-body medicine into the mainstream. *Hospital Practice,* 183–186. A review of how environmental and holistic views of health are being integrated into the traditional medical model.

Weil, A. (1997). *Healthy living: Ask Dr. Weil.* New York: Ivy Books. The famous doctor tells how to live healthier and longer.

Learning Objectives

1. Define the terms stress, stressor, eustress, distress, and stress-related illness.
2. Describe the changes in behavior, autonomic nervous system, and immune system that are caused by stress.
3. Name several physiological symptoms of stress.
4. Identify and explain the three components of stress.
5. Explain how frustration, inner conflict, and social pressures cause stress.
6. Discuss three common reactions to stress.
7. Discuss several factors that influence the degree of stress a person experiences.
8. Explain the fight-or-flight response.
9. Describe the three phases of the general adaptation syndrome.
10. Describe how stress affects the immune system.
11. Describe the relaxation response.
12. Explain how stress can be managed.

Exercises and Activities

WORKBOOK
What Are Your Stress Reactions?
How Susceptible Are You to Stress?
Do You Have Hurry Sickness?

Health and Wellness Online

 www.jbpub.com/hwonline

How Stress Contributes to Illness
Wellness Guide: Time Management
Stress and the Immune System

Chapter 2

Managing Stress: Restoring Mind-Body Harmony

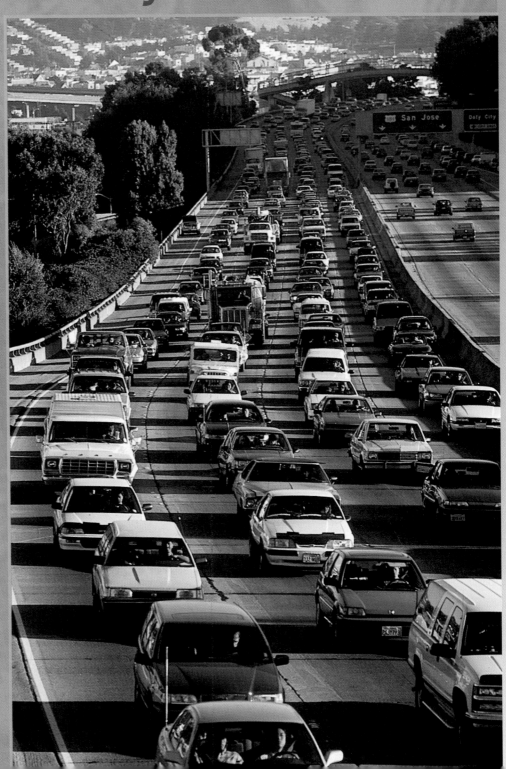

Life is filled with a never-ending array of challenges. Some of them are obstacles to accomplishing necessary daily tasks or cherished life goals. Others are opportunities for growth and positive changes in our lives. When confronted with a particular challenge—whether it be earning good grades in school, obtaining a well-paying job, becoming a parent, becoming involved in a social relationship, or living with an uncompromising roommate—we may feel excited, anxious, sad, depressed, angry, or afraid. Such feelings may cause symptoms like sleeplessness, gastrointestinal upset, headache, and muscular tension, all of which signal a disruption of psychobiological balance. Usually this disruption is brief, because we find ways to meet the challenge and to restore our well-being. Confronting and resolving a challenge often becomes a positive growth experience. Other times, however, disruption in mind-body harmony is prolonged or severe, and we are said to be "under stress" or "stressed out." Prolonged, unresolved stress can contribute to the development of several kinds of disorders.

> Anyone can do any amount of work provided it isn't the work he is supposed to be doing.
>
> ROBERT BENCHLEY,
> THE ALGONQUIN WIT

The Definition of Stress

Although most people have at some time considered themselves "under stress" or "stressed out," it is important to take note of the difference in how the word *stress* is used. When someone is "under stress," stress refers to the *cause* of the disruption of mind-body harmony; for example, "She was under stress from having to take five exams in 2 days." On the other hand, "stressed out" refers to the *experience* of the disruption in mind-body harmony; for example, "During final exams she was so stressed out that she suffered from stomach cramps, diarrhea, and insomnia."

Because it is confusing to use the word *stress* to represent both causes and results of challenging or disruptive life experiences, we use the term **stressor** in this chapter to refer to circumstances and events that produce disruptions in mind-body harmony. We use the term **stress** to refer to the symptoms resulting from stressors.

Defining stress in terms of a person's response focuses attention on an individual's experience rather than on external factors (the stressors). By doing this, the avoidance or prevention of stress is under the control of the individual, and it is suggested that stress-related illnesses can be prevented. In many instances, people can minimize their interaction with or even

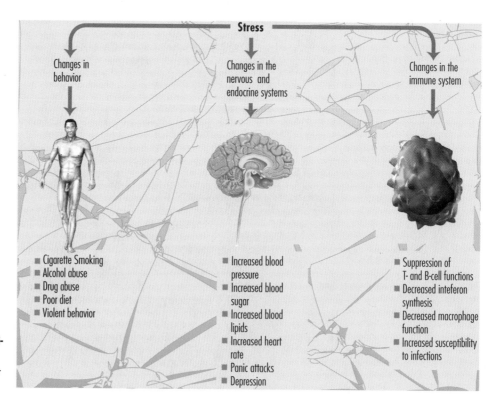

FIGURE 2.1   Stress Causes Physiological Changes Relationships between stress and changes in the nervous, endocrine, and immune systems.

avoid a stressor. They can change how they perceive a challenging situation and thereby lessen their degree of distress. And they can use physical, mental, and social resources to help them meet the challenge without incurring a stress-related illness.

 ## How Stress Contributes to Illness

When we experience a challenging situation, the nervous, endocrine (hormone), and immune systems respond to meet the challenge. These responses are aspects of normal physiology that are meant to deal with short-term stressful situations. Illness arises when the body's stress-response mechanisms are continually activated. Then, organs wear down and become diseased, and lowered immunity leads to increased susceptibility to infections and other diseases (Figure 2.1).

Stress also contributes to illness by fostering unhealthy behaviors. To manage stressful feelings, for example, some people smoke cigarettes, drink alcohol (or take other drugs), overeat, undereat, or overwork. Furthermore, people with high levels of stress may not engage in health-promoting activities, such as exercising regularly, eating properly, and getting enough sleep.

Stress has three components (Figure 2.2):

1. *Activators:* occurrences, situations, and events that are potential stressors
2. *Reactions:* interpretations of activators as taxing or exceeding one's mental, physical, and social resources to cope with them successfully. For example, taking six courses in a school term becomes an activator when the student interprets that course load as potentially overwhelming and becomes anx-

ious about completing the work successfully. This work load would not be an activator of stress to someone who did not interpret it as overwhelming.

3. *Consequences:* the psychobiological effects of a reaction to stress. These can include attempting to change the stressful situation; quelling stressful feelings with alcohol, drugs, cigarettes, tranquilizers, overwork, or other unhealthy behaviors; or, if the person is unable or unwilling to alter interaction with the activator or reaction, facing the possibility of a stress-related illness.

Stress Activators

Activators are situations that have the potential to disrupt a person's emotional or mental state. Activators or stressors can be major external events (war, flood, famine), unpleasant interactions with people (divorce, job loss), or they may result from changes in the body resulting from accidents, disease, or aging. An unmet emotional need or happy events such as marriage or winning a lottery can also activate stress.

Terms

stressor: any physical or psychological event or condition that produces stress

stress: the sum of physical and emotional reactions to any stimulus that disturbs the organism's homeostasis

activators: potential stressors; occurrences, situations, or events perceived as stressful

reactions: interpretations of activators as taxing or overwhelming

consequences: the effects of one's action; the effects of stress response

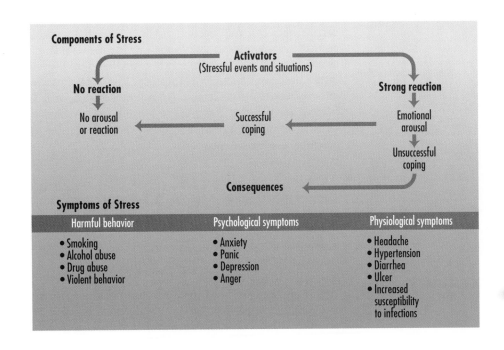

FIGURE 2.2   The Stress-Illness Relationship It is through one's reaction that a given situation is experienced as stressful.

Life Changes as Activators

Stress researchers have developed a variety of methods to identify and measure the potential for life experiences to be stress activators. One of the most common of these is the Social Readjustment Rating Scale (SRRS), which lists 43 common life events and, for each event, a corresponding number of life change units (LCUs) (Holmes and Rahe, 1967). LCUs represent the relative amount of psychological and physiological adjustment required to meet the challenge produced by the particular life event. For example, in the SRRS, the death of a spouse requires the most adjustment, with an arbitrary numerical LCU value of 100. Marriage carries a value of 50 LCUs, and a vacation has a value of 13 LCUs. Notice that both positive (marriage, vacation) and negative (death of spouse) events are on the scale.

Research has shown that accumulating more than 150 LCUs on the SRRS within 6 months correlates with a high probability that a person will experience a negative health change. The nature of the health change cannot be predicted, only that one is likely to occur. Negative health changes include heart attacks, accidents, infectious diseases, worsening of a previous illness, injuries, and metabolic disease.

The Recent Life Changes Questionnaire (RLCQ) (Table 2.1), is an updated version of the SRRS (Miller and Rahe, 1997). (Most published studies still refer to the SRRS.) The RLCQ contains 74 life events that are representative of the stressors of people living in American society today. Accumulation of more than 300 LCUs within 6 months or 500 LCUs within 1 year is indicative of a high degree of recent life stress.

Daily Events as Activators

Stress results from the cumulative effects of daily hassles, which irritate us, cause us to worry, and create psychic and bodily tension. Hassles include frustrations, inner conflicts, and social pressures.

Frustration Frustration is the feeling resulting from being blocked from attaining a personal goal, like getting stuck in a traffic jam when you're trying to get somewhere. Besides being uncomfortable, frustration produces potentially illness-causing physiological changes (increased heart rate, changes in hormone levels, and lowered immune function). Frustration can lead to feelings of aggression (the motivation to overcome an obstacle). Acting on feelings of frustration and aggression, a stuck motorist might honk the horn, yell at other stopped motorists, be angry with himself or herself for choosing this particular route, or pound on the steering wheel. None of these actions are likely to get traffic moving again; instead, they are likely only to increase frustration. It would be healthier to reduce frustration by changing the importance of the goal ("The world won't end because I'm late for work") or changing the goal to something that can be accomplished ("I'm stuck so I'm going to listen to this relaxation audiotape or enjoy a few minutes of meditation.") Releasing frustration healthfully is better than "bottling it up inside," which tends to make people sick.

Inner Conflict Inner conflict is represented by having to choose between two incompatible goals. The choice can be between two desired goals (approach-approach conflict), two undesirable goals (avoidance-avoidance conflict), or a goal that has both desired and undesired outcomes (approach-avoidance conflict). Having to choose between two desired goals, like deciding which film to see or what toppings to put on a pizza, causes little stress. Having to choose between two undesirable goals—"being between a rock and a hard place"— is very stressful.

Approach-Avoidance Approach-avoidance situations often produce vacillation, inaction, or procrastination. For example, someone wanting to ask someone out may vacillate because of fear of rejection. To get unstuck from approach-avoidance conflict, psychologists generally advise lessening focus on the negative ("Rejection might hurt but I'm still a nice person") and increasing focus on the positive ("It'll be great if she or he says yes"). Procrastinators can stop judging themselves

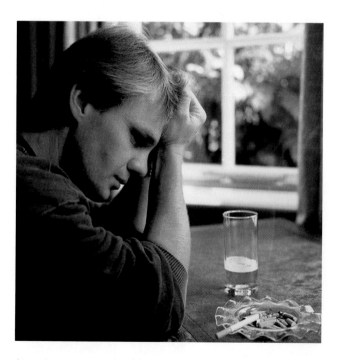

Stress can cause unhealthy behaviors, such as drinking and smoking.

TABLE 2.1   The Recent Life Changes Questionnaire

Life event	Life change units Men	Women	Life event	Life change units Men	Women
Death of son or daughter	135	103	Moderate illness	47	39
Death of spouse	122	113	Loss or damage of personal property	47	35
Death of brother or sister	111	87	Sexual difficulties	44	44
Death of parent	105	90	Getting demoted at work	44	39
Divorce	102	85	Major change in living conditions	44	37
Death of family member	96	78	Increase in income	43	30
Fired from work	85	69	Relationship problems	42	34
Separation from spouse due to marital problems	79	70	Trouble with in-laws	41	33
Major injury or illness	79	64	Beginning or ending school or college	40	35
Being held in jail	78	71	Making a major purchase	40	33
Pregnancy	74	55	New, close personal relationship	39	34
Miscarriage or abortion	74	51	Outstanding personal achievement	38	33
Death of a close friend	73	64	Troubles with co-workers at work	37	32
Laid off from work	73	59	Change in school or college	37	31
Birth of a child	71	56	Change in your work hours or conditions	36	32
Adopting a child	71	54	Troubles with workers whom you supervise	35	34
Major business adjustment	67	47	Getting a transfer at work	33	31
Decrease in income	66	49	Getting a promotion at work	33	29
Parents' divorce	63	52	Change in religious beliefs	31	27
A relative moving in with you	62	53	Christmas	30	25
Foreclosure on a mortgage or a loan	62	51	Having more responsibilities at work	29	29
Investment and/or credit difficulties	62	46	Troubles with your boss at work	29	29
Marital Reconciliation	61	48	Major change in usual type or amount of recreation	29	28
Major change in health or behavior of family member	58	50	General work troubles	29	27
Change in arguments with spouse	55	41	Change in social activities	29	24
Retirement	54	48	Major change in eating habits	29	23
Major decision regarding your immediate future	54	46	Major change in sleeping habits	28	23
Separation from spouse due to work	53	54	Change in family get-togethers	28	20
An accident	53	38	Change in personal habits	27	24
Parental remarriage	52	45	Major dental work	27	23
Change residence to a different town, city, or state	52	39	Change of residence in same town or city	27	21
Change to a new type of work	51	50	Change in political beliefs	26	21
"Falling out" of a close, personal relationship	50	41	Vacation	26	20
Marriage	50	50	Having fewer responsibilities at work	22	21
Spouse changes work	50	38	Making a moderate purchase	22	18
Child leaving home	48	38	Change in church activities	21	20
Birth of grandchild	48	34	Minor violation of the law	20	19
Engagement to marry	47	42	Correspondence course to help you in your work	19	16

Source: Adapted with permission from M. A. Miller and R. H. Rahe (1997). "Life changes scaling for the 1990s." *Journal of Psychosomatic Research, 43,* 279–292.

as inferior and instead focus on lessening the reason they avoid pursuit of their goal.

Pressure Pressure is the expectation or demand that we behave in a certain way. Pressure can be external (social or peer pressure) or internal (the perfectionist inside you). Pressure is stressful because it increases anxiety. Failure to conform risks rejection from the group, and failure to perform risks loss of self-esteem.

Antidotes to the negative effects of daily stressors are daily uplifts from the things in life that give you pleasure: spending time with a friend, having fun, enjoying a movie, or taking a walk.

Reactions to Activators

Reactions depend largely on the individual's personality and emotional makeup and not on the nature of the activator. Everyone interprets the world and events differently. Each of us is born with a capacity for certain behaviors, which are greatly modified and shaped by what we learn and experience. Each of us reacts to a particular situation according to individual values, beliefs, and attitudes.

Because of these differences, a situation that may be stressful and upsetting to one person may not even bother another. Experiencing stress requires that an individual interpret a given situation as significant ("This situation is important to me") and that he or she decide what to do with the situation ("What can I do about it?"). For most people, situations that are interpreted as stressful include (a) harm and loss, (b) threat, and (c) challenge.

Harm-and-loss situations include the death of a loved one, theft or damage to one's home, physical injury or loss of an organ, physical assault, or loss of self-esteem. Harm-and-loss situations create stress because an important physical or psychological need is not satisfied. Emotions that signal harm or loss include sadness, depression, and anger. Eight of the first ten items on the RLCQ involve harm and loss.

Threat situations are perceived and interpreted as likely to produce harm or loss whether any harm or loss actually occurs. The experience is one of continually warding off demands that tax one's abilities to cope with life. Emotions associated with threat include anger, hostility, anxiety, frustration, and depression.

Challenge situations are perceived and interpreted as opportunities for growth, mastery, and gain. Very often such situations involve major life transitions such as leaving one's family to start life on one's own, graduating from college, or getting married. Even though they are interpreted as good, life transitions can be stressful because they require considerable psychological and physical adjustment. Often a life transition involves both sadness and excitement: sadness for the loss of what is familiar and excitement in anticipation of the new. Psychologists refer to the stress that comes from positive challenges as **eustress** and the stress associated with negative life challenges or the anticipation of them as **distress.**

Interpreting a situation as threatening or challenging often leads to asking oneself, "what can I do about it?" The degree of stress may depend on your answer. Believing we can manage a stressful situation is more likely to lessen stress than believing that the situation is overwhelming. In laboratory experiments, for example, animals given the opportunity to avoid or delay a mild electric shock develop only slightly more ulcers than do animals who receive no shock at all. People who work in jobs that involve a lot of pressure to perform but allow little opportunity for deciding how the tasks of the job are to be accomplished experience greater stress than do workers who have more control over decision-making (Karasek and Theorell, 1989). Efforts to manage a situation are called **coping.**

Several factors influence the degree of distress a person experiences. Among them are predictability, control, belief in the outcome, and social support.

Predictability Research shows that knowing when a stressful situation will occur produces less stress than not knowing. Individuals may be just as stressed when the event occurs, but knowing when it will occur allows them to relax afterward. Knowing that something stressful may occur but not knowing when (like a "pop" quiz in a class) puts the individual on constant alert. For example, during World War II, London was bombed every night, but the London suburbs were not. Londoners had fewer ulcers than suburbanites, presumably because they knew bombings would occur.

Control Individuals who believe they can influence the course of their lives (internal locus of control) are likely to suffer less stress than individuals who believe their destiny is influenced largely by factors out-

Terms

harm-and-loss situations: stressful events that include death, loss of property, injury, and illness

threat situations: events that cause stress because of a perception that harm or loss may occur

challenge situations: positive events that may involve major life transitions and may cause stress

eustress: stress resulting from pleasant stressors

distress: stress resulting from unpleasant stressors

coping: attempts to manage a stressful situation

Wellness Guide

Time Management

A major cause of college student stress is the sense that there's too much to do and not enough time to do it. Since you can't make more time, the way to ease this pressure is to make the best use of the time you've got. Here are some tips for time management:

- *Perform a time audit.* For at least 3 representative days in your week (a whole week is better), write down everything you do during each of the 24 hours. Make a chart. Identify "windows" of time that could be put to better use and alter your activities accordingly.

- *Be energy efficient.* Schedule important activities for the times of the day when you are most alert and attentive. For example, if you're a morning person, take morning classes and study in between them. Schedule exercise and socializing for the afternoon. Night people might do the opposite.

- *Keep a to-do list.* At the beginning of each day, or the night before, write down all the things you have to do.

- *Prioritize tasks: first things first.* Classify tasks according to their *urgency* and *importance,* and do them in this order: (a) urgent and important;

(b) not urgent but important; (c) urgent but not important; and (d) not urgent or important. Distinguishing the urgent and important tasks from the urgent but not important tasks is often difficult because urgency is a state of mind that makes everything seem important. Before prioritizing the items on your to-do list, take a few minutes to become mentally and physically quiet. This will allow you to place truly urgent and important items at the top of your to-do list.

- *Don't sweat the small stuff.* Eliminate unimportant tasks from your list. Don't do, worry about, or think about anything that doesn't match your most important values or long-term life goals.

- *Control interruptions.* Discourage drop-in visiting; don't answer the pager or the phone (if it's important, the person will call back); stay away from TV, computer games, and the Internet.

- *Schedule time for you.* Even if it's only a few moments a day, take time for activities that you find meaningful, e.g., reading, prayer, meditation, journal writing, letter writing, musical or artistic pursuits. This will keep you from burning out.

- *Schedule time for fun.* Don't forget to play and socialize.

- *Sleep.* Not sleeping enough is like overdrawing money from a bank account: eventually you have to pay it back. Furthermore, when "overdrawn" at the sleep bank, you function at 50% to 70% efficiency, which makes school work take longer and adds to the sense that there isn't enough time.

- *Tame any tendencies toward perfectionism.* Don't try to make everything perfect. Every task has a point of diminishing returns—when the time and energy you put in is out of proportion to what you can reasonably hope to get back.

- *Understand any tendencies to procrastinate.* Procrastination often grows out of the fear of failure or exposure (people seeing you or your work and judging it harshly). When you hear your litany of excuses for not working at a task, ask yourself what you fear. Be your own best friend and encourage yourself to move ahead. Break the task into smaller parts and take them on one by one. Reward yourself when each one is finished.

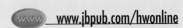 **www.jbpub.com/hwonline**

side of themselves (external locus of control). The crucial factor is not whether the locus of control is internal or external, but the belief that one can influence one's destiny.

Belief in the Outcome People who believe that things are improving (optimistic) experience less stress than do people who believe that things are getting worse (pessimistic).

Social Support Having someone to talk to and believing that that person can be supportive with physical, emotional, and intellectual resources lessens stress. For example, patients who talk with their surgeons about their fears before surgery require less anesthetic during the operation and have a smaller stress response than patients who go through such procedures feeling uninformed and unsupported.

The Consequences of Our Reactions

Although the human mind interprets a given situation as harmful, threatening, or challenging, the nervous and endocrine systems, which link the brain and the rest of the body, bring about the changes in physiology that lead to harmful behaviors or to disease. The feelings associated with stressful experiences (fear, anger, sadness, etc.) activate the nervous and endocrine systems, which in turn produce changes in the immune system and in physiology. Illnesses arise when the nervous and endocrine systems are continually activated or overstimulated. Anxiety, sadness, frustration, and other emotions alter the functions of the heart, blood vessels, immune system, and other organs. If prolonged, such alterations can produce heart disease, high blood pressure, and an increased susceptibility to infectious disease and, possibly, cancer (see chapters 9 and 10).

The Fight-or-Flight Response

The challenge-response systems activate the **fight-or-flight response.** All mammals, including humans, are capable of displaying this particular response when confronted with challenges they interpret as frightening or a threat to survival. The response is characterized by a coordinated discharge of the **sympathetic nervous system** and portions of the **parasympathetic nervous system** and by the secretion of a number of hormones, especially **epinephrine** and **cortisol.** When a person (or other animal) experiences a threatening situation, the associated emotions (usually fear or rage) that arise in the limbic system portion of the brain are translated automatically into the appropriate physiological responses through nervous and hormonal pathways mediated by the **hypothalamus.**

As Figure 2.3 shows, some prominent aspects of the fight-or-flight response are an elevation of the heart rate and blood pressure (to provide more blood to muscles), constriction of the blood vessels of the skin (to limit bleeding if wounded), dilation of the pupil of the eye (to let in more light, thereby improving vision), increased activity in the reticular formation of the brain (to increase the alert, aroused state), and liberation of glucose and free fatty acids from storage depots (to make more stored energy available to the muscles, brain, and other tissues and organs).

Everyone is capable of the fight-or-flight response; it is part of the human biological makeup. Individuals display this reaction to some extent when they narrowly escape from a dangerous mishap or when they get angry or frustrated and lose their tempers. The heart rate quickens, the person becomes more alert and tense, and he or she experiences a rush of excite-

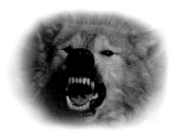

Heart
Increase in heart rate

Blood
Constriction in abdominal skeletal muscles

Eye
Contraction of the iris

Intestines
Relaxation of sphincters

Skin
Contraction of muscles and sweat glands

Spleen
Contraction

Brain
Activation

FIGURE 2.3   **The Fight-or-Flight Response**   All humans display this response when confronted with challenges they interpret as frightening or threatening.

ment from increased secretion of epinephrine into the blood. In short, the person becomes ready to take action to deal with the situation.

In our modern civilized society, however, literally fleeing from a threatening situation or engaging in physical combat is often an inappropriate—and sometimes impossible—response. Social norms dictate that people handle many difficult situations "civilly." Moreover, many threats are symbolic. The fear of losing a job, social status, or a lover is not the same as being confronted by a ferocious animal or thug, but the anxiety can produce similar stress-related physiological responses. Thus, one of the consequences of having a highly evolved brain with the ability for symbolic thought and the intellectual capacity to produce a "civilized" society is the existence of social norms that make people unwilling or unable to take direct action when confronted with threatening situations.

The General Adaptation Syndrome

Hans Selye, a pioneer in stress research, found that continued physiological responding to stressors led to a characteristic response called the General Adaptation Syndrome (GAS). The GAS is a three-phase response to a stressor (Figure 2.4). The three phases are stage of alarm, stage of resistance, and stage of exhaustion.

1. *Stage of alarm:* A person's ability to withstand or resist any type of stressor is lowered by the need to deal with the stressor, whether it is a burn, a broken arm, the loss of a loved one, the fear of failing a class, or losing a job.

2. *Stage of resistance:* The body adapts to the continued presence of the stressor by producing more epi-

Terms

fight-or-flight response: a defensive reaction that prepares the organism for conflict or escape by triggering hormonal, cardiovascular, metabolic, and other changes

sympathetic nervous system: a division of the autonomic nervous system that reacts to danger or challenges by almost instantly putting body processes into high gear

parasympathetic nervous system: a division of the autonomic nervous system that tones down the excitatory effects of the sympathetic nervous system; slows metabolism and restores energy reserves

epinephrine: a hormone secreted by the medulla (inner core) of the adrenal gland; also called adrenaline

cortisol: a steroid hormone secreted by the cortex (outer layer) of the adrenal gland

hypothalamus: a part of the brain that activates, controls, and integrates the autonomic nervous system, the endocrine system, and other bodily functions

posttraumatic stress disorder (PTSD): physical and mental illnesses resulting from severe trauma.

At least five heart attacks occur every year on the floor of the New York Stock Exchange, making it one of the highest-density heart attack zones in the U.S. The Exchange has installed a defibrillator near the bank of phones used to place orders for stock trading, and it has trained workers to use the defibrillator and perform CPR when a heart attack occurs.

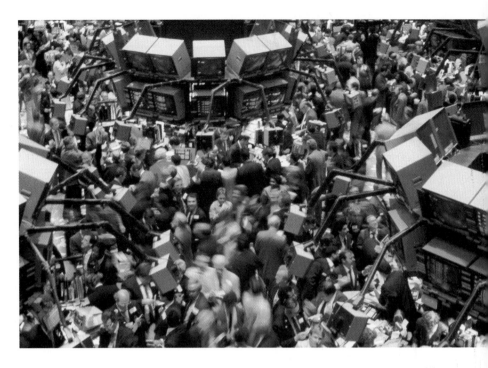

nephrine, raising blood pressure, increasing alertness, suppressing the immune system, and tensing muscles. If interaction with the stressor is prolonged, the ability to resist becomes depleted.

3. *Stage of exhaustion:* When the ability to resist is depleted, the person becomes ill. Because many months or even years of wear and tear may be required before the body's resistance is exhausted, illness may not appear until long after the initial interaction with the stressor.

Posttraumatic Stress

Some forms of stress are so severe that they produce a serious, long-lasting psychological condition called **posttraumatic stress disorder (PTSD)**. This condition can result from the stress produced by combat in war,

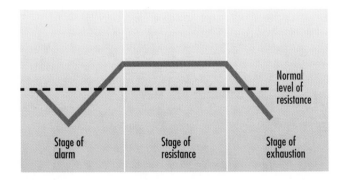

FIGURE 2.4   **The Three Phases of the General Adaptation Syndrome**   In the stage of alarm, the body's normal resistance to stress is lowered from the first interactions with the stressor. In the stage of resistance, the body adapts to the continued presence of the stressor and resistance increases. In the stage of exhaustion, the body loses its ability to resist the stressor any longer and becomes exhausted.

living through a natural disaster, such as a devastating hurricane or tornado, as well as rape, physical assault, or life-threatening illness. About 2% of the U.S. population are estimated to have PTSD as a result of traumatic and terrifying experiences. Some of the diagnostic criteria for PTSD include: (1) flashbacks to the traumatizing event(s) or recurrent thoughts and dreams of the experience; (2) difficulty sleeping, outbursts of anger, and being hyperalert and easily startled; and (3) little interest in daily activities, feeling cut off from others, and a sense of having a limited future.

PTSD came into prominence among combat veterans of the Vietnam war, and even 20 years later many of the veterans diagnosed with PTSD have an excessively high rate of circulatory, digestive, respiratory, and musculoskeletal disorders, as well as susceptibility to infectious diseases (Boscarino, 1997). How the severe stress of wartime combat, natural disasters, and physical and sexual abuse produces these illnesses is not understood. But PTSD does show that severe or prolonged stress can initiate biological changes that result in serious diseases.

Not everyone who is exposed to life-threatening or traumatic events will develop PTSD; some persons are able to cope better or are genetically or psychologically less susceptible to PTSD. Although there are several theories as to what causes PTSD, none really explains the array of psychological and biological symptoms in PTSD patients. However, any of several forms of psychological counseling can help individuals who have PTSD to cope with their traumatic experiences. What seems to matter most is not the form of psychological therapy but the rapport between the patient and the counselor. Antidepressant and sedative

Managing Stress

Progressive Muscle Relaxation

In the technique called progressive relaxation, you lie on your back in quiet, comfortable surroundings with your feet slightly apart and palms facing upward. Before beginning the exercise allow the thoughts of the day and any worries to leave your mind. Then you are ready to begin.

1. Close your eyes; squeeze your lids shut as tightly as you can. Hold them shut for a count of five; then slowly release the tension. Notice how your eyes feel as they relax. Keep your eyelids lightly closed; breathe slowly and deeply.

2. Turn your palms down. Bend your left hand back at the wrist, keeping your forearm on the floor. Bend your hand as far as it will go until you feel tension in your forearm muscles. Hold for a count of five; then release the tension. Notice the warm, relaxed sensation that enters your wrist. Repeat with your right hand.

3. With palms up, make a tight fist in your left hand by tightening the muscles of the arm and fingers. Hold for a count of five; release the tension. Notice the tingling, relaxed sensation in your hand and arm. Repeat with your right hand.

4. Focus your attention on your left leg; slowly bring the top of your foot as far forward as you can while keeping your heel on the floor. Notice the tension in the muscles of your lower leg. Hold for a count of five; release the tension. Repeat with your right leg.

5. Point the toes in your left foot away from you as far as you can. Notice the tension in your calf muscles. Release the tension slowly. Repeat with your right foot.

Similar exercises can be performed to tense and relax other muscles.

drugs also may be prescribed to alleviate symptoms while the person is learning to cope with the traumatic experiences.

The Relaxation Response

In 1975 Herbert Benson and his colleagues at Harvard Medical School (Benson et al., 1975) studied the effects of various relaxation techniques on human physiology. They discovered that hypnosis (**meditation,** in which the person focuses on breathing, a sound, or an image) and **yoga** (a combination of physical movements and mental focusing) produce similar physiological responses. They found that persons practicing these techniques had lower blood pressure and heart rate, reduced oxygen consumption, more relaxed muscles, and reduced perspiration.

Mediation is not what you think.
KRISHNAMURTI

Benson called the sum of these physiological effects the **relaxation response.** He found that, regardless of the relaxation technique used, the relaxation response embraced four common elements: (1) a quiet environment; (2) repetition of a specific word, phrase, or exercise that focuses on the mind's attention; (3) a passive, accepting mental state; and (4) a comfortable physical position.

Recently, Dr. Benson has expanded the scope of the relaxation response to include prayer as a key component of healing. He has come out strongly for prayer and a belief in God as the essential elements for promoting wellness and healing (Benson and Stark, 1996). Dr. Benson has championed the idea that human beings are "hard-wired" for God; this idea allows him to bridge the scientific gap between biology and belief.

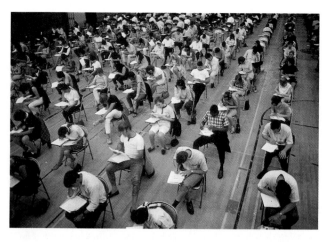

Academic pressures and test taking can produce anxiety and stress.

Terms

meditation: relaxed state of mind produced by focusing the mind on internal images, sounds, or passing thoughts

yoga: a combination of physical movements and mental exercises that relax the mind and the body

relaxation response: the physiological changes in the body that result from mental relaxation techniques

Managing Stress

Visualization Reduces Exam Anxiety

The following exercise can reduce the stress and anxiety of taking exams. It can result in improved scores and a reduction in symptoms produced by stress.

1. Find a comfortable place in your house or room and a time when you will not be disturbed by other people. Sit in a comfortable chair or lie down on a couch or floor. The main thing is to get physically comfortable. If music helps you relax, play some of your favorite music softly.

2. Close your eyes and ask your mind to recall a place and time where you felt contented. It might be a vacation time, being with someone, or being alone in a beautiful environment. Use your imagination and memory to reconstruct the scene where you felt happy and healthy. Notice that you had no concerns there at that time. Let yourself become involved with the scene. The process is similar to having a day-dream or a fantasy. While your mind is focused on pleasurable memories, your body automatically relaxes.

3. When you feel quite relaxed, refocus your mind on the upcoming exam. See yourself taking the exam while feeling relaxed and confident. Because your mind and body are relaxed and comfortable, your mind automatically associates the same feelings with the image of taking the exam. Visualize the exam room, the other students, yourself answering the questions; let your mind focus on as many details as possible.

4. Now project your mind into the future to the actual day and place of the exam. Notice how relaxed you feel as you take the exam; the anxiety you used to experience seems to have vanished. Continue with the visualization until you see yourself turning in the exam and feeling confident and pleased with your performance.

5. Do this exercise for several days prior to any exam that causes anxiety. You will be surprised at the absence of nervousness and stress on exam day. You will be even more pleased at the improvement in your grades.

Stress and the Immune System

A variety of studies have shown that stress can impair the functions of the immune system. For example, students who experience considerable stress prior to taking exams show reduced blood levels of immune system cells, thus making exam stress a risk factor for colds and flu (Van Rood et al., 1993). Stress also slows the body's ability to mount an immune response to a vaccine (Glaser et al., 1992). Men whose wives have recently died have lower-than-normal levels of immune cells. This finding may explain the observation that among older adults a surviving spouse has a higher-than-expected risk of death during the period of bereavement. Unhappily married, never married, and recently divorced people also have reduced immune functioning, as do individuals experiencing job loss. The immune system responds negatively to stress; it responds positively to relaxation.

Managing Stress

The best way to manage stress is to replace stressful ways of living with beliefs, attitudes, and behaviors that promote peace, joy, and mind-body harmony. That does not mean you must become reclusive or try to eliminate all sources of conflict and tension from your life. People need tension to be creative and grow psychologically and spiritually. It may mean, however, changing some self-harming ways of thinking and behaving. Seeking help from a teacher, counselor, psychotherapist, clergyman, or coach can help you recognize sources of stress and ways to deal with them.

One way to manage stress is to alter or eliminate interaction with the stressor, for example, by changing jobs, changing a college major, accepting that a career that makes you happy is more important than one that promises a large income. Because stress is mediated by beliefs and attitudes, another way to manage it is to alter your perception of the situation. Ask yourself, "Am I seeing this potentially stressful situation realistically? And even if I am, is it really that threatening?" By perceiving a situation as less difficult (turning a mountain into several molehills), you lessen the chance of feeling overwhelmed.

You grow up the day you have your first real laugh at yourself.
ETHEL BARRYMORE

Another way to lessen stress is to change beliefs and goals. Winning may be an athlete's highest goal, but worrying about losing may bring about an illness. The solution is not to give up sports but to change

Wellness Guide

Ten Tips for Managing Stress

Once you have recognized the fact that you are under too much stress, you are well on your way to coping with it. Although there are no pat answers, no instant solutions, no one-day stress-off programs, there are a number of ways you can manage stress.

1. *Work off stress.* If you're angry or ready to blow up, physical activities are a terrific outlet. This is a time to vent that energy. Whether you go out and chop wood, take a run, wash the floor, or tackle a time-and energy-consuming project you've put off, chances are that you'll feel better and also will have accomplished something useful.

2. *Talk to someone you truly trust.* Confiding in another person and talking out your problem, even if there is no immediate solution, usually makes you feel better. If there is no one you trust, not even a relative or clergyperson, call one of the reputable hotlines that operate around the country twenty-four hours a day. They are staffed with counselors who can listen and discuss any problem with a great deal of understanding and compassion. Look them up in a telephone directory under such listings as Alcoholics Anonymous, Gamblers Anonymous, Help.

3. *Learn to accept what you cannot change.* Sometimes problems cannot be avoided or solved right now. Whether it's a serious illness in the family, a divorce, an economic setback, or a death, simply accepting what has happened will lessen the stress.

4. *Get enough sleep and rest.* Sometimes we are so busy we tend to cut down on things we need most. Sleep is a wonderful cure-all, a time to recharge your body's batteries, and usually one of the first things sacrificed to stress. Keep in mind that lack of sleep makes you cranky and irritable. If you find that you can't sleep, after a week or ten days, consult your family physician.

5. *Take time to play.* All work won't make you dull; it's more likely to make you a nervous wreck. Working extra hours tends to be counterproductive past a certain point. Make the time to relax, even if it's only to take a short nap. Schedule a sanity break. If you are too busy to take a weekend off, schedule minivacations during the day. Treat yourself to an hour or two off whether it's to play racquetball, shop for something personal, or take a walk around the block.

6. *Take one thing at a time.* Sometimes we are so overwhelmed that we try to do everything at once—and nothing gets accomplished. Take a few minutes to make a list of what has to be done, establish priorities, and tackle one project at a time, the most essential thing first. Completing the most important, pressing project will give you a sense of accomplishment, relieve some stress, and give you the strength to dive back into your workload.

7. *Plan ahead.* If you see a period of increased stress coming—a big project, holidays, vacation, moving, even a promotion—plan now to rest and be ready. Or postpone what can be delayed.

8. *If you become sick, don't carry on as if you're not.* No matter how pressing your work, don't be a martyr. Stay home. Get enough rest until you can resume your duties. If you go back prematurely, you risk a relapse. If you don't take time off, you risk a breakdown. If your work is so vital that nothing can function without you, have work sent to your home.

9. *Don't be afraid to say no.* If you are asked to do someone a favor, or complete an extra project, and it really is too much, say so. Taking on too much can in itself be the stress that breaks you down.

10. *Be realistic about perfection.* When there is a tremendous amount of work to be done, don't dwell on doing and redoing it until it is perfect. This isn't to advocate being slipshod, but to accept that a fourth or fifth draft of a report that was due yesterday is putting an unnecessary amount of stress on yourself.

Source: What You Should Know About Stress, Diet and Exercise, Now!: The RIA Guide to Feeling Good (New York: The Research Institute of America, Inc., 1984). Reprinted with permission by the Research Institute of America, 90 Fifth Avenue, New York, NY 10011.

---

priorities, perhaps by emphasizing the joy of participation and not the outcome of competition.

You can also change beliefs about yourself. Give yourself credit for things you have done that have lessened stress in your life rather than thinking it was blind luck. This will increase your sense of **self-efficacy,** the belief and confidence that you can master many situations that you encounter. Some stressful situations cannot be overcome, but be aware of tendencies toward needlessly feeling helpless in the face of a challenge.

Stress can be reduced by seeking support from people you trust. Talk to friends, teachers, counselors—whomever you believe can understand, lend a sympathetic ear, and offer sound feedback and advice if you request it.

Terms

self-efficacy: your belief that you are capable of handling the situation; self-esteem

Managing Stress

Two Monks and the River

Two monks set out on their last day's journey to their monastery. At mid-morning they came upon a shallow river, and on the bank there stood a beautiful young maiden.

"May I help you cross?" asked the first monk.

"Why, yes, that would be most kind of you," replied the maiden.

So the first monk hoisted the maiden on his back and carried her across the river. They bowed and went their separate ways.

After an hour or two of walking, the second monk said to the first monk, "I can't believe you did that! I just can't believe it! We take vows of chastity, and you touched a woman. You even asked her! What are we going to tell the abbot when we get home? He's going to ask how our journey was, and we can't lie. What are we going to say?"

Another couple of hours passed and the second monk erupted again. "How could you do that? She didn't even ask. You offered! The abbot's going to be incredibly angry."

By late afternoon the two were nearing their home, and the second monk, now filled with anxiety, said, "I can't believe you did that! You touched a woman. You even carried her on your back. What are we going to tell the abbot?"

The first monk stopped, looked at the second monk and said, "Listen, it's true that I carried that maiden across the river. But I left her at the river bank hours ago. You've been carrying her all day."

Critical Thinking About Health

1. Three groups of people were vaccinated against a test substance (one that could not make anyone sick). Group 1 consisted of students during final exams; group 2, people complaining of loneliness; group 3, people whose spouse had cancer. Each group was further subdivided into two subgroups. One subgroup in each major group was given 6 weeks of weekly support group meetings plus education about reducing the stress of their circumstance. The other subgroup in each major group was given no support or education. Below are the results of the strength of the immune response to the test vaccine.

   a. Explain the results of the experiment.
   b. Suggest a hypothesis to explain the results of the experiment.
   c. What do the results suggest about how you can better deal with stress in your life?

2. Johann Wolfgang von Goethe (1749—1832), the German author of *Faust* and other literary works, once wrote: "Things which matter most must never be at the mercy of things which matter least."

   a. What is your interpretation of Goethe's idea?
   b. How does letting things which matter most be at the mercy of things which matter least contribute to stress?
   c. How susceptible are you to stress from letting things which matter most be at the mercy of things which matter least? What could you change to reduce that stress?

3. Offer an explanation for the following: In the 1980s, researchers studied the health of adults living in two communities that were separated by a river. North River was a prosperous farming region, and South River was an industrial region in which the major employer, an auto plant, had permanently closed. The results of the research showed that children living in South River had many more doctor visits for infections and allergies than did children in North River. Also, adults in South River had more motor vehicle accidents and colds and flu during winter months than adults in the North River did. (Hint: Refer to Figure 2.2.)

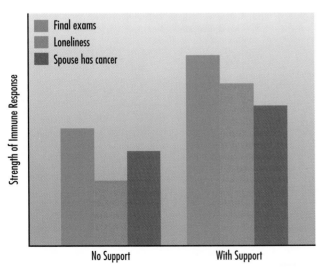

4. On the Recent Life Changes Questionnaire, the death of a child, spouse, sibling, or parent carries the highest LCU values.
   a. Offer an hypothesis to explain that result. In your hypothesis, take into account the nature of those kinds of relationships and what is lost when someone dies.
   b. What is the best way to cope with the loss of a loved one?

Health in Review

- Life presents situations that can disrupt mind-body harmony. Such situations and events are called stressors.
- Prolonged stress can impair functioning of the body's organs and immune system and may result in illness.
- Activators are situations and events that have the potential to become stressors depending on how a person interprets them.
- Responses are an individual's interpretation of activators. The nature and degree of a person's reactions depends on how threatening or challenging she or he perceives a situation to be.
- Consequences are the psychological and physiological effects of a reaction. An appraisal of how difficult it is to deal with a situation determines how well a person is able to cope.

- The onset of stress-related illness is the result of interpreting a situation as personally disruptive, threatening, or challenging and believing that personal resources to meet the challenge are insufficient.
- Stress results from the cumulative effects of daily problems, including frustrations, inner conflicts, and social pressures and demands.
- The fight-or-flight response is the body's way of dealing with the challenges it encounters.
- Stress can be reduced by disengaging from stressors, by altering perceptions and goals, and thereby reducing the potential for stress-related illness.
- Stress can be reduced by any technique that produces a peaceful state of being and the relaxation response.

Health and Wellness Online

The World Wide Web contains a wealth of information about health and wellness. By accessing the Internet using Web browser software, such as Netscape Navigator or Microsoft's Internet Explorer, you can gain a new perspective on many topics presented in *Essentials of Health and Wellness*, Second Edition. Access the Jones and Bartlett Publishers web site at http://www.jbpub.com/hwonline.

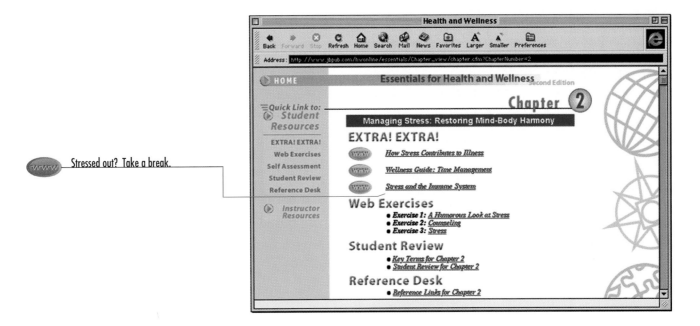

Stressed out? Take a break.

References

Benson, H., Greenwood, M., & Klemchuk, H. (1975). The relaxation response: Psychophysiologic aspects and clinical applications. *International Journal of Phychiatric Medicine, 6,* 87–98.

Benson, H., & Stark M. (1996). *Timeless healing: The power and biology of belief.* New York: Fireside Books.

Boscarino, J. S. (1997). Diseases among men 20 years after exposure to severe stress: Implications for clinical research and medical care. *Psychosomatic Medicine, 59,* 605–614.

Glaser, R. J., et al. (1992). Stress-induced modulation of the immune response to recombinant hepatitis B vaccine. *Psychosomatic Medicine, 54,* 22–29.

Holmes, T. H., & Rahe, R. H. (1967). The social readjustment rating scale. *Journal of Psychosomatic Research, 11,* 213–218.

Karasek, R., & Theorell, T. (1989). *Healthy work.* New York: Basic Books.

Miller, M. A., & Rahe, R. H. (1997). Life changes scaling for the 1990s. *Journal of Psychosomatic Research, 43,* 279–292.

Pennebaker, J. C. (1997). *Opening up: The healing power of expressing emotions.* New York: Guilford Press.

Van Rood, Y. R., Bogaards, M., Goulmy, E., & van Houweligen, H. C. (1993). The effects of stress and relaxation on the *in vitro* immune response in man: A meta-analytic study. *Journal of Behavioral Medicine, 16,* 163–181.

Suggested Readings

Benson, H., & Stuart, E. M. (1993). *The wellness book: The comprehensive guide to maintaining health and treating stress-related illness.* NY: Fireside. Harvard Medical School's renowned stress researcher offers techniques for enhancing health, reducing stress, and dealing with illness.

Covey, S., Merrill, A., & Merrill, R. (1996). *First things first.* A guide to managing your time by learning to balance your life.

Hubbard, J. R., & Edward, A. (Eds.). (1997). *Handbook of stress medicine: An organ system approach.* New York: CRC Press. An explanation of how stress causes illness and how improved care and prevention can hold down medical costs.

Kabat-Zinn, J. (1995). *Wherever you go, there you are.* NY: Hyperion. The director of the University of Massachusetts School of Medicine's Stress Reduction Program teaches the method of mindfulness meditation for managing stress.

McEwen, B. S. (1998). Protective and damaging effects of stress mediators. *New England Journal of Medicine, 338,* 171–179. A review of the long-term physiological response to stress.

Miller, E. (1980). *Letting go of stress* [cassette]. One of the best of the Emmett Miller stress management audiotapes.

Seaward, B. L. (1997). *Managing stress.* (2nd ed.). Sudbury, MA: Jones and Bartlett. A thorough text on the theory of stress and methods of stress reduction.

Exercises and Activities

WORKBOOK
Identify Your Fears or Phobias
Keep a Sleep and Dream Record

Health and Wellness Online

 www.jbpub.com/hwonline
Developing Coping Strategies
Managing Stress: Humor Therapy
Wellness Guide: If a Friend Is Considering Suicide

Chapter 3

Maintaining Emotional Wellness

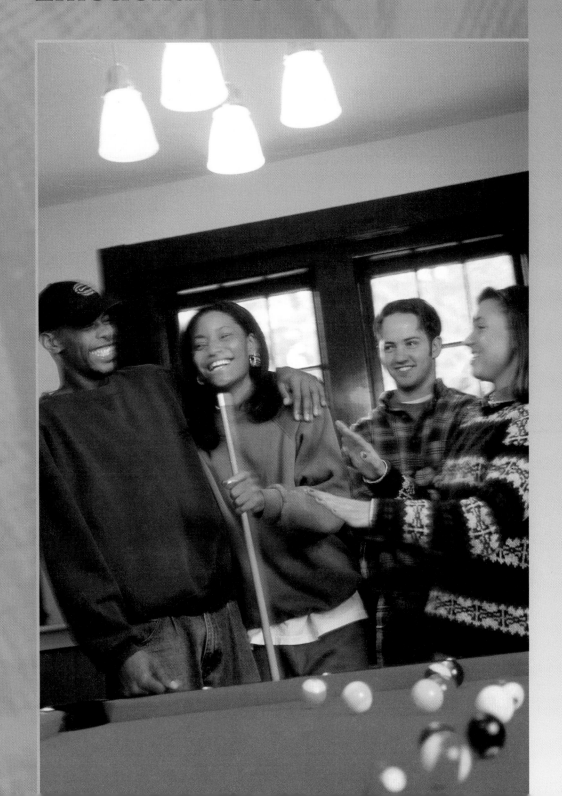

Much of human behavior is motivated by basic human needs. When individuals succeed in meeting their basic needs, they experience pleasant emotions, such as joy, pleasure, satisfaction, and contentment. When they do not, however, they experience unpleasant emotions, such as frustration, anger, sadness, grief, and shame.

> *Your health is bound to be affected if, day after day, you say the opposite of what you feel.*
>
> BORIS PASTERNAK,
> *DOCTOR ZHIVAGO*

There are two types of basic human needs: **maintenance needs** involve physical safety and survival; **growth needs** involve social belonging, self-esteem and mental, psychological, and spiritual stimulation. Mental and emotional health are functions of how successfully a person meets her or his basic needs and deals with circumstances in which these needs are not met.

According to psychologists, there is a **hierarchy of needs** that describes a process through which people navigate life. These include physiological needs, safety, love, self-esteem, and self-actualization (Figure 3.1). When the needs for food, clothing, and shelter have been met, less urgent needs become a priority. As people meet their needs, they move up the hierarchy. A person attains **self-actualization** (the highest level), by living to the fullest. People who are self-actualized have met their basic needs and reached their full human potential (Maslow, 1970).

To be emotionally healthy does not mean that we never feel angry, anxious, lonely, depressed, confused, or overwhelmed. Furthermore, being mentally healthy does not mean that we never need support, advice, or other kinds of help. In fact, inner strength is being able to recognize our limits and to seek and accept help so we can restore harmony when our mental and emotional resources are taxed.

Understanding Thoughts and Emotions

One foundation of mental health is seeing the world realistically. This perspective helps people devise strategies to meet their needs.

How we see the world is determined by the mental process called **cognition,** (from the Latin *cogito,* meaning "I know"). Cognition includes the following mental processes:

- *Perception:* interpreting data gathered by the sensory receptors (sight, smell, hearing, taste, touch, movement)
- *Learning:* integrating new perceptions with previous ones and storing them in memory as values, beliefs, and attitudes
- *Reasoning and problem solving:* formulating plans of action

Some thoughts, beliefs, and attitudes are **conscious,** which means that an individual can be aware of them. Others are **unconscious,** which means that they are not in our everyday awareness. Unconscious thoughts can be accessed through hypnosis, dreams, fantasies, and various forms of creative experience.

Cognition is usually associated with emotions. Emotions provide a sense of what is pleasant or unpleasant, which helps us evaluate an experience. This sets the stage for appropriate behavior. Emotions also provide the energy or motivation for behavior, and they play a part in evaluating the outcome of behavior.

Developing Coping Strategies

Coping strategies are ways of dealing with the emotional distress that comes from not having your needs met. In general, there are three categories of coping strategies; you can alter (a) the interaction with the cause of the distress, (b) thoughts and beliefs regarding the significance of the need that is not being met, or (c) the distressing feeling, without changing the situation or how you think about it.

To reduce emotional distress by changing your interaction with the situation, you could:

- Attack the situation head-on ("I'm anxious about asking her out, but I'll go ahead and do it").

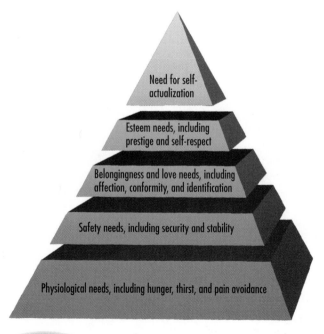

FIGURE 3.1   Maslow's Hierarchy of Human Needs

Wellness Guide

Hints for Emotional Wellness

People who have a positive self-image

. . . are not incapacitated by their emotions of fear, anger, love, jealousy, or guilt.

. . . can take life's disappointments in stride.

. . . have a tolerant attitude toward themselves and others; they can laugh at their shortcomings and mistakes.

. . . respect themselves and have self-confidence.

. . . are able to deal with most situations that come along.

. . . get satisfaction from simple, everyday pleasures.

People who feel positive about other people

. . . are able to give love and accept others the way they are.

. . . have personal relationships that are satisfying.

. . . expect to like and trust others and take it for granted that others will like and trust them.

. . . respect the many differences they see in people.

. . . do not need to control or push other people around.

. . . feel a sense of responsibility to friends and society.

People who are able to meet life's demands

. . . do something about their problems as they arise.

. . . accept their responsibilities.

. . . shape their environment whenever possible; otherwise they adjust to it.

. . . plan ahead but do not fear the future.

. . . welcome new ideas and experiences.

. . . use their natural capacities and talents.

. . . set attainable and realistic goals for themselves.

. . . get satisfaction from what they accomplish.

- Avoid the situation ("I'm too nervous about possible rejection. I'll do it some other time").
- Adapt to the situation ("I get nervous every time I ask someone out, but that's normal. So what?").

To change your thoughts and beliefs about the significance of the unmet need, you could:

- Judge your situation to be less distressing than someone else's ("At least I'm meeting people. Poor John works so much he doesn't get to meet anyone").
- See your distress as necessary or temporary ("This is the way it is," or "Eventually I'll find somebody and I won't have to go through this anymore").
- Focus on positive aspects of a situation and minimize the negative ("If she says yes, I'm sure we'll have a great time").
- Devalue the goal and believe you will do fine no matter the outcome ("If he says no, it won't be the end of the world").

Reducing emotional distress by changing or reducing the intensity of the feeling itself could involve releasing emotional energy through an alternative activity:

- Exercise helps with frustration and anger.
- Meditation helps with sadness and anger.
- Talking to a receptive and empathic person can help with grief, shame, and anxiety.

Defense Mechanisms

Defense mechanisms are strategies people use to distort the perception and awareness of reality to avoid unpleasant thoughts, memories, emotions, and situations. A common defense mechanism is denial, which is not believing a truth. An example of denial is a smoker not believing she is at risk for lung cancer even though she knows that smoking causes cancer. This person denies reality to prevent awareness of the truth, possibly to avoid the fear of death.

Defense mechanisms protect us from thoughts and beliefs that we find threatening. The distorted reality feels safe because of the distortion. Strategies for meeting needs that are based on a faulty foundation result in needs not met. This may lead to disappointment, depression, self-blame, and withdrawal or avoidance of involvement in similar situations.

Terms

maintenance needs: human needs that include physical safety and survival requirements, such as food and water

growth needs: a human need that includes social belonging, self-esteem, and spiritual growth

hierarchy of needs: a progression of human requirements, including physiological needs, safety, love, self-esteem, and self-actualization

self-actualization: a state in which a person has achieved the highest level of growth in Maslow's hierarchy of needs

cognition: the act or process of knowing in the broadest sense

conscious: knowing or perceiving something within oneself

unconscious: whatever is in the mind but out of conscious awareness

coping strategies: ways people devise to prevent, avoid, or control the emotional distress of unfulfilled needs

defense mechanisms: mental strategies for controlling anxiety

Managing Stress

Humor Therapy

On average, a person laughs about 15 times per day. This number can shrink dramatically, however, when people are influenced by emotions such as anger, fear, or grief. Just as unresolved emotions can ultimately have a negative effect on the body, positive emotions can also influence our state of health. The importance of humor on health was recognized in ancient Greece. Plato advocated humor to lighten the burdens of the soul and to improve one's health. From medieval court jesters to circus clowns, humor has long been a factor influencing mind-body healing. Now, medical science is showing that laughter is good medicine.

Thanks to the pioneering work of Norman Cousins and others, we know that our emotions can trigger physiological responses, including the release of certain neuropeptides, which seem to have a healing effect. The result of several bouts of laughter can actually bring about a sense of homeostasis to help calm the body and bring a sense of inner peace.

Here are some ways to tickle your funny bone and get your 15 laughs per day.

1. Create a tickler notebook of cartoons, stories, photographs, and other items that bring a smile to your face. Refer to it often, especially when you're down in the dumps.

2. Walk into a greeting card shop and buy five of the funniest cards you find.

3. Tell a close friend the most embarrassing event that has ever happened to you.

4. Buy 10 red roses and go to the nearest hospital or nursing home and distribute them to the first 10 people you see.

5. Over the weekend, go to a video store and pick up some comedy videos. Have a humorfest at home.

6. Read a funny story or novel.

7. Listen to a comedy audiotape or CD.

8. Hang out at a children's playground and watch little kids play for a half hour.

9. Fill your tub with hot water, bubble bath, and a rubber duck. And play!

10. Call some old friends you haven't talked to in a while, catch up on their lives; tell them a funny joke; then tell them you love them.

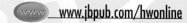 www.jbpub.com/hwonline

---

Distorting reality is not always bad. Sometimes it is necessary because of trauma or abuse. In such instances, denial helps a person cope with what would otherwise be a highly stressful psychological situation. Other times, denial can be a way to take a mental vacation. From the perspective of mental health, however, the key is knowing when you are "on a fantasy trip" and when you are not and not letting certain defensive ways of thought become habitual. You can do this by learning to observe how your mind works. Such self-knowledge is a goal of meditation, yoga, modern psychotherapies, and other practices that help to focus on awareness and engage one's consciousness.

Facilitating Coping

Even when emotions make us aware that something in our lives is not going well, we do not always know what the problem is, or what is the best way to deal with it, or how to overcome fear of change or long-standing inertia. People should not suffer in silence or believe themselves to be flawed or "crazy." Support and advice are available from trusted family members, friends, teachers, clergy, and mental health professionals, such as counselors, psychotherapists, and physicians. Reaching out to such people helps those in distress gain a new perspective on their problems and to see a workable solution.

Psychotherapists are trained professionals who help people deal with their emotional distress. Whether a person has feelings of inferiority, is troubled by painful dependency in a love relationship, or is immobilized by fear, a therapist can facilitate change that can make a person's life better. The change comes

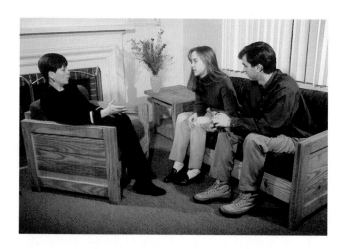

Talking with a counselor can help solve emotional problems.

Wellness Guide

Common Defense Mechanisms

Recognizing the following defense mechanisms will help you in maintaining emotional wellness.

Repression: keeping distressing thoughts and feelings unconscious

Example: A rape victim who has no memory of the assault

Projection: attributing one's own thoughts and feelings to someone else

Example: A student who dislikes her roommate but feels the roommate dislikes her

Displacement: diverting an emotion from the original target or source to another

Example: You are angry with your parents but yell at your best friends.

Reaction formation: believing and experiencing the opposite of how you really feel

Example: You are friendly to someone you dislike.

Rationalization: creating a plausible but false reason for your behavior

Example: Failing the course was due to the teacher's poor teaching methods.

Identification: imagining that someone's or some group's attributes are your own

Example: People who identify with a winning football team by wearing the team's colors, singing the team's song, and talking about the plays "we" made

Isolation and dissociation: compartmentalizing thoughts and emotions in different parts of awareness

Example: A man who gives successful and lucrative seminars to teach negotiation skills to business people, but frequently feuds with his neighbors

Denial: absolute rejection of a truth or of objective reality

Example: A college student who drinks a six-pack of beer every day but believes he has no problem with alcohol addiction

---

about not only by talking, but also by helping the distressed person adopt new behaviors and attitudes.

The value of psychotherapy, regardless of the method, is that the distressed person has faith in the professional's ability to facilitate change. This faith produces a situation of trust that enables the distressed person to be honest about himself or herself and to disclose painful and unflattering thoughts, memories, and emotions that would not likely be shared with a friend or relative.

Fears, Phobias, and Anxiety

Everybody experiences fear at some time or another. Fear is a powerful emotion that arises in situations that are interpreted as dangerous. The purpose of fear is to alert you to take protective action—usually to fight, flee, or seek assistance.

If fear is the response to a situation interpreted as dangerous, **anxiety** is the response to an *imaginary situation*—usually something in the future that has not yet happened—that is interpreted as threatening. The purpose of anxiety is to warn you of *potentially* dangerous situations.

A **phobia** involves intense fear that can seriously disrupt a person's life. Some common phobias are fear of heights *(acrophobia)*, fear of open spaces *(agoraphobia)*, fear of dirt and germs *(mysophobia)*, fear of snakes *(ophediophobia)*, and fear of animals *(zoophobia)*. Phobias produce severe, often incapacitating anxiety and even panic reactions.

Panic attacks are extreme reactions to fear. A panic attack can produce chest pain, palpitations, sweating, chills or hot flashes, trembling, shortness of breath, sensations of choking, and fear of losing control or dying. In some instances, a panic attack is a response to a life situation that seems overwhelming; for example, some people experience panic when a lover breaks up with them (separation panic). In other instances, panic attacks seem spontaneous, i.e., they happen without a situation that seems threatening.

> *To most individuals, the word Buick is not a stress, but it is to a thief who has just stolen one.*
> SEYMOUR S. KETY, MD

Panic attacks can be so debilitating that individuals require professional help to manage them. One form of therapy involves helping patients control their thoughts and breathing while experiencing a panic attack. They are also taught deep breathing to avoid hyperventilating and thus exacerbating a panic episode. If patients can identify the source of their panic, they can learn to confront their fears using imagery, followed by actual exposure to the fearful stimulus.

Terms

anxiety: the fear of an imaginary threat
phobia: a powerful and irrational fear of something
panic attacks: severe anxiety accompanied by physical symptoms

Medications can also help people manage panic attacks. Tricyclic medications (e.g., imipramine) or selective serotonin reuptake inhibitors (e.g., fluoxetine) may be effective treatment. Tranquilizers (e.g., alprazolam), while effective, are not recommended because of their potential to cause chemical dependency.

Depression

According to the National Institute of Mental Health, each day approximately one person in seven experiences **depression,** characterized by feelings of dejection, guilt, hopelessness, self-recrimination, loss of appetite, insomnia, loss of interest in sex, reduced interest in previously enjoyable activities, withdrawal from social contacts, inability to concentrate and make decisions, lowered self-esteem, and a focus on negative thoughts and the bad things in life. If asked how they feel, depressed people usually say something like, "Life's a drag" or "What's the use of doing anything?"

Depression can occur as a normal response to the loss of something that a person values or is attached to, such as a loved one, a job, good health, or self-esteem (e.g., when a person does not succeed at a task she or he deems important). When individuals experience a loss, it is "normal" for them to feel sad and depressed, and to grieve the loss. Sadness and grief are the human spirit's way to heal the hurt of loss and open the way for new attachments. When depression is associated with a loss, the depressed individual may be simultaneously aware that the experience is transitory and, along with grief, feel that there is hope for the future. This kind of depression tends to lift after the grieving ends.

In contrast to the "normal" depression that may accompany loss, some people experience a long-lasting depressive state, or periodic episodes of deep depression, that are not self-limiting and may hinder and even jeopardize a person's life. These depressions may be a response to stress, severe psychological trauma, injury, disease, biological malfunctions of some part of the brain, or a combination of factors. In some persons, major episodes of depression are accompanied by periods of excited euphoria ("mania"), resulting in a condition referred to as **bipolar disorder.**

Some individuals are susceptible to depression during the winter months because a lack of sunlight disturbs the production of neurotransmitters in the brain that affect mood. This "seasonal affective disorder" (SAD) is sometimes remedied by increased exposure to stronger-than-normal indoor lighting that mimics sunlight or relocation to southern latitudes where there is more light.

Depression can also accompany the experience of being very sick or injured. In such cases, depression results from a combination of factors, such as grieving the loss of health; coping with the stress of being sick; lack of exercise and normal routine; disruption of regular social activities; or alterations in physiology that may change brain chemistry. Medications may also make one susceptible to depression. Some people experience a mild form of depression called **dysthymia.** Like major depression, dysthymia is associated with disturbances in sleep, appetite, and the ability to concentrate.

One of the characteristics of severe depression is a considerable degree of negative thinking, characterized by severe self-criticism; negative views about the self, the world, and the future; and a variety of logic errors (Burns, 1992), including:

- *All or none thinking:* seeing things as polar extremes (e.g., all good and all bad)
- *Overgeneralizing:* interpreting one setback as evidence that *every* similar situation will *forever* turn out badly
- *Negative filtering:* focusing only on the negative while filtering out the positive
- *Disqualifying the positive:* transforming positive occurrences into negative experiences

Becoming aware of negative thoughts (often called *negative self-talk*) opens the way to adopting positive self-images and more realistic appraisals of the world. These, in turn, help to lessen the depressive state. Cognitive behavioral therapy is a very successful method for helping depressed people change their negative thought patterns.

Another characteristic of depression is that it can intensify itself, thus creating a depressive cycle. The depressed person's negative thoughts, social withdrawal, and loss of interest in pleasurable experiences serve to reinforce feelings of worthlessness, helpless-

> *In the middle of the journey of life, I found myself in a dark wood, having lost the straight path.*
>
> DANTE ALIGHIERI,
> *THE DIVINE COMEDY*

Terms

depression: a mental disorder characterized by sadness, feelings of inadequacy, and low self-esteem

bipolar disorder: major episodes of depression accompanied by periods of excitement

dysthymia: a long-lasting, mild form of depression

Global Wellness

Depression Is Worldwide

Missing my dear mother, as a son,
my liver and intestines are painfully broken!
Crying for my old mother, as a son,
my tears pour into my chest!
Thinking about my old mother, as a son,
to swallow food and tea is difficult!
Searching for my old mother, as a son,
I cannot sleep day and night!

Si-Lang, *Searching for Mother*
Tenth Century Beijing Opera

Melancholy and depression know no geographic boundaries, as this thousand-year-old Chinese aria describing the physical aspects of depression shows.

Depression has been documented in virtually all cultures, although its prevalence varies (Young, 1997). Depression in Asia, for example, is less prevalent than in North America and Europe. Rates of depression in the U.S. even vary by cultural group: The lifetime prevalence of depression among people of African and Hispanic ancestry is about 12%; among people of European ancestry, it's 17%.

Besides prevalence rates, depression manifests differently among cultures. Several Native American cultures tend to experience depression as social loneliness. A typical Caucasian North American or European is likely to experience depression in terms of psychological symptoms, such as melancholy, moodiness, and lack of interest in pleasure. However, in Asian cultures, depression tends to be experienced as physical complaints (as in the Chinese aria above), such as fatigue, loss of appetite, and sleep problems.

Help-seeking behavior for depression also varies among cultures. Latin American men and mainland Chinese tend not to seek help for depression, fearing that doing so will stigmatize them as weak. In Japan and Hong Kong, where depression tends to be experienced as a physical ailment, people tend to consult with a doctor for relief of physical symptoms. Latin American women and European-Americans are more likely to consult mental health practitioners.

ness, gloom, and doom. Recovery from depression requires both interrupting the depressive cycle and correcting the life situation that brought on the depression.

One way to deal with depression is to get life moving again. This is accomplished by establishing and achieving simple, attainable goals that can be done in a brief period of time. The goals should involve movement that restores fundamental breathing and other mind-body rhythms, which may alter the chemistry of the brain to facilitate pleasant (instead of unpleasant) moods. Many a depressed person has found relief in taking up a regular exercise program.

Also, depressed individuals should interact with people who offer support. Remaining in seclusion only reinforces feelings of loss and worthlessness. It is also helpful not to engage in long conversations with friends and family about how lousy life is. Recreational activity can divert attention from negative thinking and weaken the depressive cycle.

Several types of medication are extremely effective in helping people recover from depression. These medications are similar to ones used in panic disorder: tricyclics, antidepressants, selective serotonin reuptake inhibitors, and monamine oxidase inhibitors.

Because depression involves inactivity, withdrawal, hopelessness, and self-defeating thoughts and behaviors, it is often difficult for individuals to activate themselves on a program of self-healing. At such times, the encouragement of a caring friend or family member and the guidance of a therapist, counselor, or other helper can be invaluable. Others can help a

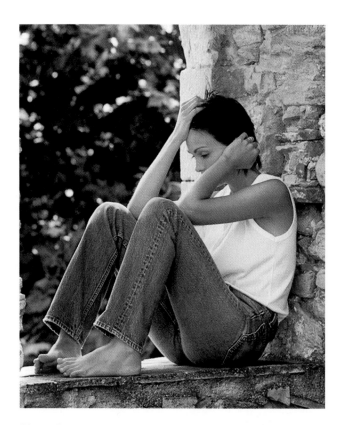

Many things may make us feel depressed temporarily.

depressed person confront the causes of the depression and become aware of and try to minimize negative self-talk—negative views about the self, the world, and the future; self-critical inner dialogue, and logic errors in the assessment of self and events.

Suicide

One of the most worrisome aspects of depression is the risk of suicide. In the United States, suicide ranks among the 10 most frequent causes of death, accounting for approximately 30,000 deaths per year. The number of reported suicides is thought to represent only 10% to 15% of suicide attempts. People over 65 make up the largest age group of suicides. Among young people (15 to 24 years old), suicide ranks third behind accidents and murder as a cause of death.

Suicide is not a disease, nor is it a disorder that can be inherited. Suicides are not caused by the weather or a full moon. Generally people consider suicide because they feel overwhelmed and painfully distressed by life and they believe suicide to be their only option. Sometimes people attempt suicide not because they really want to die but because they want to express anger at others or signal others for help. In such instances, suicide attempts are characterized by limited self-destructive acts, such as taking less than a

lethal dose of sleeping pills or arranging that the attempt be discovered in time for the person to be saved.

At the time a person contemplates suicide, life seems absolutely hopeless. But few life problems are beyond solution. Life crises improve and distressing emotions pass. Time does heal many hurts. And the experience gained by working through a distressing time of life can bring confidence, insight, and understanding. Acquiring experience and understanding, a person is better able to cope with life's problems and is better able to help others deal with their challenges.

Anger

Anger occurs when we've been attacked, blamed, hurt, or have experienced a loss; when we *imagine* we've been attacked, blamed, hurt, or have experienced a loss; when we imagine we *may* be attacked, blamed, hurt, or experience a loss; or when the pursuit of an important goal is blocked. Anger is an excitatory emotion, providing the motivational energy to protect ourselves or things we care about or to overcome obstacles to our goals. We use anger to stop physical or psychological abuse and to protect our-

Wellness Guide

If a Friend Is Considering Suicide

If you suspect that a friend is considering suicide, how can you help? You can take any of several possible courses of action. All involve you making a concrete intervention. Intervention is tough. It is much easier to tell yourself that things will get better, or tomorrow is another day. Rationalization and procrastination are not useful behaviors in a situation that involves depression or potential suicide. Let's look at some options available to you.

- Talk to your friend. Tell him or her that you are concerned. Describe the behavior that is causing you to worry. Ask if you can help (but don't give up if your friend says no).

- Ask your friend directly if he or she is thinking about suicide. You may be shocked if your friend

answers yes, but, remember, even someone who sees suicide as a potential solution always has a wish to live. If your friend admits thinking of suicide, ask if he or she has thought of a plan.

- Negotiate a "no-suicide" agreement before leaving your friend. Ask your friend to agree not to commit suicide at any time. If your friend will not agree to this contract or tries to change it to a certain time, then he or she is at increased risk. Report this situation to a professional counselor at once. Stay with your friend or arrange for someone else to stay with him or her until professional help arrives.

- If your friend agrees to a "no-suicide" pact, go to your college health service or residence hall

advisor, speak with a counselor or physician, and describe your friend's behavior. The professional will know the best way to handle the situation. And remember, even if you feel you are interfering or breaking a confidence, you may be saving a life. An intervention made now can prevent suicide.

- Talk to other friends, a residence hall advisor, or even a teacher—anyone who will assist you to verbalize your concerns and decide how to help. The most important action is to do something after you become aware of the potentially dangerous outcome.

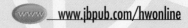 www.jbpub.com/hwonline

Wellness Guide

Some Tips for Dealing with Anger

Here are some suggestions for expressing anger constructively.

- *Recognize your anger.* Pay attention to anger in yourself when you become aware of it. Then take some time to determine which of your thoughts are causing it. Are you hurt, frustrated, frightened? What happened that made you angry?

- *Own your anger.* Try not to blame someone else for your angry feeling by means of thoughts or statements like, "It's all your fault!" or "If it weren't for you," or "If only you'd have . . ." Don't put it onto someone else unless you're sure it belongs there.

- *Find anger's origins.* Even if you are very angry, try not to act immediately on those feelings. Instead, set aside a time to think about them and how best to express them.

- *Resolve the anger.* Try not to let anger build up over time. If you do, you may become resentful, which may cause you to distance emotionally or physically or to displace the anger onto someone else, like a child or a co-worker.

- *Don't ambush.* Attacking with anger when it's least expected is unfair and invites resentment or a counterattack, not reconciliation.

- *Be specific.* When you're talking about emotional conflicts, name exactly what's causing the anger and stick to that issue. Don't bring up past hurts. Don't discuss second and third topics until the first one is settled. If other issues arise, write them down so you can discuss them later. Make it a habit to keep pencil and paper handy when issues are discussed. Don't give in to the temptation to bring up secondary issues in order to retaliate for hurt feelings or as a way to avoid resolving the issue at hand.

- *Don't hit below the belt.* Don't attack your partner with something you know will hurt because you think you're losing an argument.

- *Attack the problem, not each other.* Don't engage in character assassination with put-downs and accusations. Use "I" statements to communicate resentments. If someone attacks with a put-down, rather than retaliate, the recipient can say "Ouch, that hurt." This can be a cue to redress the attack and go on with the issue under discussion. If this doesn't happen, the discussion will probably be sidetracked from the main point to the put-down, and a fight about hurt feelings may ensue.

- *Be respectful and respectable.* When working to resolve an issue, try to maintain an attitude of respect. Try to understand the other's point of view. Ask the other person to respect you and your feelings, even though you disagree.

- *Take some time.* Sometimes you can sense that an anger-causing issue isn't getting resolved in the discussion. It's all right to acknowledge that and to take a few hours or days to reconsider things, then discuss the issue again. Sometimes emotions are too intense and it's not possible to think clearly. Sometimes you just need time to reflect and figure things out.

- *Physical affection is okay.* Sex or any other affectionate behavior before an issue is resolved is acceptable, as long as it's not taken as a sign that the issue is resolved. Both of you must understand this. Affectionate behavior shows that arguing about something can be accommodated within a caring relationship.

- *Both sides win.* After an issue has been discussed and the partners seem agreed on the outcome, if one or both feels a grudge, then the argument has produced a winner and a loser, and the relationship has been harmed. Holding a grudge is a sign that the issue is not resolved. Try again.

---

selves from the hurt of loss. Sometimes we get angry because we perceive something as threatening that really isn't. In this case, we make ourselves angry by what we think.

Many people have difficulty dealing with anger in themselves or in others. They fear the intensity of the emotion. They fear the possibility of violence that may accompany its expression. They fear retaliation or rejection.

One constructive way to work with anger is to understand the source of the emotion. For example, to deal with frustration you can reassess the merits of the goal you cannot attain or reconsider the strategy you've employed for attaining it. It may feel right to blame someone else for your troubles, but a reevalua-

tion of how you contribute to the situation may be more productive.

The next time you feel angry, take a "time out" for a few seconds, minutes, or days if necessary. Ask yourself what you've experienced that's led you to be angry. Are you really being harmed or threatened or are you making yourself angry because you've interpreted a situation as such? If you feel frustrated about not being able to accomplish a goal, is your goal realistically attainable? Have you expected too much of yourself? Have you expected too much of someone else? Is your strategy for attaining your goal workable? Is something else better? Did you communicate your goals, needs, plans, and desires to people whose help you wanted or expected?

Family arguments disrupt the emotional well-being of parents and children.

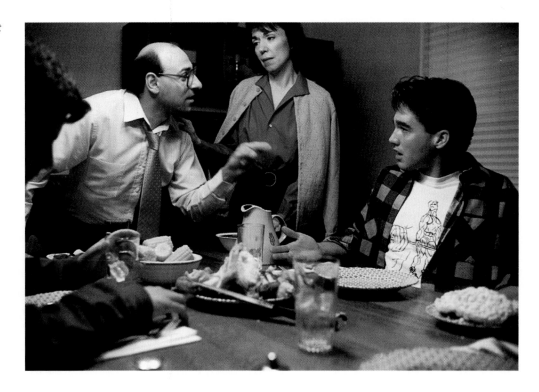

Sleep and Dreams

Everyone has a sleep-wake cycle that corresponds to their optimal degree of physical, mental, and spiritual well-being. Studies show that adequate sleep enhances attentiveness, concentration, mood, and motivation. Sleep deprivation, on the other hand, impairs a person's ability to be productive, good-humored, satisfied with life, and even to laugh at a joke! Lack of sleep can gravely impair judgment; sleeplessness is second only to drunkenness as a cause of automobile accidents. Long-term sleep deprivation can be fatal.

Sleep researchers believe that a majority of Americans are sleeping 60 to 90 minutes a night less than the seven, eight, or nine hours that would leave them refreshed and energetic during the day. Individuals "cheat on their sleep" to create time for other things in the busy schedules that characterize modern life. Sleep is considered expendable, and *not* sleeping is considered a sign of ambition and drive. Furthermore, around-the-clock TV and radio entertainment can distract people from sleeping. Before the advent of the electric light bulb about 100 years ago, people tended to sleep about nine hours a night.

Sleep Problems

Just about everyone has trouble sleeping once in a while. Experiences that commonly disrupt sleeping patterns include being sick, jet-lagged, nervous about an upcoming exam, or excited about something new; having consumed too much food, alcohol, or caffeine; or losing a loved one. Fortunately, most people tend to adjust to these situations, and their sleep rhythms return to normal (for them) in a few days. A large percentage of Americans, however, have problems with sleeping that last several weeks to years.

Insomnia

The majority of people with long-term sleep problems have **insomnia.** They have trouble falling asleep or staying asleep, or they awaken after a few hours of sleep and cannot go back to sleep. The daytime results of insomnia are fatigue, the desire to nap, impaired ability to concentrate, impaired judgment, and a lack of zest for life. Although insomnia may be related to disease or injury in the brain's sleep centers, most often it is the result of a physical illness, chronic pain,

Terms

insomnia: prolonged inability to obtain adequate sleep

narcolepsy: extreme tendency to fall asleep during the day

parasomnias: activities that interrupt restful sleep

somnambulism: sleepwalking

sleep apnea: state of troubled or interrupted breathing while sleeping

Wellness Guide

Getting a Good Night's Sleep

Here are some suggestions for getting a good night's sleep.

- *Establish a regular sleep time.* Give your own natural sleep cycle a chance to be in synchrony with the day-night cycle by going to bed at the same time each night (within an hour more or less) and arising *without being awakened by an alarm clock.* This will mean going to bed early enough to give yourself enough time to sleep. Try to maintain your regular sleep times on the weekend. Getting up early during the week and sleeping late on weekends may upset the rhythm of your sleep cycle.

- *Create a proper (for you) sleep environment.* Sleep occurs best when the sleeping environment is dark, quiet, free of distractions, and not too warm. If you use radio or TV to help you fall asleep, use an autotimer to shut off the noise after falling asleep.

- *Wind down before going to bed.* About 20 to 30 minutes before bedtime, stop any activities that cause mental or physical arousal, such as work or exercise, and take up a "quiet" activity that can create a transition to sleep. Transitional activities could include reading, watching "mindless" TV, taking a warm bath or shower, meditation, or making love.

- *Make the bedroom for sleeping only.* Make the bedroom your place for getting a good night's sleep. Try not to use it for work or for discussing problems with your partner.

- *Don't worry while in bed.* If you are unable to sleep after about 30 minutes in bed because of worry about the next day's activities, get up and do some limited activity such as reading a magazine article, doing the dishes, or meditating. Go back to bed when you feel drowsy. If you cannot sleep because of thinking about all that

you have to do, write down what's on your mind and let the paper hold onto the thoughts while you sleep. You can retrieve them in the morning.

- *Avoid alcohol and caffeine.* Some people have a glass of beer or wine before bed in order to relax. Large amounts of alcohol, while sedating, block normal sleep and dreaming patterns. Because caffeine remains in the body for several hours, people sensitive to caffeine should not ingest any after noon.

- *Exercise regularly.* Exercising 20 to 30 minutes three or four times a week enhances the ability to sleep. You should not exercise vigorously within three hours of bedtime, however, because of the possibility of becoming too aroused to sleep.

Source: Adapted from M. L. Reite, K. E. Nagel, and J. R. Ruddy, *The Evaluation and Management of Sleep Disorders* (Washington, DC: American Psychiatric Press, 1990).

---

stress, depression, anxiety, obsessive-compulsive ruminations, panic attacks, post-traumatic stress disorder, and drug or alcohol abuse.

Sometimes, as a result of insomnia, individuals have a difficult time staying awake during the day. They may feel sleepy most of the time, may "nod off" easily during a routine activity, or may nap at the slightest opportunity. Because they get insufficient sleep at night, about 20% of college students can fall asleep almost instantaneously if permitted to lie down in a darkened room. Extreme tendency to fall asleep during the day is called **narcolepsy.**

Parasomnias

Parasomnias occur in many forms and have the potential to interrupt restful sleep. Nightmares are dreams that arouse feelings of fear, terror, panic, or anxiety. Sleepwalking, or **somnambulism,** is a condition occurring primarily in children and often associated with anxiety, fatigue, or stress. The person performs motor activity, usually leaving bed and walking around, while sleeping and has no memory of it on awakening. Other vigorous behaviors, such as punching, kicking, and night terrors (episodes that begin with a loud cry followed by rapid heart rate, sweating, and feelings of

panic), will also interrupt sleep. Another abnormality is **sleep apnea,** in which individuals stop breathing while sleeping; typically, breathing resumes within 30 seconds.

Since the majority of sleep problems represent some form of disharmony within ourselves or with our surroundings, restoring harmony is a way to return to our natural rest-activity cycle. This can be accomplished by employing mind-body health practices such as meditation, exercise, and proper nutrition. For extreme sleep disorders, professional help should be sought.

Alcohol, sleeping pills, tranquilizers, and other drugs, however, offer only short-term symptomatic relief for sleep disorders. Without a holistic approach and fundamental changes in one's life-style and attitudes, relying on drugs to restore natural sleep rhythms may be harmful and may lead to physical dependency and habituation.

Understanding Our Dreams

We all dream while we sleep. Even animals dream. Some people do not recall their dreams. Others have vivid recall of the several dreams they have each night (a skill that can be learned). Dreams tend to occur in

FIGURE 3.2   Tracings of the Electrical Signals Produced During the Stages of Sleep Tiny electrodes are placed on a person's scalp and eyelids. They detect electrical signals within the brain and movements of the eyes. Notice that rapid eye movement (REM) occurs during a dream period.

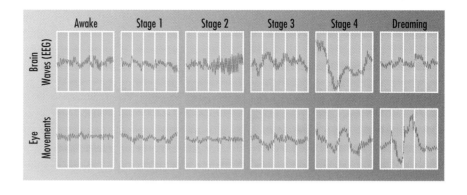

the stage of sleep called **rapid eye movement (REM) sleep** (Figure 3.2).

No one knows why we dream. Some researchers have suggested that REM sleep states are necessary for brain growth, daily information processing, and cellular rejuvenation. Others believe that dreams are the brain's way of processing and eliminating information and memories that are no longer useful. Whatever the reasons, dreams are necessary for health. Experimental subjects who were deprived of the chance to dream (they were awakened by experimenters during REM sleep) developed bizarre behaviors and psychotic symptoms. The individuals returned to normal after at least one night of catching up on the missed REM time.

For thousands of years dreams have been used in many cultures to restore mental and physical health. The temples of Asclepius were used by ancient Greeks for more than a thousand years as places where people went to have healing dreams and to have them interpreted by the priests and priestesses.

Indications that dreams can be healthy come from studies of the Senoi, a Malaysian tribe known as the "dream people." The Senoi live in a nonaggressive, noncombative, communal society. The tribe's members have a remarkable degree of mental and emotional health, which is attributed by some to the daily ritual of discussing and interpreting their dreams. Both children and adults gather each morning to recount their dreams to one another, singly and in groups. According to Senoi custom, the events, anxieties, and people in a dream are real and must be acknowledged and dealt with. Such behavior is similar to our custom of looking for meaning in dreams, especially as a component of psychotherapy.

Interpreting Your Dreams

Much dream research suggests that dreams are reflections of recent happenings, thoughts, and feelings that are not dealt with in our daily consciousness. Many people are too busy to attend to everything they experience, think, and feel. Sometimes, they purposely do not deal with reality because it is unpleasant. In a dream, however, people bring forth subtle feelings and impressions that were not attended to while awake. They engage their innermost thoughts and feelings about fears, worries, conflicts, and problems that they chose not to deal with when awake. Thus, many problems (and sometimes their solutions!) are presented in dreams.

Dreams may also be a literal representation of reality that went unattended. For example, if you dream of a mouse, perhaps you saw a mouse in your kitchen, or perhaps you noticed some movements out of the corner of your eye and thought of a mouse. In either case, your discomfort at the thought of a mouse in your house caused you to block the thought from consciousness.

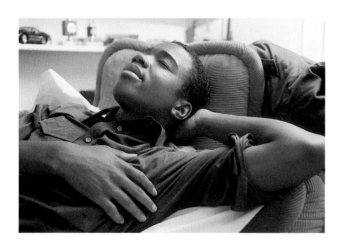

Sufficient sleep and dreams are essential to mental health.

Terms

rapid eye movement (REM) sleep: stage of sleep in which dreams occur

schizophrenia: a mental disorder that involves a disturbance in thinking, in perceiving reality, and in functioning

Mental Disorders

The brain, like all other body organs, is composed of molecules and cells whose functioning is controlled by biological processes. It is possible, therefore, for brain tissue to be affected by chemical imbalance, injury, infection, toxins, and genetic disorders. When brain injury or disease occurs, thoughts, mood, and behaviors can be impaired. In most cases, the biological basis for mental disorders is unknown.

Schizophrenia is a debilitating mental disorder characterized by hallucinations, delusions, an inability to maintain logical and coherent thought patterns, diminished emotional and social experience, and a diminished sense of purpose. Typically schizophrenia manifests in teenage years and progresses into adulthood. The disease occurs at the same rate (0.85%) in virtually all societies in the world; it is responsible for 2.5% of total U.S. health expenditures. The cause of schizophrenia is unknown, although scientists believe that biological (possibly inherited) factors are partially responsible. While medications and psychosocial rehabilitation can help lessen symptoms, there is no cure. About one third of schizophrenics become well spontaneously, but many individuals with a diagnosis of schizophrenia require ongoing medical and psychological support.

Critical Thinking About Health

1. Dr. Razmataz's book, "30 Days to Exceptional Mental Health," had been on the best seller charts for 10 weeks, but after his appearance on TV's "Inside this Week," sales went through the roof. Entertainers, business executives, professional athletes, and political leaders extolled the value of his program to lessen needless worry, improve sleep, and enhance mood, self-esteem, memory, and mental acuity.

    Dr. Razmataz based his program on 10 years of research he conducted as director of the Ersatz Mental Health Clinic. In his book and his media appearances, Dr. Razmataz explained that the type and severity of a particular mental illness was caused by either the over- or underactivity of the genes that controlled the production of the six basic neurotransmitter chemicals in the brain. The key to his method was determining a patients' genetic profile and matching it to one of six specific organic food diets.

    Questions:
    a. What factors are mentioned in the description above that might suggest to someone that Dr. Razmataz's method is credible and efficacious?
    b. Which of these factors do you find influence you when you are making a health decision?
    c. What additional information, if any, would you want before trying Dr. Razmataz's method yourself or recommending it to someone else? How would you find such information?

2. List five characteristics of a mentally healthy person. If you were a parent, how would you ensure that your child(ren) grow(s) up to manifest the five characteristics on your list? Also discuss how individuals can contribute to the mental health of people in their community.

3. John hasn't liked being Margie's supervisor since her first day of work. She just doesn't get it. And since she's the boss's niece, there is little he can do. In the past six months, whenever Margie is on John's shift-team, his finds himself so distressed that he doesn't want to go to work.
    a. The chapter describes several ways to cope with emotional distress including (a) changing the situation that is causing the distress, (b) altering the significance one places on the distressing situation, and (c) lessening the distressing emotions. Discuss how John could employ each of these coping strategies to lessen his emotional distress. Also, describe the consequences for John of implementing each coping strategy.
    b. When you experience emotional distress, which of the three coping strategies do you employ most often? Do you notice situations in which one coping strategy works better than in others?

4. Many people equate mental and emotional well-being with happiness. If they feel happy, they identify themselves as emotionally well. In your opinion, what is the relationship of emotional well-being and happiness? How do unpleasant emotions, such as sadness, grief, shame, guilt, and anger, affect one's sense of emotional well-being? Would you argue that the path to mental and emotional well-being is the pursuit of happiness? If not, in your view, what constitutes the path to mental and emotional well-being?

Health in Review

- Mental and emotional health depend on how well individuals meet their maintenance and growth needs and cope with situations in which their needs are not met.
- People understand their needs by interpreting what they sense from the environment and in their bodies. As they mature, people develop ideas about and learn strategies to meet their emotional needs.
- Emotions tell us whether we are satisfied by, and the level of satisfaction from, our experiences, plans, and outcomes of behavior.
- Emotional distress occurs when needs are not met. People cope with emotional distress by changing their modes of interaction with the environment, changing the importance of their unmet needs, or changing the distressing feelings.
- Counselors, therapists, and others can help clarify the source of emotional distress and find healthy ways to cope with it.
- Fear, anxiety, and depression are common emotional problems.
- Common phobias include acrophobia, agoraphobia, claustrophobia, mysophobia, ophediophobia, and zoophobia.

- Depression is often characterized by feelings of dejection, guilt, hopelessness, self-recrimination, loss of appetite, insomnia, loss of interest in sexual activity, withdrawal from friends, inability to concentrate, lowered self-esteem, and a focus on the negative.
- Suicide is the third leading cause of death among persons aged 15 to 24 years, of all races and both genders.
- Many of the signs of depression occur in someone suicidal. Many suicidal people talk about suicide when life appears hopeless.
- Sleep and dreams are fundamental to human health. Sleep has four stages. REM sleep, during which dreams occur, happens during the cycle of sleep from deep to lighter stages.
- Many people use their dreams to help them understand and deal with distressing situations and confusing emotions.
- Schizophrenia is a mental disorder characterized by delusions, inability to think logically and coherently, diminished social and emotional experiences, and loss of sense of purpose.

Health and Wellness Online

The World Wide Web contains a wealth of information about health and wellness. By accessing the Internet using Web browser software, such as Netscape Navigator or Microsoft's Internet Explorer, you can gain a new perspective on many topics presented in *Essentials of Health and Wellness, Second Edition.* Access the Jones and Bartlett Publishers web site at http://www.jbpub.com/hwonline.

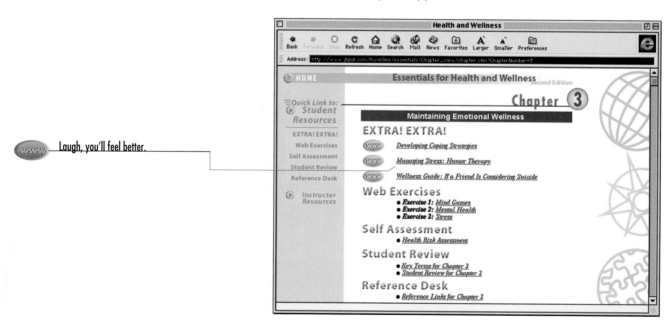

Laugh, you'll feel better.

References

Burns, D. (1992). *Feeling good.* New York: Avon.

Maslow, A. L. (1970). *Motivation and personality.* New York: Harper & Row.

Young, D. M. (1997). Depression. In W.-S. Tseng and J. Streltzer (Eds.), *Culture and psychopathology.* New York: Brunner/Mazel.

Suggested Readings

Braiker, H. B. (1989, October). The power of self-talk. *Psychotherapy Today, 23–27.* A concise guide to monitoring and eliminating inner negative self-talk and enhancing self-esteem.

Coren, S. (1996). *Sleep thieves.* New York: The Free Press. A sleep researcher gives an entertaining and highly readable account of the mysteries of sleep and the science of sleep research.

Kupfer, D. J., and Reynolds III, J. D. (1997). Current concepts: Management of insomnia. *New England Journal of Medicine, 336,* 341–345. A thorough review of the causes and management of sleep problems.

Redfield, K. (1995). *An unquiet mind.* New York: Vintage Books. A distinguished professor of psychiatry relates her personal struggles with manic-depressive illness as both scientist and poet.

Roberts, F. M. (1998). *The therapy sourcebook.* New York: Lowell House. Discusses different kinds of therapy to treat mental illness resulting from cognitive, behavioral, psychological, and biological disorders. Also lists resources.

Salmans, S. (1995). *Depression: Questions you have . . . answers you need.* Allentown, PA: People's Medical Society. Discusses all aspects of depression from causes to cures in a question-and-answer format.

Weissman, M. M. and Olfson, M. (1995). Depression in women: Implications for health care research. *Science, 269,* 799–801. Discusses current theories and research on depression in women.

Whybrow, P. C. (1998). *A mind apart.* New York: HarperCollins. A penetrating look at how the mind goes awry and becomes ill. Dr. Whybrow discusses mental illness with insight and compassion.

Making Healthy Changes

Most of us, if we were asked, "Are there any behaviors you can change that would improve your health?" would probably answer, "Yes." Everyone can improve his or her health in some way by eliminating destructive habits and by increasing healthy behaviors. Often the problem with making healthy changes is that we become overwhelmed by the sheer number of changes that should be made—getting more exercise, improving our diet, giving up cigarettes, reducing the amount of beer we drink after school or work, not being so stressed or tired all the time, not watching TV night after night while snacking constantly—the list goes on and on. Because the changes we could (or should) make seem overwhelming, we simply continue in the pattern of living to which we've become accustomed.

As with all aspects of life—school, jobs, relationships, and so forth—making changes in behaviors that will improve health takes effort, time, and learning new skills. General guidelines for healthy living are quite simple, and you probably have heard many of them from parents, teachers, or friends at various times. For example, how often have you been told the following (or said one of these to yourself)?

- Get more exercise
- Don't smoke or use drugs
- Wear your seat belt and bike helmet
- Don't get drunk
- Don't drive when drinking
- Don't keep loaded guns around the house
- Be sexually responsible
- Get plenty of sleep
- Eat your fruits and vegetables
- Take off some weight

Unfortunately, general guidelines don't affect our behaviors even though we may agree with them. Therefore, we're going to introduce a program of specific suggestions for you to follow that will improve your overall health. This program, *Making Healthy Changes*, will focus primarily on achieving emotional wellness, managing stress, increasing your level of physical activity, improving your diet, and teaching you how to be a wise consumer.

This text is divided into six parts with two or more chapters covering different aspects of improving health and preventing illness. *Making Healthy Changes* will conclude each part with specific suggestions for living healthier.

Making Healthy Changes

Now we're going to begin our program to help you make healthy changes in your life. Keep in mind that behaviors are learned and so can be unlearned and replaced by other, healthier behaviors. The key is to make changes slowly and to be patient and kind to yourself if you are not always successful in maintaining the changes. Success in making even one small healthy change, such as getting an extra hour of sleep, on average, or drinking one less can of soda a day, can put you on the path to healthier living. More importantly, each success motivates you to make another small change. Over time the small changes add up and become significant in improving your health.

The first step in the program is to keep a record of what you decide to do healthwise and of how successful you are in achieving your goals. You will need a small notebook for the record. Write in it what you've learned or accomplished each day. The record you keep can be factual and short, or it can include intimate thoughts and feelings (Figure MHC1.1). The kind of journal you keep is up to you; however, it is important that you maintain it. We'll ask you to review your journal throughout the program.

Emotional Wellness: Finding a "Safe Haven"

We all experience moments during the day when we wish we could just turn off what we are thinking about—rehashing a conversation that was insulting, forgetting to do something that we had promised to do, or feeling that there isn't time to do what we want. When you want to stop disturbing thoughts temporarily, do the following:

Close your eyes and picture an image of a place where you felt totally relaxed or comfortable in the past. It might be a place you visited while on vacation, an area by a beach or lake, or a peaceful spot you found while on a hike in the woods. It might be a favorite place in a house you lived in when you were a child:

- Just let your mind bring up any image that feels really comfortable to you.

Nov. 4

Bummer. Didn't work out again today. That's two in a row. I told myself it was because I didn't want to walk to the gym in the rain. But that's not really it. I was lazy . . . and I wanted to talk to Greg (cute!). I can't let this happen again or I will blow all the gains from the past two months. More focus.

But still it was worth it. I've wanted to talk to Greg for weeks, ever since Mary Jo introduced him to me at Kathy's. Lucky/unlucky that day. Lucky = I was so nervous I didn't get a chance to say something stupid and ruin it right away. Unlucky = it took over two months to get another chance.

It's good to be interested in guys again. Nine months is a long time. T. was pretty efficient at crushing my heart (creep). It's like all the life got stomped out of me. But now it's coming back. My heart can breathe again. Mr. Greg, I'm going to be very careful around you. Wanna work out together?

April 17

Quit-Day + 5

Today's the first day since Q-day that I have not been crazy, grumpy, spiteful, jittery, depressed, and a pain to be around. The gum? The relaxation exercise? Who cares? It's working! I still get urges but the desire to light up passes in a few seconds. I'm over the hump and I am soooooooo glad.

FIGURE MHC1.1 Sample journal entries

- Let your mind remember as much as possible about the experience and the place. What were you seeing, what were you doing, what did you smell and hear?
- Let your mind develop this image for as long as it feels comfortable.
- When you feel that your mind has explored the scene in detail, remember what you experienced and realize that this is a mental "safe haven" you can go to whenever you feel upset, stressed, or hurried. You can go to your "safe haven" while waiting in line at the checkout counter, before taking an exam, or the next time you are at the dentist's office.

Describe in your journal what your "safe haven" is like. You can have more than one, but try to stick with the one that feels the most comfortable and calming.

Stress Management: Focusing the Mind Reduces Stress

Find a place outdoors close to where you live or work that seems beautiful and peaceful to you. It might be a bench in a park, a spot in a garden, a place in a nearby woods, or simply an area in your backyard that is quiet. Go to this place several times a week and spend at least 20 minutes there. While you are there, sit in one spot and use all your senses to record every-thing you can in as much detail as possible. What does the air smell like? Notice everything on the ground around your feet—grass, flowers, insects, and anything else you see. Touch the ground and see how it feels. Is it cold or hot, dry or wet? If your thoughts start to wander, make your mind focus on this one spot. With a little practice, you will find that you can focus your mind and become very observant of everything around you. You have begun to wake up, to be aware of your surroundings instead of being "lost" in endless mental chatter.

Focusing the mind on something interesting or pleasant is a proven method for reducing stress and quieting disturbing thoughts. You should begin to feel much more centered and calm after doing this exercise a number of times. If you feel bored in a particular spot, find a new one. Record in your journal how you felt during this exercise and how you felt afterward.

A note of explanation: A small number of students may be apprehensive about mental visualization exercises or they may feel that such exercises conflict with their religious beliefs. If any exercise conflicts with something that you strongly believe in, then you should remain true to your belief. However, mental imagery and mental suggestions are a normal part of human experience. All of us daydream when we are bored (often in classes) or when we are tired of paying

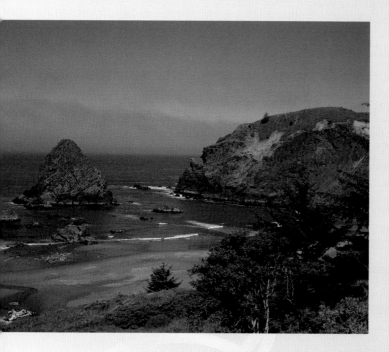

attention to someone or something. Daydreaming is a form of image visualization. In the exercises described in *Making Healthy Changes*, the suggestions are guiding your imagery, but the choice of images and the experience is yours.

It also is important to realize that no one can control your thoughts or feelings unless you allow them to. Unfortunately, many movies and TV programs would have us believe just the opposite, i.e., that our minds can be controlled by others. If you have this concern, be assured that your thoughts and feelings can never be controlled unless you *agree* to think or feel as someone tells you to. For example, we frequently say, "You made me angry." No one can make you angry. You make yourself angry because of the way you interpret a situation. In the same situation, another person might laugh. You can choose laughter over anger any time *you* choose.

The goal of advertising is to make you buy or use something that you may not need or want. We will have much more to say in *Making Healthy Changes* on how advertising can make you buy things that may have a negative effect on your health. Advertising accomplishes its goals through imagery and repeated suggestions.

The words *airplane* or *gun* are used to describe certain objects. Actually, each of us colors words based on our experiences. A person who has been shot has a very different view of the word *gun* compared to a person who has never handled a gun or been shot; a person with a fear of flying thinks differently about airplanes compared to those who enjoy flying. Similarly, the words *meditation, yoga, image visualization, relaxation response, progressive relaxation,*

stress management, and so forth are simply words. They often convey considerable benefit to those who learn what the words mean and the methods they teach.

Wise Consumer: Reducing Sugar Consumption

Unless you are that rare person, you probably consume several sodas a day. As a society, Americans drink more soda than water. There is nothing nutritious in soda (sugar is called "empty calories" because it supplies no vitamins, minerals, protein, or other nutrients), and we already obtain more sugar than is good for us in other foods. As for diet sodas, studies show that people who drink them increase their sugar intake in other foods.

We drink so much soda largely because it is promoted by companies in every way imaginable. In 1997, PepsiCo spent more than *$1 billion* advertising its sodas; CocaCola spends almost as much. In our consumer-oriented society, advertising poses a major risk to health if we let ourselves be persuaded to consume foods and drinks that have little or no nutritional value. In fact, overconsumption of sodas day after day will eventually lead to overweight and nutritional deficiencies.

Figure out how many sodas you drink each day, on average. Make a contract with yourself (write it in your journal and sign it) to give up one soda a day that you normally would drink (regular or diet, it makes no difference). Figure MHC1.2 shows an example. Reward yourself by putting the money you would have spent on the soda into a special jar marked "soda savings." Evaluate how you did after two weeks, and make a new contract to cut out two sodas a day. Again, reward yourself by depositing the money you would have spent in the jar.

Each time you consciously abstain from drinking a soda, make sure that you drink an equivalent amount of water.

Improving Your Diet: Adding Vitamins and Minerals

Most of us consume diets that are deficient in some essential nutrients. Unless your diet consists primarily of a great variety of fruits and vegetables that you eat at every meal, your body and brain probably can benefit from additional vitamins and minerals. If you do not already take vitamin supplements, begin to take a multivitamin that contains most of the essential vitamins and minerals. Multivitamins need not be expensive, although many brands sold in stores are. Look for generic brands or purchase your supplements from mail-order companies.

A gram of alcohol is chemically the same and will have the same physiological effect whether it is in beer, wine, scotch, or vodka. And the brand makes no

Personal Contract to Reduce Soda Consumption

Given that I drink, on average, three sodas per day, I will reduce my soda consumption to one per day by the end of the coming month. I will break my overall goal into two subgoals. During weeks 1 and 2, I will reduce one soda per day by eliminating the soda I have when I get home from school. During weeks 3 and 4, I will reduce two sodas per day, I will continue to eliminate the after-school soda, and I will also eliminate the late-night "study" soda, replacing it with water, tea, or juice. I will begin subgoal 1 on 3/4 and will continue until 3/18. I will begin subgoal 2 on 3/19 and will continue until 4/2. I will keep a daily diary of my soda consumption and will place the money I do not spend on sodas in a "soda savings" jar. I will use the money I save in each subgoal to buy myself a new CD. My plan for reducing soda consumption includes:

1. Not buying sodas in the store and having them around.
2. Staying stocked up on juice and tea.

I am undertaking this contract with myself because I want to be healthier and feel better.

Signed: *Stacey Mulligan*   Date: 3/1

Witness: *JoAnn Clark*   Date: 3/1

FIGURE MHC1.2   Sample "soda savings" contract

difference, either. The same is true for vitamins and minerals. Regardless of what advertisers tell you (or what you may hear at the health store), a gram of vitamin C is chemically identical to any other gram of vitamin C.

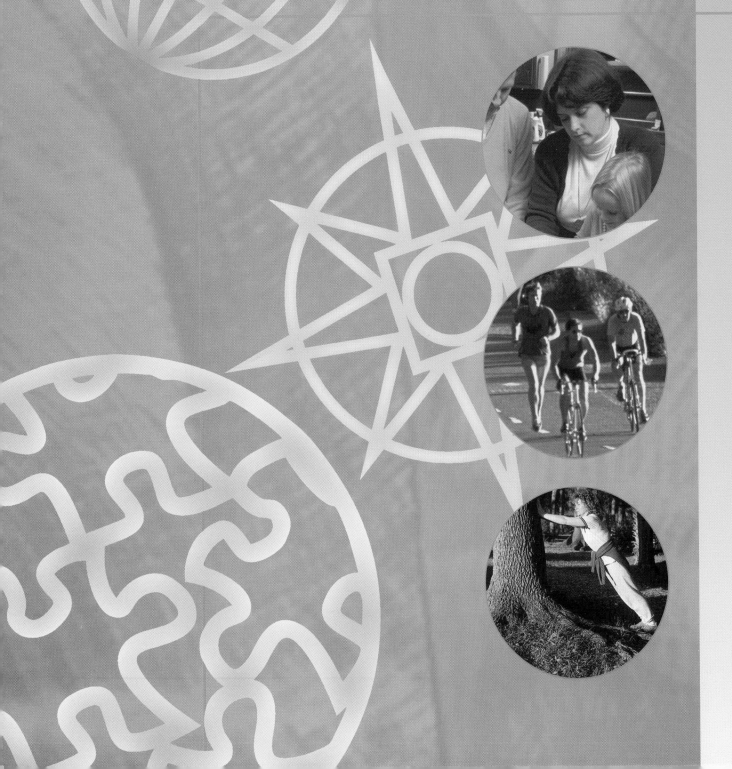

Part 2

Eating and Exercising Toward a Healthy Life-Style

Learning Objectives

1. Describe the dietary guidelines proposed by health organizations.
2. Describe which foods are at the bottom of the food guide pyramid and which are at the top and give the reasons for that placement.
3. Describe the ingredients and nutrition facts labels on manufactured foods.
4. Describe the three functions of food.
5. Define calorie.
6. List the seven components of food, and identify common foods that contain each component.
7. Describe the difference between simple and complex carbohydrates.
8. Define and identify sources of antioxidants.
9. Describe the three kinds of vegetarian diets and several reasons for vegetarianism.

Exercises and Activities

WORKBOOK
Food Diary
My Eating Habits: Some Clues to Calories
Eat for Good Nutrition
How Does Your Diet Rate for Variety?

Health and Wellness Online

 www.jbpub.com/hwonline
Dietary Supplements
Wellness Guide: Guidelines for Food Safety
Vegetarian Diets

Chapter 4

Choosing a Nutritious Diet

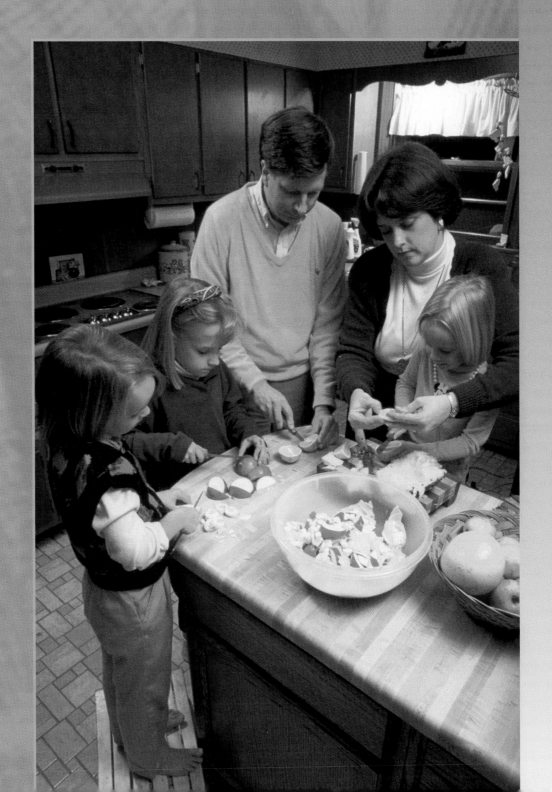

Many people are aware that good nutrition is essential for good health. But what to eat? To encourage and promote healthy dietary choices, the U.S. government, the World Health Organization, and organizations such as the American Heart Association and the American Cancer Society (Table 4.1) promote guidelines for good nutrition. These guidelines are based on the latest scientific evidence for good nutrition, obtained by examining the biological effects of specific dietary components and by comparing the dietary patterns and disease frequencies in different populations. For example, compared to the standard American diet with its associated high levels of heart disease and cancer, the high-carbohydrate, low-fat diet of rural China is associated with less heart disease and fewer cancers of all kinds (Campbell and Junshi, 1994). Seventh Day Adventists, who consume high-carbohydrate, low-fat diets, also have less heart disease and cancer than other Americans. The same is true of the people of Mediterranean countries (Greece, southern Italy), whose traditional diet is high in fruits, vegetables, and legumes and low in animal fat (Willett, 1994).

There is no sincerer love than the love of food.
GEORGE BERNARD SHAW

The U.S. Departments of Agriculture and Health and Human Services produce dietary guidelines (Figure 4.1) designed to help prevent diseases that result from poor nutrition, including:

- Heart disease, cancer of various organs, and obesity from diets high in total fat, cholesterol, and saturated fat
- Cancer of the colon from consumption of too much meat
- Diseases of the gastrointestinal tract from not consuming sufficient fiber

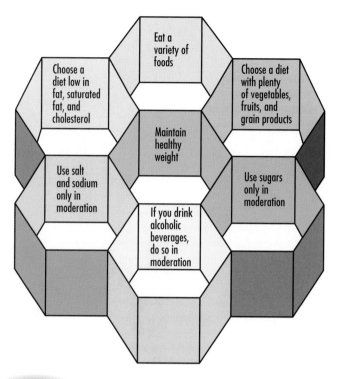

FIGURE 4.1   **Current Dietary Guidelines**   These guidelines call for moderation—avoiding extremes in diets—and reflect recommendations of nutrition authorities who agree that enough is known about diet's effect on health to encourage these dietary practices.
Source: U.S. Department of Agriculture and U.S. Department of Health and Human Services.

- High blood pressure from consuming too much salt
- Tooth decay from consuming too much sugar

The Food Guide Pyramid

To help implement the dietary guidelines, the U.S. government created the Food Guide Pyramid, which recommends diets that emphasize grains, fruits, and vegetables, with moderate to little consumption of

TABLE 4.1   American Heart Association and American Cancer Society Dietary Guidelines

American Heart Association's Dietary Guidelines with your heart in mind	*American Cancer Society's Dietary Guidelines for reducing your risk of cancer*
• Total fat intake should be less than 30% of total calories	• Maintain a desirable body weight
• Saturated fatty acid intake should be less than 10% of calories	• Eat a varied diet
• Polyunsaturated fatty acid intake should be no more than 10% of calories	• Include a variety of both vegetables and fruits in the daily diet
• Monounsaturated fatty acids should make up the rest of the total fat intake, about 10% to 15% of total calories	• Eat more high-fiber foods, e.g., whole grain cereals, legumes, vegetables, fruits
• Cholesterol intake should be no more than 300 mg/day	• Cut down on total fat intake
• Sodium intake should be no more than 3 g/day	• Limit consumption of alcoholic beverages, if any
	• Limit consumption of salt-cured, smoked, and nitrate-preserved foods

meat and dairy products, and only the sparest consumption of sweets and fats (Figure 4.2).

The Food Guide Pyramid places the most healthful foods at the bottom and the least healthful foods at the top. This arrangement helps people remember the composition of a healthful diet without having to count calories and grams. All people have to remember is to "eat low on the pyramid" by basing meals on pastas, breads, rice, fresh vegetables, and fruit. The slogan "five-a-day" was coined by nutritionists as a reminder to consume a total of five servings of fruits and vegetables each day. Vegetarians can modify their consumption of foods according to a modified food pyramid (Figure 4.3).

The typical college student's diet follows an inverted food guide pyramid; sweets, fats, and meats make up a large portion of the diet, while grains, fruits, and vegetables are virtually absent. One popular food that does conform to the food guide pyramid is pizza. The dough (made of wheat flour) is at the base, representing the grain group; the tomato sauce, mushrooms, olives, peppers, garlic, and onion represent the vegetable group; the cheese represents the dairy group; and salami, pepperoni, anchovies, and other meats represent the meat group.

The food guide pyramid has been criticized because it accommodates politically powerful meat and dairy industries and it does not offer sufficient information to guide healthy food choices. For example, meat and dairy products, which can contain high percentages of fat, are lumped together with beans and other legumes, which are high in fiber and contain little or no fat. Some products in the grain group are manufactured with considerable sugar and salt, but these additives are not reflected in the recommendations.

On the other hand, the pyramid's proponents point out that the pictorial display placing the most healthful food at the broad base and the least healthful at the tip is easy to remember. They believe it allows people to stop counting calories and grams and build diets based on foods found at the bottom of the pyramid: these include whole grains, fresh fruits, and fresh vegetables, which provide adequate nutrients and calories for good health.

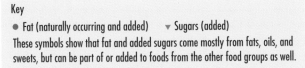

Key

● Fat (naturally occurring and added)   ▼ Sugars (added)

These symbols show that fat and added sugars come mostly from fats, oils, and sweets, but can be part of or added to foods from the other food groups as well.

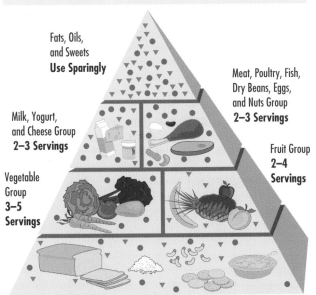

FIGURE 4.2   Food Guide Pyramid: A Guide to Daily Food Choices Each of these food groups provides some, but not all, of the nutrients you need. No one food group is more important than another—for good health, you need them all. Go easy on fats, oils, and sweets, the foods at the tip of the pyramid.

Source: U.S. Department of Agriculture and U.S. Department of Health and Human Services.

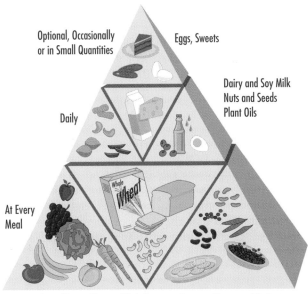

FIGURE 4.3   The Vegetarian Food Guide Pyramid. Notice that some foods are eaten at every meal, others daily, and some occasionally or in small quantities. Lactoovovegetarians can follow the regular food guide pyramid by replacing meats with two to three servings of dry beans, nuts, seeds, peanut butter, tofu, or eggs. Soy milk should be fortified with calcium and vitamins B_{12} and D. Vegans (no animal products) should consume 3 to 5 tablespoons of vegetable oil, 1 tablespoon blackstrap molasses, and 1 tablespoon of brewer's yeast daily.

Source: Cornell University, University of Rochester Medical Center, and the Human Connection.

Wellness Guide

How to Use the Food Guide Pyramid

What Counts As One Serving?

Breads, Cereals, Rice, and Pasta

1 slice of bread

1/2 cup of cooked rice or pasta

1/2 cup of cooked cereal

1 ounce of ready-to-eat cereal

Vegetables

1/2 cup of chopped raw or cooked vegetables

1 cup of leafy raw vegetables

Milk, Yogurt, and Cheese

1 cup of milk or yogurt

1-1/2 to 2 ounces of cheese

Fruits

1 piece of fruit or melon wedge

3/4 cup of juice

1/2 cup of canned fruit

1/4 cup of dried fruit

Meat, Poultry, Fish, Dry Beans, Eggs, and Nuts

2-1/2 to 3 ounces of cooked lean meat, poultry, or fish

Count 1/2 cup of cooked beans, or 1 egg, or 2 tablespoons of peanut butter as 1 ounce of lean meat (about 1/3 serving)

Fats, Oils, and Sweets

Consume sparingly.

How Many Servings Do You Need Each Day?

	No. of servings		
	Women and some older adults	Children, teenage girls, active women, most men	Teenage boys and active men
Bread group	6	9	11
Vegetable group	3	4	5
Fruit group	2	3	4
Milk group	2–3*	2–3*	2–3*
Meat group	2, for a total of 5 ounces	2, for a total of 6 ounces	3, for a total of 7 ounces

*Women who are pregnant or breastfeeding, teenagers, and young adults to age 24 need three servings.

Source: U.S. Department of Agriculture and U.S. Department of Health and Human Services, 1992.

Food Labels

The U.S. government requires that all manufactured foods carry two food labels: the **ingredients label** (Figure 4.4) and the **nutrition facts label** (Figure 4.5). The ingredients label lists the chemical composition of the food, i.e., all the substances that the manufacturer uses, including other foods (e.g., grains, eggs), natural and artificial sweeteners, natural and artificial fats, water, natural and artificial thickeners, natural and artificial flavorings, food colorings, and preservatives. The ingredients label lists foods in descending order by weight; the substance in the greatest amount is listed first and that in the least amount is listed last.

Terms

ingredient label: label on a manufactured food that lists the ingredients in descending order by weight

nutrition facts label: label on a manufactured food that lists the quantity of certain nutrients in the food and the percent daily value for those nutrients

Ingredients: Wheat flour, sugar, rolled oats, corn sweetener, molasses, partially hydrogenated safflower oil, salt, pantothenic acid, reduced iron, yellow No. 6, yellow No. 5, pyridoxine, ascorbic acid (vitamin C), BHT, riboflavin, folic acid.

FIGURE 4.4   The Ingredient Label. The government requires that food manufacturers list the substances within their products by weight from greatest to least.

The ingredients label does not specify how much—either by weight or percentage—of an ingredient is in a food, only its amount relative to the other ingredients. Also, by listing each individual substance, the ingredients label may not indicate the true relative amount of sugar or fat in the food. For example, a snack food's ingredients label could list separately sucrose, fructose, and corn sweetener, all of which are sugars.

Unlike the ingredients label, the nutrition facts label provides *quantitative* information on certain nutrients in the food (ones whose consumption should be monitored for good health) and the calorie content of the food. The amounts indicated for each nutrient and the calorie count are for a "serving," which is all or a portion of the food in the package, as determined by the manufacturer. The manufacturer's definition of

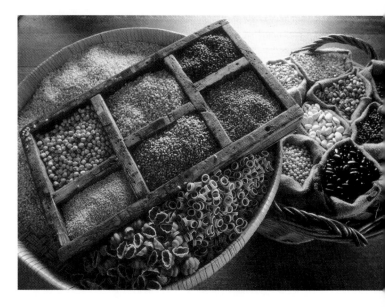

Natural, unprocessed foods provide the best nutrition.

Wellness Guide

Taking Care of Your Teeth and Gums

Taking care of your teeth and gums means adopting practices for oral health that prevent tooth decay *(dental caries)* and gum disease *(gingivitis* and *periodontitis)*. Tooth decay and gum disease are caused by the action of a variety of bacteria that live in the mouth, which produce acids by breaking down the sugars in food. The acids attack the enamel of teeth, causing tooth decay. Other bacteria are involved in the conversion of sugars and some of the material in saliva into a gelatinous substance called *plaque,* which sticks to teeth and gums and fosters more bacterial growth and decay.

Tooth and gum disease could be prevented if (a) the bacteria responsible could be removed from the mouth, (b) the sugars and other substances bacteria use to produce acids and plaque were removed from the mouth, or (c) teeth were protected from the bacterial products.

It is not yet possible to keep all tooth and gum disease-causing bacteria from the mouth or to render them harmless. So, keeping the mouth free of sugar and plaque is the best way to prevent tooth and gum problems. You can accomplish this by:

- Not eating sugar and sugar-containing foods between meals.

- Consuming sweets in liquid rather than solid form when possible.
- Avoiding sticky or slowly dissolving sweets.
- Brushing and flossing teeth after each meal.
- Rinsing the mouth with warm water when unable to brush after a snack or meal.
- Obtaining flouride (to increase resistance to tooth decay) from toothpastes, mouthwashes, and drinking water.
- Getting periodic dental checkups.

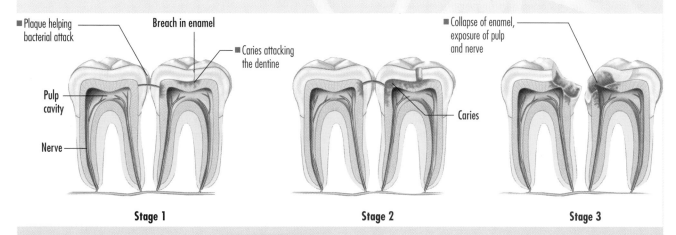

■ Plaque helping bacterial attack
Breach in enamel
■ Caries attacking the dentine
Pulp cavity
Nerve
■ Collapse of enamel, exposure of pulp and nerve
Caries

Stage 1   **Stage 2**   **Stage 3**

Total Fat

Aim low: Most people need to cut back on fat! Too much fat may contribute to heart disease and cancer. Try to limit your calories from fat. For a healthy heart, choose foods with a big difference between the total number of calories and the number of calories from fat.

Saturated Fat

A new kind of fat? No — saturated fat is part of the total fat in food. It is listed separately because it's the key player in raising blood cholesterol and your risk of heart disease. Eat less!

Cholesterol

Too much cholesterol — a second cousin to fat — can lead to heart disease. Challenge yourself to eat less than 300 mg each day.

Sodium

You call it "salt," the label calls it "sodium." Either way, it may add up to high blood pressure in some people. So, keep your sodium intake low — 2,400 to 3,000 mg or less each day. The AHA recommends no more than 3,000 mg sodium per day for healthy adults.

Daily Value

Feel like you're drowning in numbers? Let the Daily Value be your guide. Daily Values are listed for people who eat 2,000 or 2,500 calories each day. If you eat more, your personal daily value may be higher than what's listed on the label. If you eat less, your personal daily value may be lower.

For the fat, saturated fat, cholesterol and sodium, choose foods with a low % Daily Value. For total carbohydrate, dietary fiber, vitamins and minerals, your daily value goal is to reach 100% of each.

g = grams (About 28 g = 1 ounce)
mg = milligrams (1,000 mg = 1 g)

Nutrition Facts

Serving Size 1/2 cup (114 g)
Servings Per Container 4

Amount per Serving

Calories 90	Calories from Fat 30	
		% Daily Value*
Total Fat 3g		5%
Saturated Fat 0g		0%
Cholesterol 0mg		0%
Sodium 300g		13%
Total Carbohydrate 13g		4%
Dietary Fiber 3g		12%
Sugars 3g		
Protein 3g		

Vitamin A	80%	•	Vitamin C	60%
Calcium	4%	•	Iron	4%

* Percent Daily Values are based on a 2,000 calorie diet. Your daily values may be higher or lower depending on your calorie needs:

	Calories	2,000	2,500
Total Fat	Less than	65g	80g
Sat Fat	Less than	20g	25g
Cholesterol	Less than	300mg	300mg
Sodium	Less than	2,400mg	2,400mg
Total Carbohydrate		300g	375g
Fiber		25g	30g

Calories per gram:
Fat 9 • Carbohydrate 4 • Protein 4

More nutrients may be listed on some labels.

Serving Size

Is your serving the same size as the one on the label? If you eat double the serving size listed, you need to double the nutrient and calorie values. If you eat one-half the serving size shown here, cut the nutrient and calorie values in half.

Calories

Are you overweight? Cut back a little on calories! Look here to see how a serving of the food adds to your daily total. A 5'4", 138-lb. active woman needs about 2,200 calories each day. A 5'10", 174-lb. active man needs about 2,900. How about you?

Total Carbohydrate

When you cut down on fat, you can eat more carbohydrates. Carbohydrates are in foods like bread, potatoes, fruits and vegetables. Choose these often! They give you nutrients and energy.

Dietary Fiber

Grandmother called it "roughage," but her advice to eat more is still up-to-date! That goes for both soluble and insoluble kinds of dietary fiber. Fruits, vegetables, whole-grain foods, beans and peas are all good sources and can help reduce the risk of heart disease and cancer.

Protein

Most Americans get more protein than they need. Where there is minimal protein, there is also fat and cholesterol. Eat small servings of lean meat, fish and poultry. Use skim or low-fat milk, yogurt, and cheese. Try vegetable proteins like beans, grains and cereals.

Vitamins & Minerals

Your goal here is 100% of each for the day. Don't count on one food to do it all. Let a combination of foods add up to a winning score.

FIGURE 4.5   The Nutrition Facts Label

a serving is given at the top of the nutrition facts label as the "serving size."

In addition to the actual amounts of nutrients and calories, the nutrition facts label lists the **percent daily value** (PDV) for each nutrient, which is the percentage of the recommended daily amount that is contained in the food. (The percent daily value on the nutrition facts label is for someone who requires 2000 calories of food energy per day; people with higher or lower calorie requirements have a larger or smaller PDV.) Near the bottom of the nutrition facts label is the recommended daily amount of nutrients, listed by weight (in grams) for 2000- and 2500-calorie diets.

To help consumers determine health-related claims on food labels, the U.S. government requires manufacturers to adhere to certain definitions (Table 4.2).

 ## The Three Functions of Food

Food has three functions:

1. To provide the chemical constituents of the body
2. To provide the energy for life
3. To be pleasurable, including satisfying hunger; experiencing the smell, taste, sight, and texture of food; and associating food with enjoyable social activities

Body Structure and Function

Your body is made up of billions of atoms and molecules arranged in particular combinations and proportions. Most of the atoms and molecules that now make up your body were not part of you even a few weeks ago, because living things continually exchange their chemical constituents with the environment. Food provides the "raw materials" for your body's cells to manufacture the specific chemical substances that make you *you*.

Adequate amounts of 40 chemical substances, called the **essential nutrients** (Table 4.3), must be supplied continually to the body. Failure to do so can result in a nutritional deficiency disease.

Researchers have determined how much of the essential nutrients are required to prevent deficiency

Terms

percent daily value: percentage of the recommended daily amount of a particular nutrient found in a food

essential nutrients: chemical substances obtained from food and needed by the body for growth, maintenance, or repair of tissues; not made by the body; must be obtained from food

TABLE 4.2   What Words on Product Labels Mean

Calorie-free	Fewer than 5 calories per serving
Light (lite)	1/3 less calories or no more than 1/2 the fat of the higher-calorie, higher-fat version; or no more than 1/2 the sodium of the higher-sodium version
Fat-free	Less than 0.5 g of fat per serving
Low-fat	3 g of fat (or less) per serving
Reduced or less fat	At least 25% less fat per serving than the higher-fat version
Lean	Less than 10 g of fat, 4 g of saturated fat, and 95 mg of cholesterol per serving
Extra-lean	Less than 5 g of fat, 2 g of saturated fat, and 95 mg of cholesterol per serving
Low in saturated fat	1 g saturated fat (or less) per serving and not more than 15% of calories from saturated fatty acids
Cholesterol-free	Less than 2 mg of cholesterol and 2 g (or less) of saturated fat per serving
Low-cholesterol	20 mg of cholesterol (or less) and 2 g of saturated fat (or less) per serving
Reduced cholesterol	At least 25% less cholesterol than the higher-cholesterol version; and 2 g (or less) of saturated fat per serving
Sodium-free (no sodium)	Less than 5 mg of sodium per serving, and no sodium chloride (NaCl) in ingredients
Very low sodium	35 mg of sodium (or less) per serving
Low sodium	140 mg of sodium (or less) per serving
Reduced or less sodium	At least 25% less sodium per serving than the higher-sodium version
Sugar-free	Less than 0.5 g of sugar per serving
High-fiber	5 g of fiber (or more) per serving
Good source of fiber	2.5 to 4.9 g of fiber per serving

TABLE 4.3   The Essential Nutrients*

Amino acids	Fats	Water	Vitamins	Minerals
Isoleucine	Linoleic acid		Ascorbic acid (vitamin C)	Calcium
Leucine	Linolenic acid		Biotin	Chlorine
Lysine			Cobalamin (vitamin B_{12})	Chromium
Methionine			Folic acid	Cobalt
Phenylalanine			Niacin (vitamin B_3)	Copper
Threonine			Pantothenic acid	Iodine
Tryptophan			Pyridoxine (vitamin B_6)	Iron
Valine			Riboflavin (vitamin B_2)	Magnesium
Arginine[†]			Thiamine (vitamin B_1)	Manganese
Histidine[†]			Vitamin A	Molybdenum
			Vitamin D	Phosphorus
			Vitamin E	Potassium
			Vitamin K	Selenium
				Sodium
				Sulfur
				Zinc

*Must be obtained from food.

[†]Not essential for adults; needed for growth of children.

diseases. In the United States, these requirements are called the **recommended [daily] dietary allowances,** or **RDA.** The RDA is set for people in reasonably good health, i.e., not suffering from a major disease or under undue stress.

Surveys indicate that many Americans do not consume recommended RDA amounts of calcium, vitamin B$_6$, magnesium, zinc, copper, and potassium. People can determine if their diets contain the RDA of particular nutrients by consulting tables listing the composition of foods. Packaged food labels also carry information on the nutrient composition of the product.

Energy for Life

Food also provides energy to the body. The ultimate source of energy for complex organisms is sunlight, which is captured by green plants and converted to chemical energy that is stored as plant material. When humans eat plant matter or tissue of plant-eating animals, they obtain this stored chemical energy. Biological energy is used most efficiently when liberated in the presence of oxygen, which is one reason you breathe. In the process, the food material is converted to carbon dioxide, water, and other waste products and eliminated from the body in expired air, urine, feces, and sweat.

Energy transformations in living things are discussed in terms of calories. A **calorie** is the amount of heat energy required to raise 1 g of water from 14.5 °C to 15.5 °C. A **nutritional calorie,** which is what weight watchers watch, is 1000 calories, or a **kilocalorie.** Books that discuss human nutrition and physical fitness frequently use the word "calorie" when actually referring to a kilocalorie. This book follows the same convention.

Energy from food is derived from the breakdown of carbohydrates, fats, and proteins. Carbohydrates and proteins supply approximately 4 calories per gram, and fats supply approximately 9 calories per gram.

Energy is needed to support three major processes: (a) **basal** (or resting) **metabolism,** which is the energy required to keep the body alive; (b) physical activity (the things you do when you're not completely at rest); and (c) growth. The energy to support basal metabolism keeps cells functioning, maintains the body temperature within its normal limits, and keeps the heart, lungs, kidneys, and other internal organs functioning. The daily amount of energy required to support basal metabolism is called **basal metabolic rate** (BMR). The BMR for adult women is about 1100 calories per day, and 1300 calories per day for adult men.

In addition to the energy you need for basal metabolism, you use energy in physical activity: walking, running, working, and so on. The amount of energy expended for these activities depends on how strenuous the activity is, how long it is engaged in, the body's size, and the environmental temperature. It takes more energy to be active in hot weather than in moderate temperatures, and it takes more energy to maintain body temperature when the weather is cold.

Energy is also needed whenever the body produces more cells than are needed to replace ones that periodically die. Thus, all young people need additional energy for growth and physical activity. Energy is also needed to produce new cells to repair injuries.

Energy requirements for individuals vary depending on a number of factors including: body size and composition; physical activity; growth needs during adolescence and young adulthood; pregnancy or breast feeding; and injury or illness. Nutritionists recommend that carbohydrates from grains, vegetables, and fruits be the principal source of energy, supplying about 60% to 80% of total calories consumed. Fats should make up no more than 30% of total calories consumed. Protein is generally not recommended as a source of energy, but only as a source of building blocks for the body's tissues and organs.

Pleasures of Eating

Everyone has experienced the feeling of hunger and its appeasement by eating something. But hunger is not the only reason for eating in our society. Most of the time we eat because it is "time to eat," because someone has presented us with food, or simply because it feels good to be eating something—especially something sweet. The ready availability of food is unique to modern societies;

Terms

recommended [daily] dietary allowances (RDA): levels of nutrients recommended by the Food and Nutrition Board of the National Academy of Sciences for daily consumption by healthy individuals, scaled according to gender and age

calorie: the amount of energy required to raise 1 g of water from 14.5 °C to 15.5 °C

nutritional calorie: unit of energy; often used interchangeably with the term kilocalorie

kilocalorie: unit of energy; the amount of heat needed to raise one kilogram of water 1 °C, equivalent to 1000 calories

basal metabolism: the minimum amount of energy needed to keep the body alive

basal metabolic rate (BMR): the amount of energy needed per day to keep the body functioning while at rest

proteins: the foundation of every body cell; biological molecules composed of chains of amino acids

amino acids: compounds containing nitrogen, which are the building blocks of protein

essential amino acids: amino acids that cannot be synthesized by the body and must be provided by food

nonessential amino acids: eleven amino acids required for protein synthesis that are synthesized by humans and are not specifically required in the diet

a hundred years ago there were no supermarkets, fast food restaurants, or convenience stores on every block. Advertising encourages us to eat more and more often. Many of us have become addicted to trying new foods and new restaurants for pleasure. Indeed, eating has become Americans' number one pastime.

The Seven Components of Food

Food is composed of seven kinds of chemical substances: proteins, carbohydrates, lipids (fats), vitamins, minerals, phytochemicals, and water. Dietary proteins, most types of carbohydrates, and most lipids cannot be used by the body until they are broken down in the digestive system into smaller chemical units (Figure 4.6). In fact, only vitamins, minerals, a few kinds of carbohydrates, and water are absorbed into the body as is.

Proteins

Proteins make up about 20% of body mass. The main function of protein is to provide your body with the amino acids necessary for growth and maintenance of body tissues. Cells, enzymes, hormones, antibodies, muscles and blood require amino acids as building blocks obtained from protein.

Proteins are made up of chemical units called **amino acids,** which come in 20 different forms. Amino acids are classified as **essential** and **nonessential.** Eight essential amino acids are required by adults, and ten are required by infants. Animal sources of protein include milk and milk products, meat, fish, poultry, and eggs. Plant sources include breads and cereal products, legumes, nuts, and seeds. The primary sources of protein for the majority of the world's population are cereal grains and legumes.

The trouble with Italian cooking is that after five or six days you're hungry again.

HENRY MILLER

Amino acids are not stored in the body in any appreciable amounts; therefore, proper nutrition requires eating enough protein every day to meet the body's needs for essential amino acids. Adult women should consume about 45 grams per day and adult men about 55 to 60 grams. The average North American adult consumes about twice that amount; the unneeded protein is broken down by the body and excreted in urine or stored as fat.

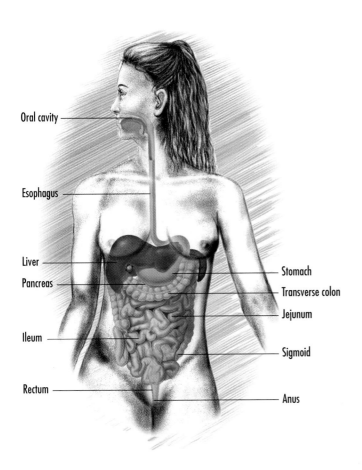

Oral cavity
Esophagus
Liver
Pancreas
Ileum
Rectum
Stomach
Transverse colon
Jejunum
Sigmoid
Anus

FIGURE 4.6   Human Digestive System
Teeth and glandular secretions in mouth help break up food, which the esophagus transports to the stomach. The stomach breaks down some of the food molecules and passes the food to the rest of the digestive tube: the duodenum, jejunum, ileum, colon, and rectum. The pancreas secretes enzymes and fluid into the duodenum to help the digestive process. The liver controls release of absorbed nutrients into the body. Undigested material is eliminated from the body at the anus.

Because the amino acid composition of most animal protein is similar, people tend to acquire adequate amounts and proportions of the essential amino acids from fish, meat, eggs, and dairy products. Most vegetable proteins, however, are deficient in one or more of the essential amino acids, so individuals who eat little or no meat or dairy products must eat foods in which an amino-acid deficiency in one food is compensated for by an amino-acid surplus in another. For example, wheat, rice, and oats contain very little lysine, but have large amounts of methionine and tryptophan. Soybeans and other legumes are relatively high in lysine, but are low in methionine and tryptophan. Meals consisting of both grains and legumes (e.g., rice and beans, corn and beans, wheat and soybeans) can supply adequate amounts of these essential amino acids.

Meat, dairy products, and eggs provide the essential amino acids, but are also high in fat, and thus contribute to the health problems associated with a high-fat diet (Table 4.4). For this reason, nutritionists recommend consuming nonfat or low-fat dairy products, using butter as a spread and not as an ingredient for cooking, being mindful of the amount of ice cream eaten, and limiting egg consumption to a few eggs per week. Nutritionists also favor trimming fat from meat before cooking, selecting meat with a low-fat content, and eating poultry (with skin removed because it contains fat) and fish, which have proportionately less fat than red meats. They also recommend using meat sparingly by adding it to grain- or bean-based dishes, rather than making it the center of the meal.

Another reason for avoiding a lot of meat is its association with colorectal cancer. Countries with the highest per capita meat consumption—New Zealand, Canada, and the United States—also have the highest rates of colon cancer. The reasons for this association are not clear. One possibility is that commercially grown and distributed meats may contain cancer causing or cancer-promoting pesticide residues (DDT), industrial chemicals (PCBs), growth hormones (DES), dyes for color enhancement, and preservatives, such as **nitrates** and **nitrites,** often found in hot dogs, ham, sausage, and other cured meats. Another possibility is that bacteria in the colon convert substances necessary for the digestion of fats (bile acids) into cancer-causing agents. A third possibility is that charring meats in cooking converts substances in the meat into cancer-causing heterocyclic amines (HCAs).

Athletes are often encouraged to increase their intake of protein, sometimes to as much as 30% of total calories—twice the recommended amount for inactive adults. Because body protein (that is, muscle tissue) can become a source of energy during exercise if carbohydrate and fat are not available, some endurance athletes may require more than the recommended amount of protein. A common recommendation for

| TABLE 4.4 | Fat and Cholesterol Content of Various Meats and Fish | | |

Food (100 g)	Total fat (g)	Polyunsaturated fat (mg)	Cholesterol (mg)
Ground beef, extra lean	16.0	600	82
Ground beef, lean	18.0	700	78
Ground beef, regular	21.0	800	87
Top round	8.8	400	85
T-bone steak	25.0	900	84
Bacon	7.0	800	48
Ham—cured, lean	4.6	400	38
Ham—cured, regular	13.0	1,400	54
Beef liver	4.9	1,100	389
Bologna (slice)	6.6	300	13
Cod	0.6	200	37
Crab	1.0	400	47
Frozen fish sticks (1 stick)	3.4	900	31
Haddock	0.6	200	49
Salmon	2.9	1,200	44
Shrimp	1.5	600	130
Tuna (in water)	.2	200	0
Tuna (in oil)	7.0	2,500	15
Chicken breast without skin, roasted	3.6	810	85
Chicken breast with skin, fried	8.7	1,900	88

Source: U.S. Department of Agriculture. Handbook Number 8.

both endurance athletes and those involved in strength training is to consume 0.6 to 0.9 grams of protein per day per pound of body weight. That protein can come from lean meat, fish, poultry, vegetables, grains, and beans. It is not necessary to consume so-called "high-protein" liquids. Regular food will do.

Carbohydrates

Carbohydrates are the principal source of the body's energy, and also are used to manufacture some cell components, such as the hereditary material, **DNA.** Because the body can manufacture them from other substances, carbohydrates are not considered essential nutrients. However, not eating enough carbohydrates, recommended by some ill-conceived reducing diets, can force the body to break down muscle tissue to supply energy necessary for life functions.

Most animals have a "sweet tooth," and humans are no exception. That's why food manufacturers often add sugars and other sweeteners to their products. Indeed, many commercial breakfast cereals are 40%

Managing Stress

Stress and Your Diet

Believe it or not, some see eating as a technique to reduce the symptoms of stress. The feeling of food in the stomach sends a message to the brain to calm down. Yet there are certain foods that can send your stress levels off the charts and most people are completely unaware of them. Moreover, repeated bouts of stress can deplete necessary nutrients, vitamins, and minerals creating a cycle of poor health. Here are some examples:

Sugar

An excess of simple sugars tends to deplete vitamin stores, particularly the vitamin B complex (niacin, thiamine, riboflavin, and B$_{12}$). White sugar and even bleached flour flushed of its vitamin and mineral content require additional B-complex vitamins to be metabolized. These and other vitamins are crucial for optimal function of the central nervous system. A depletion of the B-complex vitamin may manifest in signs of fatigue, anxiety, and irritability. In addition, increased amounts of ingested simple sugars can cause major fluctuations in blood glucose levels resulting in pronounced fatigue, headaches, and general irritability.

Caffeine

Food sources that trigger the sympathetic nervous system are referred to as *sympathomimetic agents.* There is a powerful substance in caffeine called *methylated xanthine.* This chemical stimulant with amphetamine-like characteristics triggers in the sympathetic nervous system a heightened state of alertness and arousal; it can also stimulate the release of several stress hormones. The result is an intensified alertness which makes the individual more susceptible to perceived stress. Caffeine can be found in many foods, including chocolate, coffee, tea, and several other beverages. Current estimates suggest that the average American consumes three 6-ounce cups of coffee per day. A 6-ounce cup of caffinated coffee contains approximately 250 milligrams of caffeine, half the amount necessary to provoke adverse arousal of the central nervous system.

Vitamin and Mineral Deficiency

Chronic stress can deplete several vitamins necessary for energy metabolism and for the stress response. The synthesis of cortisol requires vitamins. The stress response activates several hormones that mobilize and metabolize fats and carbohydrates for energy production. The breakdown of fats and carbohydrates requires vitamins, specifically vitamins C and the B complex. Inadequate amounts of these vitamins may also affect mental alertness, and promote depression and insomnia. Stress is also associated with depletion of calcium and the inability of bones to properly absorb calcium, setting the stage for the development of osteoporosis, which is the demineralization of bone tissue. Vitamin supplementation is a controversial issue. A balanced diet usually provides an adequate supply of vitamins and nutrients for energy metabolism. However, the majority of Americans do not maintain a balanced diet. Vitamin supplements may be useful for individuals prone to excessive stress.

---

sugar by weight. Because added sugar provides calories but no essential nutrients, sugar is usually described as contributing "empty calories" to the diet. Excess calories from added sugar are converted to fat, which in some cases may contribute to overweight problems.

There are two principal types of carbohydrates: **simple sugars,** found predominantly in fruit, and **complex carbohydrates,** found in grains, fruit, and the stems, leaves, and roots of vegetables. Simple sugars contribute about 20% of total calories in the average American diet. Except for increasing the risk of tooth decay, simple sugars in themselves are not harmful. Problems can arise when simple sugars are consumed in high-fat, low-nutrient snack foods (cakes, candies) and when they replace the more healthful complex carbohydrates in the diet.

Simple Sugars   Glucose is the most common simple sugar; it is found in all plants and animals. Glucose circulates in the bloodstream and is commonly referred to as "blood sugar." Another simple sugar is fructose, which is found in fruits and honey. **Fructose** is one of the sweetest sugars, which means you can eat less fructose than other simple sugars and taste an equivalent amount of sweetness. High fructose corn syrup is a common sweetener added to a variety of commercial food products.

Terms

nitrates: preservatives containing any salt or ester of nitric acid. Some individuals are sensitive to nitrates and may suffer from headache, diarrhea, or urticaria after ingesting them

nitrites: preservatives containing any salt or ester of nitrous acid

carbohydrates: the most economical and efficient source of energy; biological molecules consisting of one or more sugar molecules

deoxyribonucleic acid (DNA): a nucleic acid of complex molecular structure occurring in cell nuclei; carrier of the genes; present in all body cells of every species

simple sugars: a class of carbohydrates called monosaccharides; all carbohydrates must be reduced to simple sugars to be digested

complex carbohydrates: a class of carbohydrates called polysaccharides; foods composed of starch and cellulose

glucose: the principal source of energy in all cells; also called dextrose

fructose: a simple sugar found in fruits and honey

Sucrose, which is common table sugar, is a combination of glucose and fructose. Sucrose is digested by breaking down the glucose and fructose portions. Because fructose is sweeter than sucrose, you can reduce the amount of sugar in your diet without cutting out sweet tastes by replacing pastries with fresh fruit and table sugar with honey. Furthermore, you will be gaining other nutrients in the fruit and honey that are not present in refined sucrose.

Lactose, found principally in dairy products, is a sugar consisting of glucose combined with the simple sugar **galactose.** When lactose is digested, the glucose and galactose are separated and the galactose is converted to glucose. Whereas almost all babies have the capacity to digest lactose (it is the major sugar in mother's milk), many older children and adults, par-

Terms

sucrose: common refined "table" sugar; a molecule of glucose and a molecule of fructose chemically bonded together

lactose: a molecule of glucose and galactose chemically bonded together; found primarily in milk

galactose: a monosaccharide derived from lactose

lactase: enzyme secreted by glands in the small intestine that converts lactose (milk sugar) into simple sugars

starch: complex chain of glucose molecules

fiber: a group of compounds that make up the framework of plants; fiber cannot be digested

glycogen: the form in which carbohydrate is stored in humans and animals

insoluble fiber: cannot be dissolved in water

soluble fiber: can be dissolved in water

cellulose: a carbohydrate forming the skeleton of most plant structures and plant cells; the most abundant polysaccharide in nature and the source of dietary fiber

hemicellulose: substances found in plant cell walls that are composed of various sugars chemically linked together

lipids: fats such as cholesterol and triglycerides

cholesterol: a fatlike compound occurring in bile, blood, brain, nerve tissue, liver, and other parts of the body

lecithin: an essential component of cell membranes

linoleic acid: an essential fat that must be obtained from food

fatty acids: naturally occurring in fats, either saturated or unsaturated (monounsaturated or polyunsaturated)

saturated fat: generally solid at room temperature; comes from animal sources

monounsaturated fatty acid: carries one less than all the hydrogen atoms it possibly could

polyunsaturated fatty acid: carries at least two fewer hydrogen atoms than it would if saturated

trans fatty acid: an artificial fatty acid manufactured by chemically modifying monounsaturated and polyunsaturated fatty acids

ticularly of black and Asian heritage, are not able to digest it because they lack a required enzyme, **lactase,** which splits lactose into glucose and galactose. When lactase-deficient people consume dairy products, they can experience gastrointestinal upset, diarrhea, and, occasionally, severe illness. These individuals can supplement their diets with products containing lactase (e.g., Lactaid) or by eating yogurt, cheese, and other dairy products in which the lactose has been broken down by the fermentation process. Because dairy products are a major source of calcium in the North American diet, people who avoid dairy products should consume calcium-rich vegetables (e.g., broccoli and peas) and possibly take calcium supplements.

Complex Carbohydrates   These come primarily from grains (wheat, rice, corn, oats, barley); legumes (peas, beans); the leaves, stems, and roots of plants; and some animal tissue. There are two main classes of complex carbohydrates: **starch,** which is digestible, and **fiber,** which is not digestible.

Starch consists of many glucose molecules linked together. It is a way organisms store glucose until it is needed. In plants, starch is usually contained in granules within seeds, pods, or roots. Wheat flour, for example, is made by crushing wheat grain, which separates the outer husk (the bran) from the middle, starch-containing portion (the endosperm), and the inner germ. The white flour commonly used in baking is "70% extraction," which means that 70% of the original grain remains after crushing. In the milling of 70% extraction flour, many nutrients in the wheat grain are lost, so flour manufacturers add back several vitamins and minerals to produce "enriched flour." A "whole-grain flour," on the other hand, is 90% to 95% extraction and does not have to be enriched. In a reasonably varied diet, whatever nutrients not present in flour are obtained in other foods. Those wanting all the nutrients in wheat can choose whole-wheat flour.

Bread made with whole-wheat flour is brown, but not all brown bread is whole-wheat bread. Some manufacturers add molasses or honey to white-flour dough to give it a brown color, and they are allowed to label the product "wheat bread." For this reason, it is important to read the package label before buying.

Starch is also found in potatoes, which have an undeserved reputation for being fattening. Potatoes are no more fattening than any other starchy food unless they are cooked in large amounts of fat or oil, which is used in making french fries and potato chips. One large potato has about 100 calories, less than a medium-sized soft drink. French fries made from a medium potato, however, contain over 300 calories.

Animals and humans produce a starch in muscle and liver tissue called **glycogen.** When energy is needed, the glycogen breaks down and its constituent glucose molecules are liberated. Athletes sometimes eat large quantities of carbohydrates the day before competition to build up their supply of glycogen, a practice known as "carbohydrate loading." The practice of carbohydrate loading can be risky, particularly for diabetics.

Fiber is the second main class of complex carbohydrates. There are two kinds of fiber, **insoluble fiber,** which cannot dissolve in water, and **soluble fiber,** which can. Insoluble fiber is made up of **cellulose** and **hemicellulose,** substances that offer rigidity to plant material (wood; stems; the outer coverings of nuts, seeds, grains; the peels and skins of fruits and vegetables). Soluble fiber is composed of pectins, gums, and mucilages. The differences in insoluble and soluble fiber are not significant for health. Nutritionists recommend that individuals consume 20 to 35 grams of fiber daily, regardless of its type (Table 4.5).

Fiber adds bulk to the feces, thereby preventing constipation and related disorders, such as hemorrhoids and hiatal hernia, which can result from prolonged increase in intra-abdominal pressure while defecating. Fiber also facilitates the transport of waste material through the digestive tract, lessening the risk of appendicitis, diverticular disease (out-pocketings in the wall of the lower intestine), and cancer of the colon and rectum. High-fiber diets may also help to lessen the risk of heart disease and some cancers (Anderson, Smith, and Gustafson, 1994).

Lipids (Fats)

Lipids are a diverse group of substances that have the common property of being relatively insoluble in water. Some of these substances include **cholesterol** and **lecithin,** which are essential constituents of cell membranes; the steroid hormones produced by the reproductive organs and adrenal glands; vitamins A, D, E, and K; and bile acids, which aid the digestion of fats. Despite the current antifat trend, fats are an essential part of the diet. They supply calories, they provide flavor and texture to food, and digesting fat provides feelings of satiety and well-being. One kind of fat, **linoleic acid,** found in vegetable oils such as safflower, sunflower, and corn, is essential, and must be obtained in food. Deficiencies in this substance can produce skin lesions.

Much of the fat consumed in the diet is triglyceride, which is composed of **fatty acids.** These substances are further classified as **saturated, monounsaturated,** or **polyunsaturated,** depending on their chemistry. Saturation refers to the number of hydrogen atoms (and therefore the amount of energy) contained in a fatty acid. A saturated fatty acid carries all the hydrogen atoms it can. A monounsaturated fatty acid (MUFA) carries one less than all the hydrogen atoms it possibly could. A polyunsaturated fatty acid lacks two or more hydrogen atoms. A dietary fat is classified as saturated, monounsaturated, or polyunsaturated, depending on the type of fatty acids it contains in greatest quantity.

Saturated fats are found in whole milk and products made from whole milk; egg yolks; meat; meat fat; coconut and palm oils; chocolate; regular margarine; and hydrogenated vegetable shortenings. Sources of monounsaturated fats include olive oil and some nuts. Polyunsaturated fats are found in safflower, cottonseed, corn, soybean, and sesame seed oils, and fatty fish (Figure 4.7).

Diets high in cholesterol and saturated fat increase the risk of coronary heart disease, some cancers, and obesity. Many nutritionists recommend that adults consume no more than 300 mg of cholesterol per day and limit saturated fat intake to 10% or less of total calories. "Visible" dietary fats include butter, cream, and whole milk. "Hidden" dietary fats include egg yolks, nuts, seeds, olives, avocados, cakes, pies, snack foods, and even lean meat, which can be 4% to 12% fat. Conversely, polyunsaturated fats tend to lower blood cholesterol, which is why nutritionists recommend consuming vegetable oils.

Food manufacturers use a chemical process to transform natural polyunsaturated fatty acids derived from vegetable oils into artificial **trans fatty acids,** which tend to be solid at room temperature. This is how margarine and vegetable shortenings are made. Because margarine contains no cholesterol or animal fat,

TABLE 4.5   Fiber Content of Various Foods

Food	Amount	Fiber (g)
Whole-wheat bread	1 slice	1.6
Rye bread	1 slice	1.0
White bread	1 slice	0.6
Brown rice (cooked)	½ cup	2.4
White rice (cooked)	½ cup	0.1
Spaghetti (cooked)	½ cup	0.8
Kidney beans (cooked)	½ cup	5.8
Lima beans (cooked)	½ cup	4.9
Potato (baked)	medium	3.8
Corn	½ cup	3.9
Spinach	½ cup	2.0
Lettuce	½ cup	0.3
Strawberries	¾ cup	2.0
Banana	medium	2.0
Apple (with skin)	medium	2.6
Orange	small	1.2

FIGURE 4.7   Unhealthy and Healthy Fats Fats that are solid at room temperature are considered less healthy than fats that are liquid because they contain more saturated fat.

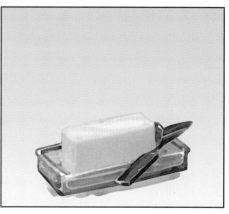
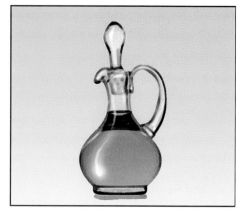

many people believe it is a healthier food than butter. In recent years, the fast-food industry switched from beef tallow to vegetable shortening for deep frying, because vegetable shortening was purported to be healthier than animal fat, and is less expensive. The bakery industry uses vegetable shortening for the same reasons to manufacture cookies, donuts, and cakes. There is no evidence, however, that margarine or vegetable shortenings are healthier than animal fats.

Indeed, analysis of dietary patterns of more than 87,000 American nurses showed that those with the highest intake of trans fatty acids (3.2% of total energy) had the highest risk for heart disease (Willett and Ascherio, 1994). While you do not need to give up eating margarine, french fries, or donuts to be healthy, you need to practice moderation. Since the amount of trans fatty acids in food products is not listed on the product label, intake of these artificial substances can be limited by using liquid vegetable oils that contain polyunsaturate fatty acids whenever possible. Moreover, vegetables oils are naturally devoid of cholesterol.

Artificial fats are chemicals that are added primarily to packaged pastries and snack foods to provide the taste of fat without contributing calories. Ingesting these substances is not without risk, however, because they may both inhibit the absorption of fat-soluble vitamins from the gastrointestinal tract and cause diarrhea. The purported benefit of artificial fat—that it contributes to weight management—apparently is overstated, because consumers tend to compensate for the lack of energy derived from fat by ingesting greater amounts of simple carbohydrates.

Vitamins

Vitamins are substances that facilitate a variety of biological processes. Vitamins do not provide building blocks for the manufacture of the body's tissues nor do they provide calories to fuel the body's functions. This is why the body requires much smaller amounts of vitamins than it does proteins, carbohydrates, and fats. The body cannot manufacture vitamins; they must be obtained from food (Table 4.6). Vitamins are classified as **water-soluble** or **fat-soluble,** depending on their chemistry.

Vitamins A (and its dietary precursor, beta-carotene), C, and E are classed as **antioxidants** because they have the capacity to neutralize the effects of chemicals called free radicals, which can damage biological structures via chemical oxidation. Consumption of antioxidants is associated with a lower risk of cancer of the upper gastrointestinal tract (vitamin C), colon (beta-carotene), breast, and lung (vitamin A). Consumption of antioxidants is also associated with lessening the risk of heart disease. Vitamins C and E protect against cataracts. Antioxidants are found in a variety of vegetables and fruits (not in beans), and can be obtained in vitamin supplements.

Folic acid (also called folate or folacin), a vitamin found in dark-green, leafy vegetables, beans, and fruits, helps prevent spina bifida and other neural tube defects in newborn babies. The diets of most American women and elderly persons of both sexes are deficient in folic acid (on average, 200 micrograms per day are consumed; 400 micrograms are recommended), so the federal gov-

Terms

artificial fat: chemicals added to packaged foods to provide the taste and texture of fat but few or no calories

vitamins: essential organic substances needed daily in small amounts to perform specific functions in the body

water-soluble vitamins: soluble in water; there are nine water-soluble vitamins

fat-soluble vitamins: soluble in fat; there are four fat-soluble vitamins

antioxidants: substances that in small amounts inhibit the oxidation of other compounds

homocysteine: a substance derived from the amino acid methionine; high blood levels increase the risk of heart disease; blood levels are reduced with adequate intake of folic acid

minerals: inorganic elements found in the body both in combination with organic compounds and alone

TABLE 4.6   Water-Soluble and Fat-Soluble Vitamins

Water-soluble vitamin	Why needed?	Primary sources	Deficiency results in
Ascorbic acid (vitamin C)	Tooth and bone formation; production of connective tissue; promotion of wound healing; may enhance immunity	Citrus fruits, tomatoes, peppers, cabbage, potatoes, melons	Scurvy (degeneration of bones, teeth, and gums)
Biotin	Involved in fat and amino acid synthesis and breakdown	Yeast, liver, milk, most vegetables, bananas, grapefruit	Skin problems; fatigue; muscle pains; nausea
Cobalamin (vitamin B_{12})	Involved in single carbon atom transfers; essential for DNA synthesis	Muscle meats, eggs, milk, and dairy products (not in vegetables)	Pernicious anemia; nervous system malfunctions
Folacin (folic acid)	Essential for synthesis of DNA and other molecules	Green leafy vegetables, organ meats, whole-wheat products	Anemia; diarrhea and other gastrointestinal problems
Niacin	Involved in energy production and synthesis of cell molecules	Grains, meats, legumes	Pellagra (skin, gastrointestinal, and mental disorders)
Pantothenic acid	Involved in energy production and synthesis and breakdown of many biological molecules	Yeast, meats and fish, nearly all vegetables and fruits	Vomiting; abdominal cramps; malaise; insomnia
Pyridoxine (vitamin B_6)	Essential for synthesis and breakdown of amino acids and manufacture of unsaturated fats from saturated fats	Meats, whole grains, most vegetables	Weakness; irritability; trouble sleeping and walking; skin problems
Riboflavin (vitamin B_2)	Involved in energy production; important for health of the eyes	Milk and dairy foods, meats, eggs, vegetables, grains	Eye and skin problems
Thiamine (vitamin B_1)	Essential for breakdown of food molecules and production of energy	Meats, legumes, grains, some vegetables	Beri-beri (nerve damage, weakness, heart failure)
Fat-soluble vitamin	Why needed?	Primary sources	Deficiency results in
Vitamin A (retinol)	Essential for maintenance of eyes and skin; influences bone and tooth formation	Liver, kidney, yellow and green leafy vegetables, apricots	Deficiency: night blindness; eye damage; skin dryness. Excess: loss of appetite; skin problems; swelling of ankles and feet
Vitamin D (calciferol)	Regulates calcium metabolism; important for growth of bones and teeth	Cod-liver oil, dairy products, eggs	Deficiency: rickets (bone deformities) in children; bone destruction in adults. Excess: thirst; nausea; weight loss; kidney damage
Vitamin E (tocopherol)	Prevents damage to cells from oxidation; prevents red blood cell destruction	Wheat germ, vegetable oils, vegetables, egg yolk, nuts	Deficiency: anemia, possibly nerve cell destruction
Vitamin K (phylloquinone)	Helps with blood clotting	Liver, vegetable oils, green leafy vegetables, tomatoes	Deficiency: severe bleeding

ernment requires that manufacturers of cereal-based foods (e.g., breads, breakfast cereals, pastas) fortify their products with it. There is debate whether the amount of folic acid in fortified foods is too low, so pregnant women are advised to ask their prenatal health care providers about taking folic acid supplements.

Folic acid also helps lower the body's manufacture of **homocysteine,** a substance derived from the essential amino acid methionine. High blood levels of homocysteine increase the risk of coronary artery disease and heart attack, so individuals are advised to obtain adequate amounts of folic acid. The best way to do this is to eat beans and fruits, and possibly take supplements (not to exceed a total of 700 micrograms of folate per day, since too much folate may be toxic).

Minerals

Many body functions require one or more inorganic elements called **minerals** (Table 4.7). Sodium, potassium, and chlorine, for example, are essential for maintaining cell membranes, conducting nerve impulses, and contracting muscle. Magnesium, copper, and cobalt facilitate certain biochemical reactions; iron is essential for the oxygen-carrying function of hemoglobin; iodine is needed to produce thyroid hormone; calcium and phosphorus make up bones and teeth. Selenium may reduce the risk of cancer, perhaps because of its activity as an antioxidant (Clark et al., 1996).

Minerals are found in almost all food, especially fresh vegetables. Women and growing young people are susceptible to iron deficiency, so they must eat iron-rich foods, such as eggs, lean meats, brans, whole grains, and green leafy vegetables. Most women and elderly people ingest too little calcium, which is found in dairy products and some green leafy vegetables (such as broccoli and turnip greens).

Many people consume too much sodium, which may contribute to high blood pressure. The amounts of sodium naturally present in almost every kind of food pose no problem; excess sodium comes from

TABLE 4.7   Essential Minerals

Mineral	Why needed?	Primary sources	Deficiency results in
Calcium	Bone and tooth formation; blood clotting; nerve transmission	Milk, cheese, dark green vegetables, dried legumes	Stunted growth; rickets, osteoporosis; convulsions
Chlorine	Formation of gastric juice; acid-base balance	Common salt	Muscle cramps; mental apathy; reduced appetite
Chromium	Glucose and energy metabolism	Fats, vegetable oils, meats	Impaired ability to metabolize glucose
Cobalt	Constituent of vitamin B_{12}	Organ and muscle meats	Not reported in man
Copper	Constituent of enzymes of iron metabolism	Meats, drinking water	Anemia (rare)
Iodine	Constituent of thyroid hormones	Marine fish and shellfish, dairy products, many vegetables	Goiter (enlarged thyroid)
Iron	Constituent of hemoglobin and enzymes of energy metabolism	Eggs, lean meats, legumes, whole grains, green leafy vegetables	Iron-deficiency anemia (weakness, reduced resistance to infection)
Magnesium	Activates enzymes; involved in protein synthesis	Whole grains, green leafy vegetables	Growth failure; behavioral disturbances; weakness, spasms
Manganese	Constituent of enzymes involved in fat synthesis	Widely distributed in foods	In animals: disturbances of nervous system, reproductive abnormalities
Molybdenum	Constituent of some enzymes	Legumes, cereals, organ meats	Not reported in man
Phosphorus	Bone and tooth formation; acid-base balance	Milk, cheese, meat, poultry, grains	Weakness, demineralization of bone
Potassium	Acid-base balance; body water balance; nerve function	Meats, milk, many fruits	Muscular weakness; paralysis
Selenium	Functions in close association with vitamin E	Seafood, meat, grains	Anemia (rare)
Sodium	Acid-base balance; body water balance; nerve function	Common salt	Muscle cramps; mental apathy; reduced appetite
Sulfur	Constituent of active tissue compounds, cartilage, and tendon	Sulfur amino acids (methionine and cysteine) in dietary proteins	Related to intake and deficiency of sulfur amino acids
Zinc	Constituent of enzymes involved in digestion	Widely distributed in foods	Growth failure

manufactured and restaurant food, to which salt is added to increase flavor, and from the overuse of table salt. Some people consume as many as 20 grams of sodium per day, which is about 10 times the 2 grams per day the body needs. Athletes are often advised to take salt tablets to replace body salt lost in sweat; this advice is misguided. Except in cases of severe fluid loss, which more often accompanies medical therapies involving diuretics than with sports, salt is readily replaced by eating food.

Phytochemicals

Plant matter contains hundreds of chemical substances, called **phytochemicals,** that positively affect human physiology. They often help the body destroy and eliminate toxins acquired from the environment or tissue-damaging substances that are byproducts of metabolism. Cruciferous plants (e.g., broccoli, cauli-

flower, kale, brussels sprouts, cabbage, mustard greens) are rich in the cancer-preventing phytochemical sulforaphane. A number of fruits, vegetables, cereal grains, and citrus oils contain substances called **isoprenoids,** which are associated with lowering cancer risk. Tea, onions, apples, and wine contain antioxidant substances called **flavonoids,** consumption of which has been associated with reducing the risk of heart disease. Barley, wheat, corn, and a variety of seeds contain **phytosterols** and **tocotrienols,** which can reduce levels of cholesterol in the blood.

Water

Water is the principal constituent of blood and is the major component of all cells. Water provides the medium in which all cell chemical activities take place.

Body water is maintained at a relatively constant level by the nervous, endocrine, and urinary systems. If body water volume is low, a person experiences thirst, which motivates drinking. A low volume of body water activates hormonal mechanisms that reduce the production of urine. Excess body water volume activates hormonal mechanisms that increase the output of urine. Increasing output is the function of diuretics, often given to reduce blood pressure, fluid volume after a heart attack, or feelings of bloatedness. Caffeine and alcohol are diuretics. The popular maxim that you

Terms

phytochemicals: chemicals produced by plants

isoprenoids: fat-soluble substances that may reduce the risk of some cancers

flavonoids: substances that may reduce the risk of heart disease

phytosterols: sterols of plant origin

tocotrienols: have some biological vitamin E activity

should drink eight glasses of water a day is partially correct. The average adult loses about that much body water through sweat, moisture in expired air, urine, and feces. This loss is partly offset by drinking water and obtaining water in other fluids and foods.

Dietary Supplements

A varied diet that contains the recommended five-a-day servings of fruits and vegetables and 55% to 80% of calories from cereals, whole grains, and legumes is likely to provide most people with the minerals and vitamins they need for good health. Strict vegetarians may need to supplement their diets with vitamin B_{12}. Supplements might also be necessary for people who eat primarily processed foods, since many nutrients are removed during manufacturing. Other people who may need supplements include those who restrict caloric intake, such as weight-conscious people; athletes concerned about body size; people who have a biological need for a particular substance; or people who consume large amounts of alcohol or coffee, which are diuretics and can increase urinary loss of vitamins and minerals. Smoking is associated with a loss of vitamin C.

Those who are concerned that their diets may be nutritionally inadequate may take vitamin, mineral, and amino acid supplements as a form of "dietary insurance." However, in massive doses (so-called megadoses), some dietary supplements can be toxic. More is not always better with vitamins A, D, K, B_3 (niacin), and B_6 (pyridoxine). In fact, when vitamins, minerals, and other nutrients are taken in large quantities for therapeutic reasons, they are considered drugs and not nutrients. This fact is rarely mentioned by proponents of megadosing, sometimes out of a sincere desire to help people and other times because of the drive to increase sales and profits. Before megadosing on vitamins, consumers should educate themselves about any possible risks.

Whether a supplement is "natural" or "synthetic" makes no difference chemically. However, there may be a difference in the purity of a substance depending on the preparation process. In 1990, thousands of Americans became ill and several died from consuming a supplement of the amino acid tryptophan because of impurities in the product.

Supplements containing enzymes, other proteins, and nucleic acids (DNA and RNA) are not absorbed intact from the digestive tract; instead, they are broken down into smaller molecules. Therefore, claims by manufacturers and sellers about the health benefits of ingesting these substances are false.

Food Additives

Manufactured foods contain a variety of additives that alter their texture, flavor, color, and stability. These additives help to increase sales appeal and lengthen shelf life.

Preservatives

About 20% of the world's food supply is lost to spoilage each year. Common preservatives include BHA (butylated hydroxyanisole), BHT (butylated hy-

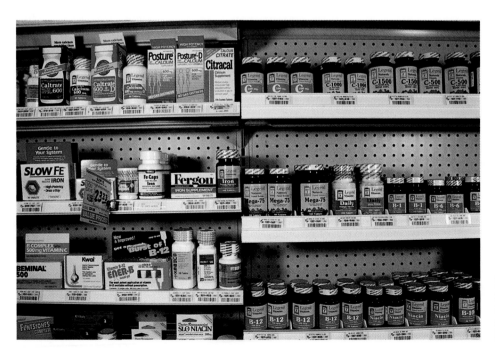

People who eat a variety of nutritious foods do not need dietary supplements; taken in excess, some supplements may be harmful.

droxytoluene), and sodium nitrite. Each of these substances can be toxic and damaging to humans if taken in excess; however, in amounts commonly consumed in food, they are presumed safe.

Sulfites in the form of sulfur dioxide, sodium sulfite, sodium or potassium bisulfite, and sodium or potassium metabisulfite are added to many foods to kill bacteria and to slow the food's breakdown. Sulfites are commonly added to wine and to dehydrated soups, vegetables, and fruit (apples, apricots, raisins, pears, and peaches). To keep vegetables looking fresh, they are also used in restaurant salad bars. Some individuals, particularly those with asthma, may be extremely sensitive to sulfite and may experience nausea, diarrhea, respiratory distress, and skin eruptions. Such problems have led to banning the use of sulfites in restaurants.

Many food additives are nutritionally unnecessary and some may adversely affect health. For example, sugar and salt are added to food to enhance taste and increase sales. Food dyes, some of which have been banned, have been implicated in human cancers and allergies. The FDA estimates that as many as 100,000 Americans are intolerant to **tartrazine,** a yellow dye added to hundreds of manufactured foods, such as frozen breakfast pastries, pill coatings, and some soft drinks.

Consumers concerned about additives should read product labels. Manufacturers must list all the additives in the order of their relative proportions in the food. Do not assume that the words "natural," "organic," or "health food" are free from additives or extra sugar and salt. The only sure way to be certain of the contents of a food is to know how it was produced.

Artificial Sweeteners

Fifty to seventy million Americans use artificial sweeteners. As a presumed ally in the continual battle against being overweight and as a theoretical help to diabetics, artificial sweeteners are in all types of foods. Their widest use, however, is in "diet" soft drinks.

The three major artificial sweeteners—cyclamate, saccharin, and aspartame—have been associated with health risks. In the 1970s, cyclamates and saccharin were linked to cancer, although the data were not strong enough to cause outright banning of these substances. Aspartame, made of the amino acids aspartic acid and a modified form of phenylalanine, has been associated with mood changes, insomnia, and seizures. Health-conscious consumers should be aware of the artificial sweeteners used in the products they ingest.

Food Safety

Outbreaks of food poisoning in the U.S. and other countries from bacterial and viral contamination of commercial beef, poultry, and fruit have raised concerns about the safety of the food supply. The U.S. Centers for Disease Control and Prevention estimates that food contaminated with the bacterium *Escherichia coli* O157:H7 is alone responsible for 20,000 cases of illness and 500 deaths per year. Each year, more than 900,000 Americans are made ill by *Salmonella* contamination in eggs. Symptoms of bacterial food poisoning are headache, nausea, and fever.

The Food and Drug Administration's 700 inspectors and the U.S. Department of Agriculture's 8000 inspectors oversee nearly 60,000 food manufacturers and processors and billions of tons of imported food. That's why it's imperative for consumers to follow food safety guidelines when they purchase, store, and prepare food.

One method of protecting food involves exposing it to **gamma irradiation** to destroy fungi, bacteria, and other microorganisms. Some opponents of food irradiation argue that the method has not been proven safe. Their concern is that irradiation may produce cancer-causing or toxic byproducts or mutant strains of toxic, radiation-resistant microorganisms. Furthermore, vitamins can be destroyed by irradiation. Nonetheless, the government has recommended that all ground meat and poultry be irradiated to destroy harmful bacteria. Irradiation *does not* make food radioactive and therefore consumers are not at risk from radiation.

Fast Food

Grabbing a fast-food meal is integral to the fast-paced life in America today. Each day approximately 46 million people, or 20% of the U.S. population, eat in a fast-food restaurant. Convenience notwithstanding,

Terms

sulfites: used as preservatives for salad, fresh fruits and vegetables, wine, beer, and dried fruit; in susceptible individuals, especially those with asthma, they can cause a severe reaction

tartrazine: a yellow food dye, referred to by the FDA as "FD&C yellow No. 5"

gamma irradiation: nonchemical method of food preservation

vegetarian: one who consumes no meat, poultry, or fish

vegan: one who excludes all animal products from the diet, including milk, cheese, eggs, and other dairy products

lacto-vegetarian: one who excludes meat, poultry, fish, and eggs, but includes dairy products

lacto-ovo-vegetarian: one who excludes meats, poultry, and fish, but includes eggs and dairy products

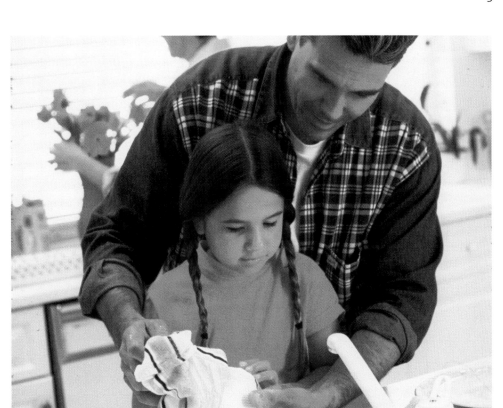

Hand washing is essential to safe food preparation.

fast-food items must be chosen carefully because many contain high quantities of saturated fat, cholesterol, and salt; few complex carbohydrates; and low levels of vitamins A and C.

The major fast-food companies have responded to consumers' concerns about nutrition by offering salads, baked potatoes, roast beef, and broiled chicken. Roast beef has less fat than hamburger, and broiled chicken breast has less fat than deep fried chicken. Be cautious, though. Fish, a low-fat food, if breaded and fried, may be 50% fat. Salads and baked potatoes can be carriers of high-fat toppings.

Vegetarian Diets

Vegetarianism has existed as long as humankind and has been advocated by such famous people as Leonardo da Vinci, George Bernard Shaw, Mahatma Gandhi, and Albert Einstein. People choose to be vegetarians for various reasons, including the following:

1. To avoid killing animals—either killing them oneself or killing by others. Some people, who have a strong affection for other animals and feel a certain biological and spiritual kinship with them, object to killing them for food.
2. To contribute to the more efficient utilization of world protein supplies. It takes approximately 10 pounds of livestock feed, usually corn or soybeans, to produce 1 pound of meat. Obviously the 10 pounds of corn or soybeans could feed more people than 1 pound of meat can. With the population of the earth doubling about every 30 years, some people feel a moral obligation to avoid overconsuming food resources in the hope that ways will be found to distribute the world food supply more equitably.
3. To live longer and healthier lives. In many cases, health benefits result from a combination of vegetarianism and nondietary life-style factors. Vegetarians, in comparison to nonvegetarians, tend to be leaner, to exercise more, to not smoke cigarettes, and to not abuse alcohol. Vegetarians have a reduced risk for heart and blood vessel disease and for colorectal cancer because of a reduced intake of cholesterol and animal fat. Their increased fiber intake also contributes to the reduced colorectal cancer risk.

There are three kinds of **vegetarian** diets: strict or **veganism,** which excludes all animal products, including milk, cheeses, eggs, and other dairy products; **lacto-vegetarianism,** which excludes meat, poultry, fish, and eggs, but includes dairy products; and **lacto-ovo-vegetarianism,** which excludes meats, poultry, and seafood, but includes eggs and dairy products.

Vegetables aren't my meat and potatoes.
YOGI BERRA, former catcher, New York Yankees

Wellness Guide

Guidelines for Food Safety

www.jbpub.com/hwonline

When Purchasing Food

1. Purchase meat and poultry products after all other groceries have been selected and keep packages of raw meat and poultry separate from other foods, particularly foods that will be eaten without further cooking. Consider using plastic bags to enclose individual packages of raw meat and poultry.

2. Make sure meat and poultry products—whether raw, pre-packaged, or cooked from the deli—are refrigerated when purchased.

3. USDA strongly advises against purchasing fresh, pre-stuffed whole birds.

4. Canned goods should be free of dents, cracks, or bulging lids.

5. Take food straight home to the refrigerator. If travel time will exceed 1 hour, pack perishable foods in a cooler with ice and keep groceries and cooler in the passenger area of the car during warm weather.

When Storing Food at Home

1. Verify the temperature of your refrigerator and freezer with an appliance thermometer—refrigerators should run at 40°F or below; freezers at 0°F. Most foodborne bacteria grow slowly at 40°F, which is a safe refrigerator temperature. Freezer temperatures of 0°F or below stop bacterial growth.

2. At home, refrigerate or freeze meat and poultry immediately.

3. To prevent raw juices from dripping on other foods in the refrigerator, use plastic bags or place meat and poultry on a plate.

4. Wash hands with soap and water for 20 seconds before and after handling any raw meat, poultry, or seafood products.

5. Store canned goods in a cool, clean, dry place. Avoid extreme heat or cold, which can be harmful to canned goods.

6. Never store any foods directly under a sink and always keep foods off the floor and separate from cleaning supplies.

When Getting Food Ready to Prepare

1. The importance of hand washing cannot be overemphasized. This simple practice is the most economical, yet often forgotten, way to prevent contamination or cross-contamination.

2. Wash hands (gloved or not) with soap and water for 20 seconds: (a) before beginning preparation; (b) after handling raw meat, poultry, seafood, or eggs; (c) after touching animals; (d) after using the bathroom; (e) after changing diapers; and (f) after blowing the nose.

3. Don't let juices from raw meat, poultry, or seafood come in contact with cooked foods or foods that will be eaten raw, such as fruits or salad ingredients.

4. Wash hands, counters, equipment, utensils, and cutting boards with soap and water immediately after use. Counters, equipment, utensils, and cutting boards can be sanitized with a chlorine solution of 1 teaspoon liquid household bleach per quart of water. Let the solution stand on the board after washing, or follow the instructions on sanitizing products.

5. Thaw meat in the refrigerator, NEVER ON THE COUNTER. It is also safe to thaw in cold water in an airtight plastic wrapper or bag, changing the water every 30 minutes until meat is thawed; Or thaw in the microwave and cook the product immediately.

6. Marinate foods in the refrigerator, NEVER ON THE COUNTER.

7. The USDA recommends that if you choose to stuff whole poultry, you must use a meat thermometer to check the internal temperature of the stuffing. The internal temperature in the center of the stuffing should reach 165°F before removing it from the oven. If you don't have a meat thermometer, cook the stuffing outside the bird. Also, don't put hot stuffing into a frozen bird. By the time it thaws, it will be contaminated inside.

When Cooking

1. Always cook thoroughly. If harmful bacteria are present, only thorough cooking will destroy them; freezing or rinsing the foods in cold water is not sufficient to destroy bacteria.

2. Use a meat thermometer to determine if your meat, poultry, or casserole has reached a safe internal temperature (145°F for roasts and steaks, 180°F for whole poultry, 160°F for ground meat, and 165°F for leftovers). Check the product in several spots to assure that a safe temperature has been reached and that harmful bacteria, such as *Salmonella* and certain strains of *E. coli,* have been destroyed.

3. Avoid interrupted cooking. Never refrigerate partially cooked food to later finish cooking on the grill or in the oven. Meat and poultry products must be cooked thoroughly the first time, and then they may be refrigerated and safely reheated.

4. When microwaving foods, carefully follow the manufacturer's instructions. Use microwave-safe containers, cover, rotate, and allow for the standing time, which contributes to thorough cooking.

When Serving

1. Wash hands with soap and water before serving or eating food.

2. Serve cooked products on clean plates with clean utensils and clean hands. Never put cooked foods on a dish that has held raw products unless the dish is first washed with soap and hot water.

3. Hold hot foods above 140°F and cold foods below 40°F.

4. Never leave foods, raw or cooked, at room temperature longer than 2 hours. On a hot day with temperatures at 90°F or warmer, this time decreases to 1 hour.

When Handling Leftovers

1. Wash hands before and after handling leftovers. Use clean utensils and surfaces.

2. Divide leftovers into small units and store in shallow containers for quick cooling. Refrigerate within 2 hours of cooking.

3. Discard anything left out too long.

4. Never taste a food to determine if it is safe.

5. When reheating leftovers, reheat thoroughly to a temperature of 165°F, or until hot and steamy. Bring soups, sauces, and gravies to a rolling boil.

6. If in doubt, throw it out.

Source: U.S. Department of Agriculture, Food Safety and Inspection Service, November 1996.

Properly planned vegetarian diets can meet the body's nutritional needs, especially by combining sources of protein to assure adequate intake of the essential amino acids. Vegans may need vitamin B_{12} (cobalamin) supplements.

How Nutrition Affects the Brain

The brain requires nutrients in order to function properly. For example, the amount of the neurotransmitter serotonin in the brain is influenced by levels in the blood of the amino acid tryptophan and by the amount of carbohydrate recently eaten. A meal containing tryptophan (derived from dietary protein) and high in carbohydrate increases brain levels of serotonin. Brain levels of the amino acid tyrosine, the precursor of the neurotransmitters dopamine, norepinephrine, and epinephrine, increase after the ingestion of tyrosine-containing protein in a meal. Ingesting choline, a component of lecithin (found in egg yolks, liver, and soybeans), increases the level of the neurotransmitter acetylcholine.

To some degree, moods, feelings of vitality, and sleep patterns depend on the amount of neurotransmitter molecules ingested and therefore depend indirectly on meals (Fernstrom, 1994). The habit of eating cookies and milk at bedtime may be a way someone increases brain serotonin to help induce a peaceful night's sleep. Some preliminary experiments indicate that tyrosine may help to relieve depression and choline may help to modify certain postural and motor disturbances.

The thoughts, moods, and body sensations of some individuals are highly sensitive to the amount of simple sugars they ingest. Shortly after consuming a couple of donuts or a candy bar, they might experience anxiety, trembling, fatigue, weakness, depression, and inability to concentrate. This response, called **reactive hypoglycemia,** is often the result of a sharp drop in blood sugar when insulin is secreted; this drop, in turn, is produced in response to the large load of sugar in the blood. Something akin to reactive hypoglycemia may be at the root of an eating pattern common to many: consumption of a high-sugar food at breakfast, followed two hours later by a reactive blood sugar low, which motivates a midmorning sugar "hit." The cycle is repeated at noon and midafternoon, and at dinner and late in the evening. To break this cycle, it helps to consume complex carbohydrates with protein and some fat, thereby moderating the rate at which simple sugars enter the body.

Terms

reactive hypoglycemia: occurring after the ingestion of carbohydrate, with consequent release of insulin

Critical Thinking About Health

1. Everyone aboard the Zoracian space vehicle XTA-9781 was thrilled when their ship's sensors indicated life forms on a small planet orbiting a medium-sized star in the Milky Way galaxy. To make contact with and explore the planet, a landing party of six underwent molecular rearrangement to take on human form in order both to survive on Earth and communicate and interact with any Earthlings they encountered.

   "When you reach the surface," explained the mission commander, "you will have about eight of their time segments before you must refuel. Energy packets can be obtained in large, stationary pods the locals call supermarkets."

   The crew of the landing party nodded. It seemed similar enough to refueling on their home planet of Zorax not to cause confusion.

   "Except for one thing," the commander cautioned. "There are thousands of kinds of energy packets, from which you will have to choose the appropriate ones."

   "Appropriate ones?" asked the assistant crew-chief.

   "Yes. None of the fuel packets are efficient. You will have to sort and select."

   The crew shifted nervously.

   "Do not worry," said the commander, handing each member of the crew a copy of the food guide pyramid. "Their leaders have prepared refueling guidelines. Take these and use them when the time comes."

   a. How would you explain to the Zoracian landing party why, with the great abundance of food choices in American supermarkets, the U.S. government advises its citizens how to eat properly?

   b. From the Zoracian's point of view, the American food supply, while abundant with many kinds of foods, is inefficient with regard to re-fueling. Explain why the American food supply is so diverse yet nutritionally inefficient.

c. What factors influence your food selection?

2. A crusading nutrition journalist points out that the food label on a soup company's best selling product indicates that a serving of the product is 32% fat. Fearing that consumers will stop buying the product, the company responds, and within weeks the label indicates that the product is 16% fat. The company has changed nothing in the product.

a. Why does the label show that the product contains half the fat?

b. What limits, if any, would you advocate be placed on what food manufacturers can put on product labels? Where would you draw the line between free enterprise, *caveat emptor* (buyer beware), and the public good?

c. How much attention do you pay to what is written on food product labels?

3. Explain how an herbicide (weed-killing chemical) could wind up in the breast milk of a woman living hundreds of miles away from the site of herbicide application. Are you concerned about pesticides and additives in the food supply?

Health in Review

- For most of us, good nutrition is a matter of informed choice and is not governed by harsh environmental and economic circumstances.

- The U.S. government commissioned nutritionists and other scientists to create dietary guidelines. These guidelines are aimed at preventing undernutrition and a variety of diseases (e.g., heart disease, many kinds of cancer), which are associated with the high-fat, low–complex carbohydrate diets of Western industrialized nations.

- The U.S. government's required food label is designed to be easy to understand. Reading the food label will help you choose foods that are healthy and that potentially reduce your risk of some diseases.

- In order to be healthy and well, people must obtain 40 essential nutrients from their food in proper amounts and proportions. Food energy, measured in calories, comes principally from sugars, carbohydrates, and fats.

- Dietary supplements can be a form of "dietary insurance" for those who are concerned their diet may be nutritionally inadequate.

- Food is composed of seven kinds of substances: proteins, carbohydrates, fats, minerals, vitamins, phytochemicals, and water. Nutritionists recommend basing our diets on complex carbohydrates and fresh fruits and vegetables to lessen the consumption of saturated fat and to ensure consumption of adequate fiber, vitamins, minerals, and micronutrients.

- Manufactured foods contain a variety of additives that alter their texture, flavor, color, and stability. Preservatives keep foods from spoiling through the use of sulfites.

- One nonchemical method of food preservation involves exposing food to gamma irradiation to destroy microorganisms.

- Artificial sweeteners are widely used, most commonly in "diet" soft drinks.

- There are several reasons for being a vegetarian, including increased interest in health, ecology, and world issues; economical issues; and the philosophy of not killing animals. A strict vegetarian, or vegan, diet eliminates all animal products, including milk, cheese, eggs, and other dairy products.

Health and Wellness Online

The World Wide Web contains a wealth of information about health and wellness. By accessing the Internet using Web browser software, such as Netscape Navigator or Microsoft's Internet Explorer, you can gain a new

perspective on many topics presented in *Essentials of Health and Wellness, Second Edition.* Access the Jones and Bartlett Publishers web site at

http://www.jbpub.com/hwonline

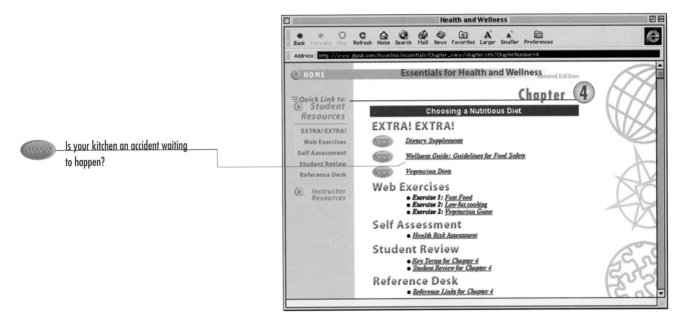

Is your kitchen an accident waiting to happen?

References

Anderson, J. W., Johnstone, B. M., & Cook-Newell, M. E. (1995). Meta-analysis of the effects of soy protein intake on serum lipids. *New England Journal of Medicine, 333(5),* 276–282.

Anderson, J. W., Smith, B. M., & Gustafson, N. J. (1994, May). Health benefits and practical aspects of high-fiber diets. *American Journal of Clinical Nutrition, 59,* 1242–1247.

Campbell, T. C., & Junshi, C. (1994). Diet and chronic degenerative diseases: Perspectives from China. *American Journal of Clinical Nutrition, 59(suppl),* 1153–1161.

Clark, L. C., et al. (1996). Effects of selenium supplementation for cancer prevention in patients with carcinoma of the skin. *Journal of the American Medical Association, 276,* 1957–1963.

Fernstrom, J. D. (1994). Dietary amino acids and brain function. *Journal of the American Dietetic Association, 94(1),* 71–78.

Kurtzweil, P. (1995). The new food label: Better information for special diets. *FDA Consumer, January–February,* 19–23.

United States Department of Agriculture. (1996). *Food safety in the kitchen.* Home and Garden Bulletin No. 232. Food Safety and Inspection Service, Washington, D.C.

Willett, W. C. (1994). Diet and health: What should we eat? *Science, 264,* 532–537.

Suggested Readings

Anderson, J., & Deskins, B. (1997). *The nutrition bible: The comprehensive, no-nonsense, guide to foods, nutrients, additives, preservatives, pollutants,* and everything else we eat and drink. New York: Quill. The title says it all.

Apple, R. D. (1996). *Vitamania: Vitamins in American culture.* New Brunswick, NJ: Rutgers University Press. Explores the scientific, social, historical, and commercial aspects of vitamin use in America. Shows how nutritional information often has been and still is twisted for commercial gain.

Clinical debate: Should a low-fat, high-carbohydrate diet be recommended for everyone? *New England Journal of Medicine, 337,* 562–567. Read how the experts slug it out over the issue of fat in the diet: how much and what kinds.

Fourteen dietary habits you can stop feeling guilty about. (1993). *Tufts University Diet and Nutrition Letter, 11(2),* 3–5. An enjoyable, simple dietary guideline to help you get through the day.

Hathcock, J. N. (1997). Vitamins and minerals: Efficacy and safety. *American Journal of Clinical Nutrition, 66(3),* 427–437. Reports on the safety and efficacy of vitamin and mineral supplements.

Karstadt, M., & Schmidt, S. (1996, March). Olestra: Procter's big gamble. *Nutrition Action Healthletter,* 4–5. Spells out the dangers of fake fats and the money to be made from them.

Liebman, B. (1996, October). Plants for supper? 10 reasons to eat more like a vegetarian. *Nutrition Action Healthletter,* 10–12. Experts explain the reasons why they eat more vegetables.

Scrimshaw, N. S., & SanGiovanni, J. P. (1997). Synergism of nutrition, infection, and immunity. *American Journal of Clinical Nutrition, 66(2),* 464S–477S. How infections affect nutritional status and how nutritional status affects immunity.

Wilkinson, S. I. (1997, November 10). Eating safely in a dirty world. *Chemical and Engineering News,* 24–33. An excellent review of foodborne illnesses and what the government is trying to do to improve food safety.

Willett, W. C. (1994). Micronutrients and cancer risk. *American Journal of Clinical Nutrition, 59(suppl),* 1162–1165. Provides an understanding of cancer risk and nutrition.

Learning Objectives

1. Describe the extent and causes of overweight in American society.
2. Describe the significance of body mass index (BMI) to health.
3. Explain the concept of fatness set point.
4. Explain why calorie-restricting weight-loss programs fail.
5. Discuss why exercise (and *not* calorie restriction) is the key to healthy weight maintenance.
6. List the psychological factors that contribute to weight problems.
7. Discuss the advantages and disadvantages of the medical treatments for overweight.
8. Describe the signs of anorexia nervosa and bulimia.

Exercises and Activities

WORKBOOK
What Are Your Weight Statistics?
Body Image

Health and Wellness Online

 www.jbpub.com/hwonline

Wellness Guide: Calculating Your Body Mass Index
Sensible Weight Maintenance
Eating Disorders

Chapter 5

Managing a Healthy Weight

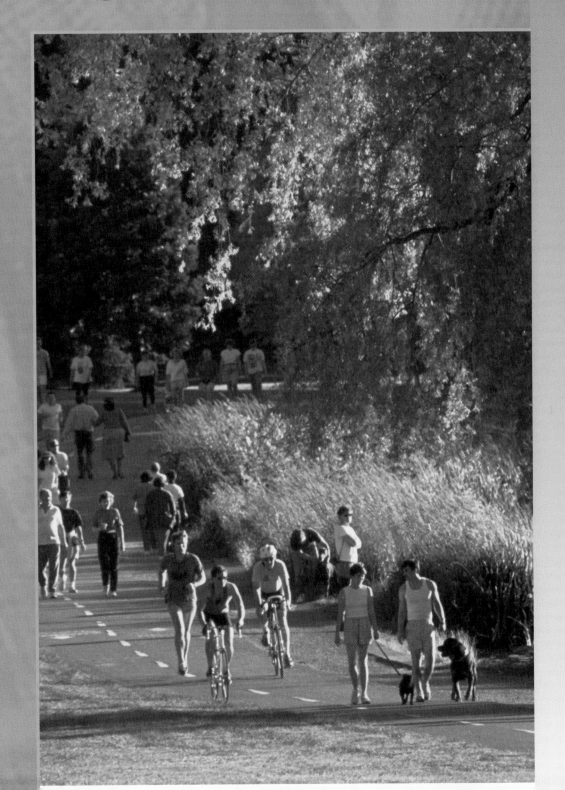

About 34% of American adults are overweight; this puts them at risk for a variety of diseases, including heart disease, stroke, high blood pressure, type 2 diabetes, and a variety of cancers. Annual health care costs related to overweight in the U.S. are approximately $70 billion.

> *A man is satisfied not by the quantity of food but by the absence of greed.*
> GURDJIEFF

Many people whose body weight does not predispose them to health problems are still weight conscious, primarily for cosmetic reasons. Their goal is to achieve a body size and shape that meets society's standards of "perfection" (generated by the fashion and advertising industries). These individuals seem to be in a continual battle with the same 5, 10, or 20 pounds, which they struggle to shed to look youthful and attractive. Concern about body weight (more typically, body *fatness*) fuels a $30 billion industry of weight-reduction programs and special foods, most of which are useless and costly in the long run.

With all the passion for being slim, it is no wonder that many people view any amount of visible fat on the body as something to get rid of. However, the human body has evolved over time in environments of food scarcity; hence, the ability to store fat easily and efficiently is a valuable physiological function that served our ancestors well for thousands of years. Only in the last few decades, and only in the wealthiest economies, has food become so plentiful and easy to obtain as to cause fat-related health problems. People no longer have to spend most of their time and energy gathering berries and seeds and hoping that a hunting party will return with meat. All we have to do nowadays is drive to the supermarket or the fast-food restaurant, where for a very low cost we can obtain nearly all of our daily calories (Table 5.1).

What Is Desirable Weight?

In most instances, concerns about being *overweight* are really concerns about being overfat. There is a difference. Some professional male athletes, for example, weigh much more than the recommended weight standards for persons of similar height. Yet as little as 1% of their body weight may be fat. Most of the body weight of a well-conditioned athlete is muscle and bone. Female body builders, who are the leanest of all female athletes, have about 8% to 13% of their total body weight as fat. This probably represents the lower limit of fat for a healthy woman.

Body fat is composed of two parts: **essential fat**—fat necessary for normal physiological functioning, such as nerve conduction—and **storage fat.** Essential fat comprises about 3% to 7% of body weight in men and about 10% to 12% of body weight in women. This gender difference, which is presumably caused by hormones, is due to the deposition of greater amounts of fat on the hips, thighs, and breasts in females. Storage fat, also called depot fat, constitutes only a small percentage of the total body weight of lean individuals and 5% to 25% of the body weight of the majority of the population (Figure 5.1). However, storage fat can account for 40% to 50% of the body weight of some persons.

Terms

essential fat: necessary and required fat in the diet; required for normal physiological functioning

storage fat: also called depot fat; energy stored as fat in various parts of the body

body mass index: a measure of body fatness, calculated by dividing body weight (in kilograms) by the square of height (in meters)

TABLE 5.1   Percentage of Daily Calories Provided by Typical Fast-Food Meals

Meal	Percentage of daily calories for three different daily calorie levels		
	1600 calories/day	2000 calories/day	2500 calories/day
Quarter Pounder French fries Milkshake	73	58	47
Whopper French fries Diet soft drink	66	54	43
Two slices of pizza Diet soft drink	33	25	20

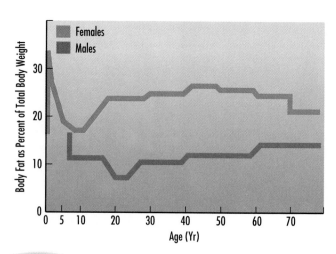

FIGURE 5.1   Body Fat Percentage The average percentage of total body weight that is body fat for U.S. men and women, by age.

Wellness Guide

Calculating Your Body Mass Index

Body mass index (BMI) is obtained by dividing your weight in kilograms by the square of your height in meters.

To convert to kilograms, divide your weight in pounds (without clothes) by 2.2: _____

To convert to meters, divide your height in inches (without shoes) by 39.4, then square it: _____

Divide your weight by your height (squared).

BMI = _____

Example:

Manuel weighs 182 pounds (without clothes) and is 5 feet 10 inches tall (without shoes), or 70 inches.

Manuel's weight in kilograms = 182 lbs./2.2 = 82.72 kg

Manuel's height in meters = 70 in./39.4 = 1.79 m

Manuel's BMI = $wgt/h^2 = 82.72/(1.79)^2 = 25.8$

www   **www.jbpub.com/hwonline**

Standards for the most "desirable" or "ideal" body weight or body composition (fat percentage) vary. For example, in some cultures, women with significant storage fat are considered physically attractive and sexually desirable, and fatness in children is considered a sign of robust health. In the United States, attitudes about desirable body configuration fluctuate and are often keyed to fashion trends. During the 1950s, for example, large body size, characterized by "full-figured" women and "he-men," was considered desirable, whereas today "slim is in."

Indexes of desirable body weight are given in tables of "ideal weight for height" issued by both government agencies and insurance companies and are based on statistics for longevity (Table 5.2) and the **body mass index** (BMI), which is calculated by dividing a person's weight in kilograms by his or her height in meters squared. Studies show that good health is associated with weighing no more than 5% below or 20% (for men) and 30% (for women) above the weight-for-height standards, or having a BMI between 19 and 25 (Lamon-Fava et al., 1996; Seidell et al., 1996)

TABLE 5.2   Metropolitan Life Insurance Company Weight-for-Height Tables

Women (with clothing)				Men (with clothing)			
Height (with shoes, 2-inch heels)	Small frame	Medium frame	Large frame	Height (with shoes, 1-inch heels)	Small frame	Medium frame	Large frame
4'10"	92–98	96–107	104–119	5'2"	112–120	118–129	126–141
4'11"	94–101	98–110	106–122	3"	115–123	121–133	129–144
5'0"	96–104	101–113	109–125	4"	118–126	124–136	142–148
1"	99–107	104–116	112–128	5"	121–129	127–139	135–152
2"	102–110	107–119	115–131	6"	124–133	130–143	138–156
3"	105–113	110–122	118–134	7"	128–137	134–147	142–161
4"	108–116	113–126	121–138	8"	132–141	138–152	147–166
5"	111–119	116–130	125–142	9"	136–145	142–156	151–170
6"	114–123	120–135	129–146	10"	140–150	146–160	155–174
7"	118–127	124–139	133–150	11"	144–154	150–165	159–179
8"	122–131	128–143	137–154	6'0"	148–158	154–170	164–184
9"	126–135	132–147	141–158	1"	152–162	158–175	168–189
10"	130–140	136–151	145–163	2"	156–167	162–180	173–194
11"	134–144	140–155	149–168	3"	160–171	167–185	178–199
6'0"	138–148	144–159	153–173	4"	164–175	172–190	182–204

Source: Metropolitan Life Insurance Company. Used by permission.

(Figure 5.2). Above the upper limits of these measures, people have higher risks for diabetes, gallbladder disease, varicose veins, arthritis, heart disease, stroke, high blood pressure, breathing problems, and accident proneness (because of a large body). People who are extremely overweight often face stigmas, such as job discrimination, lower social acceptance, and lower self-esteem.

Another health-related index of body size is the waist-to-hip ratio, which is calculated by dividing the circumference of the waist by the circumference of the hips. For example, someone with a 28-inch waist and 37-inch hips would have a waist-to-hip ratio of 0.75. Health-problems are less likely in women whose waist-to-hip ratio is less than 0.8 and in men whose waist-to-hip ratio is less than 0.95. In other words, it is healthier for a body to be pear-shaped than apple-shaped, and it's healthier *not* to have a beer belly (Figure 5.3).

The Regulation of Body Fat

The main principle of healthy weight maintenance is that you will store fat if you take in more calories than you expend. Calories enter the body as food: four calories per gram of protein or carbohydrate, seven calories per gram of alcohol, and nine calories per gram of fat. Calories leave the body as energy expended: to fuel basal (resting) metabolism, physical activity, growth, and injury repair and control body temperature. Calories from food that are not used right away are stored either as **glycogen,** a carbohydrate that is found in liver and muscle, or as **triglyceride,** a fat that is found in adipose tissue located on the body in

all-too-familiar places. At nine calories per gram, fat is the most efficient form of energy storage (one pound of fat will fuel a 40-mile walk), and fat has other biological advantages: it's lightweight, compact, spongy, and a good thermal insulator.

The Fatness Set Point

The body has an extremely complex fatness-control mechanism that maintains fatness within narrow limits called the **fatness set point.** Just as house temperature is maintained by a thermostat, the amount of body fat is maintained by the nervous system and a particular group of hormones. In your house, when the temperature drops below the "set point" on the thermostat, the heater starts to return the house to the pre-set temperature. When the house temperature rises, the air conditioner starts.

The same feedback principle applies to body fatness. If the amount of body fat decreases below the fatness set point (perhaps because an individual goes on a calorie-restricting diet), the nervous and hormone systems counter the loss by increasing appetite and conserving energy. If the amount of body fat exceeds the fatness set point (perhaps because an individual overeats), the nervous and hormone systems counter the gain by decreasing appetite and increasing energy use.

The fatness set point is controlled in a region of the hypothalamus of the brain referred to as the **appestat,** because it controls appetite and eating behavior. When your body needs calories, nerves and hormones signal the appestat and you feel hungry. When the body has sufficient calories, nerves and hormones signal the appestat and you feel full. Many situations and factors influence the appestat.

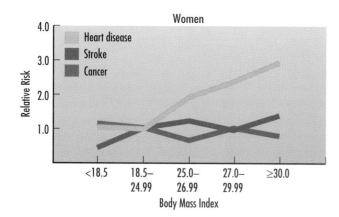
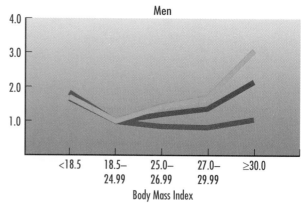

FIGURE 5.2   Relative Health Risks of Various Body Mass Indexes (BMIs) The relative risks for persons with various BMIs of death from coronary heart disease, cardiovascular disease, and cancer, as well as death from accidents, suicides, and other causes have been standardized to the BMI range 18.5 to 24.99. The higher relative risk of a BMI of < 18.5 is possibly related to smoking and weight loss from poor mental health.

Source: Data from Seidell, J. C., et al., (1996). Overweight, underweight, and mortality. *Archives of Internal Medicine, 156,* 958–963.

Apples   **Pears**

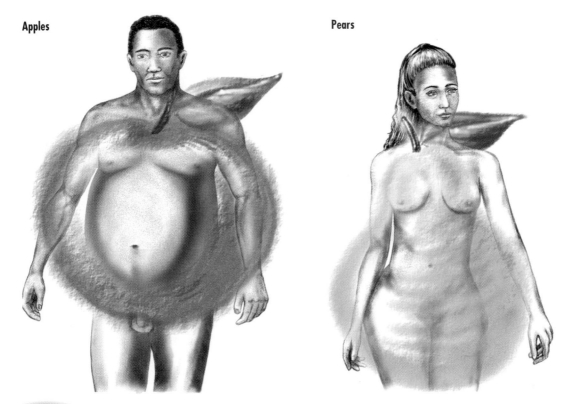

FIGURE 5.3   **Apple or Pear?**   Apple-shaped people carry much of their body fat above the waist. Pear-shaped people carry their body fat on the hips and thighs. Studies show that it's healthier to be pear-shaped than apple-shaped.

Appestat Turn-Ons

- *The amount of available energy in your body:* You haven't eaten in several hours and your blood glucose level is low.
- *Eating habits:* It's your usual dinner time and you expect to eat whether or not you are hungry.
- *Food triggers:* You walk into the mall and smell freshly baked chocolate chip cookies and can't resist one.

Appestat Turn-Offs

- *Gastric distention:* You've just overeaten and you feel as though your stomach is going to explode.
- *Food palatability:* A friend orders a pizza with toppings that you don't like and suddenly you're not hungry.
- *Social circumstances:* You invite a new love interest to dinner and are too distracted by your emotions to eat.

As long as you are generally healthy, the appestat is working properly, *and you are paying attention to it,* you are unlikely to develop a weight (fat) problem since your calorie intake will pretty much equal your calorie output; this is called being in a state of **energy balance.** However, you only have to exceed energy bal-

ance a little bit to develop a weight problem over time. Consider this example:

> Marci is a 26-year-old woman at normal weight with a BMI of 23 who recently changed jobs. Previously the solo office manager in a small real estate company, she now works as an executive assistant in a much larger firm. Two consequences of this change are: (a) Marci now spends more time sitting at her desk typing and answering the phone than in her former job, where she moved around for *every* office task, and (b) she now goes to lunch with office mates. The combination of less movement and fast-food lunches has increased Marci's daily calorie intake over expenditure an average of 10%.

Terms

glycogen: a storage form of carbohydrate

triglyceride: a storage form of fat

fatness set point: the physiologically regulated amount of fat on the body

appestat: region of the hypothalamus that controls appetite and eating behavior

energy balance: when energy consumed as food equals the energy expended in living

What's 10%? That's about 160 calories per working day, or 3200 calories a month. At 3500 calories per pound, that's enough for Marci to gain about 10 pounds per year. You can see what a few years at this job might do to Marci's waistline. When the office crew goes to lunch, often their intention is to socialize and get away from the stress of the office; they don't intend to consume a big lunch. However, the desire to be social, the smell of food, and the size of the portions make it easy to ignore satiety signals from the appestat and to overeat.

Of course, Marci could prevent gaining those 10 pounds a year by being more mindful of her lunchtime eating behaviors and walking an extra 20 minutes every day (four calories per minute). If she doesn't, however, her body is likely to store those excess calories as fat, and in a couple of years she is likely to find herself with a BMI of near 30 and in need of a new wardrobe. And if that happens and she decides to lose that extra fat, she's likely to discover—as many of us do—that it will take effort to slim down, and without a permanent change in exercise and eating habits, it will be very difficult to keep the lost weight (fat) from returning.

> *You never know what is enough unless you know what is more than enough.*
> WILLIAM BLAKE
> *The Marriage of Heaven and Hell*

That's because the body doesn't like to let go of fat it has accumulated, or as scientists say, the body defends against fat loss. Remember that the body has a fatness set point and that it is designed to store fat easily, in case you ever have to go without food for several days as your ancient ancestors did. Of course, that almost never happens to modern people, but those built-in, efficient fat-storage mechanisms are still present. So once fat is deposited, it's very hard to lose.

Another reason it is hard to lose fat is that a decrease in body fat triggers an increase in the efficiency with which the body uses energy. The resting metabolic rate decreases, and the efficiency with which muscles do work increases (Leibel et al, 1995).

Another way the body defends against fat loss is through the action of a hormone called **leptin,** which is manufactured by fat cells. When fat cells are laden with triglyceride, they secrete leptin into the bloodstream, where it finds its way to the appestat, causing a decrease in appetite and an increase in energy use.

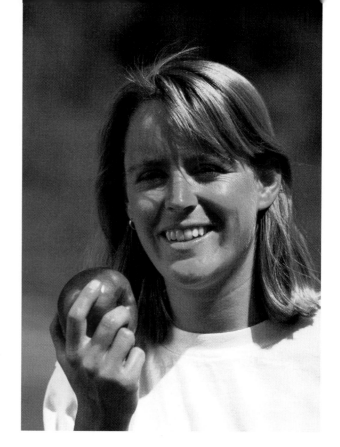

When you snack, choose healthy foods such as fruits and vegetables.

When fat cells are relatively devoid of triglyceride, leptin secretion diminishes, and appetite increases. If someone does not produce sufficient leptin, or if someone's appestat does not respond to leptin, then that person may be susceptible to becoming overfat. Genetic (inherited) variations in the leptin regulatory system may explain the susceptibility of some people to overfatness (Schwartz and Seeley, 1997).

This susceptibility explains why many a dieter's most ardent attempts to lose weight (fat) by lessening the intake of food result in failure. Calorie restriction puts a person in a state of semi-starvation, which triggers the array of biological mechanisms designed to conserve both body fat and energy expenditure. Moreover, calorie restriction is no fun. Often people become bored eating the same required foods or frustrated with not being able to eat the kinds and quantities of food they want. They become obsessed with food, and after a time they give up their diet and return to their former eating habits. And when they gain weight, they blame themselves for being weak-willed failures.

Sensible Weight Maintenance

Many advertisements suggest that a healthy body is one that is slim and muscular. However, research

Terms

leptin: a hormone that controls appetite

Wellness Guide

Weight-Management Suggestions

Control your home environment in these ways:

1. Do all at-home eating at the kitchen or dining room table.

2. Eat without reading or watching TV.

3. Keep tempting foods out of sight, hard to reach, and bothersome to prepare.

4. If you must snack, have low-calorie foods accessible, visible, easy to reach, and ready to eat.

5. Store tempting foods in containers that are opaque or difficult to open.

6. Give other family members their own snack-food storage areas.

7. Don't do non-food-related activities in the kitchen; stay out of the kitchen as much as possible.

Control your work environment in these ways:

1. Do not eat at your desk or while working. Eat at some place designated (by you) for eating only.

2. Do not keep tempting food near your workplace.

3. Prepackage low-calorie snacks and take them with you to work.

4. Carry no change to use at vending machines.

5. Use exercise instead of food when you need to take a break from work.

6. If you eat in a cafeteria, plan your order in advance and bring only enough money to cover your order.

Manage your daily food sources:

1. Do not shop when hungry.

2. Shop from a list prepared beforehand.

3. Shop quickly.

4. Avoid buying large sizes of hard-to-resist high-calorie foods.

5. Prepare foods during periods when your control is highest.

6. Try to prepare several meals at once (lunches with dinners).

7. Remove leftovers from sight as soon after mealtime as possible (use opaque storage devices).

Control your mealtime environment:

1. Do not keep serving bowls at the table.

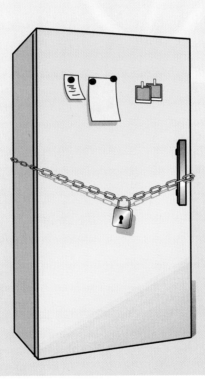

2. Use smaller plates, bowls, glasses, and serving spoons.

3. Remove the plate from the table as soon as you finish eating.

4. Practice polite refusal when extra food is offered to you.

Eat slowly:

1. Put down the eating utensil, sandwich, drink, or chicken leg between bites.

2. Swallow what is in your mouth before preparing the next bite.

3. Cut food as it is needed rather than all at once.

4. Stop eating a few times during the meal to control your eating rhythm.

5. Make each second serving only half as large as the usual amount.

Control snacking:

1. Instead of snacking, do an activity incompatible with eating.

2. Instead of snacking, do something you like to do or a small task around the house or office.

3. Instead of snacking, do a short burst of intense activity or a relaxation exercise.

4. Brush your teeth or use mouthwash to curb the urge to eat.

5. Make snacks difficult to get.

6. Drink a large glass of water before snacking.

7. Have low-calorie snack foods on hand rather than high-calorie foods.

Source: J. Waltz, *Food Habit Management* (Seattle, WA: Northwest Learning Associates, Inc., 1978).

---

shows that a variety of body sizes, shapes, and fat compositions are healthy. For example, a woman who is 5 feet 4 inches tall can weigh between 110 pounds (BMI = 19) and 156 pounds (BMI = 27) and still have a healthy body weight. What would be unhealthy is striving for an unattainable body shape and then criticizing oneself for failing to attain it. This is not good for self-esteem or mental health, and it defeats a sensible weight maintenance program.

It is true that individuals with BMIs of 30 or more should reduce their body fat percentage to avoid a variety of health problems. But instead of setting the unrealistic goal of slimming to a BMI of 20 and blaming themselves when that goal is not met, they should try to reduce their body weight by 10%, which often puts them in the range of good health.

Those who are not clinically overfat but wish to be slim for cosmetic reasons should realize that the

Exercise is essential to effective weight management.

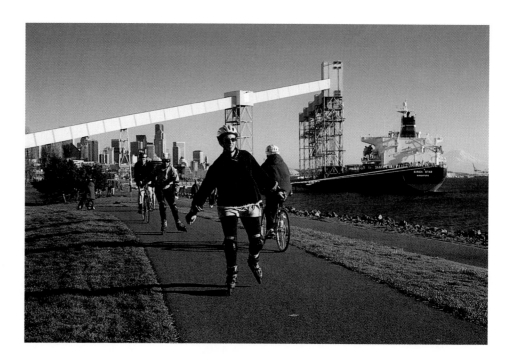

stereotypes of attractiveness are very difficult to attain without a predisposing genetic makeup or a visit to the cosmetic surgeon. Sensible weight management begins with being aware of social pressures toward unattainable goals and not succumbing to advertising and fashion trends.

No calorie-restricting weight-loss program has ever been shown to be effective over the medium-to-long term, regardless of advertising claims to the contrary. Programs lasting 2, 6, 12, or 24 weeks that are based on particular foods and portions can produce considerable weight loss, but 67% of people regain that weight within 1 year, and 95% regain it within 5 years. Improved nutrition, regular exercise, and a desire to feel good are the ways people who lose considerable weight are able to maintain the new, healthful body weight for many years (Klem, et al., 1997).

Since calorie-restricting diets by themselves don't work, what does? Unless you have a fat-storage disease, you can do it by living healthfully and letting your body find the weight that's natural for it, which involves:

- *Eat only when hungry.* Pay attention to hunger and satiety signals from your appestat. Be aware of habits and customs that influence your eating behavior: Do you eat at predetermined times of day (mealtime, between classes, on the way to work) regardless of your state of hunger? Do you eat *everything* on your plate? Do you work or study while eating?
- *Eat low on the food pyramid.* Base your diet on breads, pasta, vegetables, fresh fruits, and grains. This will keep you from overconsumption of calo-

ries, because you will more easily feel full. Also, you are less likely to consume fat calories that are "hidden" in manufactured foods to make them palatable.

- *Exercise.* Move your body around for at least 20 minutes per day, three to four times a week. And don't subscribe to the myth that exercising will increase appetite and food consumption. In fact, except for individuals who expend enormous amounts of energy (e.g., lumberjacks, football players), the opposite is true. Appetite and food consumption tend to decrease as physical activity increases.
- *Limit mindless snacking.* Mindless snacking is the kind we do when we are ravenously hungry, stressed, or zoned-out on watching TV. We wish that bag of chips were bottomless. TV advertisers encourage mindless snacking. They know that when you're watching TV you're in a state of autohypnosis, and they bank on your susceptibility to their images of beer, snack foods, candy, and soft drinks. Instead of mindless snacking, it's better to focus on the food you are eating. Be aware of satiety signals from your appestat. Learn to say to yourself, "That's enough for now."
- *Consume little or no alcohol.* Alcohol contains seven calories per gram (about 100 calories per 12-ounce beer, 4-ounce glass of wine, or one shot of distilled liquor). A couple of beers per day without a compensatory reduction in food intake or increase in exercise could lead to an excess of body fat rather quickly.
- *Be aware of eating triggers.* Many of us are susceptible to environmental cues that trigger eating. For

example, some people cannot pass a candy or soft-drink machine without feeding it money in exchange for it feeding them. At some worksites, well-meaning supervisors provide pastries and candy for their staff members, who may have a difficult time resisting, especially when stressed or fatigued.

- *Don't feed your feelings.* Stress, anxiety, loneliness, boredom, and anger can all motivate overeating. Many people derive emotional comfort from food. One possible explanation is that, as children, we learn to associate eating (particularly nursing as infants) with receiving love, affection, and comfort. Another possibility is when we consume certain foods, particularly those containing sugar and fat, they contribute to feelings of calm.

The energy equivalent of 1 pound of body fat is 3500 calories. If you want to adopt a weight-reducing program that results in a loss of 1 pound a month, plan your dietary and physical activities so you can produce a net daily deficit of 120 calories. Walk a little more each day or cut out a soft drink or a couple of cookies (Table 5.3). If you want to lose one pound a week, plan for a net daily deficit of 500 calories that includes at least a 300-calorie expenditure per day of exercise (Table 5.4). The number of calories is not nearly as important as *making a plan to which you can realistically adhere over the long haul.* Here are some other suggestions:

- Keep a diary of your weight-loss activities and modify things in your plan that do not work.
- Keep faith with your intention to attain a healthful weight. Don't let the inevitable setbacks demoralize you.

TABLE 5.3   Activity Equivalents of Calories in Some Foods (in Minutes)

Food	Walking	Cycling	Swimming	Running	Yoga
Apple	20	12	9	5	20
Can of beer	30	18	13	8	30
Piece of cake	70	45	35	20	70
Two cookies	20	12	9	5	20
One doughnut	30	18	13	8	30
Double-scoop ice cream cone	40	25	18	11	40
Piece of pie	70	45	35	20	70
Piece of pizza	35	22	16	10	35
20 french fries	60	40	30	17	60
10 potato chips	20	12	9	5	20
8-oz. soft drink	25	15	11	7	25
Hamburger	70	45	35	20	70

TABLE 5.4   Approximate Energy Expenditures During Various Activities

Light exercise (4 calories per minute)		
Cycling 5 mph	Slow dancing	Ping-pong
Walking 3 mph	Volleyball	Yoga
Canoeing	Softball	T'ai chi ch'uan
Housecleaning	Golf	
Moderate exercise (7 calories per minute)		
Tennis	Basketball	Snowshoeing
Fast dancing	Swimming 30 m/min	Walking 4.5 mph
Cycling 9 mph	Heavy gardening	Roller skating
Heavy exercise (10 calories per minute)		
Jogging	Mountain climbing	Skiing
Climbing stairs	Cycling 12 mph	Ice skating
Football	Handball and racquetball	

- Don't count calories or constantly weigh yourself; focus on feeling good.
- Ignore food advertising.

The Medical Management of Overweight

The medical term for overweight is **obesity,** a condition in adults defined as having a BMI of more than 30 or a body-fat percentage of more than 20% for men and 30% for women. People with this condition face two problems: (a) carrying a large amount of fat on the body predisposes the person to a variety of major illnesses, such as heart disease, high blood pressure, type 2 diabetes, degeneration of the joints (due to excess weight), and obstructive sleep apnea (cessation of breathing while asleep); and (b) reducing a large-sized body is difficult because the body defends against fat loss. This is why doctors strongly recommend that people eat healthfully and exercise regularly to try to maintain a BMI of 25 or less and that people with BMIs greater than 30 realize that maintaining a healthy body size is likely to be a lifelong effort.

Techniques that health professionals use to help patients reduce their BMI to a more healthful range include counseling and hypnosis, surgery, and medications.

Terms

obesity: the condition of having a BMI of more than 30 or weighing more than 20% (men) or 30% (women) of the recommended weight-for-height

Managing Stress

Treating the Underlying Emotional Causes of Obesity

Mrs. Johnson made an appointment with a psychologist to discuss being overweight. She is 40 years old, 5 feet 5 inches tall, and weighs 180 pounds. She works as a nurse at a community hospital and has no serious medical problems. She is married, her husband is unemployed, and she has three teenage children at home. Her take-home pay is modest, and the family never has enough money to pay bills. She eats mostly "junk food" from fast-food restaurants and does not exercise.

Since appropriate weight depends on *both* a healthy diet *and* exercise, the counselor must look for barriers to those two goals (Foreyt, 1997). The counselor must help the patient discover the causes of stress and negative emotions that underlie the weight problem. These generally include job or family stressors, depression, anger, loneliness, or boredom. Sometimes adult obesity has its roots in childhood sexual abuse (i.e., having a large body makes one sexually unattractive and is therefore protective).

Social aspects of being overweight also have to be explored. What are the barriers to obtaining healthy food? Does the job require a lot of travel or sitting for extended periods? How can exercise be incorporated into the daily life-style?

In Mrs. Johnson's case, she has a high-stress, low-paying job, a distressed marriage, and children at a challenging stage of development. Her life-style is out of control. With the counselor's help, Mrs. Johnson adopted a low-fat diet and began jogging in the morning before work. Later, she added weight training to her exercise program. After a few months she obtained a better-paying job with regular hours. She and her husband went to a marriage counselor and eventually decided to divorce. After about a year, Mrs. Johnson's weight stabilized at 130 pounds. She has maintained her low-fat diet and continues to exercise. She has found new friends and has begun going out on dates with men.

Many overweight people have problems similar to Mrs. Johnson's. Counseling, diet changes, exercise, and social support can help most overweight people who are willing to change their lives.

Counseling and Hypnosis

Counseling for weight loss using cognitive behavioral therapy involves helping patients examine the reasons for their unhealthful eating and exercise behaviors and develop ways to behave more healthfully. Hypnosis has been shown to increase the benefits of counseling (Kirsch, 1996).

Surgery

Surgery is indicated only for people with a BMI over 40 or people with a BMI between 35 and 40 who have severe weight-related medical conditions, such as heart problems or diabetes, and who have not responded to supervised diet and exercise regimes or drug therapy. The rationale of surgical treatments for obesity is to alter the anatomy of the gastrointestinal tract so that only a fraction of food ingested in a meal is absorbed into the body.

Medications

Medications to produce weight loss include **appetite suppressants** and agents that block the absorption of ingested fat into the body. Appetite suppressants work by altering the level of neurotransmitters in the appestat. "Uppers" (amphetamines, benzphetamine, phentermine, mazindol, phenylpropanolamine) affect the dopamine neurotransmitters in the central nervous system. Ingesting any of these agents blocks the sensation of hunger. Selective serotonin reuptake inhibitors (SSRIs), antidepressants that also act as appetite suppressants, including fluoxetine (Prozac), paroxetine (Paxil), and sertaline (Zoloft), increase the amount of the neurotransmitter serotonin, which creates feelings of satiety and thus reduces appetite. Appetite suppressants, used either alone or in combination (e.g., phentermine plus fenfluramine is "phen/fen"), are effective, although stopping the drug results in a rapid regaining of any lost weight. Also, some of these drugs are dangerous. They increase the risk of pulmonary hypertension, a fatal condition, and damage to heart valves. In September 1997, the U.S. government banned the use of "phen/fen" and similar agents because of their health risks.

Weight-Control Fads and Fallacies

"Lose weight effortlessly, even as you sleep!" "New diet discovery lets you lose excess pounds in just one week!" So claim advertisements for products and eating regimens that are directed to chronic dieters and others concerned about being overfat.

Unfortunately for consumers, nearly all of the claims made by heavily advertised weight-control regimens and products are exaggerated and misleading. By themselves, these programs are not likely to produce a significant reduction in body fat over any long-term period. The only way to reduce body fat and maintain healthy body weight is life-style modifications that include changing eating behaviors and increasing the level of physical activity.

Three ineffective, weight-control products or schemes are: (a) body wraps, (b) chemicals, (c) and diet programs.

Body Wraps

Body wraps are plastic or rubber garments, ranging from waist belts to entire body suits, that are worn during exercise, routine daily activity, or sleep in order to produce weight loss. Body wraps do result in weight loss and a reduction in body size. The catch is that the weight lost is body water and not body fat. These garments increase perspiration; they do not diminish the body's fat stores. The lost body water is quickly regained and so is the lost body weight. Because these products cause a loss of body water, they make dehydration a potential danger. Some athletes have died from exercising while using body wraps.

The appeal of body wraps stems from the common misconception that fat can be eliminated from the body by heat. The phrase "burning off fat" is part of the professional physiologist's jargon and contributes to this false notion. The process by which body fat is reduced does not involve heat. (Human body temperature is uniformly maintained at 37°C.) The "burning" that physiologists speak of is a chemical breakdown of fat molecules requiring oxygen, not the liquefaction and evaporation that one would expect from high temperatures. Hence, the claim that body wraps reduce body size by "melting away fat" is quite misleading.

Chemicals

A number of products that contain drugs and "natural" substances are sold as weight-loss remedies. Often these products are used in conjunction with dieting, modification in eating behavior, and exercise programs, so they appear effective to the naive consumer. However, no single product by itself has been shown to reduce weight.

Phenylpropanolamine (PPA) is an amphetamine-like substance that is the principal ingredient in several weight-loss products sold over the counter (Dexatrim, Acutrim). PPA is thought to be an appetite suppressant, but the doses recommended in commercial preparations are probably not effective, and higher doses (more than 75 mg/day) are likely to cause nervousness, nausea, insomnia, headaches, and elevated blood pressure.

Benzocaine, an anesthetic, is found in candies, lozenges, and chewing gums sold as aids to weight reduction. Benzocaine is supposed to help produce weight loss by numbing the sense of taste and thereby reducing the desire for food. There is no scientific evidence, however, that temporarily reducing the sense of taste leads to weight loss. Because benzocaine is intended as a topical anesthetic, these products are useful (if at all) only if they are not swallowed.

Bulk-producing agents, such as methylcellulose, psyllium, and agar, are supposed to produce a sense of fullness in the gastrointestinal tract, thus suppressing appetite. These agents swell when mixed with water and are much more effective as laxatives than as weight reducers. Glucomannan, a bulk-producing starch derived from konjac tubers, is often touted by health food enthusiasts as a "natural" weight-loss method. There is no evidence that glucomannan or any other bulk producer aids weight loss.

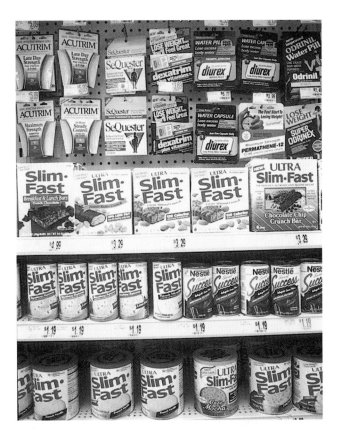

Diet aids will help you lose your money—not your excess pounds.

Terms

appetite suppressants: drugs that diminish the sense of hunger

phenylpropanolamine (PPA): active ingredient in over-the-counter weight-control products

benzocaine: an anesthetic sometimes used in over-the-counter weight-control products to numb the sense of taste

bulk-producing agents: agents used to promote a sense of fullness in the gastrointestinal tract, thus suppressing appetite

Hormones, such as human chorionic gonado-tropin (HCG) and thyroid hormone, are occasionally offered by unscrupulous clinics as aids for weight loss. Neither of these hormones is effective as a weight reducer. Moreover, because hormones are regulators of the body's homeostatic mechanisms, it is never wise to take them unless monitored closely by a well-trained clinician.

Vitamins, minerals, and some amino acids (including arginine, ornithine, tryptophan, and pheny-lalanine) are occasionally sold as weight-loss agents. For example, spirulina, a product made from blue-green algae, is claimed to be effective in reducing weight because it contains the amino acid phenylala-nine, which supposedly regulates the body's appetite. Vitamins, minerals, and amino acids have not been shown to be effective in causing weight loss. And in very high doses, some of these substances, although "natural," can be harmful.

Diet Programs

If you want to make some money, get involved in publishing a book that describes a "revolutionary" new diet for weight loss. So many people make a hobby of trying fad diets that the book is virtually guaranteed to sell many copies. Be sure that the diet you invent requires no exercise, is based on some "new" dietary or nutritional discovery, carries an air of authoritativeness, and promises a rapid reduction in body weight, although not necessarily a reduction in body fat. It doesn't matter a bit if the lost weight is regained in a short time. In fact, it's probably better for the weight-loss industry if your diet does not produce permanent weight loss, since that would reduce the sales of the next crop of diet books.

> *He who doesn't mind his belly will hardly mind anything else.*
> SAMUEL JOHNSON

Many of the weight-loss diets that have come and gone have been based on altering the usual proportions of protein, fat, and carbohydrate. Hence, the high-fat, low-fat, high-carbohydrate, low-carbohydrate, high-protein, and low-protein diets have all had their day. Occasionally diet regimens require the ingestion of only certain kinds of foods, such as fruits (grapefruit or papaya), cottage cheese, or steak. Fortunately, most of these unusual diets are too expensive, too boring, or too fatiguing to maintain for long, and people give them up before the nutritional deficiencies they can produce cause irreparable harm. Unfortunately, that is not always the case, and a few people have died from unsound dieting practices (such as unhealthy liquid diets).

A variety of weight-loss programs not only tell clients how to lose weight, but also supply packaged foods and, sometimes, social support to bolster the weight-loser's efforts. Many of these programs are based on severely calorie-restricted regimens. Some plans use "real" food but control the portion size and others are based on liquid diets containing sufficient protein, vitamins, and minerals to prevent the loss of lean body tissue. As with other special efforts to lose weight, the dietary plans often fail because they are difficult or expensive to maintain, and also because they often do not include life-style changes that promote maintaining a healthy body weight.

Body Image

Body image is a person's mental "picture" of her or his body. Nearly everyone has a body image. Nearly everyone judges that image as good, or less good, by comparing her or his body image to a standard of the "ideal body" communicated to individuals by their culture and people who are important to them, such as lovers, family, and friends.

Many people are excessively concerned about their body image and believe themselves to be overweight. Books, films, TV, and popular magazines (especially women's magazines) consistently send messages that our society esteems thin people and disdains heavy ones. Whereas maintaining appropriate body size is associated with good health, attempting to achieve an unrealistic ideal of slimness is oppressive to many. Failure to meet unrealistic standards leads many people to judge themselves as unattractive and lowers their self-esteem.

The current emphasis on slimness is partly fad—there have been times when thinness was associated with being sickly and a full body was a sign of health and sexual attractiveness—and partly desire to be healthy and fit. A lean body is associated with high status, sexual attractiveness, youthfulness, and a

Terms

hormones: complex chemicals, produced and secreted by endocrine glands, that travel through the bloodstream

body image: a person's mental image of his or her body

anorexia athletica: athletes who restrict their food intake to stay slim or lean

anorexia nervosa: emotional disorder occurring most commonly in adolescent females, characterized by abnormal body image, fear of obesity, and prolonged refusal to eat, sometimes resulting in death

bulimia: serious disorder, especially common in adolescents and young women, marked by excessive eating, often followed by self-induced vomiting, purging, or fasting

demonstration of the personal power to be fit and trim in a culture in which sedentary habits and overeating are common.

For the most part, standards of attractive and healthful appearance are set by companies seeking to sell products and increase profits. Advertisements try to convince women that they fall short of an ideal and that, by purchasing a product, dieting, or exercising to change their body size and shape, they can improve themselves and their lives. These messages cause some to judge themselves on how they look and cause others to judge people largely by their physical appearance. Overconcern about body image and weight can have adverse health consequences, including:

- Depression from low body esteem and low self-worth
- Poor nutrition from extensive dieting
- Inadequate calcium and iron intake from under-nutrition
- Anorexia or bulimia
- Musculoskeletal injuries from overexercising
- Risks associated with cosmetic surgery
- Cigarette smoking to reduce body weight

 ## Eating Disorders

Using slimness as a measure of social achievement has become an oppressive standard for many, particularly for young people. In some instances, individuals develop such a morbid fear of becoming fat that they adopt unhealthy eating behaviors.

Athletes may also be susceptible to an inordinate fear of fatness. Most serious athletes are encouraged to be as lean as possible, and some overreact to the expectations of parents and coaches by restricting their food intake to excessively low amounts. This behavior, called **anorexia athletica,** affects both males and females. According to Nathan J. Smith, an expert in sports medicine, "losing fat becomes a challenge in which the athlete promises himself uncompromised success. Hunger pains become gratifying signals of accomplishment, and food becomes the opponent in a contest that he is dedicated to win by an overwhelming score" (Smith, 1980). Counseling and reassurance that athletic goals can be met without such drastic eating behavior usually alleviate the condition.

Although abnormal eating behavior can be caused solely by the fear of becoming fat, there are instances when a compulsive desire to be slim is a manifestation of more complex psychological stress. Two of the most common eating disorders are **anorexia nervosa,** a voluntary refusal to eat, and **bulimia,** binge eating and immediate purging of the ingested food either by vomiting or by using laxatives.

Anorexia Nervosa

Anorexia nervosa is characterized by a relentless pursuit of thinness resulting in progressive weight loss

Wellness Guide

Elite Athletes Are at Risk for Eating Disorders

In 1988, at age 16, Christie Henrich missed making the U.S. Olympic team in women's gymnastics by less than two-tenths of a point. At her performance peak, Christie weighed 93 pounds. During one of the international competitions in 1988, a judge told her that she needed to watch her weight if she wanted to be a champion. According to her coach, Christie perceived herself as being too fat to be an Olympic competitor, so she began to starve herself (anorexia) and to vomit when she did eat (bulimia). By 1990, she was too weak to compete, even though she was ranked among the top 10 women gymnasts in the U.S. In 1994, Christie Henrich died; she weighed less than 60 pounds.

If someone you know seems to have an eating problem, here are some ways to help.

- Express your concern about any apparent weight loss. Even if the person denies that anything is wrong, your concern may alert him or her that something is wrong.

- Encourage the person to talk about his or her feelings concerning problems or worries, even if they are not food-related. Listen without making judgments.

- Suggest that the person see a health counselor, physician, or mental health professional.

- Express your own concerns to a professional counselor who may be able to intervene and help.

While eating disorders are estimated to occur in 1% to 3% of the general population, they occur in 15% to 62% of female athletes (Tofler, et. al., 1996). Many ambitious female athletes suffer from what is called the "female-athlete triad," which is characterized by eating disorders, menstrual dysfunction, and osteoporosis. Coaches, parents, and athletes themselves need to pay much more attention to their health and to make sure that athletic goals do not lead to severe illness and even death.

Anorexia and bulimia are very serious disorders and require professional help.

and metabolic disturbances. Most of those affected are young women. Anorexia is not caused by any known disease-causing agent but by self-induced starvation, which can lead to serious illness and even death.

Elizabeth Barrett Browning (1806–1861), one of England's most famed poets, is thought to have had anorexia nervosa. As a teenager, Elizabeth was nagged by her parents to eat and gain weight, yet she stubbornly refused to eat much more than toast. When she met her future husband, poet Robert Browning, she weighed only 87 pounds. Apparently the Barrett family possessed characteristics found in other families with an anorectic member: overprotectiveness, overinvolvement with each other, and inability to express or resolve intrafamilial conflict.

Stubbornness and irony are characteristics of anorexia nervosa. For example, persons with anorexia nervosa are likely to defend their emaciated appearance as normal and will insist that weight gain makes them feel fat. Besides distortions in normal body image, anorectic people tend to have a fanatical preoccupation with food. They may spend an inordinate amount of time planning and preparing elaborate meals for others, while they themselves eat only a few bites and claim to be full. Often they will not eat in the presence of others; when they do, they may dawdle over their food. Some anorectic persons resort to self-induced vomiting or frequent use of diuretics or laxatives to reduce their body weight. These practices may lead to severe depletion of body minerals, which can precipitate abnormal heart rhythms and even cardiac arrest. Despite the low intake of calories, anorectic persons are remarkably energetic and tend to be hyperactive.

Another characteristic of anorexia nervosa is a paralyzing sense of powerlessness. Persons with anorexia see themselves as responding to demands of others rather than taking initiative in life. Children with anorexia tend to be obedient, dutiful, helpful, and excellent students. Some psychologists interpret the intense preoccupation with weight loss as an expression of an underlying fear of incompetence. Control of eating and body weight becomes a way of demonstrating general control and competence.

One theory seeks to explain anorexia as a preoccupation with extreme slimness (and associated absence of menstruation) in an attempt to remain a child who is cared for and fed by others, who can be stubborn and obstinate, and who has no sexual identity or desires. Another theory suggests that anorexia is the manifestation of a struggle for a sense of identity and personal effectiveness through controlling the environment; the resulting stubborn, rejecting behavior then becomes reinforced by the attention received from others. Yet another theory sees anorexia as a manifestation of impaired family interaction. The family of the anorectic person becomes so engrossed with the symptoms that they avoid dealing with conflicts among themselves.

Three goals characterize the treatment of anorexia nervosa: (a) weight gain, (b) changed attitudes toward food and eating, and (c) resolution of underlying personal and family conflicts. Unfortunately, therapeutic intervention is not always successful and the condition may persist for years. Anorexia nervosa has a 15% to 20% mortality rate.

Bulimia

Bulimia is marked by a voluntary restriction of food intake followed by a binge-purge cycle: extreme overeating, usually of high-calorie junk foods, immediately followed by self-induced vomiting, use of diuretics or laxatives, or intense exercise. Like anorexia nervosa, bulimia occurs primarily in young women with a morbid fear of becoming fat, who pursue thinness relentlessly. Most bulimic persons are model individuals: good students, athletes, extremely sociable, and pleasant. Fearing discovery of their bulimic behavior, they frequently carry out their binge-purge episodes in private. Bulimic persons usually are aware that their binge-purge behavior is abnormal; however, they are unable to control it. Many feel guilty and depressed about their problem, which leads to a tendency to hide the behavior. Bulimia can pose a serious risk to health for many of the same reasons that anorexia does.

Several theories have been proposed to explain bulimia. One is that bulimia is a maladaptive way of dealing with anxiety, loneliness, and anger. Another suggests that bulimia is a manifestation of the drive to become the "ideal" woman, achieving the societal norm of slimness. Bulimic persons tend to have low self-esteem and a weak sense of identity.

Recovering from bulimia includes stopping binge-purge cycles and regaining control over eating behavior. Persons with bulimia must also establish more appropriate ways to handle unpleasant feelings and discomfort with close relationships, and their self-esteem must be improved. Often psychological counseling is helpful.

It's in Your Hands

Successful weight control involves reducing intake of calories (often by recognizing the social and psychological reasons that cause overeating) and increasing the level of physical activity. Heavily advertised reducing schemes, such as body wraps, diet pills, and fad diets, are almost totally ineffective in producing permanent fat reduction and weight loss.

The primary reason that people are overfat is that their life-styles do not include sufficient physical activity to use up the calories ingested in food. You can begin today to consciously watch what you eat and how much you exercise. You need not start out with an all-out diet or exercise regime; start slowly. When offered a cookie, decline. When you have the choice between the elevator and stairs, take the stairs. These efforts, which appear to be small, can make a difference when made daily and over an extended period of time.

Critical Thinking About Health

1. Jordana couldn't stand herself anymore, so she went to the campus health center's peer nutrition counseling program for help.

   "I disgust myself," she told her counselor. "I'm fat, fat, fat and no matter what I do I can't change it. I jog, I don't eat ice cream. I suck."

   While not ready for a starring role on "Baywatch," Jordana wasn't fat, according to her counselor. Her BMI calculated out to 28.4. "It's a little on the high side," said the counselor, "but you're not in the danger zone."

   "Tell that to my Dad," Jordana snapped. "And my boyfriend. When they look at me, their eyes go right to my stomach. It's like that's all I am—a stomach on legs!"

   a. What expectations regarding body size and shape do you experience as a member of your sex?

   b. How were these expectations transmitted to you and by whom (or by what social institution)?

   c. How are these expectations enforced in your peer group, and what are the social penalties for not meeting such expectations?

   d. To what lengths do people go to meet these expectations? Are any of these practices extreme or unhealthy?

2. Sam: Oh, man, not Roni. She's too wide!
   Mick: No, she's not. She's real nice. Call her.
   Sam: Nah.
   Mick: You're a dweeb, sucker. You didn't like Nan because her face was too round. You didn't like Carla because she was too tall. You didn't like Evy because . . . why didn't you like Evy, anyway? I forget.
   Sam: Thunder thighs.
   Mick: You're going to wind up one lonely dude, dude.

   a. Is Sam really destined to be lonely or is he being smart to wait for someone who matches his ideal of the perfect body?

   b. In your peer group, are there examples of people being attracted to people who *do not* resemble the ideal? Can you explain that discrepancy?

   c. What is the social purpose of an ideal body size and shape?

3. It is likely that in the near future there will be many drugs that are moderately effective in producing weight (fat) loss. It is also likely that these drugs will carry some risks to health.

   a. Do you think that such drugs should be made available to anyone who wants them, or should such medications be restricted to people whose weight puts them at serious risk for health problems and premature death?

   b. Besides potential harm from side effects, is it appropriate for people to depend on drugs for weight maintenance instead of modifying dietary and exercise habits and learning to reduce stress?

4. How have eating disorders touched your life?

Health in Review

- Approximately one-third of the U.S. population is overfat and at risk for a variety of illnesses, including heart disease, diabetes, hypertension, and gallbladder disease.

- Obesity is defined as having a body weight 20% (for men) and 30% (for women) over recommended weight for height or a body mass index greater than 30.

- Health problems are less likely when the waist-to-hip ratio is less than 0.8 (women) or 0.95 (men).
- Body fatness is maintained around a set point, which is maintained by neural and hormonal signals acting on the "appestat" in the brain, which controls feelings of hunger and satiety. Many physiological, psychological, social, and environmental factors affect the appestat and thus body weight.
- Healthy body weight corresponds to having a body mass index between 19 and 27. There are a variety of ways to achieve a healthy body weight. Starvation dieting is *not* one of them.

- Counseling, surgery, and medications can help some overweight people lose body fat and maintain a healthy body weight.
- People eat for reasons other than hunger, such as social interaction, recreation, and relief from stress.
- Successful weight control involves changing eating and exercise habits.
- There are three major ineffective weight control schemes: body wraps, diet pills, and diet programs.
- Two common eating disorders that occur primarily among young people today are anorexia nervosa and bulimia.

Health and Wellness Online

The World Wide Web contains a wealth of information about health and wellness. By accessing the Internet using Web browser software, such as Netscape Navigator or Microsoft's Internet Explorer, you can gain a new perspective on many topics presented in *Essentials of Health and Wellness, Second Edition*. Access the Jones and Bartlett Publishers web site at http://www.jbpub.com/hwonline.

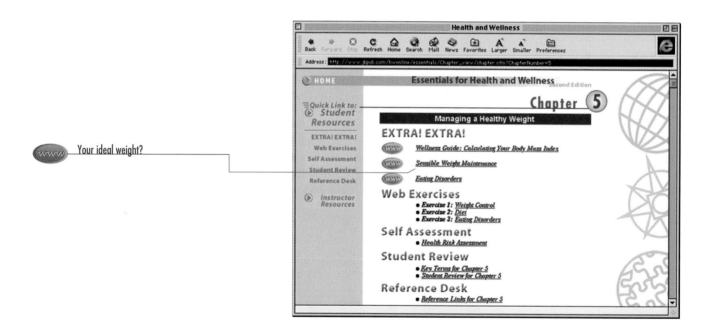

References

Foreyt, J. P. (1997, August 15). An etiological approach to obesity. *Hospital Practice,* 123–148.

Kirsch, I. (1996). Hypnotic enhancement of cognitive-behavioral weight loss treatments. *Journal of Consulting and Clinical Psychology, 64(3),* 517–519.

Klem, M. L., Wing, R. R., McGuire, M. T., Seagle, H. M., & Hill, J. O. (1997). A descriptive study of individuals successful at long-term maintenance of sub-stantial weight loss. *American Journal of Clinical Nutrition, 66,* 239–246.

Kuczmarski, R. J., Flegal, K. M., Campbell, S. M., & Johnson, C. L. (1994). Increasing prevalence of overweight among U.S. adults. *Journal of American Medical Association, 272(3),* 205–211.

Lamon-Fava S., Wilson, P. W., & Schaefer, E. L. (1996). Impact of body mass index on coronary heart disease risk factors in men and women. *Arteriosclerosis, Thrombosis, and Vascular Biology, 9,* 1509–1515.

Leibel, R. L., Rosenbaum, M., & Hirsch, J. (1995). Changes in energy expenditure resulting from altered body weight. *New England Journal of Medicine, 332,* 621–8.

Schwartz, M. E., & Seeley, R. J. (1997). Neuroendocrine responses to starvation and weight loss. *New England Journal of Medicine, 336,* 1802–1811.

Seidell, J. C., Verschuren, W. M. M., van Leer, E. M., & Kromhout, D. (1996). Overweight, under-weight and mortality. *Archives of Internal Medicine, 156,* 958–963.

Smith, N. J. (1980). Excessive weight loss and food aversion in athletes simulating anorexia nervosa. *Pediatrics, 66,* 139–142.

Tofler, I. R., et al. (1996). Physical and emotional problems of elite female athletes. *New England Journal of Medicine, 335,* 281–83.

Wickelgren, I. (1998). Obesity: How big a problem? *Science, 280,* 1364–1367.

Suggested Readings

Eldredge, K. L., Agras, W. S., & Arnow, B. (1994). The last supper: Emotional determinants of pretreatment weight fluctuation in obese binge eaters. *The International Journal of Eating Disorders, 16(1),* 83. A study of obese binge eaters' self-reported tendency to binge eat because of negative emotions of anger, anxiety, and depression.

Emery, E. M., Schmid, T. L., Kahn, H. S., & Filozof, P. P. (1993). A review of the association between abdominal fat distribution, health outcome measures, and modifiable risk factors. *American Journal of Health Promotion, 7(5),* 342–353. Examines the relationship between abdominal fat distribution and specific health outcomes, modifiable risk factors, and intervention efforts.

Foreyt, J. P. (1997, August 15). An etiological approach to obesity. *Hospital Practice,* 123–148. Discusses how to take into account emotional and social factors when trying to reduce body weight.

Fraser, L., & Weger, D. (1993). Nothing to lose. *Health, 7(7),* 60. Discusses the idea of letting the body decide when it's hungry rather than eating at set times during the day.

Kassirer, J. P., & Angell, M. (1998). Losing weight—An ill-fated New Year's resolution. *New England Journal of Medicine, 338,* 52–54. Puts the issue of weight loss for health reasons in perspective and cautions against overconcern about body size.

Regulation of body weight. (1998, May 29). *Science,* 1363–1390. This issue contains a series of up-to-date articles on the causes of obesity, treatment options, and research strategies for finding ways to prevent or treat obesity.

Rosenbaum, M., Leibel, R. L., & Hirsch, J. (1997). Obesity. *New England Journal of Medicine, 337,* 396–406. This is a thorough discussion of research on the causes and treatment of obesity.

Schwartz, M. E., & Seeley, R. J. (1997). Neuroendocrine responses to starvation and weight loss. *New England Journal of Medicine, 336,* 1802–1811. A very clear explanation of how the nervous and endocrine systems control body fatness.

St. Jeor, S. T. (1993). The role of weight management in the health of women. *Journal of the American Dietetic Association, 93(9),* 1007–1012. Discusses hormonal, psychological, and environmental influences that place women at an increased risk for overall weight concerns.

Exercises and Activities

WORKBOOK
Determine Your Fitness Index
Determine Your Flexibility Index

Health and Wellness Online

 www.jbpub.com/hwonline

Fitness and Conditioning
Making Physical Activity a Priority

Chapter 6

Physical Activity for Health and Well-Being

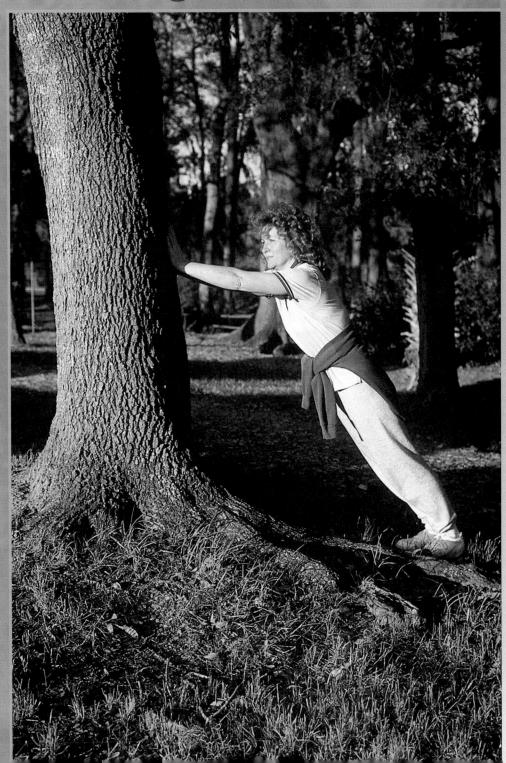

Many studies indicate that regular physical activity, whether it is work-related or recreational, contributes to health and well-being and lowers the risk of many diseases, including heart disease, high blood pressure, stroke, diabetes, osteoporosis, obesity, and colon cancer. Also, regular physical activity increases your ability to overcome fatigue, cope effectively with stress, and fight off colds and other infections by boosting the immune system. Furthermore, regular physical activity puts into life the good feelings and enjoyment that come from movement.

> *If you want to run a mile, then run a mile. If you want to experience another life, run a marathon.*
>
> EMIL ZATOPEK
> Marathon runner,
> 1952 Olympic gold medal

What Is Physical Activity?

The health club and exercise equipment industries and the advertising and TV infomercials that support them can easily lead people to think that exercising for health requires considerable time, energy, equipment, special clothing, and money. These investments can seem so overwhelming that some people forego exercising altogether.

Fortunately, physical activity does not require special equipment or spending a lot of money. Physical activity is anything you do when you are not sitting or lying down. Besides jogging, swimming, cycling, and aerobic dancing, physical activity includes yoga, tai chi ch'uan, martial arts training, gardening, and walking. For instance, regular walking strengthens muscles, increases aerobic capacity, clears and quiets the mind, reduces stress, expends calories, and causes few injuries, if any. Other than appropriate shoes, walking requires no special clothing, equipment, or money, and it can be worked into a busy schedule.

When you have physical activity in your life, other healthy behaviors often follow, such as improved eating habits and a reduction in alcohol consumption. Also, physical activity may lessen stress so that undesirable stress-reducing behaviors, such as cigarette smoking, overeating, or drug consumption, stop.

If none of these points convinces you of the many benefits of exercise, think of it as setting aside time and attention for *you.* Many people feel overwhelmed by the demands of school, job, and family. Just taking a few minutes several days a week to exercise can give you the chance to relax, reflect, and indulge your imagination.

Physiological Benefits of Physical Activity

Research shows that moderate, and not necessarily extensive, exercise is sufficient for good health (Surgeon General's Report, 1996, and Figure 6.1). An almost-daily brisk walk of 30 to 60 minutes will do. Running several miles or working out for an hour or two in the gym every day is unnecessary. In fact, high levels of exercise often increase the risk of injury.

The Health Benefits of Physical Activity

Hundreds of studies have uncovered many health benefits of physical activity. Among them are: Increased strength of the heart muscle; increased flow of blood to the heart; increased bone mass and resistance to osteoporosis; decreased amount of fat in the blood; decreased heart rate; increased longevity; maintenance of normal blood pressure and reduction in blood pressure in people with hypertension; maintenance of body weight within generally accepted normal limits; prevention and alleviation of chronic low-back pain; improved sleep; greater energy reserve for work and recreation; improved posture, which leads to improved physical appearance and the ability to withstand fatigue; greater ability of the body to cope with illness or accidents.

If you exercise regularly, your overall risk of a heart attack is about 50% less than if you are inactive.

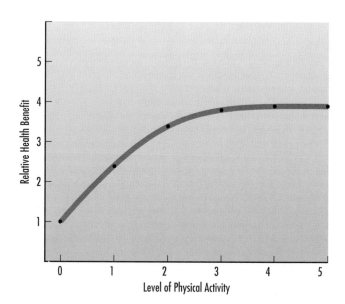

FIGURE 6.1   Health Benefit of Physical Activity The graph is a composite from many studies that demonstrate the positive effect of physical activity on health. Notice that the graph is not linear; the largest benefit comes from changing from a sedentary lifestyle to one with low-to-moderate levels of physical activity. High levels of physical activity do not produce corresponding gains in health. Health benefits include lessened risk of morbidity and mortality from cardiovascular disease, cancer, hypertension, and type II diabetes. Each level of physical activity (e.g., walking, running, cycling) corresponds to between 500 and 1000 calories per week of activity.

Source: Adapted from Blair et al, 1992.

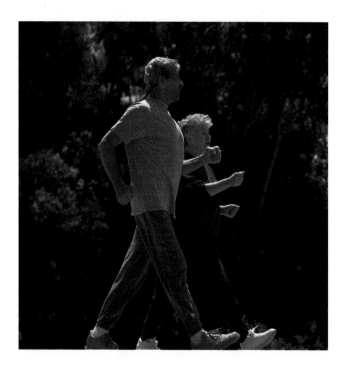

Walking is an excellent form of exercise at any age.

With routine exercise you can reach a level of physical fitness comparable to an inactive person 10 to 20 years younger. Exercise increases the size of your coronary arteries and reduces clogging due to atherosclerosis (see chapter 10). Exercise also increases the efficiency of your blood's oxygen-carrying capacity and your muscles' uptake of oxygen.

Exercise has been linked to increased levels of high-density lipoprotein (good) cholesterol and decreased low-density lipoprotein (bad) cholesterol and triglyceride levels (see chapter 10). After exercising regularly for 6 to 12 months, lowered cholesterol levels can mean as much as a 30% reduction in the risk of coronary artery disease. The Centers for Disease Control and Prevention and the American College of Sports Medicine recommend 30 minutes of physical activity at least 5 days a week (Pate et al., 1995). They define physical activity as anything from raking leaves to playing with the kids. Also you don't have to do all your activity at once. You can break up those 30 minutes into smaller segments; say, three 10-minute walks. Or, you can mix a little walking with taking the stairs instead of the elevator, doing a little gardening, or washing the car (Table 6.1).

Psychological Benefits of Physical Activity

Regular physical activity can result in periods of relaxed concentration, characterized by reduced physical and psychic tensions, regular breathing rhythms, and increased self-awareness. This effect is often compared to meditation and is the aim of all Eastern body work, including hatha yoga (Figure 6.2), t'ai chi ch'uan, and many martial arts practices. This effect also results from any physical activity in which one focuses the mind to produce a loss of self-consciousness through total concentration on various body movements. T'ai chi ch'uan instructor Sophia Delza (1996) explains:

> The goal of t'ai chi ch'uan is the achievement of health and tranquillity by means of a "way of movement," characterized by a technique of moving slowly and continuously, without strain, through a varied sequence of contrasting forms that create stable vitality with calmness, balances strength with flexibility, controlled energy with awareness. The calmness that comes from harmonious physical activity and mental perception, and the composure that comes from deep feeling and comprehension are at the very heart of this exercise.

Several hypotheses have been offered to explain the psychological benefits of exercise:

1. Exercise becomes a means for autohypnosis, which increases the tendency for creative visualization.

TABLE 6.1   **Calories Used by Everyday Activities**
Use an average of 200 calories a day by doing these activities and decrease your risk of disease and live longer, without ever going near a gym or treadmill.

| | Calories used in 10 minutes* | |
Activities	Women	Men
Walking fast	45	60
Painting	45	60
Weeding	45	60
Washing a car	45	60
Playing tag with a child	50	67
Mowing the lawn	55	73
Square dancing	55	73
Scrubbing floors	55	73
Hiking off-trail	60	80
Biking to work	60	80
Shoveling snow	60	80
Moving furniture	60	80
Walking upstairs	70	93
Cross-country skiing	80	106
Backpacking	80	106
Running upstairs	150	200

*Figures are for a 132-pound woman and a 176-pound man. All values are approximate and will vary from person to person.

FIGURE 6.2   The Sun Salute
This hatha yoga exercise is a series of twelve postures or asanas, intended to be done in one flowing routine. Each of the twelve postures is held three seconds.

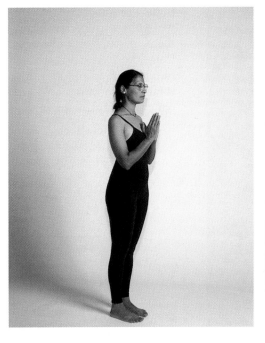

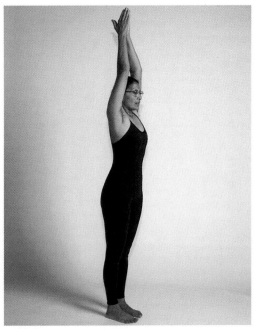

Position 1   Stand erect with your feet hip-width apart and palms together in front of your chest. Inhale and exhale slowly and calmly.

Position 2   Inhaling, raise your arms above your head, palms facing in. Lengthen through the spine, but do not arch your back.

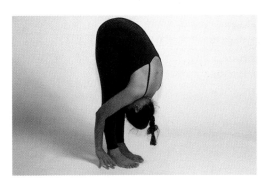

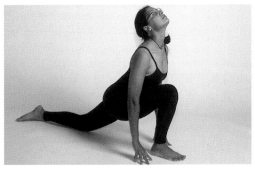

Position 3   Exhaling, bend forward from the hips, keeping your arms extended and your head hanging loosely between them. Keep your legs slightly bent and relax your neck and shoulders.

Position 4   Inhaling, bend both knees and place your palms flat on the floor by the outsides of your feet. Extend your right leg back. Stretch your chin toward the ceiling.

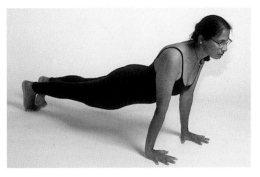

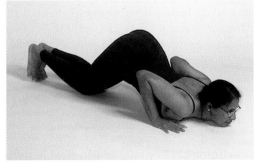

Position 5   Continue while holding the breath if you can—don't strain. Reach your forward leg back next to the other leg. Hold your body straight, supported by your hands and toes, with ankles, hips, and shoulders in a straight plane.

Position 6   Exhaling, lower your knees, chest, and chin or forehead to the floor, keeping your hips up and toes curled under.

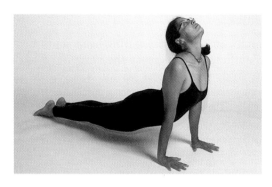

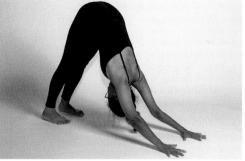

FIGURE 6.2   The Sun Salute (cont'd)
The entire routine should be done at least twice in succession, alternating the leg positions you use. The sun salute is an excellent way to stretch the body every morning or any time you may need to relax tense muscles and restore deep regular breathing. To view a video of the complete exercise visit

www   **www.jbpub.com/hwonline**

Position 7   Inhaling, bring the tops of your feet to the floor, straighten your legs, and come up to straight arms, opening the chest and stretching your chin toward the ceiling. Be careful not to overarch your lower back.

Position 8   Exhaling, curl your toes under and raise your hips into an inverted "V." Push back with your hands and lengthen your spine by reaching your hips upward. Keep your head hanging loosely.

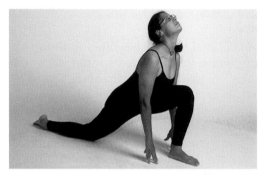

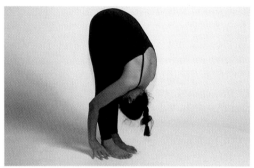

Position 9   Inhaling, lift your head and bring your right leg between your hands, keeping the left leg back. Raise your chin toward the ceiling.

Position 10   Exhaling, bring your left foot forward so your feet are together. Bend forward from the hips, keeping your legs slightly bent and your upper body relaxed. If you can, touch your head to your knees and place your palms beside your feet.

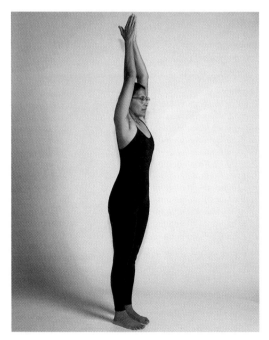

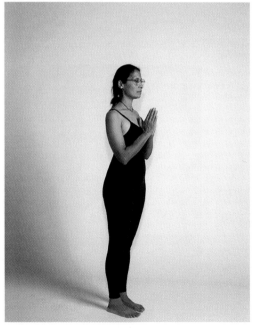

Position 11   Inhaling, slowly straighten up with your arms extended above your head. If you have any lower back pain, be sure to bend your knees.

Position 12   Exhaling, bring your hands together in front of you. Close your eyes for a moment and feel the sensations in your body.

2. Exercise increases the body's output of **epinephrine,** which produces feelings of euphoria.

3. Exercise changes the pattern of the secretion of brain neurotransmitters, particularly **norepinephrine,** which produces changes in mood.

4. Exercise increases the secretion of **endorphins** and **enkephalins,** hormone-like substances that can facilitate feelings of inner peace.

 ## Fitness and Conditioning

Sports physiologists define **fitness** as (a) adequate muscular strength and endurance to accomplish one's individual goals, (b) reasonable joint flexibility, (c) an efficient cardiovascular system, and (d) body weight and percent body fat within the normal range.

Because modern life-styles do not require much physical movement, few adults in industrial societies are fit. Rather, achieving fitness requires a commitment of time and energy to regular activities other than school, work (particularly sedentary work), and family responsibilities. To be fit, you must engage in activities that challenge the mind and body beyond what is required by a sedentary life-style.

There are a wide variety of conditioning programs or training regimens to improve fitness, but they tend to fall into two major categories: **aerobic training,** which increases the body's ability to use oxygen and improves endurance, and **strength training,** which enhances the size and strength of particular muscles and body regions.

Aerobic Training

Aerobic exercise involves stimulating heart and lungs for a period sufficient to increase the amount of oxygen that the body can process within a given time. Changes in physiology resulting from aerobic exercise are collectively called the **training effect.** Inducing the training effect involves exercising so that heart rate increases to between 60% and 80% of its theoretical maximum.

Three to four days of aerobic exercise per week is sufficient to produce a training effect. Two days per week may suffice for people already in good condition. One day a week does little to improve fitness and may increase the chances for injury. Also, exercise more than 5 days a week does little to increase fitness. It does expend calories, but it also makes one susceptible to injuries.

To obtain optimal training benefits you should exercise within your training heart-rate zone. The simplest method of computing this is to subtract your age from 220 to determine your maximum heart rate (MHR) and then multiply by 60% and 80%. While you exercise, your heart rate per minute should fall between these two values. For a 21-year-old, the target heart rate range would be 120 to 160 beats per minute (Table 6.2).

To measure your exercise heart rate, you should stop about 5 minutes into the aerobic part of your exercise to check your heart rate. Your heart rate should gradually increase during your warm-up, reach maximum level during your aerobic exercise, and gradually decrease during your cool-down exercises. Many activ-

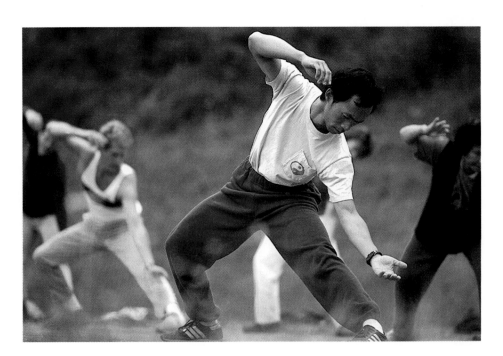

T'ai chi exercises help maintain physical fitness and mind-body harmony.

TABLE 6.2   Maximum and Target Heart Rates Predicted from Age
Take your pulse for 15 seconds immediately after exercising, and multiply by four. If heart rate is in the target range for your age, optimal training benefits have been obtained. If below target range, step up activity. If above the maximum, take it easier during workouts and gradually increase intensity.

Age (in years)	Predicted maximum heart rate (in beats per minute)	Target heart rate range (in beats per minute)
20	200	120–160
25	200	117–156
30	194	114–152
35	188	111–148
40	182	108–144
45	176	105–140
50	171	102–136
55	165	99–132
60	159	96–128
65	153	93–124

ities can provide aerobic conditioning, including walking, running, bicycling, swimming, cross-country skiing, rowing, basketball, racquetball, and soccer.

Strength Training

Strength training involves repetitively moving muscles against resistance, commonly applied by weights, such as barbells, dumbbells, and exercise machines, but also by simple pushing against an immovable object (**isometric training**). A stronger body is better able to combat fatigue; in sports, strength can improve athletic performance and reduce the likelihood of injury. For some, "pumping iron" helps release stress-induced muscle tensions.

Many people are drawn to strength training for cosmetic reasons. In their desire to look attractive, individuals may not receive adequate instruction in strength-training methods and may injure themselves. It is essential to build strength gradually with proper techniques.

Compared to most aerobic exercise, strength training produces only a modest improvement in cardiovascular fitness. The time spent exercising is insufficient to increase the heart rate long enough to produce a training effect. The energy expended during strength training is about four calories per minute, nearly the same as for walking or swimming at a comfortable pace.

A common myth associated with strength training is that consuming high-protein foods and special vitamin supplements will increase muscle mass. This assumption is incorrect. Muscle tissue responds to the demands of work, not to food. In a progressive strength-training regime, sufficient protein to build new muscle tissue will be obtained in a well-balanced diet. Excess protein and vitamins are simply excreted.

Drugs and Athletic Training

The saying "better living through chemistry" has invaded the gymnasium and practice field as some athletes turn to drugs (so-called "ergogenic" aids) to bulk up, increase strength and endurance, and enhance athletic performance. **Anabolic steroids** (testosterone and testosterone-like substances) are among the most abused substances by athletes. These drugs, however, are extremely dangerous. While they do increase muscle strength in both women and men, they also increase the risks of heart attack, stroke, liver damage, and cancer. Human growth hormone is another drug used by some athletes to increase muscle strength. Studies show, however, that this hormone is ineffective in increasing muscle mass. Any drug taken by injection carries the risk of transmitting HIV and hepatitis virus.

Creatine, a natural substance in muscle tissue required for muscle contraction, can be purchased as a nutritional supplement. Because creatine supplementation can delay the onset of fatigue in skeletal muscles and increases work capacity, many athletes use it to increase muscle mass and stamina. Laboratory studies show that creatine supplementation is more

Terms

epinephrine: hormone secreted principally by the adrenal medulla with a wide variety of functions, such as stimulating the heart, making carbohydrates available in the liver and muscles, and releasing fat from fat cells

norepinephrine: hormone that has many of the same effects as epinephrine

endorphins and **enkephalins:** morphine-like substances that are secreted by the brain that mitigate pain; produced during strenuous exercise and childbirth

fitness: the extent to which the body can respond to the demands of physical effort

aerobic training: exercise that increases the body's capacity to use oxygen

strength training: the use of resistance to increase one's ability to exert or resist force for the purpose of improving performance

training effect: beneficial physiological changes as a result of exercise

isometric training: another term for strength training

anabolic steroids: synthetic male hormones used to increase muscle size and strength

creatine: a natural substance in skeletal muscle tissue, which also can be taken in dietary supplement to enhance muscle performance

Managing Stress

Stages of Exercise-Induced Relaxed Concentration

Exercise is a great way to relieve stress. It reduces muscle tension; stimulates regular, deep breathing; increases blood levels of endorphins; and creates an opportunity to free the mind from worries. The next time you exercise, see if you can become aware of these four stages of *stress relief through exercise:*

Stage 1: Paying Attention

At the beginning of an exercise session, you focus your mind on the activity and allow any thoughts that arise to pass out of your mind. When you notice them, simply say to yourself, "Oh, I have a

thought," and bring yourself back to focusing on your activity.

Stage 2: Interested Attention

After a period of concentrating and letting go, you no longer have to concentrate on eliminating distractions, and you sense a flowing with the activity.

Stage 3: Absorbed Attention

Absorption with the activity is so great that it is very difficult for you to be distracted by what is going on around you. You may experience altered perceptions

of space and time, and your mind may move through thoughts and images without your direction. The experience can be dreamlike, except you are entirely awake and attentive.

Stage 4: Merging

You no longer are aware of any separation between you and what you are doing. The experience of union is complete: physical, mental, and spiritual. You attain a complete loss of self-consciousness, and even though you may be working your body very hard, mentally and spiritually you feel very calm.

---

effective on untrained individuals than on trained athletes, perhaps because the muscles of trained individuals are already working near peak efficiency without

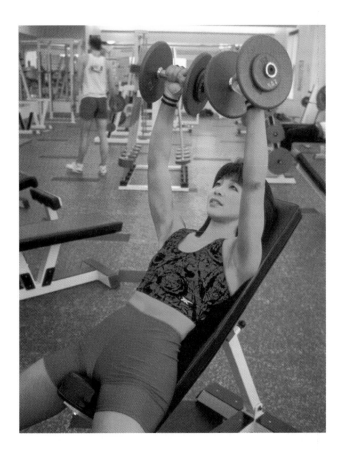

Weight-lifting builds muscle strength.

the supplement (Mujika and Padilla, 1997). In doses commonly used (3 to 5 g/day), creatine apparently is not harmful.

Making Physical Activity a Priority

For many people, the mere mention of physical activity conjures up unpleasant images of painfully boring exercises or rough competitive sports whose proposed beneficial effects on health and character development rarely seem to meet the promises made by enthusiastic players and coaches.

Part of the idea of physical activity is to incorporate a playful or joyful activity into your life for its own sake. Americans are highly product-oriented; we tend to value what we do on the basis of outcome. With physical activity the *process of doing* is itself the reward. So choose activities that you will enjoy. If you like to be around people, join an exercise class or organize some friends to work out with you. After you have accomplished a difficult task, reward yourself with praise. And remember, physical activity, even active sports, does not have to involve competition unless you want it to.

Choosing the Right Exercise

Once you have decided to begin exercising, it is tempting to do what others are doing (e.g., roller blading, jogging, racquetball). But before you go out and buy expensive running shoes and that new outfit, you must decide what exercise is right for you. First you may want to ask yourself what your goals are in an exercise program. Some goals may be: stress reduction; a healthy heart; weight control or weight reduction;

Wellness Guide

Getting into Shape

Undertake a program to increase aerobic conditioning by following these guidelines:

1. Frequency: you should exercise three to five times a week.

2. Intensity: you should exercise within 60% to 80% of your exercise heart rate.

3. Duration: you should exercise within your target zone for 20 to 60 minutes each time.

4. Type of exercise: appropriate exercises are rhythmic and continuous and use the large muscles of the legs and hips. Such exercises include walking, jogging, bicycling, swimming, cross-country skiing, and aerobic dancing.

5. Warm up and cool down. It is optimal to raise the body's core temperature about 1°F to 3°F by doing the warm up and stretching activities before the aerobic workout. After the aerobic workout, you should slow your heart rate and cool down for 30 to 60 minutes. Optimal time to stretch is when the muscles are warmed (i.e., after aerobic exercise).

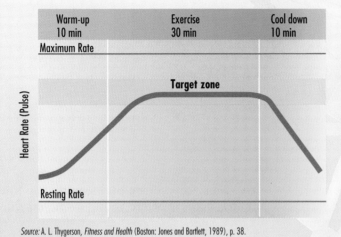

Source: A. L. Thygerson, *Fitness and Health* (Boston: Jones and Bartlett, 1989), p. 38.

greater strength; building muscles; greater stamina; or relaxation.

After you have determined your goals, you want to make sure that the activities you adopt go along with your goals. You may choose swimming as your main exercise. Swimming is good for weight maintenance, but not for body building. Other important factors when selecting your exercise of choice are: motivation; realistic expectations; comfort; convenience; and cost factors.

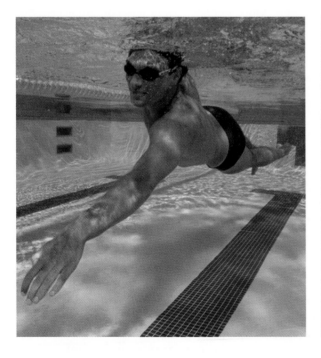

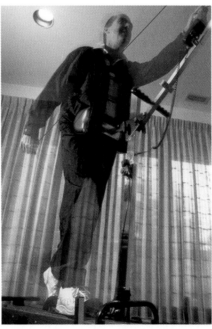

When choosing an exercise, pick one that's fun and convenient for you.

Wellness Guide

What's Your Excuse? Changing the Attitudes That Block Exercising

Excuse	New Attitude
Exercise is work.	I'm going to do something active that I enjoy and that makes me feel good.
I don't have time.	I can always find 5 or 10 minutes here and there to move my body, even if it's just for a short walk.
I'm too tired.	I don't feel like it now, but I know that after I exercise I always feel better.
I'll fail.	If I start slowly and do what I can, that is success enough. Being healthy and well is not a contest.
I'm too old.	Too old for what? I just want to enjoy myself.
I'm too heavy.	I always feel better after I move my body.
Exercise is boring.	I can make exercise interesting by choosing an activity I like, and doing it with a friend or while listening to the radio.
It's too cold (icy, rainy, hot, etc.).	I'll exercise at home by stretching out, or maybe I'll take a walk at the mall.

To be sure you can commit to an exercise class, take a trial class before signing up for several months. Make sure you enjoy the exercise. You should be able to enjoy working out and getting in shape at the same time. The more you enjoy what you are doing, the more likely you will stay motivated and continue to exercise and meet your fitness goals.

If you have never exercised or are not in good shape, do not expect to see results overnight. Achieving physical fitness takes time and consistency. Changes will most likely be seen in the first month; however, achieving total physical fitness will take months of constant exercise.

> *Beware all enterprises that require new clothes.*
> HENRY DAVID THOREAU

For some people, a fitness club or recreation center can be intimidating if everyone else is in good shape. Some find more informal "shaping-up" classes better for them. However, for others, being surrounded by a lot of physically fit people in a fitness club is motivating. Some may wish to stay at home and exercise. You need to decide in what environment you feel comfortable exercising.

Make sure whatever activity you choose is convenient. Don't choose one that requires you to drive 30 minutes, because before you know it you will be saying "it's too far." Choose an activity within a convenient distance.

Decide how much money you can afford to spend. Remember to include the cost of equipment, proper clothing, and transportation. Look into exercise classes that allow you to pay as you go; or find a fitness club that will allow you to join for a one-month trial program. Both options are good if you are still unsure about which exercise program is right for you.

Types of Beneficial Exercises

Different kinds of exercises provide different benefits. After you have determined your goal(s) and your method of exercise, you must make sure the exercise provides the type of benefit you wish to achieve. There are exercises that help relieve stress, aid the heart, control weight, define muscles, improve strength, increase power and **endurance,** and maintain **flexibility.** You may choose one or more of these; you decide.

Exercising for Stress Reduction   Exercise is a form of positive stress; one of its effects is to cancel the negative emotional stresses that accumulate daily. Almost any exercise where you work out for at least one-half hour is effective. Pleasant surroundings also help in relieving stress. Swimming is soothing and relaxing for many people; others enjoy jogging.

Exercising for Your Heart   Aerobic exercises are considered the most effective in terms of increasing heart capacity. Thirty minutes is what most studies believe is the magic number to produce maximum benefits

Terms

endurance: the ability to work out over a period of time without fatigue

flexibility: the ability of a joint to move through its range of motion

warm-up: low-intensity exercise done before full-effort physical activity to improve muscle and joint performance, prevent injury, reinforce motor skills, and maximize blood flow to the muscles and heart

cool-down: light or mild exercise immediately following competition or a training session; the primary purpose is to speed the removal of lactic acid from the muscles and allow the body to gradually return to a resting state

Wellness Guide

A Plan for Fitness

Here are some guidelines to keep in mind when incorporating any kind of physical activity into your life:

1. **Have a plan.** Before beginning any body work program, you need to develop a plan and commit yourself to it for a reasonable amount of time. To make a plan that will help you achieve your personal goals, you can consult a high school or college coach, attend an exercise class, or follow the plan in one of the "how to" books that have been written for almost every activity.

2. **Get a physical checkup.** If you have been inactive for many months or have concerns about your body's ability to perform at the level you would like, you may want to have a physician check you over.

3. **Accomplish goals.** The goal of any body work program is attainment of complete mind-body harmony. This can be done by progressively attaining higher and higher goals. It is customary in our culture to measure progress by "how far" and "how fast." Such goals might be suitable for competitive athletes, but they are unsuitable for people who engage in body work activities for the purpose of receiving greater enjoyment from living. For most of us, personal goals based on such questions as "Does this level of activity make me feel good?" or "Does this help me toward my goal of losing weight?" make more sense than blind adherence to a stopwatch.

4. **Progress slowly.** Slow, deliberate progress gives you the opportunity to integrate your body work activity into your normal life routine. Begin slowly; don't impulsively try to run a long distance the first day.

5. **Warm up and cool down.** All body work activity should be preceded by a brief period of stretching, breathing, and relaxation to prepare your mind and body to receive the utmost benefit and pleasure from body work. This is a good time to focus attention on how your body feels. When you have finished your body work activity, it is a good idea to let your body cool down slowly. If you have been involved in strenuous aerobic exercise, slowly reduce the pace of your activity until your heart rate and breathing return to almost normal. By slowly reducing your activity level you help prevent muscle cramps that sometimes occur when strenuous activity is suddenly stopped. You can prevent later muscle stiffness by doing a few stretching exercises to loosen the muscles that have worked hard during exercise. While cooling down, try to focus your attention on the sensations that your body work has brought you.

---

from aerobics (this 30 minutes does not include the **warm-up** or **cool-down** periods).

Exercising to Maintain Weight Regular physical activity carried out consistently over many months (indeed, for life) is the key to weight management and weight reduction (see chapter 5). When you exercise regularly, not only do you expend calories, but you also tend not to use food to relieve stress-related mental tension: you tend to eat less in general. It requires the expenditure of 3500 calories to lose one pound of body fat. That is the equivalent of walking for about 14.6 hours (walking expends 4 calories per minute) or jogging about 8 hours (jogging expends about 7 calories per minute). Anyone on a weight-loss program needs both to reduce the consumption of needless calories and increase significantly the time devoted to physical activity. This is why achieving *and maintaining* weight loss takes time and perseverance.

Exercising for Strength Body building generally means weight training with light barbells, dumbbells, and weight machines. In strength training, you use many of the same techniques as those for building muscles. The difference between muscle building and strength building is that less weight and more repetitions are used with strength building. In other words, instead of lifting 100 pounds 10 times, you might lift 10-pound weights 50 times: the same amount of body work builds strength instead of bulk muscle.

Exercising for Endurance and Power Endurance is your body's ability to withstand stress over a period of time, and power is your muscles' ability to perform over an extended period of time. Endurance is built by gradually increasing the length of time of strenuous activity, whereas power is achieved by short bursts of strenuous activity followed by rest periods. Sports not suitable for strength and endurance are softball and golf.

Exercising for Flexibility Calisthenics and yoga are great for flexibility. Keep in mind that flexibility should not be confused with fitness; flexibility is part of fitness, but flexibility exercises alone do not make a person physically fit. Almost all sports and exercises will increase flexibility. Stretching exercises should be incorporated into all sports activities and workouts (Figure 6.3).

Text continued on p. 118

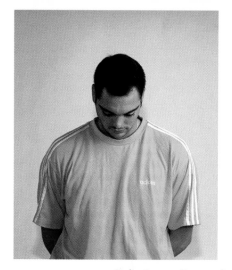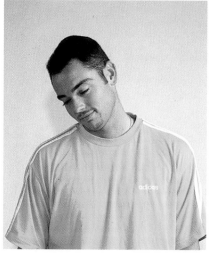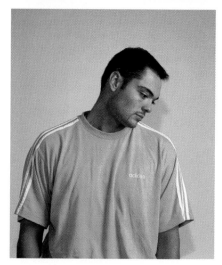

Neck   Drop your chin to your chest. Turn your head as far right as you can without moving your shoulders and hold. Repeat to the left. Tilt your head toward the left ear without bending your torso or hunching your shoulders and hold. Repeat to the right.

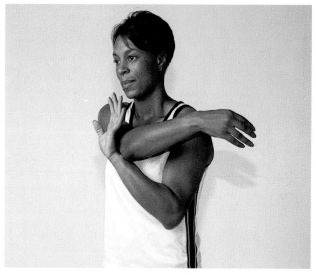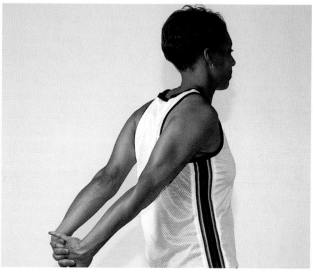

Shoulder Stretch 1   With your left hand, grasp your right elbow and pull your arm across your chest, keeping it bent at a 90° angle. Alternate arms.

Shoulder Stretch 2   Standing, grasp both arms behind your back and raise them up as far as you can.

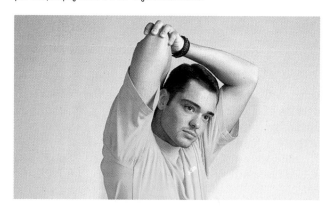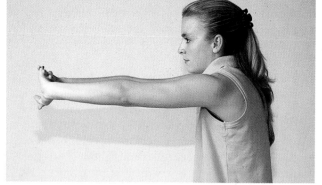

Triceps Stretch   Grasp the opposite elbow and pull the arm behind the head and down until a stretch is felt in the back of the arm. Hold and then repeat for the other arm.

Upper-back Stretch   Clasp your hands in front of your body, and press your palms forward.

FIGURE 6.3   **Flexibility Exercises**   It is best to do stretching exercises when the muscles are warm. You should stretch to the point of *mild* discomfort, but stop immediately if you experience pain—particularly in the lower back or knees. Hold all stretches for 15–30 seconds, rest for 30–60 seconds, and then repeat the stretch, trying to go a little further. For all standing stretches, legs should be hip-width apart, with knees slightly bent, back straight, and weight evenly distributed from the front to the back of the feet. To view a video of the exercises visit

   www.jbpub.com/hwonline

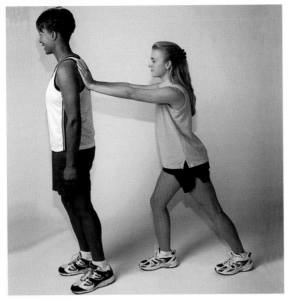

Calf Stretch   Stand approximately 2 to 3 feet away from a wall, tree, or stretching partner. Move one foot in close to the wall, while keeping the back leg straight behind you with the foot and heel flat on the ground. Slowly move your hips forward, bending the forward knee and keeping the back foot on the ground. You should feel a slight stretch in your calf muscles. Repeat with the opposite leg.

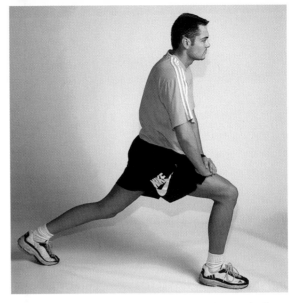

Lunge Stretch   Step forward and bend your forward knee, keeping it directly above your ankle. Stretch your other leg back behind you but don't lock your knee. Press your hips forward and down to stretch. Your arms can be at your sides, on top of your knee, or on the ground for balance. Repeat on the other side.

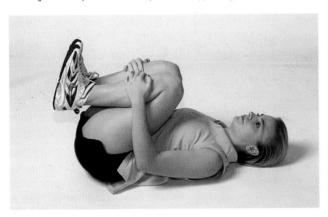

Low Back Stretch   Lie on your back and pull both knees in to the chest. Keep your lower back on the floor.

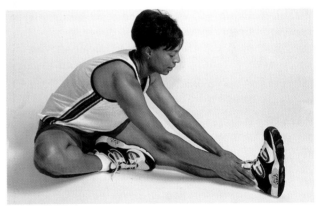

Modified Hurdler   Sit with your right leg straight out in front of you and your left leg tucked close to your body. Reach toward your right foot as far as possible. Do not curve your back. Go only as far as you can with a straight back. Repeat for the other leg.

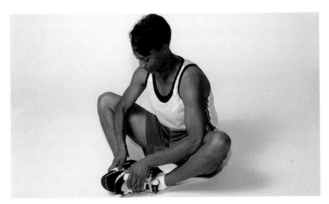

Groin Stretch   Sit with your back straight (don't slouch; you may want to put your back against a wall) and bend your legs, with the soles of your feet together. Try to get your heels as close to your groin as is comfortably possible. For a passive stretch, push your knees to the floor as far as you can (you may use your hands to assist but do not resist with the knees) and hold them there. This can be hard on the knees so please be careful. Now, keep your knees where they are, and then exhale as you bend over, trying to get your chest as close to the floor as possible.

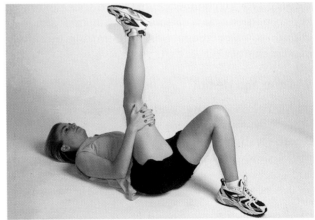

Supine Hamstring Stretch   Lie on your back and pull one leg up to a stretched position. The leg should remain as straight as possible. The opposite leg should be bent with the heel on the floor; keep your lower back on the floor. Alternate legs.

Wellness Guide

Common Overuse Injuries

Strain: Commonly referred to as "pulled muscles" or "pulled tendons." Caused by overstretching, tearing, or ripping of a muscle and/or its tendon

Tendonitis: Inflammation of a tendon caused by

chronic, low-grade strain of a muscle-tendon unit

Bursitis: Inflammation of the lubricating sac (*bursa*) that surrounds a joint caused by repeated low-grade strain of the joint's supporting tissues

Sprain: Overstretching or tearing of ligaments

Blisters: Fluid-filled swellings on the skin caused by friction from the rubbing of skin against shoes, clothing, and equipment

Don't ask your muscles to do more than they can. Relishing the pain of overexertion—"going for the burn"—is dangerous. This pain is the body's message that something is wrong, not that the exerciser is lazy. If you want to increase your performance, build muscle strength slowly, following a supervised regime. Also, preactivity and postactivity stretching helps to prevent damage to muscles and joints. Injuries are more likely if equipment such as weights and other kinds of apparatus are improperly used or are in disrepair.

Most people participate in physical activity because (a) they want to have fun, (b) they want to gain a sense of accomplishment by doing something well, and (c) they want to feel physically and psychologically better. While pursuing these goals, no one wants to be hurt. It turns out that maximizing the "have fun, do well, feel good" aspects of exercise and minimizing the potential for injury go together. Physical activity is most satisfying when you are totally absorbed in it, when your body responds readily to your commands, when you run or play with confidence, and when your equipment and conditions are optimal. Take sports seriously enough to enjoy them, while minimizing the likelihood of injuries.

> *When I feel a desire to exercise, I lie down until it goes away.*
> W. C. FIELDS

Walking and Health

If jogging, swimming, cycling, aerobic dancing, and other strenuous activities aren't for you, try walking. Regular walking contributes many of the health benefits of other activities. And walking has advantages that other activities do not: other than appropriate shoes, no special clothing or equipment is required, and walking can be fit easily into a busy schedule.

Walking contributes the most to health when it is done regularly (about four times a week) for a minimum of 20 minutes each day. How strenuous the walk should be depends on the desires and physical abilities of the walker. Most of the benefits can be derived by walking between two and four miles per hour. Aerobic capacity can be increased by walking briskly enough to increase the heart rate.

Exercise Abuse

Although few would argue that being fashionably healthy and attractive are desirable goals, many people are so zealous in pursuing these goals that they harm themselves. For example, some individuals place higher priority on running or other fitness activities than they do on work, family, interpersonal relationships, and even their own health. Some are unwilling to stop exercising (even for a day!) to attend to other matters in life or to allow an exercise injury to heal properly. In their attempts to attain the "perfect body," a large number of women exercise and lose weight to such extremes that they stop menstruating (**athletic amenorrhea**) or develop anorexia or bulimia (see chapter 5).

The most common form of exercise abuse is exercising a body part or the entire body beyond its biological limit, to the point of injury. Such injuries are referred to as **overuse syndromes.** Between 25% and 50% of athletes visiting sports medicine clinics may have sustained an overuse injury. Commonly, overuse injuries affect the skin and muscles, tendons, ligaments, and joints, which are constructed of fibrous bands of protein. These fibers can be torn if they are overloaded, as when lifting a heavy weight or running at top speed, or when forced to perform when fatigued. Damage can also occur by repeated small injuries that lead over time to a more serious problem. The common causes of overuse injuries are excessive exercising, faulty technique, and poor equipment.

Terms

athletic amenorrhea: irregular or cessation of menstruation due to excessive participation in athletics

overuse syndromes: injuries to muscles, tendons, ligaments, and joints resulting from too much exercise

All bodies are not anatomically capable of the same degree of physical exertion, especially the high performance exhibited by marathon runners or triathletes. The architecture of the body, the alignment of the legs, the capacity of the lungs, the size and strength of the bones and muscles, and other anatomical factors set limits on an individual's physical ability. Few people have the biological endowment to perform at championship levels. Physical activity can be much more enjoyable when you respect, accept, and appreciate your body's biological limits.

Critical Thinking About Health

1. Another Christmas Day at Grandma's. Well, almost. After everyone had eaten all they possibly could and all the children had ripped open their Christmas gifts, Suzanne's Uncle Ron sat next to her on the couch.

   "I understand that you're taking a health class at school," he said.

   "That's right," Suzanne replied.

   "Then tell me," Uncle Ron continued, "What's the best exercise? My New Year's resolution is to get back in shape, and I want to do it right this time. I'm joining the gym on January 2. What workouts do you recommend?"

   a. What advice should Suzanne give her uncle? Take into account that Uncle Ron has tried working out before, apparently without success. Uncle Ron is a 39-year-old telecommunications engineer who works long hours at a computer terminal when he's at his office. His job also requires him to travel, so he eats a lot of fast food. He is married and has three young children.

2. What are the effects on society and on organized sports of athletes using performance-enhancing drugs, even when such substances are legal?

3. How far? How fast? How much? How might questions such as these affect a person's attitude and approach to physical activity for health (i.e., not competition)? List a new set of questions that illustrate a noncompetitive perspective on physical activity for health.

Health in Review

- Being physically active helps us to be both physiologically and psychologically well.
- Physiological benefits from physical activity include increased efficiency and strength of heart, lungs, and muscles; more effective weight control; reduced fatigue and increased energy; a higher level of immunity; lower blood cholesterol levels; improved sugar metabolism; lower blood pressure; and improved posture.
- Psychological benefits from physical activity include: reduced fatigue and better sleep patterns; a more positive mental outlook; less stress; release of tension and anxiety; and improved self-image and self-confidence.
- Fitness is the extent to which the body can respond to the demands of physical effort. Aerobic training and strength training are major fitness categories.
- Aerobic conditioning may be achieved through walking, running, bicycling, swimming, cross-country skiing, rowing, basketball, racquetball, and soccer.
- Aerobic exercise strengthens the heart. Strength training produces only a modest improvement in cardiovascular fitness, but builds muscle strength, unlike aerobic conditioning.
- Goals for an exercise program may include stress reduction; a healthy heart; weight control or maintenance; greater strength; muscle-building; greater stamina; or relaxation.
- The most common form of exercise abuse is exercising a body part or the entire body beyond its biological limit to the point of injury. Common injuries include strain, tendonitis, bursitis, sprain, and blisters.

Health and Wellness Online

The World Wide Web contains a wealth of information about health and wellness. By accessing the Internet using Web browser software, such as Netscape Navigator or Microsoft's Internet Explorer, you can gain a new perspective on many topics presented in *Essentials of Health and Wellness, Second Edition.* Access the Jones and Bartlett Publishers web site at http://www.jbpub.com/hwonline.

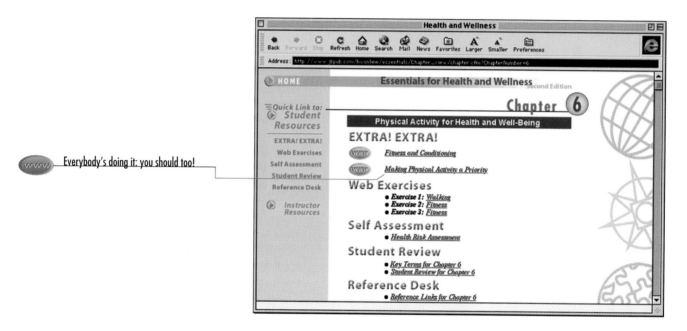

References

Blair, S. N., Kohl, H. W., Gordon, N. F., & Paffenbarger, Jr, R. S. (1992). How much physical activity is good for health? *Annual Review of Public Health, 13,* 99–126.

Blair, S. N., Kohl, H. W., Paffenbarger, R. S., Clark, D. G., Cooper, K. H., & Gibbons, L. W. (1989). Physical fitness and all cause mortality: A prospective study of healthy men and women. *Journal of the American Medical Association, 262(17),* 2395–2401.

Delza, Sophia. (1996). *The tai chi chuan experience: Reflections and perceptions on body-mind harmony.* New York: State University of New York Press.

Hakim, A., Petrovitch, H., Burchfiel, C. M., Ross, G. W., Rodriguez, B. L., White, L. R., Yano, K., Curb, J. D., & Abbott, R. D. (1998). Effects of walking on mortality among nonsmoking retired men. *The New England Journal of Medicine, 338,* 94–9.

Mujika, I., & Padilla, S. (1997). Creatine supplementation as an ergogenic aid for sports performance in highly trained athletes. *International Journal of Sports Medicine, 18,* 491–496.

Pate, R. R., et al. (1995). Physical activity and public health: A recommendation from the Centers for Disease Control and Prevention and the American College of Sports Medicine. *Journal of the American Medical Association, 273(5),* 402–407.

U.S. Department of Health and Human Services, Centers for Disease Control and Prevention, National Center for Chronic Disease Prevention and Health Promotion, & President's Council on Physical Fitness and Sports. (1996). *Physical activity and health: A report of the Surgeon General* (017-023-00196-5). Washington, DC: U.S. Government Printing Office.

Suggested Readings

Applewhite, M. P., Jansen, G. R., Marriot, M. M., & Breen, V. M. (1994). The effects of diet on performance—an initial review. *Journal of the American Medical Association, 271(2),* 98–99. A review of the literature to determine the effects of diet on performance. The article discusses The Institute of Medicine's Food and Nutrition Board's review of diet and performance.

How fit are you? (1997). *Consumer Reports on Health, 9(7),* 27–31. How to improve your strength, aerobic capacity, flexibility, and balance.

Jaret, P., & Fahey, V. (1994). The old advice: Work out. The new advice: Walk the dog and take the stairs. *Health, 8(5),* 62. Discusses how the definition of physical activity and exercise has changed. It includes anything from raking the leaves to roughhousing with the kids.

Optimal workouts. (1997). *UC Berkeley Wellness Letter, 13(7),* 6–7. Advice on the best workout programs.

U.S. Department of Health and Human Services, Centers for Disease Control and Prevention, National Center for Chronic Disease Prevention and Health Promotion, & President's Council on Physical Fitness and Sports. (1996). *Physical activity and health: A report of the Surgeon General* (017-023-00196-5). Washington, DC: U.S. Government Printing Office.

Walk away pounds. (1997). *Weight Watchers Magazine, 30(2),* 64–66. Walking instructions and advice on proper shoes and clothing.

Making *Healthy Changes*

Eating is one of the great pleasures in life. Because of the enormous variety of foods that are available to us, most of us overeat, especially foods that do not contribute to a nutritious diet and to health. Our cells, organs, and bodies require dozens of different elements and thousands of different molecules to perform the chemical reactions that keep us alive and well. All of the essential chemicals *must* come from the diet. If even one essential mineral, vitamin, amino acid, or lipid is in short supply, your body cannot function optimally. If one of these components is completely missing or present in less than needed amounts for extended periods of time, disease results.

I recall an experiment that was done in one of my grammar school classes more than half a century ago. Such an experiment cannot be done today because it is unethical and probably illegal. But it taught me something important about food and health. The teacher brought in a couple of mice in a cage. For several weeks, we all gathered around the cage every morning to observe the activity of the mice on an exercise wheel, to watch them eat, and to clean and fill their water dish.

After several weeks, the teacher asked us to make a list of our favorite foods. The list included candy, sodas, cake, chips, popcorn, and other goodies. Then the teacher asked us what we thought would happen if we changed the diet of the mice from the prepared pellets that they had been eating to a diet of our favorite foods. Nobody in the class knew, although one girl guessed that the mice would get cavities. So the teacher proposed an experiment and explained that experiments were performed by scientists to answer questions such as the one the teacher had posed.

The next day, each child brought in a supply of his or her favorite food. The teacher replaced the pellets with a mixture of our favorite foods. We were delighted to watch the mice gobble up the foods we liked to eat. Each day we gathered around the cage to watch the mice. After about a week, they were not using the exercise wheel and just lay around most of the time. After another week, their fur began to fall out. One morning when we came in, one mouse was dead. The other mouse died a few days later.

The teacher explained what had happened. The mice did not starve to death; in fact, they had too much to eat. But the foods that they were eating did not contain nutrients essential to life. That's how we were taught about the importance of fruits and vegetables in our diet and what the term "junk food" really means.

Wise Consumer: Become Aware of the Power of Advertising

Because a significant portion of everyone's income is used to purchase food and beverages, companies spend billions of dollars each year to convince us to buy their cereal, soda, potato chips, cookies, pizza, and so forth. Often, the advertised food is a high-profit item low in nutritional value, such as potato chips. Potatoes cost about $0.60 a pound in the supermarket or about $0.30 a pound wholesale. An 8 oz bag of potato chips contains less than $0.15 worth of potatoes. If you pay $1.50 for the bag, most of the money goes to packaging, advertising, and profit. In general, you will be healthier (and wealthier) if you spend your money on unprocessed, fresh foods.

The greater the variety of foods in the diet, the more nutritious the diet. Whole grains, fresh fruits and vegetables, nuts, seeds, milk, cheese, soy products, along with fish and a moderate amount of meat will ensure a varied diet and improved health. Buying heavily advertised food products means that most of what you pay goes to advertising agencies and to corporate profits—not to improving your health.

You can find out the complete nutritional value of almost any food or food product by contacting the USDA Nutrient Database at www.nal.usda.gov/fnic/foodcomp. Make a list of 10 advertised foods that you eat regularly and find out their nutritional content by using the USDA database. Try to find similar unprocessed foods that you could eat instead of the advertised products and compare their nutritional values. Describe in your journal any changes in diet that you make as a result of using the USDA Nutrient Database.

Improving Your Diet: Add Color to Your Diet

Most of us eat a limited variety of fruits and vegetables—bananas and oranges, lettuce and cucumbers, potatoes and tomatoes. But there are literally hundreds of different fruits and vegetables that are offered in today's markets, especially if you have access to farmer's markets or to Asian markets. Colors of fruits and vegetables range from purple (eggplant, pomegranate, purple sweet potatoes, grapes) to red (beets, red peppers, rhubarb, red grapefruit) to orange (pumpkin, can-

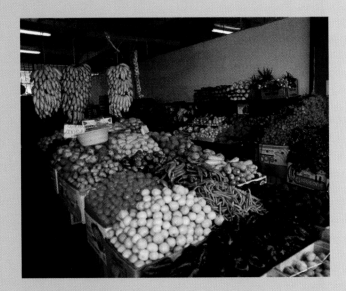

teloupe, oranges, carrots) to yellow (mango, papaya, squash, onion, yellow peppers) to every shade of green.

Make a list of five fruits or vegetables, each of a different color, that you seldom or never eat. Buy enough of each for a few servings. Add one new color to your diet for five consecutive days. If the fruit or vegetable needs to be cooked, consult a cookbook to find ways to prepare it. (Many vegetables such as eggplant, zucchini, onion, tomato, and so forth are delicious if marinated overnight and grilled over hot charcoal. Also, stir frying is a great way to cook a mixture of vegetables.) If you're eating in a dining hall, select different fruits and vegetables in side dishes. Eat more often from the salad bar.

Describe in your journal the new fruits and vegetables that you chose and how they were prepared. Describe your reaction to these new foods. If there were some that you did not like, find another of the same or similar color. The importance of having differently colored fruits and vegetables in the diet is that they contain different essential chemicals that contribute to the body's overall nutrition and health.

Physical Activity: Beginning to Exercise (For Those Who Do Not)

If you are overweight or physically inactive, or both, then this is a good way to begin increasing your physical activity: walking, just walking. You don't need special shoes or clothes, and you certainly don't need a Walkman plugged into your ear to cut you off from experiencing the environment. When you exercise, you become aware of your body's movements, discovering where it is stiff or uncomfortable. You become aware of your breathing and muscles that have not been used in some time.

Pick a route near home, school, or work that you can walk briskly in 15–20 minutes—away from traffic if possible. Find a convenient time four or five times a week when you can perform this walk and do it faithfully. While you are walking (not running yet), be aware of your surroundings and notice as many details along the way as you can. The movement and the mental attention will help to reduce stress and give you energy for other tasks.

Once you have begun to walk on a regular basis, find other occasions in your daily activities where you can increase your physical activity. For example, stop taking elevators if you have to go up or down only a few floors. Perhaps there are occasions when you could walk to do an errand rather than drive. Describe in your journal how you feel on your walk and any other changes in physical activity that you have made, such as not using an elevator or using a bike to run errands.

Wise Consumer: Beware of Weight Loss Advertising

Because so many Americans eat excessive amounts of food, about one-third of the population is overweight and has increased health risks. Two enormous industries profit from the excessive American appetites: food companies and diet companies. Food companies urge you to buy and eat their products often, especially snacks and "fast foods." Some restaurants offer an "all you can eat" menu, thereby urging you to eat more than you need or want. After you have been encouraged to overeat and overconsume, the diet industry is eager to take the rest of your money by selling you weight reduction schemes and devices.

The fact is that *no* innovative diet, *no* weight-loss device, and *no* appetite-suppressant pill can produce sustained weight loss. Consuming less food and exercising more is the *only* way to lose weight permanently.

To appreciate how advertising appeals to peoples' desire to lose weight effortlessly, following are excerpts from a newspaper advertisement showing how overweight consumers are enticed into wasting their money on weight-loss pills.

The biggest headline in the advertisement is "guarantees rapid weight-loss." This tells you what you want to hear—losing weight is fast and guaranteed. Next, the magic weight-loss pill "contains no drugs" (so, of course, it's safe) and comes from the exotic East. Then comes the "medical tests and scientific studies," which prove the magic substance in the pill really works. And, of course, weight loss should be accomplished without effort, so the "weight-loss pill does all the work."

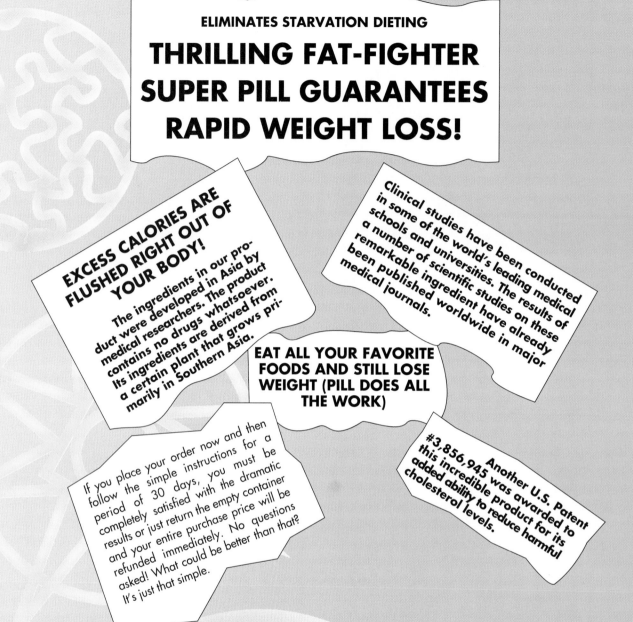

ELIMINATES STARVATION DIETING

THRILLING FAT-FIGHTER SUPER PILL GUARANTEES RAPID WEIGHT LOSS!

EXCESS CALORIES ARE FLUSHED RIGHT OUT OF YOUR BODY!

The ingredients in our product were developed in Asia by medical researchers. The product contains no drugs whatsoever. Its ingredients are derived from a certain plant that grows primarily in Southern Asia.

Clinical studies have been conducted in some of the world's leading medical schools and universities. The results of a number of scientific studies on these remarkable ingredient have already been published worldwide in major medical journals.

EAT ALL YOUR FAVORITE FOODS AND STILL LOSE WEIGHT (PILL DOES ALL THE WORK)

If you place your order now and then follow the simple instructions for a period of 30 days, you must be completely satisfied with the dramatic results or just return the empty container and your entire purchase price will be refunded immediately. No questions asked! What could be better than that? It's just that simple.

Another U.S. Patent #3,856,945 was awarded to this incredible product for its added ability to reduce harmful cholesterol levels.

And why not also get money from people with normal weight but who have high cholesterol levels? That's accomplished by the U.S. patent, which suggests to you that the government is impressed by the usefulness of this product. Finally, to make you rush your order is the "unconditional money-back guarantee if you're not satisfied after 30 days."

Most people are too embarrassed to ask for their money back—they figure it's their fault the product didn't work for them. Those who do ask for their money back probably will find that the phone number has been disconnected or they will be put on hold until next Christmas.

It's easy to make fun of weight-loss advertising, but millions of overweight Americans are desperate enough to pay billions of dollars every year to try anything that promises to help them lose weight without much effort. Describe in your journal any diet or weight-loss products you have purchased. Did any of them help you?

Soda Update

Write an update in your journal on how you are doing with cutting back or eliminating sodas from your diet. How much money is in your anti-soda fund? Here's a calculation that might motivate you: If you are 18 years old now and take $2 a day that you would spend on sodas and put it into a savings account earning just 2% interest compounded quarterly, by age 65 you would have $56,283.45. If you put the same amount into stocks or bonds with an estimated annual return of 8%, at age 65 you would have accumulated $352,235.16. Does that make your soda fund worth the effort to quit?

Emotional Wellness: Imagine Yourself Thin

Stress at home, school, or work can lead to poor diet and increased intake of fattening foods. Although it is true that you *must* expend more calories than you take in to lose weight over a period of time, there also is no question that the mind plays an essential role in how much you eat and the kind of foods you purchase. The mind usually ignores direct negative suggestions such as, "I will not overeat. I will not smoke anymore. I will not be so lazy or inactive." However, the mind does accept subtle suggestions, which can produce a significant change in behavior and health. The following imagery and mental suggestions can help you lose weight if you are overweight.

Many people enjoy shopping for clothes. Women know what size dresses they usually wear; men know what waist measurement they need to look for in selecting pants. A person who is overweight frequently tries on clothes that are too small, hoping that they will fit. Here's where imagery can help.

Find a quiet, comfortable spot. Sit or lie down. Close your eyes. Let your mind go to one of your favorite stores where you shop for clothes. Let your mind find some jeans or another garment that you really like. But as you hold the garment up to see how it

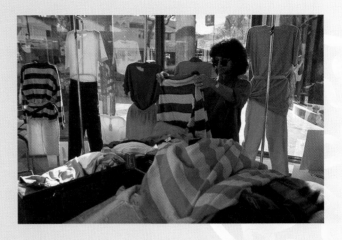

might look on you, notice that "large," which is the size that you normally wear, seems too big; "medium" seems as if it would be a better fit. Notice that you are picking clothes off the rack that are one to two sizes smaller than you usually wear. Notice how good you feel to be able to wear a smaller size than before. As you look at the clothes, notice what your body feels like now that you have lost weight and can fit into smaller sizes. You can make this image as detailed as your mind wants; be creative in the clothes you are choosing or the stores where you shop.

This mental visualization exercise should be repeated every day for at least 5 to 10 minutes. A longer time is fine if your mind is enjoying your mental shopping trip. You may want to bring along a friend who comments on how nice you look since you lost weight. If you practice this exercise, describe in your journal any changes in weight, exercise, or eating behaviors that you noticed.

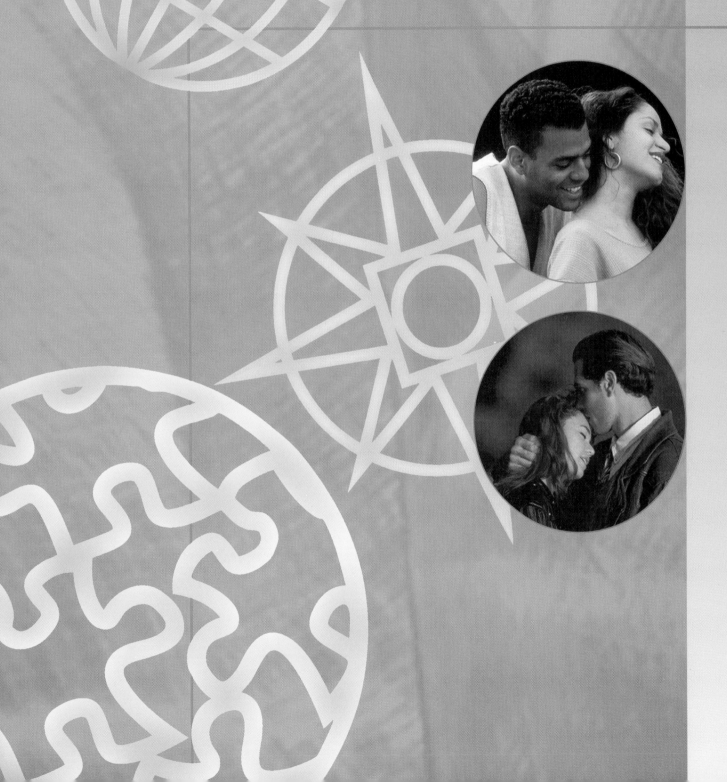

Building Healthy Relationships

Exercises and Activities

WORKBOOK
An Assessment of Sexual Communication
Gender Roles in Society

Health and Wellness Online

 www.jbpub.com/hwonline

Sexual Arousal and Response
Developing Positive Sexual Relationships
Pregnancy
Infertility
Adoption

Chapter 7

Understanding Sexuality and Pregnancy

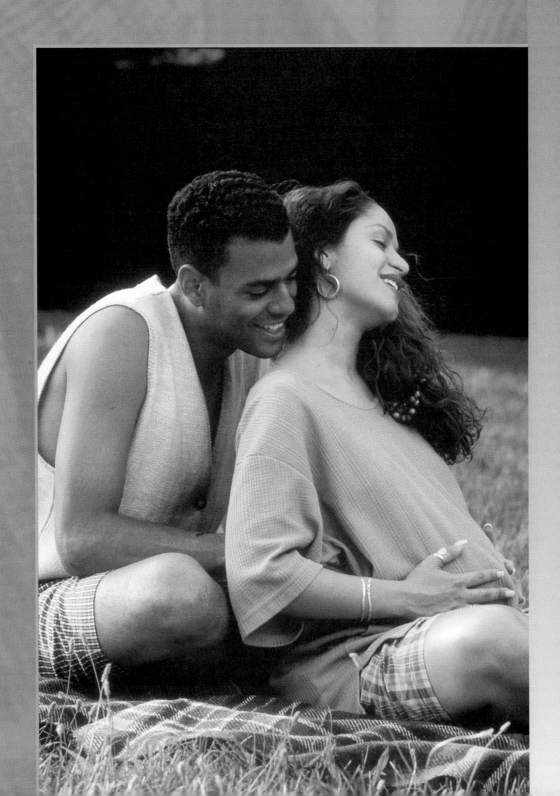

Sexuality represents a truly holistic aspect of living, for it involves the simultaneous expression of mind, body, and spirit—the whole self. Although sexuality is commonly represented in advertising and other media as having to do solely with physical gratification, most people are aware that sexuality involves much more than the stimulation of the body's sex organs. Sexuality involves thoughts, feelings, and identity. Sexuality is also a powerful form of communication between people.

> *Love is a great exaggeration of the worth of one individual over the worth of everybody else.*
> GEORGE BERNARD SHAW

From the standpoint of personal health, sexuality is an area over which you have considerable individual control. You choose when and with whom you wish to have sex, and which feelings you wish to express in sexual ways. With some fundamental knowledge of sexual biology, you can conduct your sexual life responsibly, thus avoiding unnecessary illness and exercising a choice of whether and when to have children.

Defining Sex and Sexuality

Sex

Sex can refer to (a) an individual's classification as male or female as determined by the presence of certain anatomical and physiological characteristics, (b) a set of behaviors, and (c) the experience of erotic pleasure.

At the most fundamental biological level, sex refers to the mating of two anatomically distinct individuals, a male and a female, each of which manufactures specific cells, or **gametes,** which fuse to become the first cell of a new individual. To facilitate the fusion process (called **fertilization**), males and females possess specific organs and display certain behaviors that are intended to bring about the union of gametes.

Often the word *sex* is used to denote aspects of an individual's personal characteristics that are thought to derive from her or his biological classification. Thus, the biological property of "femaleness" is associated with the social quality of "femininity," and the biological property of "maleness" is associated with the social quality of "masculinity." Although most modern dictionaries still define sex as having to do with personality characteristics, this concept is more accurately referred to as *gender* to distinguish its origins in culture rather than biology.

Besides biological classification, sex is also associated with certain behaviors that are defined as **sexual.** These activities usually involve touching in various ways certain anatomical regions of the body, such as the genitalia and breasts, and sexual intercourse.

Sex can also mean erotic pleasure, a certain kind of experience with unique and identifiable qualities that distinguish it from other kinds of pleasure, such as the satisfaction of hunger or the enjoyment of music. A variety of circumstances and events has the potential to activate the erotic pleasure centers, including certain kinds of tactile stimulation (e.g., touching, kissing) of certain body regions (e.g., mouth, breasts, genitals); certain kinds of visual, olfactory, and auditory stimulation; and fantasy. Potentially erotic stimuli become actual erotic stimuli when other centers in the brain interpret them as erotic. That is why not every touch, kiss, or potentially sexual situation is erotically arousing.

Sexuality

Sexuality, as distinct from sex, consists of the aspects of a person's sense of self that are used to create sexual experiences. Another term for sexuality is the sexual self, which has several dimensions:

1. The *physical dimension* refers to any region of the body to which an individual gives sexual meaning, including the organs and organ systems that one employs to create erotic experiences (e.g., the skin, genitals). It also includes the physical features that define oneself to oneself and to others as a sexual being.

2. The *psychological dimension* refers to emotions and conscious and unconscious beliefs that guide the interpretation of experience. This aspect of sexuality generates strategies for actions that are intended to satisfy the individual's wants and needs.

3. The *social dimension* refers to sexual attitudes and behaviors that affect an individual's interactions with members of the social groups to which she or he belongs.

4. The *orientation dimension* refers to the tendency to feel most "naturally" sexually attracted to, and the ability to emotionally bond with, members of a particular gender. About 85% to 90% of Americans are oriented to members of the opposite sex; the rest of the population orients to individuals of either sex (bisexuals) or, more often, exclusively to members of the same sex (homosexuals). Individuals do not choose their sexual orientation; it develops as a fundamental aspect of a person's personality. Scientific studies are being undertaken to determine any genetic, hormonal, metabolic, or psychological mechanisms underlying sexual orientation.

5. The *developmental dimension* is the evolution of oneself throughout a lifetime. This evolution includes the body, belief systems, and the ways sex is employed to create and maintain intimacy.

6. The *skill dimension* speaks to the physical and social skills that affect how well one meets one's sexual wants and needs.

Gender Identity and Gender Role

Although anatomy and physiology explain the biological bases of human sexuality, most people's sexual experiences also involve beliefs, thoughts, feelings, and social behaviors. How individuals come to think and behave sexually is almost entirely a product of what they learn as children about the kinds of behaviors that are expected of members of one sex or the other. Studies of psychosexual development indicate that the development of gender identity and the subsequent expression of sex-specific behaviors begins with the sex typing of newborn infants. When a child is born, almost the first thing noticed is its biological sex as determined by the appearance of its external genitals. If the infant is born with a penis, those attending the birth will exclaim "It's a boy!" Similarly, "It's a girl!" follows the observation of a newborn's female external genitals.

Having been sex typed at birth, the infant is thereafter treated by adults in a manner they think is appropriate for a child of that sex, and eventually the infant incorporates into his or her self-image the awareness of being a male or a female. This awareness, called **gender identity,** refers to our own personal, subjective sense that "I am a male" or "I am a female." **Gender role** refers to a collection of attitudes and behaviors that are considered normal and appropriate in a culture. Gender roles establish sex-related behavioral expectations that people are expected to fulfill. By about the age of two, a child's gender is fixed for life.

Defining Sexual Orientation

A person's **sexual orientation** is his or her attraction toward and interest in members of one or both genders. A **heterosexual** is a person who is attracted to someone of the opposite gender. A **homosexual** is attracted to someone of the same gender. Therefore, a homosexual's gender identity agrees with his or her biological sex. That is, a homosexual person perceives himself or herself as male or female, respectively, and feels attraction toward a person of the same sex. A **bisexual** is someone who is attracted to members of both genders. The terms heterosexual and homosexual do not imply normalcy or a type of sexual act; they simply describe a person's preference with regard to one gender or another. The concept of sexual orientation and identity has evolved over time, as views of masculinity and femininity have changed. Today we view masculinity and femininity as a set of characteristics, which vary among both men and women.

A recent study of sexual practices in the United States tried to address the question, "How many people are homosexual?" (Lauman, Gagnon, Michael, and Michaels, 1994). Researchers asked a sample across the United States to self-report whether they considered themselves homosexual or heterosexual. About 1.4% of women and 2.8% of men reported same-gender sexuality. However, 6.2% of the heterosexual men reported being somewhat attracted to men, and 4.5% indicated the idea of sex with another man was appealing. Of the women, 5.6% reported finding the idea of sex with a woman appealing, and 4.4% reported sexual attraction to women.

Recent research has provided evidence for genetics as a basis for sexual orientation. Simon LeVay's research, in which he dissected and studied brains of 41

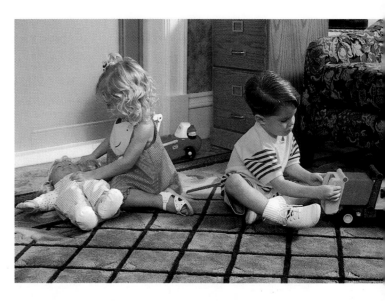

Often, children are taught early on how to "act" female or male.

Terms

sex: has several definitions: (a) an individual's classification as male or female based on anatomical characteristics; (b) a set of behaviors; (c) the experience of erotic pleasure

gametes: sex cells, either sperm or ova, that fuse at fertilization; gametes carry a complete set of genetic information from each parent that is passed on to the child

fertilization: the fusion of a sperm cell and an ovum

sexual: characterized by or having the qualities of sex; the opposite is asexual

sexuality: a person's sense of self that is used to create sexual experiences

gender identity: awareness of being male or female

gender role: behaviors specific to a gender

sexual orientation: attraction toward and interest in members of one or both genders

heterosexual: someone who is attracted to people of the opposite gender

homosexual: someone who is attracted to people of the same gender

bisexual: someone who is attracted to members of both genders

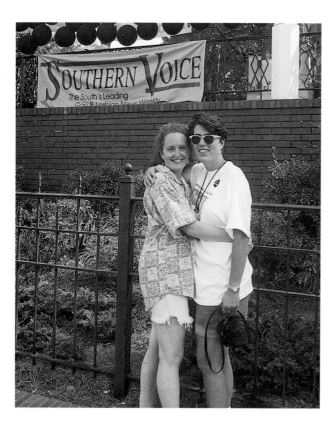

Intimate relationships between couples of the same sex are increasingly accepted in our society.

men and women who had died, showed a minute but measurable difference between the brains of homosexual and heterosexual men. This difference was in a tiny cell cluster known as the third interstitial nucleus of the anterior hypothalamus, or INAH3, which is "deeply involved in regulating male-typical sexual behavior" (Nimmons, 1994).

In another study, researchers looked at 108 sets of female twins in which one or both twins was a lesbian (Bailey, Pillard, Neale, & Ageyi, 1993). In 48% of the sets of identical twins, both twins were lesbian; among the nonidentical twins, only 16% were both lesbian. Similar results were found in studies of twin males. Although these results may suggest a genetic component to sexual orientation, other influences may also come into play because the identical twins were not always the same orientation.

Sexual Biology

One of the fundamental roles of sexuality is biological reproduction. The reproductive role of the male is to produce reproductively capable sperm and to deposit them in the female reproductive tract during sexual intercourse. The reproductive role of the female is to provide reproductively capable eggs, called **ova**, and to provide a safe, nutrient-filled environment in which the fetus develops for the 9 months of pregnancy.

Male or female reproductive biology is genetically determined at conception. The fusion of an X-bearing egg with the X-bearing sperm produces a female (XX); fusion with the Y-bearing sperm produces a male (XY). Once the chromosome pattern is set, the development of the sexual anatomy follows from the precise instructions of the genes contained in the chromosomes. A particular chromosome set determines whether the as yet immature sex cells that appear at about the fifth week of development will eventually produce sperm or ova. The sex chromosomes determine whether the fetus will ultimately develop the male sex organs—testes, sperm ducts, semen-producing glands, and penis; or the female organs—ovaries, fallopian tubes, uterus, vagina, and external female genitals.

The genetic determination of sexual anatomy also specifies the pattern of male or female steroid hormone production, which in turn affects the **secondary sex characteristics** that distinguish males and females: the extent and distribution of facial and body hair; body build and stature; and appearance of breasts.

Female Sexual Anatomy

A woman's internal sexual organs consist of two **ovaries,** which lie on either side of the abdominal cavity, the **fallopian tubes,** the **uterus,** and the **vagina;** together these structures make up a specialized tube that goes from each ovary to the outside of the body (Figure 7.1). The function of the ovaries, which are about the size and shape of almonds, is to produce fertilizable ova as well as sex hormones, which control the development of the female body type, maintain normal female sexual physiology, and help regulate the course of a normal pregnancy. The fallopian tubes gather and transport the ova that are released from the ovaries (about one each month). The two fallopian tubes connect to the uterus, an organ about the size of a woman's fist, which is situated just behind the pelvic bone and the bladder. The uterus is part of the passageway for sperm as they move from the vagina to the fallopian tubes to effect fertilization; after fertilization, it provides the environment in which the fetus grows. It is the inner lining of the uterus that is shed each month in menstruation.

The lower part of the uterus is the **cervix,** and the cavity of the uterus is connected to the vagina by means of a small opening called the cervical os. The cervix secretes mucus, which changes in consistency depending on the phase of the menstrual cycle. Some women learn to estimate the time of **ovulation** (ovum release) by examining their cervical mucus.

The vagina is a hollow tube that leads from the cervix to the outside of the body. The nonaroused

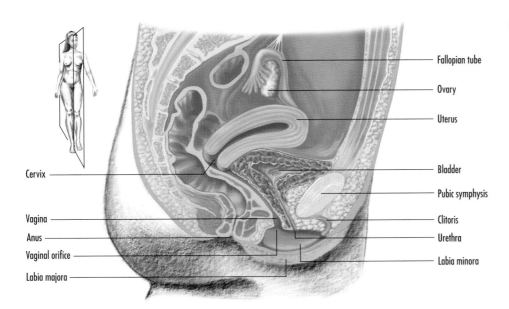

FIGURE 7.1   A Cross-section of the Female Sexual-Reproductive System

Fallopian tube

Ovary

Uterus

Bladder

Pubic symphysis

Clitoris

Urethra

Labia minora

Cervix

Vagina

Anus

Vaginal orifice

Labia majora

vagina is approximately three to five inches long. Normally, the vaginal tube is rather narrow, but it can readily widen to accommodate the penis during intercourse, a tampon during menstruation, the passage of a baby during childbirth, or a pelvic examination.

The **vulva** encompasses all female external genital structures—the hair, the folds of skin, the **clitoris,** and the urinary and vaginal openings (Figure 7.2). The smaller, inner pair of folds are called the **labia minora,** and the larger, outer pair are called the **labia majora.** The clitoris, a highly sensitive sexual organ, is situated above the vaginal opening. Although other sexual organs have additional functions of reproduction or the elimination of waste material, the only purpose of the clitoris is sexual arousal.

The opening of the **urethra,** which is the exit tube for urine, is located at the vaginal region just below the clitoris.

In addition to the primary sex organs, women have secondary sex characteristics, including the **breasts.** The breasts consist of a network of milk glands and milk ducts embedded in fatty tissue, and are influenced by pregnancy, nursing, or birth control pills, as well as the different phases of the menstrual cycle. The variation in breast size among women is due to differing amounts of fatty tissue within the breasts. There is little variation among women in the amount of milk-producing tissue; thus, a woman's ability to breast feed is unrelated to the size of her breasts.

The Menstrual Cycle

Each month or so, women usually produce one ovum that is able to be fertilized. During each period of this ovum production—the menstrual cycle—a woman's body undergoes several hormonally induced changes

that prepare her body for pregnancy if the ovum is fertilized. One of these changes involves the thickening of the lining of the uterus, the **endometrium,** to support the first stages of pregnancy. If conception does not occur, the lining sloughs off and is discharged as menstrual flow. In addition, certain blood vessels in the uterus increase in size. Their role is to bring the maternal nutrients to the fetus via the placenta if

Terms

ova: a term for female eggs (singular, *ovum*)

secondary sex characteristics: anatomical features appearing at puberty that distinguish males from females

ovaries: a pair of almond-shaped organs in the female abdomen that produce egg cells (ova) and female sex hormones

fallopian tubes: the usual site of fertilization; a pair of tube-like structures that transport ova from the ovaries to the uterus

uterus: the female organ in which a fetus develops

vagina: a woman's organ of copulation and the exit pathway for the fetus at birth

cervix: the lower, narrow end of the uterus

ovulation: release of an egg (ovum) from the ovary

vulva: the female external genital structures

clitoris: small, sensitive organ located above the vaginal opening; center of sexual pleasuring

labia minora: a pair of fleshy folds that cover the vagina

labia majora: a pair of fleshy folds that cover the labia minora

urethra: a tube that carries urine from the bladder to the outside

breasts: secondary sex characteristics; a network of milk glands and ducts in fatty tissue

endometrium: the inner lining of the uterus

FIGURE 7.2 **External Female Sexual Reproductive Organs**

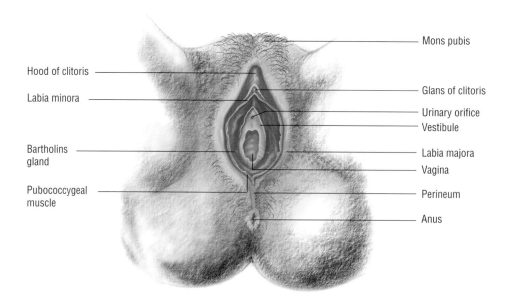

pregnancy occurs. This produces a loss of about 15 to 45 milliliters (about two or three tablespoons) of blood, mucus, and endometrial membranes, which leaves the body through the vagina over the course of 3 to 6 days. This discharge is **menstruation. Menarche** is the first menstruation a young woman experiences.

Terms

menstruation: the regular sloughing of the uterine lining via the vagina

menarche: the beginning of menstruation

gonadotropin-releasing hormone: hormone that directs the release of pituitary sex hormones

follicle-stimulating hormone: stimulates ovaries to develop mature follicles (with eggs); the follicle produces estrogen

luteinizing hormone: stimulates the release of the ovum (egg) by the follicle; the follicle produces progesterone

prolactin: hormone that promotes milk production

oxytocin: hormone that promotes release of milk; also can cause muscles in the uterine wall to contract

menopause: the cessation of menstruation in mid-life

testes: a pair of male reproductive organs that produce sperm cells and male sex hormones

penis: the male's organ of copulation and urination

copulation: sexual intercourse

scrotum: the sac of skin that contains the testes

seminal vesicles: sac-like structures that secrete a fluid that activates the sperm

prostate gland: gland at the base of the bladder providing seminal fluid

Cowper's glands: small glands secreting drops of alkalinizing fluid into the urethra

semen: a whitish, creamy fluid containing sperm

foreskin: a fold of skin over the end of the penis

The average age for menarche is between 12 and 13 years of age, although it can occur as early as 10 years of age or as late as 19 years of age.

The length and regularity of the menstrual cycle vary from woman to woman. Most women experience cycles of approximately 28 days, with cycle lengths between 24 and 35 days being the most common. Shorter and longer cycles are possible, but they are regarded as irregular cycles. Irregular cycles can occur monthly, with the number of days between menstruations varying from cycle to cycle. Irregular cycles are common when females first begin to menstruate and also when they stop producing ova later in life.

The menstrual cycle is controlled by a number of hormones. Hormones from the hypothalamus in the brain, called **gonadotropin-releasing hormone** (GnRH), are secreted and influence the release of other hormones from the pituitary gland. The pituitary gland produces two gonad-stimulating hormones, **follicle-stimulating hormone** (FSH) and **luteinizing hormone** (LH). The other hormones released by the pituitary gland are **prolactin** and **oxytocin.** These hormones circulate throughout the woman's bloodstream and induce changes necessary to support pregnancy. The preparation of the lining of the uterus for pregnancy is only one function of estrogen and progesterone. The menstrual cycle is regulated so that if fertilization does not occur, the hormonal support of tissue growth in the uterus stops, and the uterine tissue is lost in a menstrual discharge.

Menopause

Menopause is the gradual cessation of ovulation and menstruation. It is a time when the ovaries stop producing ova and the ovaries' production of hormones wanes considerably. Therefore, the two principal bio-

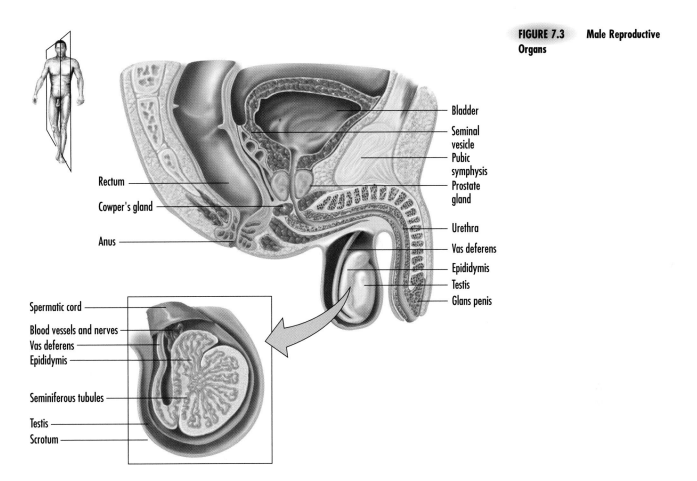

FIGURE 7.3   **Male Reproductive Organs**

Labels (upper figure): Bladder, Seminal vesicle, Pubic symphysis, Prostate gland, Urethra, Vas deferens, Epididymis, Testis, Glans penis, Rectum, Cowper's gland, Anus

Labels (lower figure): Spermatic cord, Blood vessels and nerves, Vas deferens, Epididymis, Seminiferous tubules, Testis, Scrotum

logical consequences of menopause are: a woman no longer is capable of becoming pregnant, and her body may undergo some changes from the diminished production of ovarian hormones, like estrogen. There is a wide range of age for menopause. Many women experience menopause between ages 50 and 52; however, it can occur as early as age 35 and as late as age 55. The age at which menopause occurs may be affected by hereditary, social, and nutritional factors. There is no relation between the age at which menopause occurs and the age at which a woman first begins to menstruate.

Male Sexual Anatomy

The principal reproductive role of male sexual organs is to make numerous viable sperm cells and to deliver them into the female reproductive tract during sexual intercourse. The male sexual and reproductive system consists of two **testes,** the sites of sperm and sex hormone production; a series of connected sperm ducts that originate at the testes, course through the pelvis, and terminate at the urethra of the penis; glands that produce seminal fluid; and the **penis,** the organ of **copulation** (Figure 7.3).

The penis consists of nerves, blood vessels, fibrous tissue, and three parallel cylinders of spongy tissue. It does not contain bone, nor does it possess an abundance of muscular tissue, contrary to some people's beliefs. However, there is an extensive network of muscles around the base of the penis that help to eject both semen and urine through the urethra.

The testes are located in a flesh-covered sac, the **scrotum,** that hangs outside the man's body. In the embryo, the testes develop inside the body, but just before birth they descend into the scrotum. Inside the scrotum, the testes are kept at a temperature a few degrees cooler than the internal body temperature, a condition that is apparently necessary for the production of reproductively capable sperm.

When a man ejaculates, sperm are propelled through the sperm ducts and out of the penis by contractions of the smooth muscles that line the ducts and the muscles of the pelvis. As they move out of the male body, the sperm mix with secretions of seminal fluid from the **seminal vesicles, prostate gland,** and **Cowper's glands** to form **semen.** The semen, which is the gelatinous milky fluid emitted at ejaculation, contains a mixture of about 300 million sperm cells and about 3 to 6 milliliters of seminal fluid. The seminal fluid contributes 95% or more of the entire volume of semen.

All men are born with a fold of skin, the **foreskin,** that covers the end of the penis. For centuries, Jewish and Moslem families have surgically removed the foreskin from male children for religious reasons. This procedure is called **circumcision.** Although there is no clear medical indication that circumcision is beneficial, removal of the foreskin does eliminate the buildup of **smegma,** a white, cheesy substance that can accumulate under the foreskin. The belief that circumcision leads to an increase in sexual arousal because it exposes the glans and the related belief that circumcision produces an inability to delay ejaculation are myths. For most men, circumcision has no effect on sexual arousal and sexual activity.

Sexual Arousal and Response

Sexual arousal and response are often thought of in terms of genital stimulation, genital responses, and orgasm. But in reality, sexual experience is a holistic process involving one's body, mind, emotions, spirit, and relationship with the partner.

Sexual Arousal

Because sex is a whole-person experience, sexual interaction involves a change from a nonerotic to an erotic state of being, one in which erotic experience—for whatever reasons—is expected and sought. The change from a nonerotic to an erotic state usually involves these elements:

1. *Sexual interest:* openness to erotic arousal
2. *Desire or motivation:* energizing oneself toward creating an erotic experience
3. *Decision:* offering or accepting invitations for sex
4. *Participation:* engaging in behaviors that produce erotic arousal

   Although in our society people are expected to be highly and frequently interested in sex, in reality the desire for sexual activity varies among individuals and couples, changes over time, and is influenced by interpersonal and psychological factors. For example, many

couples report a higher degree of sexual desire at the beginning of their relationship than after the relationship has matured. Alternatively, couples who have been together for many years may experience an increase in sexual interest when the childrearing phase of the family life cycle is completed. Various physical and psychological situations can affect sexual interest as well. For example, many women report a transient loss of sexual interest during the first few weeks after childbirth. And depression is sometimes associated with loss of interest in sex.

   Having sexual desire does not necessarily mean that a person will behave sexually. Human sexual behavior is not "reflexive;" activity does not occur automatically whenever one feels "horny" or one is presented with a sexual opportunity. Instead, sexual activity is the result of a decision (except in instances of sexual coercion and assault) that is based on desire to conform to social norms, personal values, and physical and psychological needs.

   Creating a sexual experience involves two kinds of decisions. The first concerns context, that is, the social situation in which sexual activity takes place. Societies have rules and norms that govern sexual activity. Individuals are not permitted to have sex with just anyone or in any social setting. For example, most people have sex only in the bedroom, not in the living room or kitchen or dining room.

   The second type of decision concerns participation in a sexual episode. Even in a situation or relationship in which sexual activity is acceptable, and opportunities to have sex are present, a person can decide "yes," "no," "not yet," or "maybe" whenever a sexual opportunity occurs. The decision is made by evaluating how one feels physically and emotionally at the time, one's personal criteria for being sexual within the presenting situation, and one's expectation of how having sex at that time will affect one's self-esteem and the relationship.

   There is no formula for creating sexual arousal. Everyone has preferences. In situations and circumstances that they deem appropriate for sex, most people respond sexually to being touched in certain ways. Certain regions of the body are highly sexually sensitive in nearly all people. These are the classic erogenous zones—the genitals, the breasts, the anus, the lips, the inner thighs, and the mouth.

The Sexual Response Cycle

When a person becomes sexually aroused, the brain and nervous system prepare the body for sexual activity. Impulses from the brain are transmitted by the spinal nerves to various parts of the body and cause physiological changes. These changes include: the tightening of many skeletal muscles (**myotonia**);

Terms

circumcision: a surgical procedure to remove the foreskin from the penis

smegma: a white, cheesy substance that accumulates under the foreskin of the penis

myotonia: muscle tension

vasocongestion: the engorgement of blood vessels in particular body parts in response to sexual arousal

sexual response cycle: the physiological response in both men and women as described in four phases

masturbation: self-induced sexual stimulation

celibacy: sexual abstinence

changes in the pattern of blood flow or **vasocongestion** (especially an increase in blood flow in the pelvis); increases in heart rate, blood pressure, and respiratory rate; increase in the general level of excitement; and increase in erotic feelings.

Increased pelvic blood flow in the male produces erection of the penis. The penis enlarges because the spongy tissues within it fill with blood. In the female, increased pelvic blood flow produces lubrication of the vagina and swelling of the clitoris and vaginal lips. Vaginal lubrication is produced by the release of fluids from the walls of the vagina. Swelling of the clitoris and vaginal lips is due to the filling with blood of spongy tissues within them. In some women the changes in blood flow due to sexual arousal also produces a swelling of the breasts.

Regardless of the type of sexual stimulation, the physiological response in both men and women is similar and follows a pattern called the **sexual response cycle**, which consists of four phases as identified by Masters and Johnson (Figure 7.4):

- *Phase 1:* Excitement, in which the person experiences sexual arousal from any source and the body responds with specific changes: erection of the penis in males; vaginal lubrication and swelling of the clitoris and genitalia in females; and sex flush in both males and females.
- *Phase 2:* Plateau, in which the physiological changes of the excitement phase level off, although subjective feelings of sexual arousal may increase.
- *Phase 3:* Orgasm, in which the tensions that build up during excitement and plateau are released.
- *Phase 4:* Resolution, in which the body returns to the physiologically nonstimulated state. In addition, Masters and Johnson include a refractory period (a recovery stage in which there is a temporary inability to reach orgasm) in the male resolution phase.

There is considerable variation in the extent and duration of the sexual response cycle among individuals of either sex. There is even variation in the nature of the response in the same person, for each sexual encounter is different. Masters and Johnson (1966) found more variation in the sexual response cycle for women than for men.

Masturbation

Masturbation is self-stimulation to produce erotic arousal, usually to the point of orgasm. While social and religious attitudes in many cultures consider it improper, immoral, or perverse, masturbation is nevertheless practiced widely throughout the world and even among other animal species.

Many people find masturbation a rewarding variation in their sex lives. People masturbate for many of the same reasons that they have partner sex: to experience erotic pleasure; to relieve physical tensions; to produce a sense of relaxation; to induce sleep; and when done with a partner, to create feelings of intimacy and bonding. Often, people find masturbation to be valuable as a means of self-exploration so they can better understand what pleases them sexually.

A number of personal harmful effects have long been rumored to result from masturbation. Among them are hair loss, insanity, pimples, warts, unhappy personal relations, and the inability to have children. There is no evidence that any of these claims are true. Physically, masturbation is harmless as long as it is not injurious to the stimulated organs.

Sexual Abstinence

Although for most people interest in and desire for sex is relatively constant, some people choose to abstain from sexual activity. For religious reasons certain people practice lifelong sexual abstinence (sometimes called **celibacy,** which literally means remaining unmarried). Some individuals refrain from sexual intercourse until they marry. Still others avoid sexual interaction because they fear the closeness and intimacy implied by sex or they have strong negative feelings regarding sex.

Individuals not wishing to practice lifelong sexual abstinence may nevertheless benefit from a sex "time out." For example, recovery from a physical or emotional illness may include sexual abstinence. No sex is a sure way to avoid an unintended pregnancy or a sexually transmitted infection. Some people find abstaining helpful while recovering from the break-up of a love relationship. The healing of the emotional wound seems to proceed more smoothly without the emotional intensity that often accompanies sexual interaction.

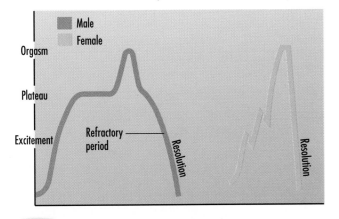

FIGURE 7.4   **Sexual Response Cycle as Identified by Masters and Johnson**

Sexual abstinence can also provide an opportunity to develop a new set of personal and relational experiences. By avoiding the intimacy that accompanies a lot of sex, abstinence provides a way to discover new dimensions in interpersonal relationships. Without the diversion of sex (or the search for sex partners) an individual can focus on self-development, career, or school and put energy into long-time friendships. New romantic relationships can develop without the pressure for sex early in the relationship, thus permitting the partners to develop trust and caring before becoming sexual.

> It's been so long since I made love, I can't remember who gets tied up.
>
> JOAN RIVERS

For some, sexual abstinence seems like a hardship because their sexual needs and their needs for touching, physical contact, and emotional closeness may not be met. During a period of sexual abstinence, the need for touching and physical contact can be met through professional (nonsexual) massage, or hugging among friends and between parents and children. Masturbation can relieve sexual tensions. And intimacy needs can be met by deepening one's ongoing friendships, giving oneself to others through volunteer work, increasing one's level of self-awareness and self-development, or involving oneself in spiritual and religious activity.

Sexual Dysfunctions

Many individuals expect sex always to be exciting and satisfying; anything less is cause for concern. Life is full of changes, however, and the demands of career or parenting or occasional physical illness can sometimes produce a temporary loss in interest in sex or the ability to engage in sex. Such changes in sexual interest and ability are normal and usually resolve themselves eventually. Persistent difficulties with sex may signal that consulting a therapist would be helpful. Lack of interest in sex may be connected to many factors, including failure to communicate likes and dislikes; boredom; stress, fatigue, and depression; alcohol and drugs; pregnancy and children; hostility and anger; change in physical appearance; and physical illness.

A recent national survey showed that sexual dysfunctions are highly prevalent in both men and women, ranging from 10% to 52% of men and 25% to 63% of women (Laumann, Paik, & Rosen, 1999). Overall, sexual dysfunction is more prevalent for women (43%) than men (31%). Sexual dysfunction is associated with age and education level and highly associated with negative experiences in sexual relationships and a lack of overall well-being.

Erectile Dysfunction Difficulty in achieving or maintaining an erection can be the result of an injury or disease. It can also be due to alcohol, heroin, and other recreational drugs and some medications for high blood pressure. More often, however, erection problems are the result of fear of sexual performance (including anxiety about one's ability to get an erection) or the wish not to be sexual with a particular partner. Also known as *impotence*, an estimated 20 million men in the United States are affected, with less than 10% receiving treatment.

Ejaculatory Disorders It is impossible to define "rapid" or "premature" ejaculation in terms of minutes; however, some therapists define it as absence of voluntary control of ejaculation. Ejaculation is a reflex activity that a man can learn to control just as he does bladder function. The key to controlling ejaculation is awareness of the bodily sensations that signal the onset of ejaculation, followed by modulating arousal according to one's desires.

Vaginismus In women, painful intercourse can be caused by vaginal infections, insufficient vaginal lubrication before intercourse (usually the result of not being sufficiently sexually aroused), and anxiety-produced spasms of the muscles surrounding the vagina, which makes vaginal penetration painful. Another source of pain associated with intercourse is a deep, aching sensation in the pelvis for women occurring during sex. This condition is caused by the congestion of blood in the pelvic region brought about by sexual arousal. Orgasm often reverses the congestion, but lack of orgasm can cause blood to remain and cause discomfort and pain.

Lack of Orgasm Both men and women can have difficulty experiencing orgasm. Most often this difficulty is the result of insufficient sexual arousal, perhaps because of aversion to a particular partner, fear of pregnancy or sexually transmitted diseases, fear of letting go, lack of trust, or negative attitudes about sexual pleasure.

Developing Positive Sexual Relationships

We all need intimacy—that feeling of closeness, trust, and openness with another person that tells us that our innermost self can be shared without fear of attack or emotional hurt and that we are understood in the deepest sense possible.

Intimate relationships can have an enormous impact on one's sense of vitality and well-being. When an intimate relationship is flowing smoothly, it can produce rich emotional satisfaction unparalleled by any other experience. Those who are involved in genuinely supportive and caring relationships tend to feel confident about the potential of life to be harmonious and beautiful. On the other hand, when an intimate relationship is not going well, those involved can be overwhelmed by moroseness, and unable to think of anything but their misery. They can be angry, depressed, anxious, or distraught, sometimes to the point of being unable to function at work or at school.

A lack of intimacy in life can adversely affect physical health as well as emotions and feelings. Studies indicate that married people are in better physical health than divorced, separated, and widowed people. The association between intimacy and physical health is suggested by the finding that recently widowed people suffer increased mortality during the first few months after the death of their spouse. Apparently these people do indeed die of a "broken heart."

What Is Intimacy?

Many people mistakenly equate genuine intimacy with sexual intercourse. This happens because love and affection are feelings associated with intimacy, and in our culture there is much confusion about love and sex. But intimacy is a feeling, not an act. It is the *quality* of a relationship between two people—a shared experiencing of their personal lives. People who have an intimate relationship may or may not choose to express their closeness with sex.

Many kinds of intimacies are possible. There are intimacies between other-sex peers, same-sex peers, children and parents, members of a family, neighbors, close friends, and even co-workers. Each intimacy has its unique and distinctive quality depending on the people involved, on the extent to which their personal histories are similar, and on the facets of themselves they choose to share with each other.

Yet intimacies possess certain common characteristics. They are relationships of mutual consent. One person cannot be intimate with another unless both agree that that is what they want. Intimacies tend to grow deeper and richer over time; partners need to share meaningful experiences in order to establish genuine trust and caring. Intimacies also carry the feeling that the personalities of the intimates are interconnected in some complex way. This is not the same as the feeling of having their identities merge so they become "one," but rather that they feel both joined and separate at the same time in some way.

The Life Cycle of Intimate Relationships

Intimate relationships tend to develop through the stages of (a) selecting a partner, (b) developing intimacy, and (c) establishing commitment.

Selecting a Partner   Factors that influence the choice of intimate partners include:

- *Proximity.* People are most likely to become intimate with someone with whom they are in physical proximity.
- *Similarity.* Similar age, religion, race, education, social background, attitudes, values, and interests affect the possibility for intimacy in two ways: 1) they influence proximity and 2) they reflect social norms for permissible peer intimacies. Note, for example, biases against interracial and older-younger intimacies. Colleges and universities provide students with relatively easy access to a "pool of eligibles" because they bring together individuals of similar age, religion, intelligence, expectations, and values.

> *Personally, I think if a woman hasn't met the right man by the time she's twenty-four, she may be lucky.*
> DEBORAH KERR

- *Physical appearance.* Physical appearance provides cues that indicate who among the pool of eligibles is a desirable intimate partner. Those who are judged "attractive" tend to be thought of as kind, understanding, and affectionate ("what is beautiful is good"). Pairing with someone who is considered

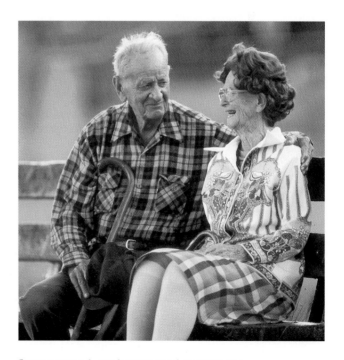

Intimacy is a basic human need at every age.

physically attractive enhances one's social status and self-esteem.

Developing Intimacy Most people want their intimate relationships to develop feelings of closeness, positive regard, warmth, and familiarity with the other's innermost thoughts and feelings. This deep knowledge of each other comes from sharing the most important and often secret aspects of one's personality—one's goals, aspirations, strengths, weaknesses, and physical and sexual desires. The sharing of such private information is called **self-disclosure.**

When relationships begin, little intimate information is usually disclosed. People talk about the weather, the stock market, or politics. They gossip about professors, students, or other people they know. And they ask each other the classic leading questions: Where are you from? What do you do? What's your major?

Intimacy develops through a progressive, mutual revealing of innermost thoughts. Psychologists compare people's personalities to onions—having many layers from an outer surface to an inner core. As acquaintances gain more and more knowledge about each other, they penetrate deeper and deeper through the layers of the other's personality, which establishes their intimacy. Another view compares intimate development to the peeling of an artichoke. Resistance and barriers to sharing information about oneself are like the leaves of the artichoke; as intimacy progresses, intimates peel away the leaves to get to the other's "heart."

Self-disclosure leads to the development of intimacy in two ways. First, you tend to be affected either positively or negatively by the information that is disclosed. If you make a positive judgment, you are likely to want to continue interacting with that person, for you believe that future interactions will be equally or even more positive. The same logic applies to negative assessments. If your reaction is unfavorable, you are likely to terminate the relationship, or perhaps maintain it on a lesser level of intimacy.

The second way that self-disclosure leads to intimacy is the *act* of self-disclosure, which, regardless of the information offered, often leads to reciprocal self-disclosure. By sharing important information, you communicate that you trust the other person, and usually that person accepts your trust and becomes more willing to disclose information. In this way intimacy progresses by a cycle of self-disclosure leading to trust, which brings about self-disclosure, which leads to more trust, and so on.

Establishing Commitment After a period of self-disclosure, individuals may sense that their relationship has progressed to a state of "us-ness," that it has become a special friendship, a love relationship, or a marital-type relationship. This state of "us-ness" is one of commitment, which has three aspects.

- *An action, pledge, or promise.* One makes a promise and thus announces one's intention explicitly, even if it is only to the partner. Various social values and norms regarding keeping promises and the guilt and loss of self-esteem that come with breaking promises are among the "push" factors that keep a person committed. If the promise involves a social ritual (i.e., marriage ceremony, getting pinned), then family, friends, and the state become additional "push" factors.

- *A state of being obligated or emotionally compelled.* This state involves a cluster of emotions such as love, comfort, caring, and relief from separation anxiety and loneliness.

- *An unwillingness to consider any partner other than the current one.* The rewards of the current relationship outweigh the costs of exploring other opportunities for intimacy.

Endings

Everything in the universe (even the universe itself!) has a beginning and an end. Close relationships have a beginning and an end also. Sometimes a relationship lasts for only a few minutes; sometimes it lasts until one of the partners dies (and even then the relationship may still be "alive" in the imagination of the surviving partner). Sometimes the structure of a close relationship persists but the closeness and the dynamism wane, creating a "shell" relationship without vitality. Sometimes a relationship goes through cycles of birth and death within the structure of its ongoingness. When a close relationship ends, some or all of its structure, exchange of resources (e.g., love, caring, financial support), and feelings of attachment and emotional bondedness end also.

Endings occur for a variety of reasons. Partners' feelings of attachment and bondedness may be absent or weak. Life goals, values, or interests may no longer be shared. One or both partners may be unwilling or unable to invest personal resources such as greater time shared with the partner, or to commit to an exclusive relationship. Whether partners continue in a relationship also is affected by their assessment of other options such as another potential partner or singlehood. Without suitable alternatives, leaving a relationship may seem difficult, unwise, or impossible.

Occasionally the seeds of an ending are sown into a relationship at its beginning. For example, partners

Terms

self-disclosure: sharing personal experiences and feelings with someone

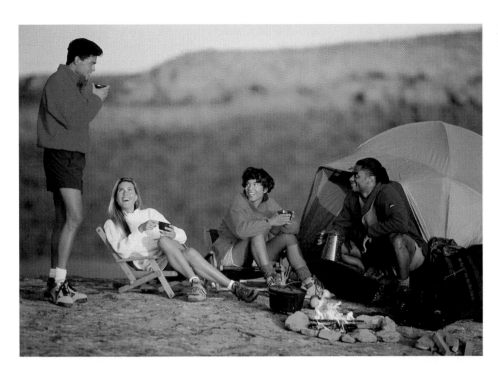

Intimacy begins by doing fun things together.

may seek closeness as a way to cope with or avoid personal problems. They may feel rejected and lonely because of the break-up of a previous relationship. They may feel that they cannot take care of themselves. They may be afraid of leaving home or school. If, as often happens, a partner or relationship does not turn out to be the solution to a personal problem, a disappointed, angry, or frustrated partner may seek alternative ways of coping. These alternatives, such as drug or alcohol abuse, extra-relationship affairs, or physically or emotionally abusing the partner (or other family members) (see chapter 13), may very well be destructive to the relationship.

When a break-up does occur, individuals may feel tired, lethargic, lonely, sad, depressed, angry, resentful, and guilty. They may be unable to sleep or eat, may miss class, or be unable to work. They may withdraw from friends. They may find concentrating difficult, because they are continually thinking about the partner and what happened in the relationship. They may feel helpless ("what will become of me?") and hopeless ("I'll never find a true love") or skeptical and cynical ("love can never work out").

Some partners feel relaxed, hopeful, and relieved that what they identify as a bad or going-nowhere relationship has ended, and they are free to pursue personal goals or find a relationship partner who is better suited to them. Sometimes individuals feel euphoric and self-confident. They say that the separation was for the best, and they become more active and outgoing. This positive outlook may alternate with emotional distress.

When a person is emotionally (and sometimes physically) wracked with the pain of an ending, he or she may have difficulty seeing any good in that experience, but often endings mark the start of a new and better future. A study of remarried people showed that many had learned a lot about themselves and the nature of close relationships from a previous marriage(s) and found that their current marriage was much more satisfying. Guiding principles for enhanced relationships are patience and experience.

Communicating in Intimate Relationships

Communication is a symbolic process of creating and sharing meaning. At the heart of communication is an individual act, which involves imparting a message to another person to share information or feelings, to coordinate behavior with an individual or group of people, or to persuade someone to do something.

A communication act begins as a mental image; an idea, a wish, or a feeling (or some combination of all three). If humans were capable of mind reading, senders could impart mental images directly to receivers. Few people can read minds, however, so communication requires that thoughts be transformed into symbols that can carry information. Those symbols make up the message. The most common symbols in communication are:

- *Words:* spoken, printed, or shouted
- *Visual images:* paintings, sculpture
- *Posture or body language:* gaze, touch, smile, physical proximity, folding arms, frowning, turning away
- *Objects:* flowers, gifts, food

- *Behaviors:* doing a favor, giving a kiss, ignoring an appointment

The sender's encoding of her or his mental images into the symbols that make up the message is only half of a communication act. The other half is the receiver's reactions: this involves taking in the symbols that make up the message and decoding them into her or his own mental images. Thus, a communication act requires two transformations: in the sender, the transformation of mental images into symbols; in the receiver, the transformation of symbols into mental images.

> *The image of myself which I try to create in my own mind in order that I may love myself is very different from the image which I try to create in the minds of others in order that they may love me.*
>
> W. H. AUDEN, poet

Every communication act carries two types of message or potential meaning. The first is the **literal message,** which is the message conveyed by the symbols themselves, as in the words "it's raining." The second is the **metamessage** ("meta" is the Greek word for "beyond," "additional," or "transcendent"), which carries implicit messages about the reason for the communication, how the message is to be interpreted, and the nature of the relationship of the sender and receiver. Most metacommunication occurs unconsciously.

The basis for effective sexual communication is **mutual empathy**—the underlying knowledge that each partner in a relationship cares for the other and knows that the care is reciprocated.

Sending Clear Messages

A clear message is one in which the symbols represent as closely as possible the sender's intent. Clear messages are best delivered with **I-statements;** these are sentences that begin with (or have as the subject) the pronoun "I." I-statements clearly identify the sender as the source of a thought, emotion, desire, or act: I think . . . . I feel . . . . I want (need) . . . . I did (will do) . . . .

You-statements, which begin with (or have as the subject) the pronoun "you," as in "You always . . . ," "You never . . . ," "You are . . . ," or the interrogatives, "Why don't you . . . ?" or "How could you . . . ?" often are put-downs or character assassinations. They imply that the receiver is not-OK. Very often the not-OK message is explicit, as in "You're incompetent" or "You're stupid"—just about any negative adjective will do. People often respond to the metamessage in a you-statement, which is "I think you're no good," by feeling attacked, which can lead to hurt feelings and counterattacks or withdrawal.

Effective Listening

Effective communication requires both sending and receiving, both talking and listening. Effective listening is important because the receiver not only takes in the sender's message, but also helps establish the physical and emotional context for the communication. The listener also must communicate to the sender that the sender's message was received. This is called **feedback.** Some techniques for effective receiving are: giving the sender your full attention; making eye contact; listening; being empathic; being open for receiving the message; giving verbal feedback; acknowledging the sender's feelings; praising the sender's efforts; and being unconditional.

Give the Sender Your Full Attention Don't fake it. If you can't pay attention because you are tired, hungry,

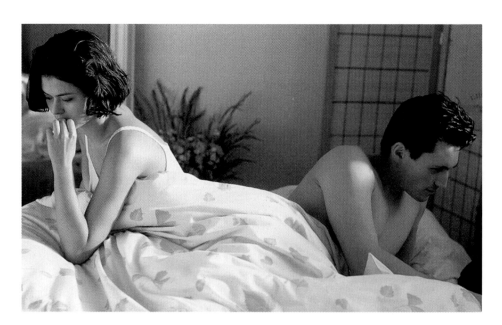

When communication breaks down, stress and tension ensue.

Managing Stress

Pillow Talk

When problems arise among intimate couples, virtually every incident can be traced back to some misinterpretation in communication. "I thought you said this!" "I thought you meant that." Although not all communication styles are verbal, the amount of communication expressed through words leads to most of the difficulty in relationships. Poor communication in any relationship, and in particular sexual relationships, can lead to stress.

There are many issues involving sexual intercourse that can act as stressors. These include, but are not limited to, contraception, fertility control, risk of pregnancy, infertility, STIs, vaginismus, molestation, celibacy, guilt, rape, self-respect, abortion, impotency, premature ejaculation, intimacy, ability to reach orgasm, homosexuality, and sexual satisfaction. This incomplete list is quite long and each item weighs heavy as a stressor for those who experience them. In addition, problems of this nature do not go away once a couple has initiated sexual relations. To the contrary, if communications are poor at the start of a relationship, they tend to get worse as the relationship continues. Sex counselors advocate that *before* and *after* each and every act of sexual intimacy there should be a thorough conversation airing these and other issues. As any AIDS patient or woman with an unwanted pregnancy will tell you, the short-term pleasures of sex are surely not worth risking your life, nor are they worth the days, months, and years of agony that may follow unresolved sex-related problems. The stakes of sexual encounters are high. Make it a point to include a healthy conversation as a requirement in all sexually intimate encounters.

Here are some suggestions for conversation with someone you become intimate with.

- Learn to become comfortable with words about sexual intimacy, such as erection, penis, orgasm, and condom. The inability to articulate your feelings and preferences creates additional stress in relationships.

- If you are anxious about explaining your feelings, rehearse a conversation in which you ask your partner how he or she feels about you, where he or she likes to be touched, or tell him or her that you wish to date him or her exclusively (specific aspects of this degree of intimacy).

- Learn to ask your partner what pleases him or her and what they don't like. Conversely, feel assertive enough to make known your preferences to your partner. Don't assume that he or she knows.

Open channels of communication are vital to the health of intimate relationships, whereas poor communication only adds to the stress of a relationship. In uncomfortable moments, your first reaction may be to avoid confronting issues of intimacy. At these times, rather than giving in to reactions of avoidance or silence, we must respond with an open heart.

---

distracted, angry, or whatever, tell the sender how you feel and ask if it's OK to talk after you rest, or eat, or go to the bathroom, or just talk at another time.

Make Eye Contact   Try to assume similar postures (i.e., both sitting or both standing) to create a sense of equal status. Making eye-to-eye contact allows the receiver to feel comfortable as well as conveying that you are listening to her and taking in the complete message.

Just Listen   Don't interrupt until you have a signal that the sender is finished or until the sender has asked for a response, unless you don't understand what is being communicated. You can acknowledge that you are actively listening with gestures, nods, and vocalizations like "uh-huh," "yes," "go on," "I see," and so forth.

Be Empathic   Try to "hear" the sender's feelings as well as the words. Be open to the sender's intentions and motivations as well as her or his ideas. Ask yourself, "What is this person feeling right now?"

Be an Open Channel for Receiving the Message   Don't judge or evaluate the sender or the message while the sender is talking. Try not to correct the sender or, if the sender is being critical of you, to think of a defense.

> *If I could tell you what it meant, there would be no point in dancing it.*
> ISADORA DUNCAN, dancer

Give Verbal Feedback   Don't mind read. Summarize in your own words your understanding of the sender's thoughts and emotions. This way the sender can find

Terms

literal message: a message that is conveyed by symbols

metamessage: how the message is interpreted between sender and receiver

mutual empathy: both partners care about and understand each other

I-statements: statements beginning with "I"; positive communication skill

you-statements: statements beginning with "You"; negative communication skill

feedback: response of the receiver of a message to let the sender know he or she received the message and what the message was

out if the message that was intended was actually received. If so, then you can respond. If not, then the sender can try again.

Acknowledge the Sender's Emotions "It seems to me that you're feeling . . ." and if you're not sure, add "do I have that right?" By acknowledging or providing feedback, you are sharing what you believe are the sender's emotions. If you are incorrect, the sender can relay that to you.

Praise the Sender's Effort Acknowledge the sender's efforts for investing the time, energy, and care to communicate with you, especially if the communication was a difficult one.

Be Unconditional Let the sender know that you respect him or her even if you are uncomfortable with the messages that are being communicated. Assure the sender that even though things may be difficult, you are willing to continue talking and working through difficult feelings.

Expressing Anger Constructively

Disagreements and conflicts are inevitable in any close relationship. The notion that people in intimate relationships shouldn't have to fight because love makes them see eye to eye on everything and the idea that you can't possibly be angry with someone you love are romantic myths. By expressing anger constructively, intimates fight for the success of their relationship as well as for their individual needs.

In constructive fighting, there should be no "winner" and no "loser." Good fights are efforts of individuals to be heard and to improve the relationship. The best fights occur when the people involved feel that they have gained something.

Here are some suggestions for expressing anger constructively:

- Try not to let anger and resentment build up over time. Express feelings when you become aware of them.
- Agree on a time, a place, and the content for fights. It is certainly acceptable to get mad spontaneously if that is how you feel, but it is better to set aside a specific time for the resolution of an issue rather than trying to deal with it when you or your partner may not be psychologically or physically ready to argue. Be sure that the person you are angry with knows what the issue is before the fight.
- Be specific as to what you are angry about and stick to the issue. Don't bring up old hurts. Try not to discuss second and third topics, especially as a means of retaliation.

- Attack the problem, not each other. Don't denigrate the other's personal qualities. Use I-statements to communicate resentments. I-statements tell how you feel. You-statements are often received as personal attacks. At the same time, express appreciation for your partner as a person. This acknowledges that we can be angered by our partners' behaviors and feel loving toward them as people at the same time.
- Try to resolve the issue with an air of compromise and respect. Try to understand the other's point of view.
- Know when it is time to stop. Sometimes you can sense that the argument isn't getting resolved. It is okay to acknowledge that and to take a few hours or days to reconsider things and to discuss the issue again. Sometimes emotions are too high and it is not possible to think clearly. That may be the time to stop the fight until tempers cool.
- Engaging in sex or any other affectionate behavior before an issue is resolved should not be taken as a sign that everything is forgotten. Such behavior shows that the fight fits into what is believed to be healthy relationship.
- Don't hold grudges.

Understanding Pregnancy and Parenthood

Many people are awed by the idea that the union of one of their body's cells with a cell from their mate can bring forth a unique human being whose well-being is highly dependent on the physical and emotional foundations they provide. There is a tremendous responsibility in being the best kind of parent so that both the child and society benefit.

People want children for a variety of reasons. A couple may believe that a child is an expression of their love and that having children adds to their sense of bonding. Some see a child as a way to leave a legacy to the world or to carry on the family name. Some couples may feel pressured by their families or by societal or religious expectations to have children, and others may hope that having children will improve their marriage. Being a parent can make some people feel important, needed, or proud. Parenthood may reinforce the ideals of feminine and masculine roles. Prospective parents may also see children as adding fun, excitement, love, and companionship to their lives.

Choosing Whether or Not to Be a Parent

Not everyone chooses to become a parent. About 5% of fertile American married couples do not become

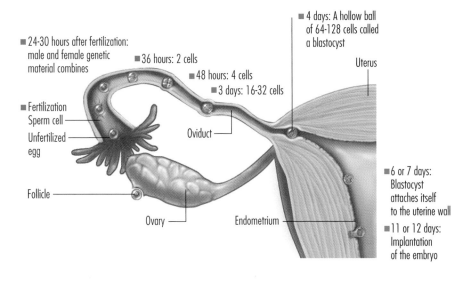

- 24-30 hours after fertilization: male and female genetic material combines
- 36 hours: 2 cells
- 48 hours: 4 cells
- 3 days: 16-32 cells
- 4 days: A hollow ball of 64-128 cells called a blastocyst

Uterus

- Fertilization
Sperm cell
Unfertilized egg

Oviduct

Follicle

Ovary

Endometrium

- 6 or 7 days: Blastocyst attaches itself to the uterine wall
- 11 or 12 days: Implantation of the embryo

FIGURE 7.5   Fertilization and Early Development of the Embryo   Joining of sperm and egg in fertilization. After fertilization, zygote travels down fallopian tube to uterus. Implantation of zygote begins approximately 6 days after fertilization.

parents. Some see parenthood as infringing on their career goals or as an unnecessary or unwanted addition to their intimate partnership. Some may have doubts about their psychological or economic abilities to nurture or support children. Others may know or suspect that their children might inherit a genetic disease. Still others may feel that they do not want to contribute more children to an already overpopulated world.

Giving birth to and raising a child requires major adjustments in the parents' lives. The career plans of one or both parents and the distribution of family resources—time, energy, physical space, and money—may change. First-time parents may feel overwhelmed by their responsibilities. The decision to parent should not be taken lightly. The years of parenting are often intense. However, you will never experience such responsibility, hard work, and intimacy as that involved in the growth and development of another human being.

Becoming Pregnant

A typical pregnancy lasts 40 weeks, with the baby's due date calculated from the mother's last menstrual cycle. Every pregnancy begins with **fertilization,** which is the fusion of a father's sperm cell with a mother's ovum to form the first cell of their child, called the fertilized egg, or **zygote.** When a man ejaculates during sexual intercourse, hundreds of millions of sperm cells are released into the vagina. Propelled by the swimming motion of their long tails, these tadpole-like cells make their way through the uterus and into the fallopian tubes, the usual site of fertilization (Figure 7.5). Only one of the many sperm cells actually fertilizes the egg. After fertilization, the zygote moves to the uterus, where it implants in the inner lining and proceeds to develop as an **embryo.**

During the first 3 days after fertilization, the cells of the embryo replicate at about daily intervals, and the embryo moves along the fallopian tube toward the uterus. By about the fourth day after fertilization, the embryo, now comprised of between 50 and 100 cells, arranged as a fluid-filled sphere, enters the uterus. On about the sixth day after fertilization, the embryo attaches to the lining of the uterus; shortly thereafter, it implants in the uterus by eroding the uterine lining.

 ### Pregnancy

Soon after the embryo implants in the uterus, it secretes a hormone unique to pregnancy, called **human chorionic gonadotropin (HCG)** into the maternal bloodstream (Figure 7.6). Under the influence of HCG, the mother's ovaries are stimulated to increase the production of estrogen and progesterone, which in turn forestalls the next menstrual period and permits the pregnancy to continue. Increases in the levels of estrogen and progesterone bring about the first noticeable signs of pregnancy: absence of the next menstrual period, occasional nausea and vomiting referred to as "morning sickness," enlarged and tender breasts, increased frequency of urination, fatigue, and enlargement of the uterus.

> *If you want a baby, have a new one. Don't baby the old one.*
> JESSAMYN WEST

Both clinical and home pregnancy tests are based on

Terms

fertilization: the fusion of a sperm cell and an ovum

zygote: the first cell of a new person, formed at fertilization

embryo: the developing infant during the first two months of conception

human chorionic gonadotropin (HCG): a hormone produced during the first stages of pregnancy; it is used as a basis for pregnancy tests

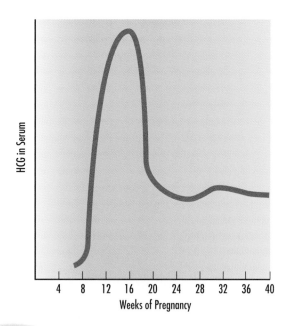

FIGURE 7.6 *Pattern of Human Chorionic Gonadotropin (HCG) Secretion During Pregnancy*

analyzing a woman's urine for the presence of HCG. Such tests are about 80–90% accurate. The most frequent type of inaccuracy is a false negative result—reporting no pregnancy when one actually exists.

On rare occasions, the fertilized egg implants outside the uterus, usually in a fallopian tube where its passage is blocked by tubal malformation or scarring or twisting from an earlier infection, often gonorrhea or chlamydia. A pregnancy in which the fertilized egg implants somewhere other than in the uterus is called an **ectopic pregnancy.**

The Developing Fetus

The 9-month span of pregnancy is customarily divided into three 3-month segments called trimesters. Characteristic changes occur in each trimester.

First Trimester

Day 1: The sperm joins with the ovum (egg) to form one cell, which is smaller than the head of a pin. The embryo has inherited 23 chromosomes from each parent, 46 total, which contain the complex genetic blueprint for every detail of development.

Days 3 to 4: The fertilized egg journeys down the fallopian tube to the uterus, where the lining is now prepared for implantation.

Days 5 to 9: During this time, the fertilized egg implants itself in the rich lining of the uterus and begins to draw nourishment.

Days 10 to 14: The developing embryo signals its presence through placental chemicals and hormones, preventing the mother from menstruating.

Day 20: An early brain, spinal cord, and nervous system has already developed.

Day 21: The heart begins to beat.

Day 35: Five fingers are visible on the hand. The eyes darken as pigment is produced.

Day 40: Brain waves can be detected and recorded.

Week 6: The embryo's liver is producing its own blood cells, and the brain controls movements of muscles and organs. The mother has missed her second period and has probably confirmed that she is pregnant.

Week 7: Teeth buds can be seen on the newly formed jaws. New eyelids close to protect the sensitive developing eyes. The eyes will not reopen until the end of the sixth month and beginning of the seventh month.

Week 8: The embryo is now officially called a fetus (Latin for *young one* or *offspring*). Everything that can be found in a human adult is now present in the fetus. The stomach produces digestive juices and the kidneys have begun to function. Forty separate sets of muscles are operating. Testicles begin to form in the male; ovary formation occurs a little bit later in the female. The fetus responds to touch, but the body is so small (about 1/2 inches long) that the mother is not yet able to feel any movement.

Week 9: Fingerprints are already evident on the skin. The fetus will curl its fingers around an object placed in the palm of its hand.

Week 10: The uterus has now doubled in size. The fetus can squint, swallow, and wrinkle its forehead.

Week 11: The fetus now sleeps, wakes, and exercises its muscles energetically—turning its head, curling its toes, and opening and closing its mouth. The fetus breathes amniotic fluid to help strengthen its respiratory system.

Second Trimester

Month 4: The ears are functioning, and the fetus hears the mother's voice and heartbeat as well as external noises. The eyebrows and eyelashes become visible. The fetus' entire body structure is formed, and the skin is covered with fine down-like hair. The sex of the fetus can be identified by ultrasonography, which uses high-frequency sound waves to create a visual image (sonogram).

Month 5: The mother can feel movement now, often referred to as the *"quickening."* If a sound is especially loud or startling, the fetus may jump in reaction to it. The scalp hair is visible. The skin has a bright pinkish hue and is covered by a cheese-like substance that will remain until after birth. The fetus is now 8 inches long and weighs about 11 ounces.

Month 6: Oil and sweat glands are functioning. Eyelids have separated and are open and skin is wrinkled and red. The fetus is 10 to 12 inches long and weighs 1 to 1½ pounds. About 4 out of 10 babies born now will survive.

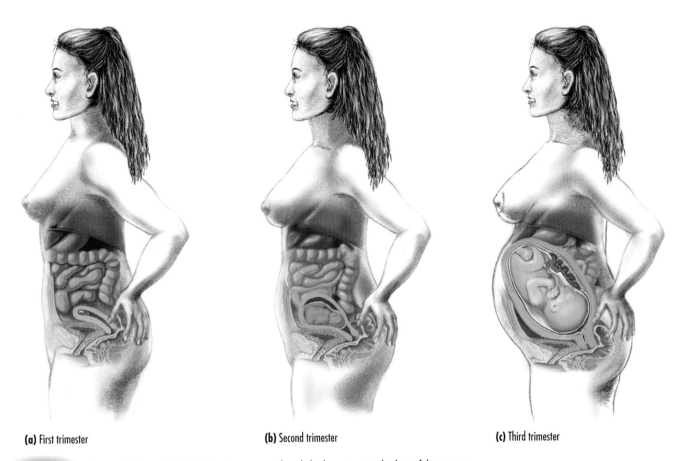

(a) First trimester   **(b)** Second trimester   **(c)** Third trimester

FIGURE 7.7   **Changes in Woman's Body During Pregnancy**   Through the three trimesters, the shape of the pregnant woman's body changes dramatically.

Third Trimester

Month 7: The baby uses four senses, all but touch, and can recognize the mother's voice. By the end of this month, the head and body are more proportionate, and the eyes are open. The testes of the male have descended into the scrotum. The baby has rotated and repositioned with the head downward toward the cervix of the uterus and now weights 2½ pounds and is about 11 to 13 inches long. About 9 out of 10 babies born now will survive.

Month 8: By the end of this month, the baby weighs 3½ to 4 pounds and is 14 to 16 inches long. Almost all babies born now will survive.

Month 9: The skin has lost its wrinkled appearance as a result of the accumulation of body fat. Toward the end of this month, the baby is ready for birth. Healthy fetuses born after the normal 266-day gestation period weigh between 5 and 10 pounds (The First 9 Months Fetal Development, 1998).

Fetal development and growth take place with the fetus enclosed in a fluid-filled membranous sac called the **amnion,** which forms during the second week of development. As it develops in the **amniotic fluid,** the fetus is able to grow unimpeded by the mother's internal organs. The amniotic fluid also protects the fetus from potentially damaging jolts when the mother changes her body position. The amnion ruptures just before birth, sometimes called "breaking of the bag of waters."

The growth and development of the fetus are supported by the **placenta,** an organ unique to pregnancy. The placenta manufactures many hormones needed to sustain pregnancy and is responsible for transporting oxygen and nutrients from the mother to the fetus and waste products from the fetus to the mother.

A number of changes occur in a pregnant woman's physiology (Figure 7.7). For example, the blood plasma increases in volume as much as 50% over her non-pregnant levels; the heart beats 10% faster and with

Terms

ectopic pregnancy: a pregnancy occurring outside the uterus, usually in the fallopian tubes

amnion: the inner membrane that forms a fluid-filled sac surrounding and protecting the embryo and fetus

amniotic fluid: fluid of the amnion

placenta: the flat circular vascular structure within the pregnant uterus that provides nourishment to and eliminates wastes from the developing embryo and fetus and is passed as afterbirth after the baby is born

20% to 30% greater output per minute; the number of red blood cells increases; and breathing becomes deeper and slightly faster. One of the most striking changes during pregnancy is the growth of the uterus. The nonpregnant uterus is approximately 7 to 8 centimeters long (2¾ to 3½ inches) and weighs about 60 to 100 grams (2 to 3½ ounces). By the end of pregnancy, the uterus is approximately 30 centimeters long (12 inches) and weighs nearly 1,000 grams (2.2 pounds).

Health Habits During Pregnancy

Every child deserves to be born as healthy as possible. It is only fair to the unborn child—who did not ask to be conceived—that all the genetic potential to develop a healthy body and mind be given the opportunity to be fully expressed. Few of us are as careful about maintaining proper health habits as we could be. Most people live with whatever risk might be associated with nonhealthy behaviors and are presumably willing to accept the consequences of those behaviors. But when a woman is pregnant, disregarding fundamental health practices endangers her child as well as herself, and perhaps more so, because the developing baby's body and mind are extremely vulnerable to damage. A mother-to-be must make every effort to practice good health habits.

Nutrition

Throughout pregnancy, the fetus' cells and physiological capacities are developing. Perhaps more than at any other time of life, an ample supply of nutrients is required so that the formation of new cells and the development of organs proceeds optimally. All fetal nutrients come from the mother via the placenta. Therefore, a pregnant woman directly influences the nutritional status of her baby, and she must be sure her diet contains adequate nutrients for herself and for her baby. Mothers-to-be who eat highly nutritious diets during pregnancy are more likely to give birth to healthy babies than are mothers whose diets are nutritionally poor. Pregnant women should increase their intake of essential nutrients and calories. For some women it is advisable to supplement a generally well-balanced diet with extra iron and folic acid. Remember that early in the pregnancy, the developing fetus inside of the mother is tiny and only requires about 300 calories a day. Later, as the mother's metabolism speeds up, she may need more than the 300 calories for her baby.

Many pregnant women are concerned with the amount of weight they gain. While it is never good to weigh too much, current obstetric practice allows a mother-to-be to gain a reasonable amount of weight, about 28 to 30 pounds by the end of pregnancy, most of which comes in the last two-thirds of pregnancy. About 7 of these pounds are contributed by the fetus. The enlarged uterus accounts for another 2 pounds, and the placenta and amniotic fluid contribute 1 pound each. About 4 to 8 pounds of fluid are added to the maternal system as extra blood and extracellular fluid. And the mother may gain about 4 pounds of body fat.

Physical Activity and Exercise

There are special benefits to being physically active during pregnancy. Some women feel lethargic during pregnancy. In just a few weeks, their bodies take on unfamiliar proportions and they have to carry up to 20% more weight than when they are not pregnant. They may feel uncomfortable, unattractive, and clumsy. Through movement and exercise, a pregnant woman can become accustomed to the temporary changes in her body and accept pregnancy as a positive and fulfilling time of her life. Physical activity also helps prepare the mother's body for childbirth, which is often physically demanding. By keeping active, a pregnant woman can improve her circulation and thereby reduce swelling and formation of varicose veins in the lower legs, which can be common in pregnancy. Well-conditioned women who engage in aerobics or run regularly have (as a group) shorter labors and fewer cesarean deliveries. Exercise during pregnancy can tone a woman's muscles so that her body returns more quickly to its original shape after delivery. Perhaps the greatest benefit from physical activity during pregnancy is maintaining the habit of being active. That way, after the baby is born, the mother can lose body fat gained during pregnancy and return her body to a firm nonpregnant state.

Emotional Well-Being

Pregnancy can be a time of intense feelings, not only for the mother-to-be but also for her partner and others who are close to her. Enthusiasm, excitement, anticipation, fear about the baby's condition, uncertainties about one's suitability as a parent, and a desire for more (or less) love, affection, and sex are all natural. Recognizing that intense feelings are normal in pregnancy and accepting them with patience and understanding are the keys to a rewarding experience.

Perhaps the best way to deal with intense feelings at any time in life, including pregnancy, is to take time each day to quiet the mind and body with meditation, yoga, or other relaxation methods. Massage is also beneficial, and it fulfills some of the desires of those who feel more sensual during pregnancy. Some couples feel increased desire for sexual intercourse during pregnancy, which is all right unless the woman has a medical problem that would be worsened by sex. In that event couples can engage in the many forms of pleasuring that do not involve sexual intercourse.

Prenatal Care

Pregnancy involves several profound biological changes. Not only does the fetus develop from a single cell to a 7- or 8-pound newborn infant (composed of many millions of cells) but the mother's body also undergoes a number of anatomical and physiological changes in order to support fetal development. Moreover, the fetal-maternal relationship is maintained by the placenta, an organ that develops only during pregnancy and is expelled from the mother's uterus after the baby is born. Any rapidly changing system is vulnerable to errors and problems, and so it is with pregnancy and fetal development. That is why it is recommended that mothers-to-be receive professional prenatal care.

A number of studies have shown that the more prenatal care a woman receives, the fewer problems she will have during pregnancy and childbirth and the more likely that her infant will be born healthy. Professional prenatal care can help a mother-to-be avoid the consequences of a number of pregnancy-specific illnesses, such as toxemia, pregnancy-induced diabetes, and infection. These illnesses can threaten both the mother's health and the proper development and delivery of her baby. Professional prenatal care can also help manage problems resulting from a malfunctioning placenta and can educate a mother about proper nutrition and advise her on how smoking at any time during pregnancy can adversely affect her baby's development, as can consumption of alcohol. Maternal infections that are harmful to the fetus, such as rubella (German measles), syphilis, gonorrhea, toxoplasmosis, herpes, and the HIV infection, can be detected and managed. Another reason for prenatal care is to be sure the maternal and fetal blood cells are immunologically (Rh factor) compatible.

Drugs Both legal medications (prescription and over-the-counter) and street (illegal) drugs taken by a woman or her partner can significantly affect her and her fetus during pregnancy. Especially critical are drugs that, if taken during the embryonic period (from week 2 through week 8), can cause developmental malformations.

Aspirin and other drugs that contain salicylate are not recommended for use during the last 3 months of pregnancy unless under a physician's supervision.

Wellness Guide

Healthy Eating Tips During Pregnancy

- Protein is a must during pregnancy; at least 60 to 75 grams daily are essential for proper fetal development.

- Vitamin C helps in tissue repair and other healing processes; try for two servings daily. Also, vitamin C is used by your baby for strong teeth and bones.

- Calcium is necessary to ensure your baby grows healthy and strong. Calcium aids in the development of bones, teeth, muscles, heart, and nerves. Aim for at least four servings of calcium daily.

- Vitamins A and E help your baby develop healthy skin, eyes, and bones. Indulge in three servings daily of yellow fruits and green leafy vegetables.

- Vitamin B, zinc, magnesium, and selenium can be found in whole wheat breads, pasta, cereals, beans, and rice. Have five servings daily.

- Iron is essential to the fetal blood supply and the mother's as well. Iron supplements can be taken after the twelfth week of pregnancy.

- Extra fluids for the mother during pregnancy help to reduce constipation, rid the body of toxins, reduce urinary tract infections, and keep skin hydrated. Eight glasses of fluids should be consumed daily.

- Avoid foods such as sweets, cakes, cookies, fried foods, high-cholesterol and high-fat foods, pork, lamb, and beef.

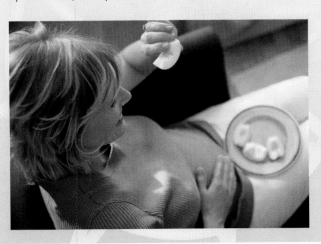

Staying physically active during pregnancy has many benefits.

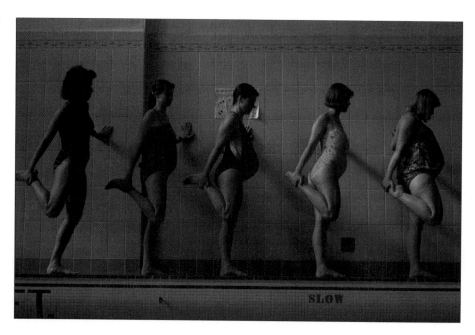

Acetylsalicylate, found in many painkillers, can prolong pregnancy and cause excessive bleeding before and after delivery.

Cocaine used by a pregnant woman subjects the fetus to a higher risk of retarded growth, attention and orientation problems, a tendency to stop breathing, crib death, and malformed or missing organs, as well as increasing the risk of miscarriage, premature birth, and stillbirth.

Other illicit drugs can also adversely affect an unborn child. Marijuana interferes with the normal production of male sperm. Heroin, morphine, and other opiates can damage the chromosomes in the ovum and sperm, causing abnormalities.

Alcohol   When alcohol crosses the placental barrier, it reaches a level in the fetus equal to that in the body of the woman. Because the body of the fetus is small and its detoxification system immature, alcohol remains in fetal blood long after it has disappeared in the woman's blood. The relationship between fetal alcohol exposure and occurrence of birth defects is complex. However, scientists agree that drinking alcohol can harm the fetus, and that the risk of damage increases as the quantity and frequency of maternal alcohol consumption increases. The fetus is at risk of developing fetal alcohol syndrome (FAS) if the mother drinks six or more drinks per day during her pregnancy. The symptoms of FAS include growth retardation, facial malformations, and central nervous system dysfunctions, including mental retardation and behavioral dysfunctions. FAS is the third most common cause of mental retardation in the western world, after Down syndrome and malformations of the nervous system. This is particularly distressing because FAS can be prevented!

Cigarette Smoking   Another serious health hazard for the fetus is cigarette smoking. Maternal smoking increases the chances of spontaneous abortion and of complications that can result in fetal or infant death. Smoking reduces the amount of oxygen in the bloodstream, and this can adversely affect the fetus by slowing its growth. Infants of mothers who smoked during pregnancy often weigh less and are in poorer general condition than are infants of nonsmoking mothers. Smoking may be teratogenic, causing cardiac abnormalities and anencephaly (absence of a cerebrum). Maternal smoking appears to be a significant factor in the development of cleft lip and palate, and a positive relationship has been shown between both cigarette smoking and inhalation of passive (secondhand) smoke and the occurrence of sudden infant death syndrome (SIDS).

Prenatal Testing

A reliable and accurate test for detecting birth defects, known as an **amniocentesis,** can be performed between the fourteenth and eighteenth week of pregnancy. The procedure consists of inserting a hollow needle with the assistance of ultrasonographic imagery through the woman's abdominal wall and into the uterine cavity to draw out a sample of the amniotic fluid (fluid surrounding the fetus). Fetal cells are cultured for chromosomal analysis and analyzed under a microscope. The procedure can detect several hundred fetal abnormalities and biochemical defects.

The test can be performed during any trimester if enough fluid is present. If done during the first trimester, it is usually for genetic studies; in the second trimester, for Rh isoimmunization studies; and in the third trimester, for assessing fetal lung maturity.

Chorionic villus sampling (CVS) is used during the first trimester of pregnancy to detect biochemical disorders and chromosomal abnormalities. Chorionic villi are threadlike protrusions on a membrane surrounding the fetus that are comprised of fetal cells. This test involves inserting a thin catheter with the assistance of ultrasonographic imagery through the abdomen or vagina and cervix into the uterus, where a small sample of chorionic villi is removed for analysis. This procedure has an advantage over amniocentesis because it can be done as early as the eighth week after the last menstrual period.

Problems During Pregnancy

Most women have uneventful pregnancies, but others encounter complications along the way. Spontaneous abortion, stillbirth, preeclampsia, and premature birth are some of the problems that pregnant women may face.

Spontaneous Abortion and Stillbirth

Spontaneous abortion, or miscarriage, occurs in the first 20 weeks of pregnancy when the fetus cannot live outside the uterus. A stillbirth is one in which there are no signs of life in the fetus at birth or after.

The majority of miscarriages occur in the first 12 weeks of pregnancy and may appear as a heavier than usual menstrual flow; miscarriages that occur later may involve uncomfortable cramping and heavy bleeding. Miscarriages increase in frequency with maternal and paternal age. An early miscarriage might be the result of an embryonic or fetal problem, such as a chromosomal or developmental abnormality. It is estimated that 10% of all pregnancies end in spontaneous abortion.

Miscarriage or stillbirth can be a significant loss for the woman or couple. She may experience feelings of anger, grief, despair, guilt, jealousy, and isolation. A woman's adjustment after a loss through miscarriage or stillbirth is not only emotional but also physical. Her body experiences the sudden withdrawal of pregnancy hormones. Friends and family can be helpful in acknowledging the loss and asking what the experience has been like for the person.

Preeclampsia

About 15% of pregnant women experience elevated blood pressure, or pregnancy-induced hypertension (PIH). If PIH is accompanied by protein in the urine and swelling in the face, hands, and feet, the condition is referred to as preeclampsia, which apparently results from impaired kidney functioning. Signs of this condition usually occur after the twentieth week: a woman's blood pressure must be checked during each prenatal visit. In severe cases, painful headache and blurred vision may occur (eclampsia). If preeclampsia is evident, the woman should be admitted to the hospital for observation.

I was so ugly when I was born, the doctor slapped my mother.
HENNY YOUNGMAN

Premature Birth

The best indicator of adequate fetal growth and development is birth weight. An infant weighing 5½ pounds or less at birth is considered a premature infant. Several factors influencing birth weight include gender (male babies weigh more than female babies), birth order (firstborns weigh less), race (white babies weigh more at term than African American babies), age of the mother (under age 17 or over age 34), socioeconomic status (poverty), marital status (unmarried), education (uneducated), and prenatal care (lack of access).

Premature and low-birth-weight babies have had a significantly higher chance of survival in recent years as a result of the development of neonatal intensive care units, which include control of oxygen, temperature, humidity levels, and intravenous feeding until the infant maintains a healthy weight. Care can be expensive, and often there are long-term severe mental and physical handicaps in low-birth-weight babies.

Childbirth

For the parents, the moment of childbirth can bring a mixture of feelings that might include great joy, relief that the 9 months of waiting are over, and surprise at the baby's appearance. All in attendance may experience concern for the condition of the mother and baby and awe and wonder at the miracle of new life.

Childbirth Preparation

A variety of programs and organizations provide education for parents-to-be in preparation for the childbirth experience and parenthood. These are usually 6- to 8-week courses, sometimes called "natural childbirth," "Lamaze," or simply childbirth preparation.

Terms

amniocentesis: a procedure that involves aspiration of amniotic fluid from the uterus to detect certain abnormalities in the fetus

chorionic villus sampling (CVS): a method to detect biochemical disorders and chromosomal abnormalities in the fetus

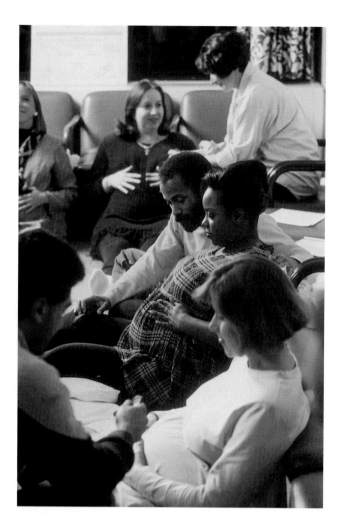

Childbirth preparation classes help ensure a healthy baby.

Childbirth preparation classes can enhance the intimate relationship of the expectant couple and increase their confidence and self-esteem. In addition, women who participate in childbirth preparation are likely to have less pain and discomfort in childbirth, to require less medication, and to have fewer complications. Prepared women are also more likely to have positive attitudes toward childbirth and parenting. Fathers who attend childbirth preparation classes tend to feel more comfortable about sharing the birth experience with their partners and about helping them during it. They are also more likely to be interested and involved in parenting after the baby is born.

Almost all childbirth preparation courses teach prospective parents the basic biology of pregnancy and childbirth. They also teach breathing and relaxation exercises, and some teach imagery and affirmations, all intended to make the delivery of the baby proceed more smoothly and comfortably.

Giving Birth

A few weeks before the onset of childbirth, or **labor,** the fetus becomes positioned for birth by descending in the uterus, a process called **lightening.** When this happens the pressure on some of the mother's internal organs is relieved and she may find it easier to breathe, stand, and digest food. In about 95% of all births the fetus is in a head-down position. When not head-down, the fetus may be head-up, referred to as a breech position. In nearly all instances, the fetus' legs are tucked up against its abdomen in the "fetal position."

There are three generally recognizable stages in the process of childbirth (Figure 7.8). Before the first stage begins, the cervix has already effaced (flattened and thinned) and dilated slightly. The **first stage** of labor starts with the beginning of uterine contractions and lasts until the cervix is fully dilated. Another indication of first-stage labor may be the "bloody show," the discharge of the mucous plug from the cervix. The first stage is the longest of the three stages, usually lasting 10 to 16 hours for the first childbirth and 4 to 8 hours in subsequent deliveries. This stage lasts until the cervix is dilated 10 centimeters.

The **second stage** of labor begins when the cervix is fully dilated and the infant descends farther into the vaginal birth canal (normally, head first). This stage lasts from 30 minutes to 2 hours. During this time the woman can actively push with each contraction until the infant is expelled. The remaining amniotic fluid gushes out. The infant is cleaned and its vital signs, such as breathing and color, are quickly checked. The umbilical cord is clamped off several inches from the navel, and the baby soon begins to breathe.

The **third stage** of labor lasts from the time of birth until the delivery of the placenta, or **afterbirth.** With one or two more uterine contractions, the placenta usually separates from the uterine wall and is expelled from the vagina, generally within 30 minutes after the baby is born. During this time, the uterus begins returning to its original size.

Options for Controlling Discomfort

Intense discomfort or pain can accompany labor, especially in the later phases of the first stage and the early stages of the second. The intensity of feeling is caused by stretches and strains on the uterine muscle tissue, effacement of the cervix, and stretching of the perineum. Pain relief methods include relaxation techniques, deep breathing, acupuncture, hypnosis, massaging and supporting of the perineum by the birth attendant, medications that block pain awareness (analgesia), and medications that block the pain sensations (anesthesia). The most common anesthesia used during labor is a regional anesthetic to diminish sensation only in the pelvic region. This leaves the mother conscious during labor so that she can actively "bear down" to help push the baby out. General anesthesia (complete unconsciousness) is used only in

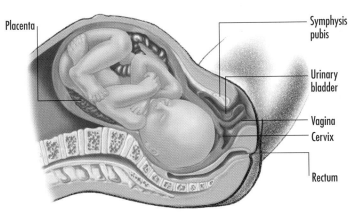

Placenta — Symphysis pubis

Urinary bladder

Vagina
Cervix

Rectum

(a) Early first-stage labor

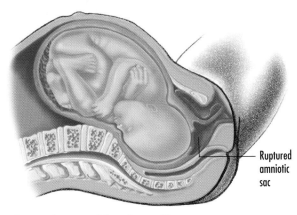

Ruptured amniotic sac

(b) Later first-stage labor: the transition

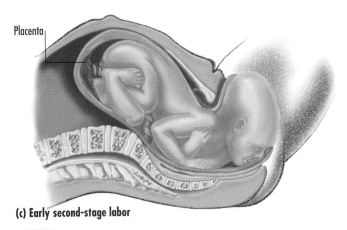

Placenta

(c) Early second-stage labor

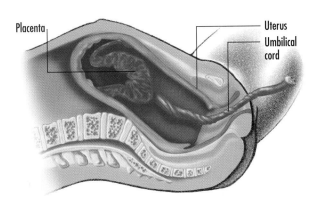

Uterus
Umbilical cord

Placenta

(d) Third-stage labor: delivery of afterbirth

FIGURE 7.8 **Childbirth** The stages of labor. **(a)** First stage: The cervix is dilating. **(b)** Late first stage (transition stage): The cervix is fully dilated, and the amniotic sac has ruptured, releasing amniotic fluid. **(c)** Second stage: The birth of the infant. **(d)** Third stage: Delivery of the placenta (afterbirth).

cases of difficult births and interventions, such as cesarean sections.

Besides the administration of medications, an **episiotomy,** an incision in the perineum from the vagina to the anus, is often done late in the first stage of labor before the head of the infant emerges. The procedure may be necessary when the infant's head is too large for the opening, when the infant is in distress or in an irregular position, when there is need for a forceps delivery, or when the perineum has not stretched sufficiently. Episiotomies are performed on the majority of first-time mothers in the United States.

The benefits of episiotomies are that they speed up birth time, prevent tearing, protect against incontinence, protect against pelvic floor elevations, and heal more easily than tears. Although these are valid reasons for an episiotomy, reported side effects of the procedure include infection, increased pain, increase in third- and fourth-degree vaginal lacerations, slower healing, and increased discomfort when intercourse is resumed. If a woman is concerned about having an episiotomy, she should talk to her doctor, because much of the time episiotomies are not necessary.

Cesarean Section

When a normal vaginal delivery is considered dangerous or impossible, a fetus is removed through an incision made in the abdominal wall and uterus, in a surgical procedure called a **cesarean section,** or **C-section.** Cesarean births may be recommended in a variety of

Terms

labor: the process of childbirth

lightening: the positioning of the fetus for birth by descent in the uterus

first-stage labor: the beginning of labor during which there are regular contractions of the uterus

second-stage labor: the stage during which the baby moves out through the vagina and is delivered

third-stage labor: the stage during which the afterbirth is expelled

afterbirth: placenta and fetal membranes

episiotomy: an incision in the perineum to facilitate passage of the baby's head during childbirth, while minimizing injury to the woman

cesarean section: delivery of the fetus through a surgical opening in the abdomen and uterus

situations, including a fetal head that is too large for the mother's pelvic structure, maternal illness, active herpes infection in the vaginal tract, fetal distress during labor, or birth complications such as breech-fetal presentation (feet or bottom coming out of the uterus first).

The Postpartum Transition and Breast-Feeding

After the child is born, the mother goes through several weeks of postpartum transition called the **puerperium.** During this time, the physiological changes of pregnancy slowly reverse and the vagina and the surrounding structures recuperate from labor. Uterine tissue that is no longer needed is discharged for the first month or so after childbirth. The discharge, called lochia, at first resembles a heavy menstrual flow, then typically tapers off after a week or two. Following delivery, estrogen and progesterone levels, which were high during pregnancy, drop rapidly, reaching almost zero about 72 hours after birth.

During this period the mother and her partner begin to adjust to their often demanding new life situation. Childbirth and infant care are exhausting. Many women experience the "baby blues," which are transitory mood changes involving tiredness, depression, loneliness, or fear. These feelings usually abate in the weeks following childbirth, but a minority of women experience postpartum depression severe enough to be disabling and require professional help. Postpartum mood changes are so common that experts suggest they may be related to the massive changes in hor-

mone levels that accompany childbirth. Others, while not denying the effects of hormonal changes, point out that childbirth is a life transition that brings many changes and psychological adjustments for the woman, her partner, and other family and household members.

The preparation of the breasts for nursing begins in the early weeks of pregnancy with an increase in the number of milk ducts and the deposit of fat in the breast tissue. This growth causes breast tenderness early in pregnancy. In addition to the increase in breast size, the nipples enlarge and often deepen in color. About midway into pregnancy, the breasts begin to manufacture **colostrum,** a yellowish precursor to actual mother's milk. For the first few days after birth, colostrum is the major substance emitted from the breasts. As the newborn nurses, colostrum is drained from the breasts and is replaced by mother's milk. Colostrum contains nutrients and is especially high in antibodies that protect the infant against infection. Mother's milk contains specific milk proteins, antibodies, lactose, fat, and water. The synthesis of milk is controlled by the pituitary hormone **prolactin,** the levels of which rise tremendously during pregnancy and are maintained as long as the mother continues to nurse.

A mother can nurse for many months. As long as the baby is sucking and the breasts are regularly drained of milk, the hormonal stimulation of milk production will continue. Without such stimuli, milk production stops.

Although there are advantages to breast-feeding, this does not mean that bottle feeding is not wholesome. Many healthy, well-adjusted people were bottle-fed infants. Some women are physically unable to

Breast milk provides a baby with essential nutrients and helps prevent infections.

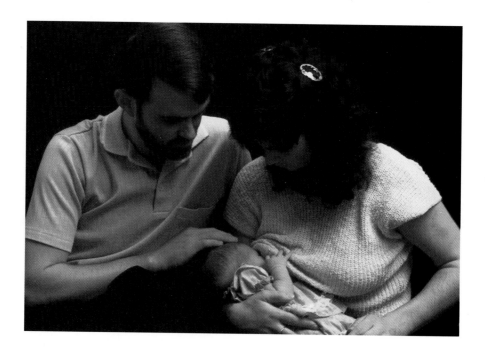

breast-feed. Some mothers choose not to breast-feed because work, family, and other responsibilities make it inconvenient. Breast-feeding in public or at work is, unfortunately, still not acceptable in many communities or places of employment. Some women choose not to breast-feed because they fear that changes in the shape of their breasts will decrease their sexual attractiveness.

Some women breast-feed their infants for several weeks or months and then gradually substitute bottle feedings for breast feedings until the child is completely **weaned,** that is, has stopped nursing altogether. More important than whether the milk comes from the breast or a bottle is the physical contact and loving the infant receives while being fed.

Infertility

Approximately one in five of all American married couples of childbearing age are **infertile,** which means that they are unable to become pregnant after a year of trying. Male factors are responsible for infertility in about 40% of infertile couples; female factors in another 40% to 50%. In about 10% of infertile couples, no cause can be determined. With professional help, about half of all infertile couples can eventually have children. A significant percentage of couples medically determined to be infertile eventually have children without medical interventions.

In both sexes, infertility can be caused by a variety of conditions that adversely affect the functioning of an otherwise normal reproductive system. For example, ill health, cigarette smoking, chronic alcohol use, marijuana and other drug abuse, exposure to radiation or toxic chemicals, malnutrition, anxiety, stress, and fatigue can lessen a person's reproductive capabilities. Medical treatments or changes in life-style can often restore fertility.

Obstacles to Fertility

Because sperm and ovum production and the functions of the male and female reproductive tracts are absolutely dependent on adequate hormone production, hormonal problems are a common cause of infertility in both men and women. Infertility can also be caused by anatomical abnormalities or damage to the male or female reproductive systems. A common cause of damage is scarring and subsequent blocking of the fallopian tubes and, less frequently, the epididymis, by gonorrhea or chlamydia infections (see chapter 8). The scar tissue from such diseases blocks the tubes and prevents the passage of sperm and ova. Growths and tumors in the reproductive tract can also block the passage of sperm and ova. Sometimes surgical repair of blocked or damaged tubes can restore fertility.

Problems with **insemination** and sperm transport can also cause infertility. For example, a man may have difficulty getting and maintaining an erection or ejaculating into the vagina. A woman may produce very thick or voluminous cervical mucus, which can block entry of sperm into the uterus. Sometimes a couple has trouble conceiving because they are not having intercourse near the time of ovulation.

Enhancing Fertility Options

A variety of medical interventions are available to help infertile couples become pregnant. For example, if a male partner produces too few sperm, but those he does produce are healthy, conception is unlikely to occur. For conception to occur, more than 20 million healthy sperm need to be deposited in the vagina. Fertilization can be facilitated by introducing semen obtained from the man directly into the cervix with a syringe. This is called **artificial insemination.** If the male partner cannot produce sufficient numbers of healthy sperm even for artificial insemination, the couple may become pregnant by artificial insemination with semen from a donor.

Another way to overcome infertility is ***in vitro fertilization (IVF),*** which involves obtaining several ova from the ovaries and fertilizing them in a laboratory dish. The resultant embryo is placed into the woman's uterus. *In vitro* fertilization is employed when a woman's fallopian tubes do not function correctly. GIFT (gamete intrafallopian transfer) and ZIFT (zygote intrafallopian transfer) are similar to *in vitro* fertilization. With GIFT, the ova are placed in equal numbers in each of the fallopian tubes and semen is introduced directly into the tubes. With ZIFT, eggs are fertilized *in vitro* and an embryo is placed in the fallopian tube. These procedures are successful between 10% and 20% of the time.

Terms

puerperium: the 6 weeks after childbirth, also called postpartum period

colostrum: yellowish liquid secreted from the breasts; contains antibodies and protein

prolactin: a hormone produced by the anterior lobe of the pituitary gland that stimulates milk secretion

weaned: to discontinue breast-feeding, using other means to provide nutrients

infertile: unable to become pregnant or to impregnate

insemination: introduction of semen into the uterus or oviduct

artificial insemination: introduction of semen into the uterus or oviduct by other than natural means

***in vitro* fertilization (IVF):** a procedure in which an egg is removed from a ripe follicle and fertilized by a sperm cell outside the human body; the fertilized egg is allowed to divide in a protected environment for about 2 days and then is inserted back into the uterus

For some couples, the prospect of not being able to have a child is devastating. Many of these couples embark on lengthy efforts, which may cost thousands of dollars and consume much of their emotional energy, to become pregnant and have a healthy baby. Such couples may be asked to keep careful records of the woman's fertility cycle and to time intercourse for maximum likelihood of conception. They may be counseled to have intercourse at certain times after hormone treatments. They may make repeated visits to fertility clinics to undergo IVF or other medical interventions.

About 40,000 infertile couples in the United States attempt to have a child using IVF techniques each year. However, for most of these couples repeated attempts to conceive end in failure. For women under age 35, the success rate is approximately 20%; for women over age 40, the success rate is under 10% (Begley, 1995). In addition to the poor success rate, couples pay approximately $10,000 for each attempt to become pregnant and health insurance generally does not cover any IVF costs.

> When my kids become wild and unruly, I use a nice, safe playpen. When they're finished, I climb out.
>
> ERMA BOMBECK,
> columnist

 ## Adoption

There are many reasons why adults may want to raise children who are not biologically their own. They may be partially motivated by a concern with overpopulation and a desire to give homeless children love and security. Another common reason is that a couple is unable to have children because of infertility. One alternative for couples, or even single people and gay couples, is adoption. Many adoptions bring the happiness anticipated to otherwise childless couples.

There are three avenues to pursue when couples would like to adopt a child. Most commonly, adoptions are handled through state-licensed *private* or *public adoption agencies,* usually nonprofit social services, which handle approximately 70% of all adoptions. An agency adoption may be the best option for adopting an older child, a minority child, or a child with special needs, although agencies also help in the adoption of infants and foreign children. Signing up with an adoption agency can be a lengthy process, often lasting several years.

Another way to adopt a child is through an *independent* or *private adoption.* The individuals wishing to adopt a child make arrangements with a woman who wants to give up custody of her child, often with an attorney, physician, or cleric serving as an intermediary. Every state has its own laws concerning independent adoption, and the prospective parents should know the laws in their state as well as the state of the birth mother. In all independent adoptions, the birth parents can give consent for adoption only after the birth of the child.

A third avenue to pursue is an *international adoption.* This is becoming an increasingly popular avenue for prospective parents. Both state and federal requirements must be met in international adoptions; however, the waiting period is not as lengthy as it is in private or public adoptions.

Critical Thinking About Health

1. Think about the small children in your immediate or extended family. How did your family gender-type these children (e.g., clothes, toys, decoration of rooms, playmates)? How does the media contribute to gender-typing of children? Does gender-typing continue as we grow older? (Give examples to back up your answer.)

2. Communication is critical to negotiating condom use, whether for birth control or prevention of sexually transmitted infections. There are many reasons why men and women do not want to use a condom, but you must be prepared in advance to respond thoughtfully and respectfully to ensure a condom will be used. Describe how you would respond to the following statements:

   Condoms are too expensive.
   Sex isn't pleasurable with a condom.
   I'm Catholic; I'm not allowed to use a condom.
   I can't believe that you think I have an STI.
   If you really loved me, you wouldn't ask me to use a condom.

3. List all the people (e.g., parents, siblings, friends, boyfriends or girlfriends, spouses) that you are currently "intimate" with. (Remember that "being intimate" does not mean "having sex.") Describe what each of those relationships means to you and discuss how they all contribute to your health and happiness.

4. You have recently found out you are 6 weeks pregnant (or that your girlfriend is pregnant). You have been dating for 6 months and have discussed marriage. But neither of you has finished college and you both want to go to graduate school.
   a. List the options available to you. Identify the pros and cons for each option.
   b. Of the options listed, which would you do given the above circumstances? Why?

5. We know that drugs, alcohol, and smoking are dangerous to a developing fetus. Imagine that you are working as a server in a restaurant.
   a. What would you do if a customer who was pregnant ordered a glass of wine? Would you serve her?
   b. What would you do if a customer who was pregnant was smoking a cigarette? Would you say something?
   c. How do the woman's rights compare to the fetus' rights?

Health in Review

- Sex refers to one's biological classification as male or female and to the experience of creating erotic pleasure.
- Sexuality consists of the aspects of oneself that affect sexual experience: the physical, psychological, social, orientational, developmental, and sexual skill dimensions of the whole self.
- One's sexual biology is determined by genetic makeup, which in turn determines the nature of sex organs: the testes, sperm ducts, semen-producing glands, and penis in the male; and the ovaries, fallopian tubes, uterus, vagina, and external genitalia in the female.
- One's sexual psychology is rooted in gender identity, which guides gender role behaviors.
- Sexual arousal and response involves four phases: excitement, plateau, orgasm, and resolution.
- Sexual dysfunctions include erectile dysfunction, ejaculatory disorders, vaginismus, and lack of orgasm.
- Intimate relationships involve sharing one's innermost self. They develop through three stages: selecting a partner, developing intimacy through self-disclosure, and commitment.
- Effective communication is crucial for developing and maintaining relationships.
- Fertilization is followed by cleavages of the embryo as it moves into the uterus. About the sixth day after fertilization the embryo implants in the lining of the uterus, and for the next 266 days or so the fetus develops. After 40 weeks of pregnancy a baby is born.

- Health habits during pregnancy, such as good nutrition, seeking prenatal care, exercise and physical activity, and emotional well-being are particularly important for the development of a healthy fetus.
- Taking drugs, consuming alcohol, and smoking cigarettes during pregnancy can cause fetal damage or birth defects. Tests, such as amniocentesis or chorionic villus sampling, are available to determine whether or not birth defects are present.
- Optimal childbirth can be achieved by attending childbirth preparation classes, ensuring emotional support for the mother during childbirth, and making wise choices about medical interventions, such as episiotomy and pain management.
- Childbirth is divided into three stages. The first stage starts with the beginning of labor and lasts until the cervix is fully dilated. The second stage is the birth of the baby. The third stage is the delivery of the placenta.
- Approximately 20% of American married couples are infertile. Some of these couples can be medically assisted to become pregnant; pregnancy also may occur with *in vitro* fertilization or artificial insemination.
- Adoption is an alternative for childless couples. Children can be adopted through a private or public adoption agency or in an independent or private adoption or an international adoption.

Health and Wellness Online

The World Wide Web contains a wealth of information about health and wellness. By accessing the Internet using Web browser software, such as Netscape Navigator or Microsoft's Internet Explorer, you can gain a new perspective on many topics presented in *Essentials of Health and Wellness, Second Edition*. Access the Jones and Bartlett Publishers web site at http://www.jbpub.com/hwonline.

Everything you always wanted to know about sex—from the experts.

Dealing with the expected and the unexpected.

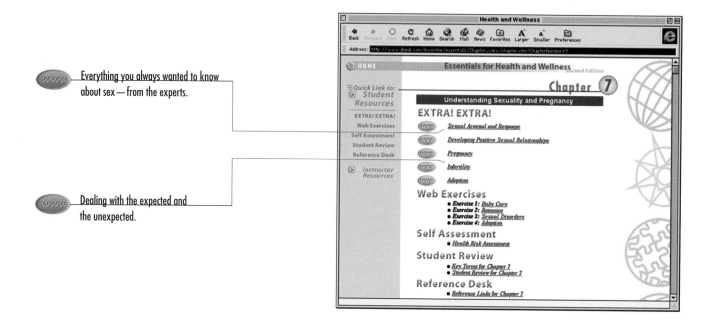

References

Bailey, M., Pillard, R., Neale, M., & Agyei, Y. (1993). Heritable factors influence sexual orientation. *Archives of General Psychiatry, 50,* 217–223.

Begley, S. (1995, September 4). The baby myth. *Newsweek.*

Laumann, E. O., Paik, A., & Rosen, R. C. (1999). Sexual dysfunction in the United States: Prevalence and predictors. *Journal of the American Medical Association, 281*(6), 537–544.

Laumann, E. O., Gagnon, J. H., Michael, R. T., & Michaels, S. (1994). The social organization of sexuality: Sexual practices in the United States. Chicago: The University of Chicago Press.

Masters, W., & Johnson, V. (1996). *Human sexual response.* Boston: Little, Brown.

Mayo Foundation for Medical Education and Research. (1997, October 30). Episiotomy still common, but not always necessary. *Mayo Health Oasis,* URL: http://www.mayohealth.org/9710/htm/episioto.htm

Nimmons, D. (1994, March). Sex and the brain. *Discover,* 64.

Suggested Readings

Blum, D. (1998, April). What made Troy gay? *Health,* 82–86. Troy believes he was born gay, and so do his mother and ex-wife. There is evidence today that may support what Troy believes.

Conti, J., Abraham, S., & Taylor, A. (1998). Eating behavior and pregnancy outcome—What do we know? *Journal of Psychosomatic Research, 44*(3–4), 465–477. The article studies the relationships among clinical eating disorders, maternal body weight, shape, eating concerns, and pregnancy outcomes. Certain pregnancy outcomes of concern include low-birth-weight infants.

Gersberg, C. O. (1998). Pregnant pleasures. *Parents Magazine,* 89–90. This fact-filled article offers advice and guidelines for sexual pleasure during pregnancy.

Gittleman, A. L. (1998). *Before the change: Taking care of your perimenopause.* New York: HarperCollins Publishers. An easy-to-read, well-documented book that provides guidelines for a healthy passage into menopause and beyond.

Handy, B. (1998, May 4). The Viagra craze. *Time,* 50–57. The magic bullet for impotency, Viagra has become a household word. This article explains how Viagra works to produce erections as well as its limits in treating sexual dysfunction.

Jones, M. (1998). *Motherhood after 35: Choices, decisions, options.* Tucson, AZ: Fisher Books. For women between 35 and 45 who are trying to have a baby or who have already conceived, this book evaluates the advantages and the risks of later motherhood.

Longman, P. J. (1998, March 30). The cost of children. *U.S. News & World Report,* 51–53. The average cost of raising a child to adult age is $1.45 million according to the author. This figure may not be so far off once conception, feeding, housing, clothing, toys, and college are considered, not to mention all the incidentals.

Lutz, E. (1998). *Baby maneuvers.* New York: Macmillan General Reference. A humorous book on how to stay active, how to keep doing everyday things, and how to travel with children.

McCarthy, E. (1998). *Male sexual awareness.* NY: Carroll & Graf. This book will guide both men and women toward emotional cooperation and satisfaction, while debunking the myths of rigid male roles and unrealistic performance demands.

Michael, R. T., Gagnon, J. H., Laumann, E. O., & Kolata, G. (1994). *Sex in America.* Boston: Little, Brown. Findings from a national study of adult sexual behavior. Book is intended for the general audience.

Sanders, S. A., & Reinisch, J. M. (1999). Would you say you "had sex" if . . .? *Journal of American Medical Association, 281*(3), 275–277. What does having "had sex" mean to you? This article reports that Americans hold widely divergent opinions about what behaviors do and do not constitute having "had sex."

Schnarch, D. (1998). *Passionate marriage.* NY: Henry Holt and Co. This respectful, erotic, uplifting, and spiritual guide shares how couples can—and must—simultaneously break through the sexual and emotional blocks that hold them back from total satisfaction.

The Boston Women's Health Book Collective. (1998). *Our Bodies, ourselves for the new century: A book by and for women.* NY: Touchstone. This book reflects the vital health concerns of women of diverse ages, ethnic and racial backgrounds, and sexual orientation—a must-read for every woman.

Learning Objectives

1. Identify the advantages and disadvantages for the following fertility control methods: male condom, female condom, spermicides, diaphragm, cervical cap, hormonal contraceptives, Norplant, Depo-Provera, intrauterine device, abstinence, sterilization, withdrawal, and postcoital methods.
2. Identify the most effective and least effective fertility control method.
3. Determine the best fertility control method for your sexual lifestyle.
4. Explain why some sexually active people do not use fertility control.
5. Define abortion and describe the different types of abortion procedures.
6. Describe the impact of sexually transmitted infections (STIs) on society.
7. List the risk factors for contracting an STI.
8. Identify the causative agent, symptoms, and treatment for the following diseases: trichomonas vaginalis and gardnerella vaginalis, chlamydia, gonorrhea, syphilis, genital herpes, genital warts, pubic lice, scabies, and AIDS.
9. Identify several "safer sex" practices.

Exercises and Activities

WORKBOOK
Contraceptive Comfort and Confidence Scale
Knowledge of STIs

Health and Wellness Online

 www.jbpub.com/hwonline

Fertility Control
Sterilization
Common STIs
Global Wellness: HIV Infections Worldwide
Preventing STIs

Choosing a Fertility Control Method and Protecting against Sexually Transmitted Infections

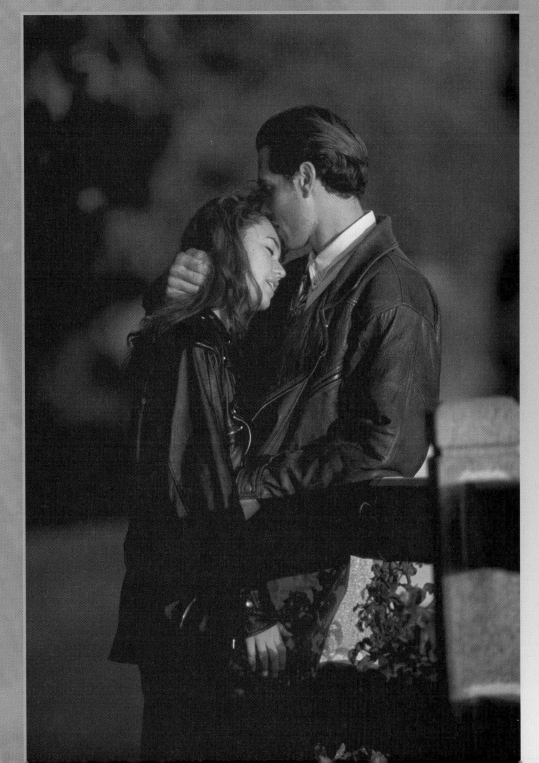

To be aware of the many facets of human sexuality—sexual values, the structure of sexual anatomy, aspects of sexual identity and sexual behavior, and sexual responsiveness—is the first step toward attaining a healthy and fulfilling sexual life. Because sexual activities nearly always involve others, our sexual decisions must also involve concern for the health and well-being of the partner. In this chapter, we discuss responsible sexual decision making as it pertains to the avoidance or termination of unintended pregnancy and the prevention of sexually transmitted (venereal) diseases.

Fertility Control

Many Americans engage in acts of sexual intercourse each year for reasons other than to produce children. Instead of procreation, people often have sex because it is pleasurable and a way to express love and affection. Given the choice, most persons would prefer to separate nearly all of their sexual experiences from conception. Unfortunately, there is no perfect, 100% effective, 100% easy-to-use fertility control method. People decide what contraceptive method to use by considering comfort, desire to use contraception independent of intercourse, how much cooperation they can expect from their partner, and whether or not they also need protection against sexually transmitted infections (STIs).

> *It goes without saying that you should never have more children than you have car windows.*
> ERMA BOMBECK

The most popular contraceptive methods in the United States are female sterilization (10.7 million people), oral contraceptive pills (10.4 million), male condoms (7.9 million), and male sterilization (4.2 million) (Hatcher, et al., 1998).

Throughout history, hundreds of methods of fertility control have been advocated; however, at no time in the past have people had available to them as many safe, reliable methods of fertility control as they have today. Unlike the ancient methods, which were often based on observing animals, their own trial and error, or rooted in superstition and folklore, today's fertility control methods are based on scientific knowledge of human reproductive biology. Some of the modern fertility control techniques are preconception methods (contraceptives). They work by preventing the development or union of sperm and ova. Other techniques are postconception methods. They inhibit in various ways the development of the fertilized ovum or embryo.

When you consider the several methods of fertility control, keep in mind that sex without intercourse is a highly effective way to prevent pregnancy. Genital (penis-in-vagina) intercourse is not the only way to give and receive sexual pleasure. Touching, kissing, and stroking can bring intense sexual enjoyment and even orgasm to both partners.

A fertility control method's effectiveness is measured in terms of its **contraceptive failure rate,** which is the percentage of women who, on average, are likely to become pregnant using a particular method for one year. Failure rates are reported in two ways: **typical use** failure rate and **perfect use** failure rate. Typical use refers to the percentage of *typical* couples who experience an unintended pregnancy during their first year of using the method. Typical users may not use every time and may use incorrectly at times. For example, a 35% typical use failure rate means 35 out of 100 typical users will become pregnant in the first year. Perfect use refers to the percentage of *perfect* couples who experience an unintended pregnancy during their first year using the method. Perfect users are those who use the contraceptive method both consistently and correctly. For example, a 25% perfect use failure rate means 25 out of 100 perfect users will become pregnant in the first year.

Another important measure of contraceptive effectiveness is the **continuation rate.** This is the number of couples attempting to avoid pregnancy who use the contraceptive method continuously for a period of one year. This is an important measure because many couples do not use a method continually or discontinue a method and do not replace it immediately, resulting in an unintended pregnancy.

Although failure rates are available for the different fertility control methods, basic effectiveness in terms of percentages is the easiest to use when making decisions about which fertility control method to use or not use. Effectiveness of fertility control methods ranges from 15% to 99.5%.

Withdrawal

The withdrawal method of fertility control (**coitus interruptus**) requires that the man withdraw his penis from the vagina before ejaculation. In theory, with-

Terms

contraceptive failure rate: likelihood of becoming pregnant if using a birth control method for one year

typical use: percentage of typical users who unintentionally become pregnant in their first year of use

perfect use: percentage of perfect users who unintentionally become pregnant in their first year of use

continuation rate: percentage of couples who use the method continually for one year who are not trying to get pregnant

coitus interruptus: removing the penis from the vagina just prior to ejaculation; also called withdrawal or pulling out

drawal prevents sperm from being deposited in the vagina and subsequently fertilizing an ovum. The male must exercise great control and restraint in order to withdraw the penis in time. Withdrawal is risky because a small emission may occur before ejaculation (pre-ejaculate), which may contain HIV or other STI bacteria or viruses. Even if no sperm are actually deposited in the vagina, pregnancy is possible if sperm are released near the vagina and enter later, perhaps inadvertently, through body-to-body contact.

Hormonal Contraception: The Pill

In 1960, the U.S. Food and Drug Administration (FDA) approved the use of oral hormonal contraceptive agents for women. The pill continues to be popular because of its convenience, low cost, reversibility, tolerable side effects (for most users), and, most significantly, its effectiveness. The pill is 95% to 99.9% effective in preventing conception, when used correctly.

Combination Birth Control Pills

The most common hormonal contraceptives contain a combination of two synthetic hormones that in many ways mimic the actions of a woman's natural ovarian hormones. One of the synthetic hormones is similar to the natural hormone estrogen, and the other is similar to the natural hormone progesterone. The progesterone-like compound is called a progestogen or progestin. Today, combination pills generally contain between 35 and 80 micrograms of estrogen and .15 and 2.5 milligrams of progestin, compared with 100 to 175 micrograms of estrogen and 10 milligrams of progestin in the pills of the 1960s. Some combination pills also have an iron supplement to help prevent iron-deficiency anemia.

Regardless of brand or dose of synthetic hormones, the method of taking the combination oral contraceptives is the same. The pills come in packages of 21 or 28 pills. In the 21-pill packets, all the pills contain a prescribed mixture of the two synthetic hormones. In the 28-pill packets, 21 of the pills contain hormones; the other seven pills are inert or contain iron and serve as a way to keep track of the days that no hormone is to be taken. The pills with the hormones are usually a different color from the inert, or iron-containing tablets. The first pill in a packet is taken on a predetermined day, and one pill is taken each day. Approximately two days after the last active pill is taken, a menstrual period should occur. Mini-pills come in 28-day packets; each pill contains active hormone. One pill is taken each day for an entire cycle, even during menstruation.

Those using pills are encouraged to take their daily pill with some routine activity, such as eating a meal, brushing their teeth, or going to bed. Taking the pill at the same time each day increases its effectiveness and decreases the likelihood of forgetting to take it. The hormones in today's birth control pills only prevent ovulation for approximately 24 hours. This is why the timing of taking the pill is important. It takes up to 1 month for the pill to become effective; thus, it is important to use a back-up method until the first packet is completed.

The effectiveness of birth control pills may be lessened when they are taken simultaneously with certain other medications, such as antibiotics, anticonvulsants, and a variety of pain relievers and anti-inflammatory drugs. Pill users should continue birth control pill use and consult their health professional about this possibility when taking other medications.

Approximately half the women using oral contraceptives experience unwanted and unintended side effects. Most of the time the side effects present little long-term risk to health, and often they disappear after several cycles on the pill. The more common of the less serious side effects are nausea, weight gain, breast tenderness, mild headaches, spotty bleeding between periods, decreased menstrual flow, increased frequency of vaginitis, increased depression, and lowering of the sex drive. Some other frequent side effects of the pill are considered beneficial by many women. Among these are lessening of acne outbreaks, diminution and even absence of menstrual cramps, decreased number of menstrual bleeding days, and absolute regulation of the menstrual cycle, which can be important for travelers and athletes.

Studies indicate that pill use may help prevent certain diseases. Women who take combination birth control pills have about one-third the chance of developing pelvic inflammatory disease, one-half the chance of developing benign (noncancerous) breast disease and ovarian cysts, nearly complete protection against ectopic pregnancy, and one-half the risk of developing iron-deficiency anemia in comparison to the general population. Data also indicate that combination birth control pills may protect against rheumatoid arthritis, endometrial cancer, and ovarian cancer.

There is no evidence that fertility is affected by taking the pill, even after many years of use. Some women, however, experience menstrual irregularities after discontinuing the pill. Despite the myth, after discontinuing the pill, women can become pregnant immediately. Studies indicate that there is no association between pill use and the possibility of birth defects in children born to pill users.

For a small percentage of women, oral contraceptives present a severe health risk. Several studies have shown that the risk of fatal blood clots and heart attack is greater for some women who take oral contraceptives than for those who do not. Women most at risk are those who are over age 35 and those who smoke cigarettes. These women should consider using a birth control method other than the pill. Any pill user who experiences severe abdominal pain, chest pain, headaches, unusual eye problems (blurred vision, flashing lights, temporary blindness), or severe calf and thigh pain should consult a physician or family planning agency immediately. The risk of developing liver disease, gallbladder disease, high blood pressure, and stroke is also slightly greater for pill users. Recent studies show that pill use carries no increased risk of developing breast cancer.

> *Whenever I hear people discussing birth control, I always remember that I was the fifth.*
> CLARENCE DARROW, lawyer

Progestin-Only Contraceptives

Progestin-only contraceptives are available as pills, injections, and implants. Progestin-only contraceptives work by inhibiting ovulation and thickening the cervical mucus, making it more difficult for sperm to reach the egg. Side effects may include menstrual irregularities, weight gain, depression, fatigue, decreased sex drive, acne or oily skin, and headaches. Progestin-only contraceptives are completely reversible. A woman returns to her previous level of fertility when she stops using any of the methods.

Depo-Provera is a 12-week supply of a hormone similar to progesterone, one of the hormones that regulate the menstrual cycle. It is called depot-medroxyprogesterone acetate (DMPA) and is injected intramuscularly by a health care provider. The hormone is released at a steady rate. At the end of the 12 weeks, a replacement injection or another contraceptive must be obtained.

Depo-Provera inhibits ovulation. If an egg is not released from the ovaries during the menstrual cycle, it cannot become fertilized by sperm and result in pregnancy. Depo-Provera also causes changes in the lining of the uterus that make it less likely for pregnancy to occur. Depo-Provera is 99.7% effective for both the typical and perfect users.

Depo-Provera is one of the most reversible methods of birth control. To stop using Depo-Provera, the woman simply does not get the next injection. Most women who get pregnant do so within 12 to 18 months of the last injection. This method can be used while breast-feeding, starting 6 weeks after delivery. The most common side effects include: irregular menstrual bleeding, amenorrhea, weight gain, headache, nervousness, stomach pain or cramps, dizziness, weakness or fatigue, and decreased sex drive. Depo-Provera is intended to prevent pregnancy only, and does not

protect against the transmission of sexually transmitted infections (STIs). Therefore, another method needs to be used in conjunction with Depo-Provera to prevent STI transmission.

Norplant, like Depo-Provera, is an extremely effective contraceptive. It consists of six thin, hormone-containing (levonorgestrel) capsules made of soft flexible material, which are placed in a fan-like pattern under the skin on the inside surface of the upper arm. After insertion, the hormone (levonorgestrel) is released into the body continuously, suppressing ovulation in at least half the cycles. One insertion is effective for up to 5 years. Norplant is nearly 100% effective in preventing pregnancy; however, it is not effective in protecting against STIs. Norplant is inserted by a trained medical professional in an office or clinic; the procedure takes about 10 to 15 minutes. Once under the skin, the capsules are invisible, but the outline of the capsules can be felt and sometimes seen. For some women, discoloration over the placement site occurs, which usually reverses when the capsules are removed, and irregular menstrual bleeding and weight gain may also occur. The removal procedure (or replacement with fresh hormone-filled capsules) is supposed to be simple. In some women, however, fibrous scar tissue builds up around the capsules, making their removal difficult and painful.

The Intrauterine Device

The **intrauterine device (IUD)** was used by approximately 106 million women worldwide in 1995, with almost 90% of users in the United States in their 30s or 40s. The IUD is a small device, containing copper or the hormone progesterone, implanted by a health care professional inside the uterus. (Figure 8.1). Currently, two types of IUD are available in the United States: Progesterone T, approved in 1976, and Copper-T 380 (CuT 380A), approved in 1984. The Copper IUD causes an increase in uterine fluids that alters how the sperm and ovum are transported, ultimately affecting egg fertilization. It is made of polyethlene with a fine copper wire wrapped around the vertical stem of the T. The Copper IUD is highly effective in preventing pregnancy, with an effectiveness rate of 99.2% to 99.4%, and can be used for at least 10 years.

Progestin IUDs have a hormonal action. The cervical mucus is thickened, which disrupts the ovulation pattern, alters the endometrial lining, and impairs tubal and uterine motility. Although studies are inconclusive, progestin IUDs probably interfere with fertilization. The Progesterone T releases 65 micrograms of progesterone daily and must be replaced annually. Its effectiveness is 98% to 98.5%.

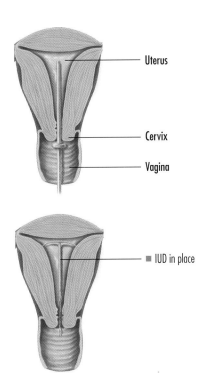

FIGURE 8.1 The IUD is inserted past the cervix into the uterus. Prior to insertion the length of the uterus is measured with an instrument called a sound. Upon insertion the arms of the IUD gradually unfold. Once the inserter is removed the threads attached to the IUD will be clipped to extend into the vagina through the cervical opening.

Research indicates that IUD use increases the risk for pelvic inflammatory diseases, uterine perforations, and increased risk of **ectopic pregnancy,** if a pregnancy occurs with the device in place. **Pelvic inflammatory disease (PID)** can damage the fallopian tubes sufficiently to make a woman infertile or to increase the likelihood of ectopic pregnancy.

Barrier Methods

Barrier methods of fertility control involve devices that physically block the path of sperm movement in the female reproductive tract and usually bring sperm in contact with a sperm-killing (spermicidal) chemical, most often nonoxynol-9. Several contraceptive methods work on this principle, including the diaphragm; the cervical cap; spermicidal foams, jellies, and creams; and the condom.

The Diaphragm

The **diaphragm** is a dome-shaped latex cup with a flexible rim, which is placed in the vagina to cover the cervix (Figure 8.2). A metal spring in the rim of the diaphragm holds the device snugly in place between the back wall of the vagina and the pubic bone in the front of the pelvis. In this position the diaphragm blocks the movement of sperm from the vagina to the uterus, although it does not fit snugly enough to keep all of the sperm out. Its primary purpose is to hold a spermicide in place next to the cervix. Correct usage requires that the rim and cup of the diaphragm be coated with a tablespoon or two of a spermicidal jelly or cream. The spermicides used with the diaphragm also help prevent the transmission of some microorganisms responsible for genital infections.

The diaphragm can be inserted up to 6 hours before intercourse, so a couple does not have to interrupt sexual pleasuring to insert the device. If a diaphragm is inserted several hours before sexual activity, however, it is advisable to put an additional amount of spermicidal jelly or cream into the vagina before intercourse. The diaphragm must be left in place at least 6 hours after last intercourse, but should not be used longer than 24 hours because of the possible risk of toxic shock syndrome.

Diaphragm purchases require a prescription and must be fitted by a family planning professional or health care provider to ensure a correct fit. Any change in a woman's body size—a gain or loss of several pounds, pregnancy, or pelvic surgery—is reason to check the fit and have a new diaphragm prescribed if necessary. A woman should not use another woman's diaphragm because the fit might be wrong, lowering the device's effectiveness.

One disadvantage of the diaphragm is the possibility of dislodgment during intercourse. Only rarely will a man feel the diaphragm during sexual intercourse if the device is inserted properly. If either the man or the woman experiences unusual sensations or discomfort during intercourse, then the diaphragm may not be inserted correctly, it may have become dislodged during intercourse, or it may be the wrong size. Other disadvantages of the diaphragm are that spermicides can be messy to use, and the diaphragm should not be used during menstruation or vaginal infection.

Terms

progestin-only contraceptives: work by inhibiting ovulation and thickening of the cervical mucus; completely reversible

Depo-Provera: injectable form of medroxyprogesterone acetate

Norplant: hormone-containing capsule inserted under the skin

intrauterine device (IUD): a flexible, usually plastic, device inserted into the uterus to prevent pregnancy

ectopic pregnancy: implanting of the embryo outside the uterus, usually in the fallopian tubes

pelvic inflammatory disease (PID): inflammation of the pelvic structures, especially the uterus and fallopian tubes; often caused by a sexually transmitted disease

diaphragm: a soft, rubber, dome-shaped contraceptive device worn over the cervix and used with spermicidal jelly or cream

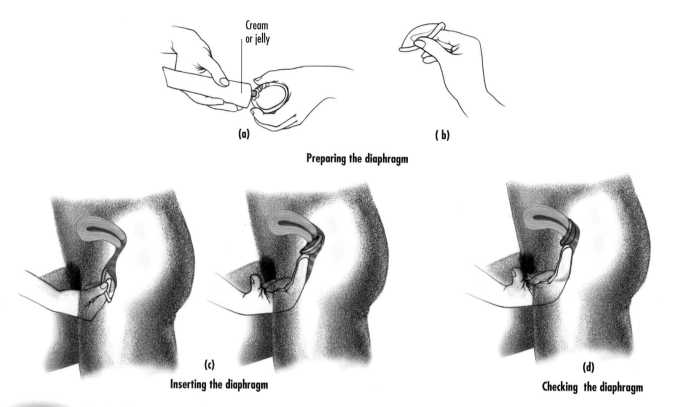

Cream or jelly

(a)   (b)

Preparing the diaphragm

(c)   (d)

Inserting the diaphragm   **Checking the diaphragm**

FIGURE 8.2   Procedure for Inserting a Diaphragm   (a) Before inserting the diaphragm coat the rim and cup with a spermicidal cream or jelly. (b) Squeeze the rim of the diaphragm together between your thumb and index finger. (c) Insert the diaphragm into the vagina with the rim facing up and push it toward the small of your back. As you let go of the diaphragm it will spring open, continue to guide it to your cervix with the tips of your fingers. (d) Be sure to check that the diaphragm completely covers the cervix.

Periodically the diaphragm should be held against a light to check for tiny holes and weak spots (where the rubber buckles). With proper care a diaphragm will last a year or two.

The Cervical Cap

The **cervical cap** is a soft, deep rubber cup with a firm round rim that snugly covers the cervix similar to the way a thimble fits on a finger. Like a diaphragm, a cervical cap needs to be coated with spermicide to be as effective as possible and remain in place for 8 hours after last intercourse. Cervical caps come in several sizes and must be fitted for each woman. One distinct difference between the diaphragm and the cervical cap is the fact that the cervical cap provides continuous contraceptive protection for 48 hours.

The principal advantages of the cervical cap are:

- Low cost and convenience
- Can be inserted any time of the day intercourse is anticipated
- Sexual activity can take place spontaneously during the ensuing 48 hours without concern about fertility control.

The major disadvantages of the cervical cap are difficulty with insertion and removal, occasional discomfort during intercourse, dislodgment during intercourse, and possibly irritation of the cervix. The cervical cap should not be left in place for more than 48 hours at a time.

Male Condoms

The male **condom,** or rubber, is a membranous sheath that covers the erect penis and catches semen before it enters the vagina. About 99% of male condoms are made of latex; the rest, so-called "skin" condoms, which are not effective against STIs, are manufactured from lamb intestines.

Condoms can be obtained in pharmacies, supermarkets, vending machines, and through mail order advertisements in newspapers, magazines, and catalogs. When stored in a cool, dry place, condoms retain their effectiveness for many years. Kept in a warm environment, such as in a wallet in the back pocket of one's pants or in the glove compartment of a car, the

Terms

cervical cap: small latex cap that covers the cervix, used with spermicidal jelly or cream inside the cap

male condom: a latex or polyurethane sheath worn over the penis; can be both a barrier method and act as a prophylactic against sexually transmitted infections

Wellness Guide

Putting On a Condom

For pleasure, ease, and effectiveness, both partners should know how to put on and use a condom. To learn without feeling pressured or embarrassed, practice on your penis or a penis-shaped object, such as a ketchup bottle, banana, cucumber, or squash.

Remember: Practice Makes Perfect

- Put the condom on before the penis touches the vulva. Men leak fluids from their penises before and after ejaculation. Pre-ejaculate ("pre-cum") can carry enough sperm to cause pregnancy and enough germs to cause STIs.

- Use a condom only once. Use a fresh one for each erection ("hard-on"). Have a good supply on hand.

- Condoms usually come rolled into a ring shape. They are individually sealed in aluminum foil or plastic. Be careful—don't tear the condom while unwrapping it. If it is brittle, stiff, or sticky, throw it away and use another.

- Put a drop or two of lubricant inside the condom.

- Place the rolled condom over the tip of the hard penis.

- Leave one-half inch of space at the tip to collect semen.

- If the penis is not circumcised, pull back the foreskin before rolling on the condom.

- Pinch the air out of the tip with one hand. (Friction against air bubbles causes most condom breaks.)

- Unroll the condom over the penis with the other hand.

- Roll it all the way down to the base of the penis.

- Smooth out any air bubbles.

- Lubricate the outside of the condom.

Taking Off a Condom

- Pull out before the penis softens.

- Don't spill the semen—hold the condom against the base of the penis while you pull out.

- Throw the condom away.

- Wash the penis with soap and water before embracing again.

Source: Planned Parenthood Federation of America, Inc. http://www.plannedparenthood.org/

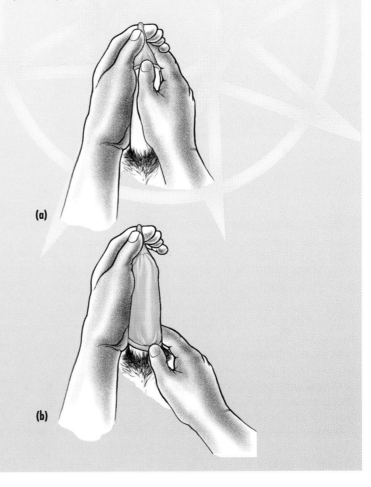

(a)

(b)

latex will deteriorate. To be effective, condoms must be used with water-based lubricants, such as K-Y Jelly, because petroleum-based lubricants will cause the latex to deteriorate.

There are many advantages to using condoms. Condoms are:

- Easy to obtain
- Inexpensive
- Free of medical risk (rarely a man or a woman may be allergic to the latex, lubricant, or spermicide)
- Reliable
- Effective
- Proven protection against STIs

A primary reason for condom failure in preventing pregnancy is error in use. The typical use failure rate for male condom use is 14%, while those who use them consistently and correctly every time have only a 3% failure rate. Used in conjunction with another barrier method, such as a diaphragm or spermicidal foam, condoms are very effective. Another advantage

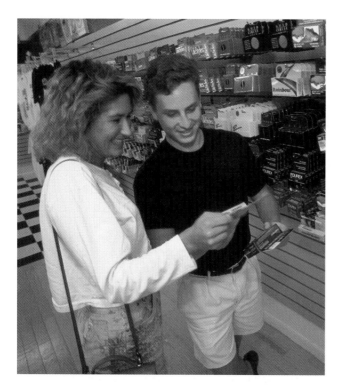

Condoms are an effective form of fertility control and provide protection against STIs. It's important that both partners take responsibility for using condoms.

is that condoms help prevent the transmission of chlamydia, gonorrhea, herpes, HIV infection, and other kinds of infections.

Some people complain that the condom diminishes pleasurable sensations, but the device does not totally block genital feeling, which, in any event, is only one of many factors that contribute to sexual arousal and pleasure. A negative attitude about condoms may diminish pleasure far more than a thin layer of latex ever could. Instead of thinking about how condoms block sensations, it might enhance lovemaking to think of them as a fun way to help make lovemaking more pleasurable because of the protection they provide.

Female Condoms

The **female condom**, the brand name of which is Reality, is a thin, loose-fitting polyurethane plastic pouch that lines the vagina. It has two flexible rings: an inner ring at the closed end, used to insert the device inside the vagina and hold it in place, and an outer ring which remains outside the vagina and covers the external genitalia. Figure 8.3 shows the insertion and positioning of the female condom. Because the device is made from polyurethane, which is 40% stronger than latex, the female condom can be used with any type of lubricant without compromising the integrity of the device.

Two advantages of the female condom are that (a) it warms up instantly to body temperature once it is inserted, thus enhancing sensation for both partners and (b) it provides protection from STIs (by covering both internal and external genitalia), including HIV, and prevents pregnancy. Also, the female condom is easy to buy in drugstores and supermarkets, an erection is unnecessary to keep the female condom in place, and it can be used by people allergic to latex or spermicide.

Some disadvantages of the female condom are that it cannot be used with a male condom, and is not as effective as a male condom. Its pregnancy failure rate is 5% for those who use it correctly every time compared with 3% for the male condom. The typical failure rate, for those who did not use it correctly every time they had sex was 21% compared to 14% for the male latex condom. Occasionally, the outer ring may be pushed inside the vagina. Other problems include (a) difficulties in insertion and removal; (b) minor irritation; (c) discomfort or breakage, which can be decreased by using enough lubrication; (d) it is not aesthetically pleasing; and (e) it costs more than male condoms.

Vaginal Spermicides

A variety of fertility control methods consist solely of a spermicidal agent (nonoxynol-9 in the United States) that acts as a surfactant that destroys the sperm cell membrane. Specific directions in the packages tell you how to insert the **spermicide** and what timing recommendations and repeat applications are necessary. These agents include foams, gels, creams, and vaginal **suppositories.** Although often displayed in stores with other feminine hygiene products, vaginal spermicides should not be confused with douches, deodorant products, or lubricants, none of which are effective fertility control methods.

Vaginal contraceptive film (VCF) is a small sheet of film that contains a spermicide and is inserted into the vagina to cover the cervical opening. It can be used alone or with a condom, diaphragm, or cervical cap. The 2" × 2" paper-thin sheet of film must be inserted at least 15 minutes before intercourse to allow time for the sheet to dissolve. Placing the film on the tip of the penis for insertion is not recommended because this does not provide adequate time for the vaginal contraceptive film to dissolve.

The effectiveness of all of the vaginal spermicides depends on a sufficient quantity of sperm-killing chemical bathing the cervix at the time of ejaculation. Among typical users, however, the failure rate is about 26 pregnancies per 100 women per year. The failure rate for perfect users is 6 unintended pregnan-

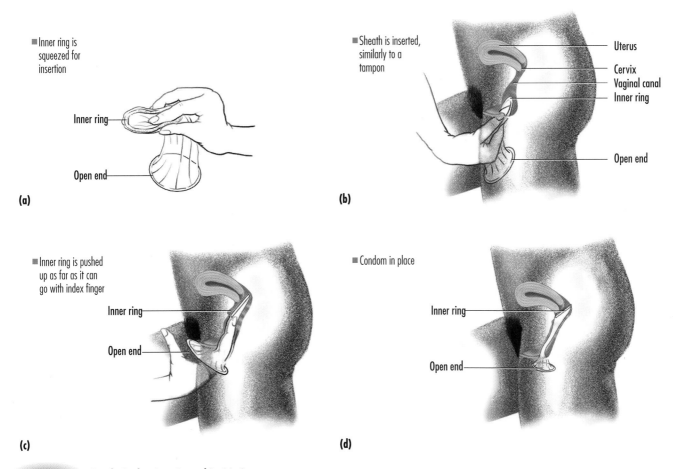

- Inner ring is squeezed for insertion

Inner ring

Open end

(a)

- Sheath is inserted, similarly to a tampon

Uterus
Cervix
Vaginal canal
Inner ring
Open end

(b)

- Inner ring is pushed up as far as it can go with index finger

Inner ring
Open end

(c)

- Condom in place

Inner ring
Open end

(d)

FIGURE 8.3   **Female Condom Insertion and Positioning**

cies per 100 women per year. Using vaginal spermicides requires dedication and competence. Users must put the spermicide in the vagina immediately before every act of intercourse and before each subsequent intercourse in the same sexual encounter.

Users of foam should be sure that the foam is frothy and bubbly, which is achieved by shaking the container about twenty times before filling the applicator. Because there is no way to know how much foam remains in a container, a spare container should be kept on hand.

Suppositories should be placed as far back in the vagina as possible so that the dissolved spermicide covers the cervix. It is important to allow enough time (from 10 to 15 minutes, depending on the product) for the suppository to dissolve completely before each act of intercourse. Vaginal suppositories have the disadvantage of the waiting period to allow the tablet to melt.

Major advantages of vaginal spermicides are:

- They are available without a doctor's prescription.
- They can be purchased in pharmacies and many supermarkets.
- The spermicidal chemicals give some added protection against STIs.

- The effectiveness of spermicidal agents increases to nearly 100% when they are used simultaneously with a condom.

Vaginal spermicides tend to be slippery, which occasionally can be a nuisance, but the moisture can augment a woman's natural vaginal lubrication and enhance sensation. These methods may also be a hindrance to oral-genital stimulation. In rare instances, someone may be allergic to a particular product. Changing brands may alleviate this problem. Some women experience irritation if the tablet has not dissolved completely before intercourse takes place.

Terms

female condom: a loose-fitting polyurethane pouch that lines the vagina; can be both a barrier method and protection against sexually transmitted infections

spermicide: a chemical that kills sperm; particularly foams, creams, gels, and suppositories used for contraception

suppositories: a medicine placed in a body orifice to dissolve and sometimes to be absorbed; birth control suppositories contain spermicidal chemicals

vaginal contraceptive film (VCF): a small sheet of film covered with spermicide inserted on or near the cervix

Some erroneously believe that spermicides cause birth defects; this belief is a myth.

 ### Fertility Awareness Methods

Fertility awareness methods of fertility control (sometimes called natural family planning, the rhythm method, or periodic abstinence) attempt to determine a woman's most fertile period; that is, when an ovum has been released from the ovary and is capable of being fertilized. In general, the time when a woman is most fertile occurs 14 days before her next period. During ovulation, the egg lives only 24 hours. If the egg is not fertilized, the woman will shed the lining of the uterus and have a period 2 weeks later. Although the egg lives only 24 hours, sperm can live 3 to 5 days inside the body waiting for the egg to mature. Therefore, it is possible to become pregnant during the 5 to 6 days of each menstrual cycle. In women who cycle every 28 days, this fertility occurs mid-cycle. Fertility cannot be predicted with absolute certainty because no two women are exactly alike and even an individual woman's cycles may vary from month to month or be affected by stress, lack of sleep, or illness. Fertility awareness methods of birth control either estimate when ovulation is most likely to occur or indicate when ovulation has already taken place, thereby telling a couple the days in the menstrual cycle not to have unprotected intercourse. Those are referred to as "unsafe days." The days when a woman is not likely to be fertile are referred to as "safe days." On unsafe days, a couple should use an alternative method of birth control, such as condoms, a diaphragm, or spermicidal foam. Other options include enjoying ways of sexual pleasuring other than genital intercourse, or complete sexual abstinence.

Couples using fertility awareness methods should realize that, even on safe days, fertilization is still possible because of natural variations in a woman's reproductive processes. Therefore, safe days are really *relatively* safe days.

Fertility awareness offers the advantages of posing no health risks and being cost-free; furthermore, some peoples' religious convictions make fertility awareness the only acceptable method of birth control. Unintentional pregnancies occur because people do not keep careful records, they find the intervals of abstinence during the unsafe days too long, and they find having to plan sex only for the safe days a hindrance to spontaneous lovemaking.

Calendar Rhythm

Calendar rhythm is a way to estimate the most likely fertile, or unsafe, days in a woman's menstrual cycle by assuming that:

1. Ovulation usually takes place 14 days (plus or minus 2 days) before the onset of the next menstrual flow.
2. An ovum is capable of being fertilized for 24 hours.
3. Sperm deposited in the vagina remain capable of fertilization for up to 3 days.

Using calendar rhythm effectively requires knowledge of the female fertility cycle and instruction in doing the calculations correctly. Family planning agencies, women's health clinics, and books on fertility awareness methods can be helpful in learning the method.

The Temperature Method

The **basal body temperature (BBT)** is the lowest temperature in a healthy person during waking hours. In 70% to 90% of women, the BBT rises approximately one degree after ovulation, presumably because of changes in hormone levels. By keeping a daily record of the BBT, a woman can determine when ovulation has occurred and therefore the unsafe and safe days for intercourse between ovulation and the beginning of the next menstrual cycle. Because the BBT method cannot predict when ovulation will occur, a woman must still estimate with another fertility awareness method (calendar method, mucus method) the safe and unsafe days before ovulation.

The Cervical Mucus Method

Certain hormone-sensitive glands in the cervix produce mucus that changes in amount, color, and consistency during different phases of the menstrual cycle. Learning to recognize the changes in cervical mucus can help determine when ovulation occurs, and safe and unsafe days for intercourse can be planned accordingly.

The mucus method requires that cervical mucus be examined frequently during the cycle. Samples of mucus may be obtained with a finger or on toilet tissue or discharge on underpants may be observed. Collection with a finger is best because it permits direct determination of the amount and consistency of mucus.

Because douching, vaginal infections, semen, contraceptive foams and jellies, vaginal lubricants, medications, and vaginal lubrication from sexual arousal can interfere with the recognition of mucus patterns, women wishing to use the mucus method should obtain instructions from an experienced user, a family planning clinic, or a health center. A woman should plan on charting her cervical mucus for at least a month to learn her individual pattern of mucus changes before relying on the method for fertility control.

The **sympto-thermal method** involves using the temperature and mucus methods simultaneously.

Ovulation Detection Methods

Chemical methods of fertility awareness measure the amount of **luteinizing hormone** in a woman's urine, which peaks at the time of ovulation. Ovulation predictor kits to measure the levels of LH can be purchased in pharmacies. Manufacturers claim that the kits have an accuracy rate of 85%.

Sterilization

Sterility is being permanently unable to have children. For people who are certain that they do not want children, or, as is more often the case, no more children, surgical methods that render a person sterile but have no effect on sexual arousal or activities may be the most desirable form of birth control. Indeed, for married couples over age 30, "permanent fertility control" (sterilization of either the male or female partner) has become the most frequently chosen method of fertility control. The popularity of sterilization as a method of fertility control stems from its nearly 100% effectiveness, the relative safety of the procedure, and its relatively low one-time cost.

Male Sterilization

The sterilization of a man is called **vasectomy.** Approximately 500,000 men in the United States choose vasectomy every year. This procedure involves the cutting and tying of each of the two vas deferentia, the tubes that connect the testes (where sperm are made) to the penis (Figure 8.4). When these tubes are cut, sperm are no longer emitted upon ejaculation because their passage is blocked. Because the cut is made "upstream" from the organs that produce seminal fluid, a man still ejaculates, but the semen contains no sperm cells. And because the sperm cells make up only a small percentage of the total volume of the semen, neither a man nor his partner is aware of any change in their sex life, except that no other form of contraception is needed.

Although vasectomy should be considered a permanent form of contraception, it is sometimes possible to reverse the condition by rejoining the cut ends of the vas deferentia. The success of vasectomy reversal as measured by the ability to have children again is about 50% although some surgeons claim much higher reversal rates.

One of the reasons vasectomy is such a popular method of contraception is that it is uncomplicated and causes few problems. The procedure is usually carried out in a doctor's office with a local anesthetic

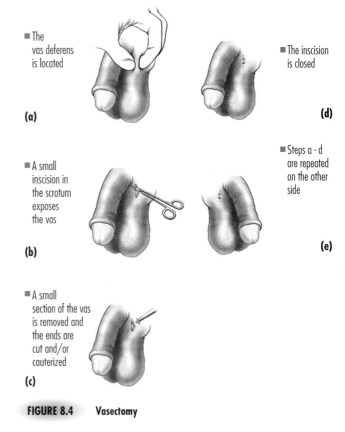

- The vas deferens is located

(a)

- A small inscision in the scrotum exposes the vas

(b)

- A small section of the vas is removed and the ends are cut and/or cauterized

(c)

- The inscision is closed

(d)

- Steps a - d are repeated on the other side

(e)

FIGURE 8.4   **Vasectomy**

in about 15 to 30 minutes. The incidence of postoperative complications is very low, and within a week most men can return to regular activities, including sex. About one-half to two-thirds of vasectomized men develop antibodies to sperm, but there is no evidence to suggest that this is harmful. A man can be fertile for several weeks, because the sperm pathway contains sperm present before the vasectomy. Once these are ejaculated the man is sterile.

Terms

fertility awareness methods: methods of birth control in which a couple charts the cyclic signs of the woman's fertility and ovulation, using basal body temperature, mucus changes, and other signs to determine fertile periods

calendar rhythm: estimation of fertile, or unsafe, days to have intercourse

basal body temperature (BBT) method: uses daily body temperature readings taken immediately after waking to identify the time of ovulation; approximately 24 hours after ovulation, the BBT increases

sympto-thermal method: using both the BBT and the mucus methods at the same time

luteinizing hormone: anterior pituitary hormone that causes a follicle to release a ripened ovum and become a corpus luteum; in the male, it stimulates testosterone production and the production of sperm cells

sterility: not being able to be impregnated or impregnate

vasectomy: a surgical procedure in men in which segments of the vas deferens are removed and the ends tied to prevent the passage of sperm

Female Sterilization

Female sterilization is a procedure that blocks the fallopian tubes. Blocking can be accomplished by cutting and tying the tubes, by sealing the tubes (cautery), or by closing them with clips, bands, or rings (Figure 8.5). Most female sterilization procedures can be done as an outpatient with local anesthesia. The incidence of post-operative complications is low.

There are two types of abdominal female sterilization: suprapubic **minilaparotomy** and **laparoscopy**. The suprapubic minilaparotomy involves a small abdominal incision above the pubic hairline. Through the incision, the fallopian tubes are grasped and occluded. For many women this incision is invisible.

The laparoscopic procedure involves making a small incision in the navel and inserting an instrument (a laparoscope) to find the fallopian tubes. Once the fallopian tubes are found, the health care provider can place rings (bands) or clips on the tubes or electrocoagulate the oviducts. Because these incisions are

> *Liberty means responsibility. That's why most men dread it.*
> GEORGE BERNARD SHAW

smaller than the incision used in the minilaparotomy procedure, this method is often less painful.

The fallopian tubes can also be reached through an incision in the vagina; this procedure is called a **colpotomy**. This gives the health care provider a direct view and accessibility to the fallopian tubes, which can be directly cut and sutured. Vaginal approaches tend to be less effective than minilaparotomy or laparoscopic approaches and have a greater risk for infection.

Sharing the Responsibility for Fertility Control

Most people engage in sexual activity because they want a joyous, rewarding experience. Because an unintended pregnancy can cause enormous hardship, birth control is an important part of every sexual relationship. Denying the possibility of pregnancy by assuming "it can't happen to me" is just gambling against the odds.

The responsibility for fertility control has two components. First, a fertility control method must be chosen, taking into consideration the nature of an individual's sexual activities or a couple's sexual relationship, the frequency of intercourse, future plans regarding children, and personal and religious values. Second, the chosen method must be used consistently and correctly.

The responsibility for fertility control can be shared in a number of ways. The most important is to discuss it. In an ongoing relationship, there are many opportunities to talk about fertility control. Couples can go to fertility control clinics together, they can read and discuss information about the advantages and disadvantages of the different methods, and they can try out various methods to find out which are best suited for them. They can share the time and the financial costs of their chosen method, or they can divide responsibilities. For example, if a woman has to take time to go to a clinic or doctor, her partner could pay for the clinic visit and the contraceptives.

Partners can also share in using their chosen method. They can discuss any difficulties or concerns they have with their method of fertility control. Partners can even remind each other to use their chosen fertility control method. A man can learn how a diaphragm is used, a woman can learn about the condom, and they can incorporate into their lovemaking preparing to use these and other barrier methods. Furthermore, partners can share the responsibility of inserting, removing, and cleaning the woman's diaphragm or cervical cap. If a woman is using fertility awareness methods, a man can share the responsibility by helping to determine the safe and unsafe days and by sharing the responsibility for abstaining from sexual intercourse.

(a) Sagittal section

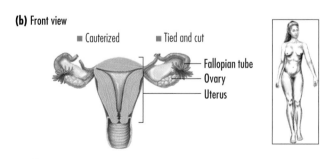

Laparoscope

Fallopian tube

(b) Front view

■ Cauterized　　■ Tied and cut

Fallopian tube
Ovary
Uterus

FIGURE 8.5 **Tubal Ligation** Female sterilization by laparoscopic ligation. **(a)** Cross section: The tubes are located using a laparoscope and cut, tied, or cauterized through a second incision. **(b)** Front view: The tubes after ligation.

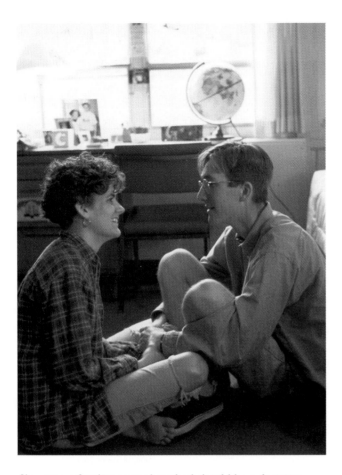

Choosing a fertility control method should be a decision made by both sexual partners and should be discussed before having sex.

Partners who share the responsibility for fertility control are more likely to use their chosen method(s) properly, which makes fertility control more effective. And reducing the fear of pregnancy makes sex more enjoyable. Another benefit of sharing this responsibility is that it tends to enhance intimacy in a relationship. The discussion of fertility control and the mutual decision making involved in choosing and using a method lead to better communication.

It is always a good idea for you to have some method of fertility control with you if you anticipate that sexual intercourse might occur. For example, both men and women can carry a condom or spermicides with them on dates or to parties if they think that sexual activity is a possibility.

Why Sexually Active People Do Not Use Fertility Control

Despite a presumed and sometimes stated desire not to become pregnant, approximately 5% of married individuals and 15% of unmarried sexually active indi-

viduals use no fertility control. Some of the major reasons that people do not use fertility control, even if they wish to avoid pregnancy, include:

- *Low motivation.* People who have mixed feelings about avoiding pregnancy are less motivated to use fertility control. For example, a couple that has decided that they want to have a child "sometime in the near future" is less likely to be motivated to use fertility control than is a couple that is absolutely certain they do not want a child until some specified time, or at all.
- *Lack of knowledge.* Lack of knowledge about the process of conception and how to use fertility control effectively can lead to an incorrect perception of the risk of becoming pregnant. For example, some people believe the myths that pregnancy is not possible if a woman has an orgasm, if she urinates after intercourse, or if she is having sexual intercourse for the first time. Sometimes a method is believed to be more effective than it really is, or the chosen method is used incorrectly. For example, some people erroneously believe that a woman is most fertile during the bleeding days of the menstrual cycle and thus practice fertility awareness at the wrong time. Some couples lose, misplace, or run out of their primary method and do not have a back-up method available.
- *Negative attitudes about fertility control.* Some people believe that fertility control is immoral, a hassle, unromantic, or harmful. One's own negative attitudes or the perceived negative attitudes of others, such as peers or parents, can inhibit one from obtaining contraceptives. People use these as excuses not to visit doctors or clinics, or they may shy away from obtaining over-the-counter contraceptives.
- *Relationship issues.* Individuals in committed relationships are better contraceptors than individuals who are not in such relationships. Involvement with a committed partner tends to lessen guilt associated with sexual activity and hence improves attitudes about contraceptive practice. People in a committed relationship tend to have sexual intercourse more often and regularly, which gives the couple opportunities to talk about contraception and to be-

Terms

minilaparotomy: female sterilization procedure in which the fallopian tubes are ligated or cauterized through a small abdominal incision

laparoscopy: a surgical incision into the abdomen used to visualize internal organs, enabling the surgeon to perform a sterilization procedure

colpotomy: a female sterilization procedure

Wellness Guide

Birth Control Guide

The following table shows common contraceptive methods used by women in the United States, the percentage of women experiencing an unintended pregnancy during the first year of typical use and the first year of perfect use, and the percentage of women continuing use at the end of the first year. Dangers, side effects, and noncontraceptive benefits are provided.

	Typical Use Failure Rate (percent)	Perfect Use Failure Rate (percent)	Continuation Rate (percent)	Dangers	Side Effects	Noncontraceptive Benefits
Withdrawal	19	4	–			
Abstinence				None known	Psychological reactions	Prevents infections, including HIV
Contraceptive Pill	–	0.5	–	CVD complications (stroke, heart attack, blood clots, HBP), depression, hepatic adenomas, possible increased risk of breast and cervical cancers	Nausea, headaches, dizziness, spotting, weight gain, breast tenderness, chloasma	Decreases in menstrual pain, PMS, and blood loss; protects against symptomatic PID, some cancers (ovarian and endometrial), some benign tumors (leiomyomata, benign breast masses), and ovarian cysts; reduces acne
Progestin only Combined	–	0.1	–			
Implant (Norplant)	0.05	0.05	88	Infection at implant site, complicated removals, depression	Tenderness at site, menstrual changes, hair loss, weight gain	Lactation not disturbed; may decrease menstrual cramps, pain, and blood loss
Injection (Depo-Provera)	0.3	0.3	70	Depression, allergic reactions, pathologic weight gain, possible bone loss	Menstrual changes, weight gain, headaches, adverse effects on lipids	Lactation not disturbed, reduces risk of seizure, may have protective effects against PID and ovarian and endometrial cancers
IUD				PID following insertion, uterine perforation, anemia	Menstrual cramping, spotting, increased bleeding	None known except for progestin-releasing IUDs, which decrease menstrual blood loss and pain
Progesterone T	2.0	1.5	81			
Copper T 380A	0.8		78			
LNg 20	0.1	0.1	81			
Fertility Awareness						
Periodic Abstinence	25					
Calendar	13					
BBT	20					
Cervical Mucus	20					
Symptothermal	13–20					

come adept at using method(s). Individuals with irregular sexual contact, either because of geographical separation or relationship problems, may have difficulties in establishing a birth control regime. In new or casual sexual relationships, there is a tendency to use no method or a poor method at first.

Emergency Contraception

Emergency contraception is designed to prevent pregnancy after unprotected vaginal intercourse. The most common option is a regimen of combined oral contraceptive pills (called ECPs, emergency contraceptive pills) within 72 hours of unprotected intercourse. Other options include the insertion of a copper-releasing intrauterine device (IUD) within five days or

the use of progestin-only minipills within 48 to 72 hours. "The mechanism of action for ECPs is to prevent pregnancy, but not to interrupt or disrupt an already-established pregnancy. ECPs inhibit or delay ovulation to prevent fertilization, and they possibly alter the endometrium to impair implantation" (Hatcher et al., 1998, p. 281). Side effects are infrequent. Nausea and vomiting are the most common, along with breast tenderness, irregular bleeding, cramping, and headache.

You may choose to use emergency contraception if:

- His condom broke or slipped off, and he ejaculated inside your vagina.
- You forgot to take your birth control pills.
- Your diaphragm or cervical cap slipped out of place, and he ejaculated inside your vagina.

	Typical Use Failure Rate (percent)	Perfect Use Failure Rate (percent)	Continuation Rate (percent)	Dangers	Side Effects	Noncontraceptive Benefits
Male Condom	14	3	61	Anaphylactic reaction to latex	Decreased sensation, allergy to latex, loss of spontaneity	Protects against sexually transmitted infections, including HIV; delays premature ejaculation
Female Condom	21	5	56	None known	Aesthetically unappealing and awkward to use for some	Protects against sexually transmitted infections
Diaphragm	20	6	56	Vaginal and urinary tract infections, toxic shock syndrome	Pelvic pressure, vaginal irritation, vaginal discharges if left in too long, allergy	Provides modest protection against some sexually transmitted infections
Spermicides	26	6	40	Vaginal and urinary tract infections	Vaginal irritation, allergy	Provides modest protection against some sexually transmitted infections
Female Sterilization	0.5	0.5	100	Infection; anesthetic complications	Pain at surgical site, psychological reactions, subsequent regret that the procedure was performed	Tubal sterilization reduces the risk of ovarian cancer and may protect against PID
Male Sterilization	0.15	0.10	100	Infection; anesthetic complications	Pain at surgical site, psychological reactions, subsequent regret that the procedure was performed	

Adapted from Hatcher, et al. (1998).

A dash in a column means no information available.

- You miscalculated your "safe" days.
- He didn't pull out in time.
- You weren't using any fertility control.
- He forced you to have unprotected vaginal intercourse.

Abortion

Abortion, in the form of the intentional, premature termination of pregnancy, is one of the oldest and most widely practiced methods of fertility control. Chinese medical writings from 2700 B.C. recommend abortion. A cross-cultural study found that all but one of 300 societies has used abortion to control the size of families. Currently, in the United States, approximately 1.5 million abortions are performed annually. This number represents about one-fourth of all pregnancies and about one-half of all unintended pregnancies.

In 1995 there was a 4.5% decrease of legal abortions reported compared to 1994. Women undergoing legal abortions tend to be young, white, and unmarried; most are obtaining an abortion for the first time. Over half (54%) of all abortions performed in 1995 were performed at less than or equal to 8 weeks of gestation, and about 88% were performed before 13 weeks. Women 24 years of age or younger are more

Terms

abortion: the expulsion or extraction of the products of conception from the uterus before the embryo or fetus is capable of independent life; abortions may be spontaneous or induced

likely to obtain an abortion later in pregnancy than are older women. Four types of abortions can be performed: medical abortions, early abortions, early second-trimester abortions, and abortion after 24 weeks of pregnancy. In very early abortion, the uterus is emptied with the gentle suction of a syringe; this type of abortion can be performed up to 49 days after the last menstrual period.

Medical Abortions

A medical abortion is done without entering the uterus. Either of two medications, methotrexate or mifepristone, can be used for a medical abortion under the guidance of a health care provider. Each of these medications is taken together with another medication, misoprostol, and either combination will end a pregnancy (National Abortion Federation, 1997). Medical abortions must take place within the first 6 weeks of pregnancy.

Early Abortions

The usual method for an early abortion is suction curettage. **Vacuum** or **suction curettage** is the safest and most commonly used abortion method; about 90% of all abortions are vacuum aspiration. The procedure takes about 10 minutes. Vacuum curettage is a two-part procedure. First, the woman is given general or (more often) local anesthesia and the cervix is gradually widened, either with a series of progressively tapered cylinders called dilators, or by insertion of slim rolls of **laminaria,** a seaweed product that expands when exposed to the liquid in cervical secretions. In the second part of the procedure, a narrow wand, called a **cannula,** is connected to a suction device, which is used to empty the uterus. Vacuum curettage is usually performed from 6 to 14 weeks after the woman's last period.

Early Second-Trimester Abortion

Abortions performed early in the second trimester can be either **dilation and curettage** (D & C) or **dilation and evacuation** (D & E). These procedures can be performed up to the twenty-fourth week.

In a "D & C," the cervix is dilated as in the vacuum method, but instead of suction, the uterus is emptied by cleaning the inner lining with a spoon-shaped scraping-instrument (the curette).

If abortion is performed between the thirteenth and twentieth weeks of pregnancy, a procedure combining vacuum and surgical curettage, called dilation and extraction, or "D & E," is usually performed.

Abortion After 24 Weeks of Pregnancy

Only one out of every 10,000 women have abortions after the twenty-fourth week of pregnancy. These are performed only when there is a serious threat to the woman's life or health or if the fetus is severely deformed. One procedure is called the induction method, which is usually done in the hospital and requires staying overnight.

The Legality and Morality of Abortion

On January 22, 1973 the U.S. Supreme Court declared that states could not make laws prohibiting abortion on the ground that they violated a woman's right to privacy, in this case, the right to decide about the outcome of a pregnancy. This decision,

Terms

vacuum (suction) curettage: removal of fetal tissue by suctioning off contents of the uterus

laminaria: a plug of sterile dried kelp (seaweed), which expands when in contact with water and can thus be placed in the cervical canal to dilate the cervix

cannula: a hollow tube for insertion into the body cavity

dilation and curettage (D & C): dilation of the cervix with use of a wand or laminaria and scraping the uterine lining; this procedure is often used during abortion

dilation and evacuation (D & E): dilation of the cervix and evacuation of the uterine contents using vacuum techniques

sexually transmitted infections (STIs): infections passed from person to person by sexual contact

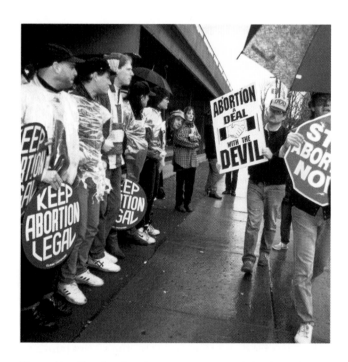

The option for abortion is a very controversial subject in our society.

known as *Roe* v. *Wade,* declared (a) that the decision to have an abortion during the first trimester (12 weeks) of pregnancy should be left entirely to the woman and her physician, and (b) during the second trimester, individual states could regulate the abortion procedure for only one purpose—to protect the woman's health.

Many people have mixed feelings about abortion. Because there is no universally accepted scientific definition of when a life begins, some individuals view abortion as murder. Some opponents of abortion believe that its availability encourages irresponsible sexual behavior or haphazard use of fertility control. Some see abortion as a threat to family life. Even the staunchest proponents of abortion rights would prefer that abortions never occur, but they argue that women must have the right to control their bodies. They believe that abortion is a necessary last resort if contraception fails, if a woman becomes pregnant because of rape or incest, if the child may suffer a birth defect, or if the woman's life and health are jeopardized by pregnancy or childbirth.

Whether pro-choice or pro-life, both positions agree on the value and dignity of human life, but are divided on when life begins, how conflicts such as religion, morals, and philosophy are to be balanced, and how human life is best preserved and enhanced. Several factors ensure that the abortion debate will continue. These factors include: (a) advances in neonatal medicine; (b) political aspects of abortion; and (c) ethical issues regarding when life begins.

Protecting against Sexually Transmitted Infections

A variety of infections can be passed from person to person through sexual contact. Traditionally, these infections have been called venereal diseases, or "VD"—the word *venereal* being derived from Venus, the mythical Roman goddess of love. To identify more clearly their origins, these diseases are now called **sexually transmitted infections,** or **STIs.**

In the United States each year, approximately 14 million people acquire an STI—a rate of infection second only to the common cold (Figure 8.6). The majority of these cases are in people under age 25; two-thirds of the cases of gonorrhea and chlamydia are in people under age 24.

The human and social costs of STIs are enormous. The human suffering and economic costs wrought by AIDS are well-known. Less well-known are the disappointment and suffering of thousands of women who are left infertile after a serious STI-related pelvic in-

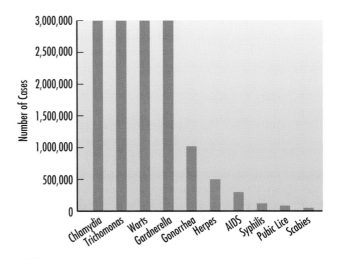

FIGURE 8.6   **Estimated Yearly Number of STIs in the United States**

fection. Women who acquire a human papillomavirus (HPV) infection (genital warts) are predisposed to cervical cancer. And the half million people who acquire genital herpes each year will be potentially infectious for their entire lives.

STI Risk Factors

Several factors increase the risk of contracting an STI. Being aware of these factors can help you decrease your risk of infection and help you to support STI prevention efforts in your community.

Multiple Sexual Partners

There is a large pool of unmarried sexually active people, because many individuals become sexually active in late adolescence and delay marriage until their mid-to-late 20s and early 30s. One-third of unmarried sexually active people report having more than one sexual partner in the previous year (Kost and Forrest, 1992).

False Sense of Safety

Using birth control pills tends to decrease the use of condoms and spermicides, which help prevent transmission of STIs. The availability of antibiotics makes many people less afraid of sexually transmitted diseases. They erroneously believe that there is a cure for every STI.

Absence of Signs and Symptoms

Some STIs have very mild or no symptoms, so that the infection can worsen and may be unknowingly passed on to others. One study showed that approximately 8% of college students were infected with chlamydia and did not know it. Another 1.5% were infected with gonorrhea and did not know it. People infected with HIV can have mild or no symptoms for years, yet still be infectious.

Untreated Conditions

Some individuals lack sufficient knowledge of the signs and symptoms of STIs to know that they are infected. Those who are not accustomed to seeking health care, or who financially cannot afford it, are less likely to seek treatment for an infection. Furthermore, many individuals with STIs do not comply with treatment regimes. When medications are not taken for the required length of time, an infection may not be completely eradicated even though symptoms may disappear. People who do not complete treatment may still be infectious.

Impaired Judgment

The use of drugs, including alcohol, can increase the risk of transmitting STIs because people with drug-impaired judgment are less likely to use condoms. Also, people in this state may be more likely to have sex with someone they do not know; they may know nothing of their partner's past sexual and drug history (Graves and Hines, 1997).

Lack of Immunity

Some STI-causing organisms, such as HIV and herpesvirus, can escape the body's immune defenses, causing individuals to remain infected and transmit the infection. This may permit reinfection and also makes the development of vaccinations difficult or impossible (see chapter 9).

Body Piercing

Piercing of the body, particularly the genitals, increases the risk of transmission of STIs. The wound from piercing gives organisms direct access to the bloodstream, and pierced genitals may impede proper use of condoms. Moreover, people with nipple, tongue, and lip jewelry may have a higher risk of infection via oral sex. People who have their bodies pierced should follow after-care instructions faithfully to prevent infection and should abstain from sexual contact in the pierced region until the hole is completely healed, which takes 3 to 6 months.

Value Judgments

Unlike nearly all other kinds of infections, STIs are associated with sinfulness, dirtiness, condemnation, shame, guilt, and disgust. These negative attitudes keep people from getting check-ups, contacting partners when an STI has been diagnosed, and talking to new partners about previous exposures. In the nineteenth century, when syphilis was a scourge of Europe, rather than trying to prevent its spread (effective treatments had not yet been invented), countries blamed the disease on the weak character or immorality of their neighbors: the English referred to syphilis as the "French disease," and the French called it the "Spanish disease." Prejudice and scapegoating helped spread the disease.

Denial

With respect to contracting an STI, many people think, "It can't happen to me," or "He is too nice to have an STI," or "She isn't the type of person who would have an STI." Because there are no vaccinations against infectious agents that cause STIs, the only way to prevent them is for sexually active individuals, who are not in life-long single-partner (monogamous) sexual relationships, to assume responsibility for protecting themselves and their partners. This means becoming aware of the signs and symptoms of the common STIs and seeking treatment when such signs occur. It means that sexually active people who have more than one partner within a year should obtain periodic (about every 6 months) STI check-ups. It also means knowing about and practicing "safer sex."

 ## Common STIs

Although many nonviral STIs can be treated with medications, the epidemic of STIs persists worldwide (Holmes, 1994). There are no vaccinations for either the bacterial or viral infections that cause the most common sexually transmitted diseases. Dealing directly and responsibly with STIs is not easy. However, we owe it to the people we care about to do so. Table 8.1 outlines the major STIs, including their symptoms and treatment.

Trichomonas and Gardnerella Vaginalis

Although not often regarded as sexually transmitted diseases, vaginal infections caused by the protozoan *Trichomonas vaginalis* and the bacterium *Gardnerella vaginalis* are transmitted during intercourse. Symptoms tend to occur only in women (vaginal itching and a cheesy, odorous discharge from the vagina), but the organisms can survive in the urethra of the penis and under the penile foreskin. A man who harbors these organisms can infect other partners or even reinfect the partner who transmitted the organisms to him. Medications can eliminate these

TABLE 8.1 Common Sexually Transmitted Infections (STIs)

STI	Symptoms	Treatment
AIDS	Flu-like symptoms followed by any of a number of diseases characteristic of immunodeficiency	New drugs may retard viral reproduction temporarily. Opportunistic infections can be treated to some degree.
Chlamydia	Usually occur within 3 weeks: infected men have a discharge from the penis and painful urination, women may have a vaginal discharge, but often are asymptomatic	Antibiotics
Gardnerella vaginalis	Yellow-green vaginal discharge with an unpleasant odor; painful urination; vaginal itching	Metronidazole
Genital warts	Usually occur within 1 to 3 months: small, dry growths on the genitals, anus, cervix, and possibly mouth	Podophyllin
Gonorrhea	Usually occur within 2 weeks: discharge from the penis, vagina, or anus; pain on urination or defecation or during sexual intercourse; pain and swelling in the pelvic region; genital and oral infections may be asymptomatic	Antibiotics
Hepatitis B	Low-grade fever, fatigue, headaches, loss of appetite, nausea, dark urine, jaundice	Rest, proper nutrition; vaccination for hepatitis B
Genital herpes	Usually occur within 2 weeks: painful blisters on site(s) of infection (genitals, anus, cervix); occasionally, itching, painful urination, and fever	None; acyclovir relieves symptoms
Molluscum contagiosum	Smooth, rounded, shiny, whitish growths on the skin of the trunk and anogenital region	Surgical
Pubic lice	Usually occur within 5 weeks: intense itching in the genital region; lice may be visible in pubic hair; small white eggs may be visible on pubic hair	Gamma benzene hexachloride
Syphilis	Usually occur within 3 weeks: a chancre (painless sore) on the genitals, anus, or mouth; secondary stage—skin rash—if left untreated; tertiary stage includes diseases of several body organs	Antibiotics
Trichomonas vaginalis	Yellowish-green vaginal discharge with an unpleasant odor; vaginal itching; occasionally painful intercourse	Metronidazole

infections, and it is essential for both partners to undergo treatment.

Chlamydia

Chlamydia is caused by the microorganism *Chlamydia trachomatis*, which specifically infects certain cells lining the mucous membranes of the genitals, mouth, anus and rectum, the conjunctiva of the eyes, and occasionally the lungs.

In the United States and other Western countries, chlamydia is the most prevalent STI. Each year approximately 3 million Americans are reported to contract chlamydia, which public health experts estimate represents only one-third of all actual cases. In as many as half of all cases, chlamydia occurs simultaneously with gonorrhea. Newborns also are susceptible to chlamydial infection if their mothers are infected at the time of delivery. The most common complications of chlamydial infection in newborns are conjunctivitis (eye infection) and pneumonia.

One reason that chlamydial infections are so prevalent is that infected individuals often have extremely mild or no symptoms. Thus infected individuals can unknowingly transmit the infection to new sex partners. When symptoms do occur, they include pain during urination in both men and women (dysuria) and a whitish discharge from the penis or vagina. Symptoms generally appear within 7 to 21 days after infection.

Chlamydia can be treated with antibiotics. Left untreated, the chlamydial bacteria can multiply and

cause inflammation and damage of the reproductive organs in both sexes. In men, untreated chlamydia can result in inflammation of the epididymis (**epididymitis**), characterized by pain, swelling, and tenderness in the scrotum and sometimes by a mild fever. Damage to the tissues in the epididymis can eventually lead to sterility. In women, chlamydial infections affect the cervix, uterus, fallopian tubes, and peritoneum. Often chlamydial infections of the reproductive tract produce no symptoms until the infection is advanced. A woman may then experience chronic pelvic pain, vaginal discharge, intermittent vaginal bleeding, and pain during intercourse. Infection of the fallopian tubes can produce scar tissue that damages the tubes' lining and partially or completely blocks the tubes. These effects may increase the risk of ectopic pregnancy or render a woman infertile; in fact, about 10,000 cases of female infertility per year result from fallopian tube damage from chlamydia (Grodstein and Rothman, 1994).

Terms

chlamydia: a sexually transmitted disease caused by the bacterium *Chlamydia trachomatis*

epididymitis: inflammation of the epididymis (a structure that connects the vas deferens and the testes)

Gonorrhea

Gonorrhea, also known as "the clap," is caused by the bacterium *Neisseria gonorrheae.* Gonorrheal organisms specifically infect the mucous membranes of the body, most often the genitals, reproductive organs, mouth and throat, anus, and eyes. *N. gonorrheae* cannot survive on toilet seats, doorknobs, bedsheets, clothes, or towels. Transmission in adults almost always occurs by genital, oral, or anal sexual contact; infection of the eyes occurs by hand (often through self-infection). Each year, about 1 million American adults are infected with gonorrhea.

Although the bacteria causing them are quite different, the symptoms of gonorrheal and chlamydial infections are very similar. Like chlamydia, many people infected with gonorrheal organisms do not develop symptoms and their infections go unnoticed. If the infection progresses, men may develop epididymitis and women may develop infections of the uterus, fallopian tubes, and pelvic region. Such infections may cause sterility. When symptoms appear, they include painful urination in both sexes and a yellowish discharge from the penis or vagina. Occasionally there is pain in the groin, testes, or lower abdomen. The first symptoms of gonorrhea usually appear within 7 to 10 days after exposure.

Gonorrhea can be treated with antibiotics. However, new antibiotic-resistant strains of the organism are constantly evolving. In nearly half of all cases of gonorrhea, chlamydia also is present. Individuals undergoing diagnosis for gonorrhea should also be tested for chlamydia.

Syphilis

Syphilis is caused by a spiral-shaped bacterium called *Treponema pallidum.* These organisms are transmitted from person to person through genital, oral, and anal contact, as well as being acquired from infected blood. Syphilis can also be transmitted from a mother to her unborn fetus, perhaps as early as the ninth week of pregnancy.

The first noticeable sign of syphilis is a painless open sore called a **chancre** ("shanker"), which can appear any time between the first week and third month after infection. If the infection is not treated within that period, the chancre will heal and the disease will enter a secondary stage, characterized by a skin rash, hair loss, and the appearance of round, flat-topped growths on most areas of the body. Left untreated, the signs of the secondary stage also disappear, and the infection enters a symptomless (latency) period, during which the syphilis organisms multiply in many other regions of the body. In the final, tertiary stage, the disease eventually damages vital organs, such as the heart or brain, and can cause severe symptoms or death. Syphilis can be treated with antibiotics at any stage of the infection.

Herpes

Herpes is caused by the Herpes simplex virus (HSV). Various strains of HSV can cause cold sores on the mouth ("fever blisters"), skin rashes, mononucleosis, and lesions on the penis, vagina, or rectum. Herpesvirus can infect the eyes, leading to impaired vision and even blindness. If the virus is present in the birth canal, newborn babies can be infected, often resulting in brain damage and abnormal development. About 500 babies are born each year with herpes, and two-thirds of infected babies who are not treated die. Pregnant women who have had herpes should tell their physicians of the previous infection in order to prevent transmission of HSV to their babies.

Each year, about 500,000 Americans acquire genital herpes infection. In the United States, 20.8% of adults, or 45 million people, have been infected with the strain *herpes simplex virus, type 2* (HSV-2). Among teenagers, the prevalence of HSV-2 infection is five times higher now than in the late 1970s; among people aged 20 to 29, the prevalence is twice as high (Fleming et al, 1997). Oral herpes infections, which are generally caused by *herpes simplex virus, type 1* (HSV-1), occur in many children, and by age 50, more than three-fourths of the adult population has experienced an oral herpes infection.

Infections with HSV-2 often are asymptomatic. Indeed, 90% of people infected with HSV-2 do not know it. Nevertheless, they are infectious and may contribute to the spread of this disease by having unprotected sex. When symptoms do occur, they include the presence of one or more blisters, which eventually break to become wet, painful sores that last about 2 or 3 weeks; fever; and occasionally pain

---

Terms

gonorrhea: sexually transmitted disease caused by gonococcal bacteria (*Neisseria gonorrhea*)

syphilis: a sexually transmitted disease caused by spirochete bacteria (*Treponema pallidum*)

chancre: the primary lesion of syphilis, which appears as a hard, painless sore or ulcer often on the penis or vaginal tissue

herpes: sexually transmitted infection caused by *Herpes simplex virus, HSV*

sexually transmitted warts: hard growths caused by an infection with human papillomavirus (HPV) that appears on the skin of the genitals or anus

human papillomavirus (HPV): a genus of viruses including those causing papillomas (small nipple-like protrusions of the skin or mucous membrane) and warts in the lower abdomen. Eventually these initial symptoms disappear, but herpesvirus remains dormant in certain of the body's nerve cells, permitting periodic recurrences of the symptoms, called "flare-ups," at or near the site(s) of the initial infection. Stress, anxiety, improper nutrition, sunlight, and skin irritation can bring on flare-ups.

There is no cure for herpes. Infected individuals remain so for life. The drug acyclovir can minimize the duration and severity of the symptoms of an initial infection or a flare-up. There is no vaccine for herpes.

Herpes is extremely contagious when a sore is present. People with open lesions should avoid sex with others until the lesions disappear. Even if no sore is present, transmission is possible, although much less likely, through the "shedding" of virus particles from the skin.

Because the herpes virus remains in the body, and because flare-ups are a persistent possibility, some people believe that infected persons can never be sexually active. This is not true. People with herpes can learn to manage the condition. In many instances, after one or two episodes, additional flare-ups never occur. Some people can anticipate a flare-up because they get a tingling sensation, itching, pain, or numbness at the site of the initial infection. This can be a signal to refrain from sexual contact. If used appropriately, condoms and spermicides can protect against the spread of herpes.

Because genital herpes is associated with a risk of cervical cancer, women with herpes are advised to have annual Pap smears to ascertain the condition of the vagina and cervix.

Sexually Transmitted Warts

Sexually transmitted warts *(Condylomata acuminata)*, also known as genital or venereal warts, are hard, cauliflower-like growths that appear in men on the penis, in women on the external genitals and cervix, and in both sexes in the anal region. Warts are caused by several of the approximately 50 varieties of **human papillomavirus (HPV).** When HPV infects skin cells and cells of the genital tract, it causes them to multiply, thus forming the wart. Infection with many varieties of HPV is often more of a nuisance than it is dangerous. However, a dozen varieties of HPV may cause or facilitate uncontrolled multiplication of cells of the cervix and, eventually, cancer of the cervix (Shah, 1997). HPV infection may also contribute to cancer of the penis, vulva, and anus (Frisch, et al., 1997).

Sexually transmitted warts usually appear about 3 months after contact with an infected person. They can be removed by coating the wart with a liquid containing podophyllin, which dries the wart. In severe cases, wart removal is accomplished by freezing the warts with liquid nitrogen or removing them with laser surgery.

Hepatitis B

Hepatitis B is a disease of the liver caused by infection by hepatitis B virus (HBV), one of several types of hepatitis viruses. Compared to other hepatitis viruses, which tend to be transmitted in fecally contaminated food, HBV is transmitted sexually and in blood, in a manner similar to HIV, the AIDS virus. About 150,000 sexually transmitted HBV infections occur in the U.S. each year; worldwide, the number of people infected with HBV is estimated at 300 million (Figure 8.7). Hepatitis B virus is sexually transmitted 100 times more effectively than HIV.

The symptoms of hepatitis B infection include low-grade fever, tiredness, headaches, loss of appetite, nausea, dark urine, and jaundice (i.e., yellowing of the white of the eyes and the skin). The first symptoms,

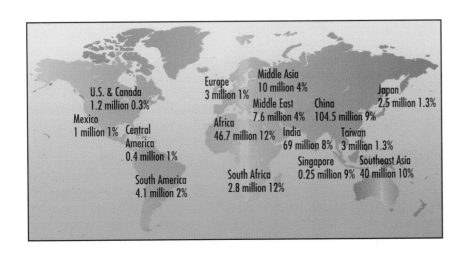

FIGURE 8.7   Hepatitis B Infection Worldwide   Number of people infected with hepatitis B virus in 1997 in the world and the percentage infected in each region.

Source: World Health Organization (1997).

which are flu-like, tend to occur 14 to 100 days after infection. Signs of liver disease (e.g., dark urine, jaundice) appear later. No specific therapy exists for HBV infection. Rest, proper nutrition, and avoidance of substances harmful to the liver (e.g., alcohol and drugs) are required for recovery, which may take many months. Long-term liver damage is possible, including liver cancer and death.

A vaccine against HBV exists and everyone is advised to be vaccinated, especially children, health workers, and others who are at high risk of exposure.

Molluscum Contagiosum

Molluscum contagiosum is caused by a virus of the same name. Fewer than 100,000 infections occur in the U.S. each year. The infection is characterized by the appearance of freckle-sized, smooth, rounded, shiny, whitish growths on the skin of the trunk and anogenital region. Generally, there are no associated symptoms. The lesions may resolve spontaneously, but it is best to have them removed by a health care provider, otherwise they may be transmitted to others or reoccur.

Pubic Lice

Pubic lice *(Phthirus pubis),* also known as "crabs," are barely visible insects that live on hair shafts primarily in the genital-rectal region and occasionally on hair in the armpits, beard, and eyelashes. The organisms' claws are specifically adapted for grasping hairs with the diameter of pubic and axillary hair, which differs in diameter from the shafts of scalp hair. Thus pubic lice are not usually found on the head. (Scalp hair is the ecological niche of the head louse, *Pediculus humanus capitis.*)

Lice feed on blood taken from tiny blood vessels in the skin, which they pierce with their mouth. Some people are sensitive to the bites and may experience itching, which is often the main symptom of infestation. The lice can also be seen; they look like small freckles. The eggs of lice are enclosed in small white pods (called "nits"), which attach to hair shafts. The presence of nits is also a sign of infestation.

Terms

pubic lice: small insects that live primarily in hair in the genital and rectal regions

scabies: infestation of the skin by microscopic mites (insects)

human immunodeficiency virus (HIV): the virus that causes AIDS; it causes a defect in the body's immune system by invading and then multiplying within the white blood cells

Transfer of lice is via physical—usually sexual—contact. They can also be transmitted via contact with objects on which eggs might have been laid, such as towels, bed linens, and clothes. An infestation of pubic lice can be eliminated by washing the pubic hair with liquids or shampoos containing agents that specifically kill lice (e.g., pyrethrins, piperonyl butoxide, and gamma benzene hydrochloride). All of an infected person's clothes, towels, and bed linens should also be washed with cleaning agents made specifically for killing lice.

Scabies

Scabies is an infestation of certain regions of the skin by extremely small (invisible to the naked eye) mites, *Sarcoptes scabiei.* The mites burrow into the skin where they live and lay eggs. The tiny lesions produced by the mites often cause intense itching, which is the major sign of a scabies infection. The mites produce tiny burrows across skin lines, which often go unnoticed. Occasionally, an infestation will produce small round nodules. The mites tend to live in the webs between the fingers, on the sides of fingers, and on the wrists, elbows, breasts, abdomen, penis, and buttocks. Rarely do mites live on the face, neck, upper back, palms and soles.

Scabies can be transmitted both sexually and nonsexually. All that is required is close personal contact. The itching and physical symptoms often take several weeks to appear. Scabies can be treated with topical agents that kill the mites and their eggs.

Acquired Immune Deficiency Syndrome (AIDS)

AIDS is caused by **human immunodeficiency virus,** or **HIV**. HIV infection causes disease by destroying immune system cells and weakening the body's immune system. Destruction of the body's immune system makes HIV-infected individuals susceptible to a variety of bacterial, viral, and fungal infections that a person with an intact immune system could readily ward off. HIV infection in the brain leads to loss of mental faculties (AIDS dementia).

HIV is mainly transmitted via blood, semen, or vaginal fluids of infected people. Sexual transmission is most common by having unprotected penis-anus sex with an infected person. Unprotected sex is exposure to sexual fluids and blood without consistent and correct use of a male or female condom.

When individuals become infected with HIV, within a few weeks they usually experience flu-like symptoms, from which they eventually recover. Their immune systems are still intact and they produce copious antibodies to HIV. The mounting of an immune response in the early phases of an HIV infection provides the basis for HIV testing. Nearly all of the tests for HIV infection detect antibodies to HIV. A positive result (seropositive) indicates that a person has been exposed to sufficient quantities of HIV particles to mount an immune response.

An HIV-infected individual may not manifest symptoms of AIDS for as many as 15 or 20 years after the initial infection. During this latency period, the infected person is contagious and can spread the infection to others, even though she or he is symptomless. The first signs of AIDS are usually mononucleosis-like symptoms (e.g., swollen lymph glands, fever, night sweats) and possibly headaches and impaired mental functioning caused by HIV infection of the brain. As the disease progresses, individuals most often suffer weight loss, infections on the skin (shingles) or in the throat (thrush), one or more opportunistic infections, and cancer.

Because there is no way to rid the body of HIV and hence cure AIDS, treatment of the disease relies on (a) medically managing the opportunistic infections that result from immune suppression and (b) attempting to suppress HIV infection within the affected person's body. Treating HIV infection involves administering combinations of different drugs, but unfortunately, the combination therapies are not a cure and not all HIV-infected individuals respond. Also, because the drugs only suppress HIV, even those who do respond must take the drugs for life lest the virus begin multiplying again. Because HIV mutates rapidly, in many cases drug resistance develops. Finally, combination drug treatments cost about $10,000 per person per year, so they are unavailable for the economically disadvantaged, who make up 90% of the more than 32 million HIV-infected people in the world.

Because many viral diseases have been conquered by vaccination, much effort has gone into developing vaccines against HIV, but without success so far. The only effective way to control the spread of AIDS is to prevent the transfer of HIV from person to person. This is accomplished by using condoms and spermicides (which destroy the virus), reducing exposure to infected individuals, and avoiding casual sex.

Reducing the Risk of HIV/AIDS   Because the first reported cases of AIDS in the United States were among male homosexuals, and because many thousands of men in that group have died from AIDS, some people mistakenly believe that only homosexual men can get AIDS. This is not so. Anyone can get AIDS. The reasons that so many male homosexual males acquired AIDS include:

- Without knowledge of the infectious agent HIV, it was impossible to take precautions.

- In the late 1970s and early 1980s, sexual mores among young people, including male homosexuals, permitted multiple sexual partners affording HIV rapid access to a large population.
- Anal intercourse provides HIV a highly efficient route of infection because microscopic tears in the rectum give the virus access to the recipient's blood. Microscopic tears in the penis also allow blood transmission and blood in semen provides a further avenue of infection.

Love is giving someone the space to be the way they are—and the way they are not.

EDMUND BURKE

After it was determined that HIV caused AIDS and once strategies were developed to stop its transmission, the frequency of new HIV infections among homosexual males declined dramatically. This decline demonstrated that educational efforts and motivation can prevent the transmission of HIV/AIDS and other STIs. Although AIDS is still a threat to male homosexuals, the majority of new cases of AIDS are among injection drug users who share their drug paraphernalia (needles and syringes) with others, and persons who engage in sexual intercourse with these individuals. AIDS is increasing among heterosexuals around the world.

Testing for HIV Infection   Health officials do not advocate that everyone be tested for HIV infection. But certainly those who suspect that they have been exposed to the virus are candidates for testing. These individuals include males who have had unprotected sex with other males and anyone who has:

- had unprotected sex with someone who is known or suspected to be infected with HIV.
- had a sexually transmitted disease.
- had unprotected sex with someone while drunk.
- had sex with someone whose AIDS-risky behaviors are unknown.
- had several sexual partners.
- shared needles or syringes to inject drugs of any kind.

Testing begins with a counseling session. You will be given materials to read before the session with a counselor or doctor. In the session, you'll be asked why you want to be tested and about your behavior and that of your sex partner(s). This will help your counselor and you to determine whether testing is appropriate. If testing is appropriate, your counselor or doctor will

Global Wellness

HIV Infections Worldwide

Of the millions of persons worldwide who are infected with HIV, about 90% live in the developing world and most of them are not aware of their infection. By the year 2000 it is projected that as many as 40 million people worldwide will be infected with HIV. In 1997, more than 2 million people around the world died from AIDS; since the AIDS pandemic began, about 12 million people have died from AIDS. Of all the persons who have died from AIDS, about 500,000 have been children and the rest of the deaths have been divided more or less equally among men and women.

Sub-Saharan Africa is the region of the world with the most infections: 7.4% of all those aged 15 to 49 are infected with HIV. The region has 90% of the world's total of children born with HIV. Unprotected sex between men and women accounts for most of the adult infections. High fertility combined with poor access to information and services for the prevention of mother-to-child transmission of HIV accounts for infections among children.

East Africa was one of the first areas to suffer a massive regional epidemic, and one country in the region, Uganda, was among the first to respond with open and concerted efforts to prevent the spread of the virus. Today, Uganda's infection rate is about one-fifth of what it was in the early 1990s.

Infection rates in Asia are lower than Africa but the numbers are large. Indeed, with between 3 million and 5 million people living with HIV, India has the largest number of HIV-infected people in the world. In China, as many as 400,000 people may be infected.

In Thailand, the number of new infections has decreased, especially among prostitutes and their

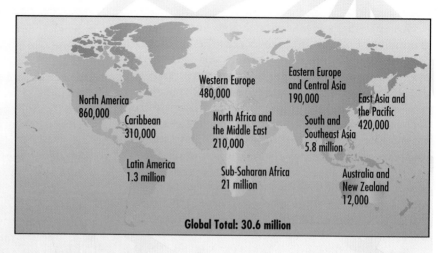

North America 860,000
Caribbean 310,000
Latin America 1.3 million
Western Europe 480,000
North Africa and the Middle East 210,000
Sub-Saharan Africa 21 million
Eastern Europe and Central Asia 190,000
South and Southeast Asia 5.8 million
East Asia and the Pacific 420,000
Australia and New Zealand 12,000
Global Total: 30.6 million

Source: World Health Organization, 1997.

clients, which account for the majority of the 750,000 persons currently infected (representing 2.3% of the adult population). The decrease in new infections is a result of prevention efforts aimed at increasing condom use, boosting respect for women, discouraging men from visiting prostitutes, and offering young women better educational and employment opportunities to discourage their entry into the commercial sex business.

In Latin America, the epidemic has taken its greatest toll on men who have sex with men and among injection drug users. In Latin America and the Caribbean as a whole, AIDS has already overtaken traffic accidents as a leading cause of death. HIV infection rates among pregnant women are 3% in some parts of Brazil, and 8% in Haiti and the Dominican Republic.

In Eastern Europe, drug injection is responsible for most HIV infections. The potential for sexual transmission also exists, since STIs are increasingly common. Increasing rates of non-HIV STIs indicate that individuals are not practicing safe sex.

Furthermore, an untreated STI makes HIV (when present) spread much more easily.

In Western Europe, North America, Australia, and New Zealand, the number of new AIDS cases has dropped considerably since 1995 because of better prevention and treatment. The fall is greatest in countries in which infection has been concentrated in homosexual men, in whom HIV infection rates began dropping in the late 1980s. Only in communities in which unsafe drug injection is the main mode of transmission do new AIDS cases show substantial rises.

Because the vast majority of people living with HIV are in the developing world, where access to prevention information, health care, and anti-AIDS medicines are often difficult or impossible to obtain, international public health officials are concerned that many of the millions of people currently infected with HIV will die within the next decade.

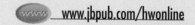 **www.jbpub.com/hwonline**

describe the test and how it is done, provide basic AIDS education, explain confidentiality issues, discuss the meaning of possible test results and what impact you think the test result will have on you, and talk about whom you might tell about your result.

The actual test involves taking a small amount of blood from your arm, which is tested in a special lab-

oratory. Results are usually returned in a few days. When your result is available, you will be asked to return to the counseling and testing center to receive the information. This is true for everyone tested regardless of the results.

HIV tests can be obtained from physicians and a variety of health agencies. There are two kinds of HIV-testing: anonymous and confidential. In the anonymous system, individuals are identified only by a self-selected number or alias, so the true identity is never recorded. In the confidential system, one's name is part of the medical record, which is supposed to be confidential. At-home HIV tests are also available. These require individuals to collect a drop or two of blood from a finger-stick and mail the sample to a laboratory for analysis and follow-up telephone counseling.

Before HIV tests became available, thousands of people were inadvertently infected with HIV as a result of receiving HIV-tainted products derived from blood or blood transfusions (for example, tennis star Arthur Ashe). In the 1980s thousands of people with **hemophilia** (a hereditary blood disease) received clotting factor derived from pooled blood that was contaminated with HIV, and many have since been stricken with AIDS. In France, a national scandal erupted when it was learned that French health officials knowingly continued to allow hemophiliacs to receive contaminated blood products. All clotting factor products used today are manufactured by biotechnology companies and are free of viral contamination. In addition, all blood donations in the United States today are tested for HIV and other viral contamination. However, new strains of HIV continually arise, and tests are not available for all of them. For any elective surgery, patients often are advised to donate their own blood beforehand should a transfusion be required.

Preventing STIs

Preventing STIs requires that societies provide continuous, widespread public health programs and services for STI education and treatment. It is also crucial that infected individuals seek prompt treatment, take responsibility for not infecting other individuals, and practice safer sex to lower their risk of infection.

The stigma associated with STIs is a great hindrance to prevention efforts. Thinking about STIs in moral terms, i.e., associating them with dirtiness and immorality, makes people reluctant to think and talk about them. It also makes society want to ignore STI epidemics. During World Wars I and II, American society supported massive gonorrhea and syphilis control programs; as a result, the incidence of these infections dropped tremendously. When the threat of a postwar STI epidemic seemed to wane, moralistic concerns thwarted the continuation of control efforts, and the incidence of STIs increased. Public health officials realize that ongoing efforts are the only way to control STIs.

Judgmental attitudes also make talking about STIs difficult. To have to tell a partner that you have an STI, or even to say that you once had an infection and are now perfectly okay, can bring feelings of guilt and shame, which can lead to the avoidance of discussion altogether. Similarly, to ask about a partner's previous STIs may be interpreted as an accusation that the person is "loose" or immoral. To avoid feeling embarrassed or risk offending a sexual partner, people are likely to avoid the topic of STIs. Prevention would be enhanced if sexually active individuals developed an open attitude about talking about STIs (and other aspects of sex) and acquired the necessary communication skills.

Practicing Safer Sex

The surest way to reduce the risk of acquiring a sexually transmitted infection is to abstain from sexual intercourse. This does not mean that one has to give up sexual interaction. There are many ways of giving and receiving sexual pleasure without engaging in sexual intercourse: touching, kissing, exchanging a massage, even sleeping together without intercourse.

Another way to reduce risk is to know a partner's sexual history, including all high-risk activities in which a partner may have engaged. Often this kind of information is difficult to gain early in a relationship, because exchanging information about sexual histories requires a certain level of trust, which takes some time to develop.

Until you have this knowledge, it is essential to protect yourself by using condoms and spermicides when having sex. Women and men who are sexually active should come to accept as standard practice with new partners the use of condoms and spermicides, since birth control pills offer no protection against STIs. Sexually active women and men should carry condoms and spermicides whenever the possibility of sex exists and use them. This requires overcoming the gender role stereotypes that women who admit to being sexual are "sluts" and men who behave the same way are "studs."

Some barriers to safer sex include:

- **Denying that there is a risk.** Many people assume that STIs happen only to "dirty," "promiscuous," and "immoral" people, and since they themselves have sex only with people who are "clean" and "nice," getting an STI is impossible. Another form of denial is to tell oneself, "I eat right. I exercise. I can't get an STI."

Terms

hemophilia: a hereditary disease (primarily in men) caused by lack of an essential blood clotting factor; results in excessive bleeding in response to any scratch or injury

- **Believing that the campus community is somehow insulated from STIs.** The truth is that about half of college students are sexually active before they enter college. As a result, students can arrive on campus with an infection. Also, on many campuses, students in the same living groups and student organizations have sex with one another. One infected person could lead to a whole chain of infections.

- **Feeling guilty and uncomfortable about being sexual.** This prevents individuals from planning sex and carrying condoms and spermicides, and talking about possible risks with new partners.

- **Succumbing to social and peer pressure to be sexual.** These pressures encourage people to be sexual in situations that are potentially risky, such as "one night stands" and brief relationships that are sexual virtually from the beginning. The risk of infection is lessened when individuals resist peer pressure to have sex with a relative stranger, and ask themselves instead, "Is this the right relationship?," "Is this the right partner?," "Am I going to feel OK about this afterwards?"

Effective Communication Skills

The pressure to be sexual early in a relationship, before the partners know each other well enough to talk about their past sexual experiences, may force partners to deny there may be a risk. A less risky strategy would be to postpone sexual interaction by saying, "I'd like to be close to you, but I'm not ready to have sex until we get to know each other better." "Not yet" and "maybe" are options when weighing an invitation to be sexual.

Even if a person is ready to talk about the sexual aspects of a new relationship, including birth control and possible exposure to STIs, it can be difficult because of fear of being rejected, offending the partner, or just spoiling the mood. Disclosing one's discomfort about talking about the subject is one way to relieve anxiety about it. A conversation could begin with one partner saying, "There's something I want us to talk about and I feel sort of uncomfortable about it, but I think it's important to both of us, so here goes."

After that introduction, the individual can offer information by saying something like, "We don't know each other very well; I'm concerned about sexual diseases. I want you to know this about me." That person should offer all of the information that he or she would like to be told. After hearing the disclosure, the other person is more likely to respond in kind. And if more information is desired, one could say something like, "Thanks for telling me all of that. I'd feel more comfortable if I knew a little more about . . ." whatever it is.

What if the other person gets offended or won't talk about this subject? Or what if the other person can't be trusted? If partners cannot discuss something as serious as STIs, it is prudent to postpone sexual interaction until the relationship has progressed to a greater level of trust. Potential sexual partners should remember that being under the influence of alcohol or other drugs can affect judgment in making decisions about what is and is not safe. Also, being drunk or

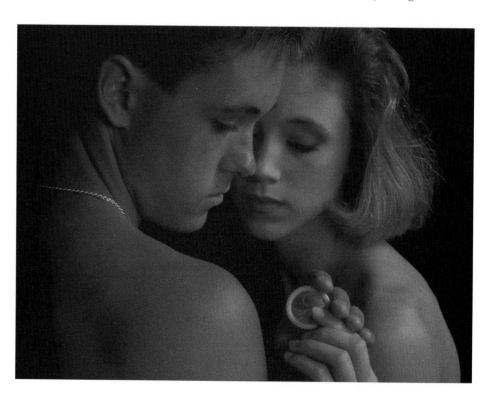

Both partners need to be responsible for practicing safe sex.

Managing Stress

Preventing STIs and AIDS: Confidence Building

Pressure from a friend to be sexually intimate when it is not your first choice to do so can result in some serious consequences. Thoughts of disease, illness, and death are almost nonexistent in the mind of a young college student. Rather, feelings of immortality and invincibility are the norm. However, in today's society, in which the risk of AIDS and sexually transmitted infections is so prevalent, no one can afford to be naive. Having the world at your feet ready to explore is a wonderful prospect, yet it can be cut short without taking precautions. Precautions don't begin with condoms. They begin with attitudes, beliefs, and values.

One attitude that is essential to dealing with the stress of sexual intimacy is confidence. Confidence is a feeling at gut level that guides your sense of willpower to make choices that make you feel comfortable, not guilty. While we all have access to confidence, some people let it atrophy like an unexercised muscle. Yet it is confidence, a belief in yourself, a feeling of security, a feeling of groundedness that guides you through times of peer pressure or undesired sexual impositions. With confidence, there is a responsibility to honor your integrity, not jeopardize it with feelings of arrogance.

Confidence, coupled with intuition and humility, proves to be a powerful inner resource that can help steer you clear of unnecessary dangers such as AIDS and STIs. When confidence acts alone, the result is often cockiness. Rather than helping you avoid potentially dangerous or unhealthy situations, this arrogance leads you straight into them.

So what are some ways to increase your sense of confidence? You can begin by telling yourself that you feel comfortable and responsible about your sexual behavior. Try it. Say to yourself, *"I feel comfortable and responsible with my sexual behavior."* When you say it to yourself, don't only think it to yourself, feel it in your stomach, at the gut level. Once you have said this, say it again. Say it to yourself enough that you feel comfortable with saying it and understand the message you are giving yourself. Then make a habit of saying this or a similar phrase to yourself every day, enough so that it becomes second nature to you, part of your own being. And when you find yourself preparing for a moment of sexual intimacy, repeat the phrase to yourself again, so that it guides you through each experience, feeling good about yourself and your partner.

It is impossible to live life without regrets, for regret teaches many of life's lessons. Yet we can also learn from others. Those who have encountered AIDS and STIs firsthand will tell you that this is one lesson you don't have to experience firsthand to grasp fully. Let your confidence and balanced solid intuition be your guides.

stoned can impair using condoms effectively—or using them at all!

Safer sex does not mean no sex. It does not mean that sex is dangerous. It does not mean that sex cannot be fun. It does mean that sex is cooperative. It means that partners are making choices together.

Critical Thinking About Health

1. Bill and Sandy have been dating for several months. One Friday evening they go out to dinner and then to a movie. After the movie they go back to Sandy's place. Bill and Sandy begin to kiss, and within 10 to 15 minutes they decide to have sexual intercourse. Neither of them has a condom or spermicide, and Sandy is not using any kind of fertility control method. Despite the fact that neither Sandy nor Bill is using fertility control or has a fertility control method with them, they have unprotected sexual intercourse that evening.
   a. What could they have done instead of having sexual intercourse?
   b. How could this situation have been avoided?
   c. Whose responsibility is it to plan for fertility control?

2. Go to your student health center and find out which fertility control options are available to students who attend your college or university.
   a. How does one go about obtaining the available methods and how much do they cost?
   b. If there are some methods that are not available, ask why and find out where in your community they are available.

3. Because she had consistently voted to support research on HIV and AIDS, it shocked many people when Congresswoman Harmas refused to vote for the $7.8 billion appropriations bill to pay for protease inhibitor medicines for the medically indigent with AIDS in both the U.S. and around the world. "I have total compassion for these people," said Harmas, "but at $10,000 a year, we cannot afford to take care of everyone who is sick. Further-

more, in our country, most of the money will go to treating injection drug users, who ought to know better than to get the disease in the first place. And for all the poverty-stricken sick people, principally in Asia and Africa, all I can say is I'm sorry, complain to your own government. We're broke." Do you agree or disagree with the congresswoman's position?

Health in Review

- A variety of safe, reliable, and effective fertility control methods are available today. These include hormonal contraception (the birth control pill and progestin-only contraceptives); barrier methods (condom, diaphragm, cervical cap, and spermicides); fertility awareness methods; the IUD; sterilization; withdrawal; and abstinence.
- A contraceptive's effectiveness is measured in terms of typical use and perfect use failure rates.
- Although most fertility control methods are designed for use in the woman's body, both partners share the responsibility for fertility control. Communication and cooperation are keys to shared responsibility.
- People who say they do not want to have a baby, yet do not use fertility control methods, tend to have low motivation, lack of knowledge of human reproduction and fertility control methods, or negative attitudes toward fertility control or are in relationships that hinder correct fertility control practice.
- Medical and surgical abortions are available.

- Abortion became legal in the U.S. in 1973 with the Supreme Court's Roe v. Wade decision.
- Sexually transmitted infections (formerly called venereal disease, or VD) are passed from person to person, most frequently by sexual contact.
- Millions of sexually transmitted infections occur each year in the United States.
- STIs are epidemic in the United States because people are uninformed about them, because they engage in high-risk behaviors, and because vaccines and cures (for several) are unavailable.
- The most common STIs in the United States are trichomonas and gardnerella vaginalis, chlamydia, gonorrhea, syphilis, herpes, genital warts, pubic lice, and AIDS.
- Preventing STIs involves supporting public health efforts to inform the populace about STIs and their prevention and treatment. It also requires individuals to practice "safer sex" and to comply with treatment when they are infected.
- PREVENTION is the key!

Health and Wellness Online

The World Wide Web contains a wealth of information about health and wellness. By accessing the Internet using Web browser software, such as Netscape Navigator or Microsoft's Internet Explorer, you can gain a new perspective on many topics presented in *Essentials of Health and Wellness, Second Edition.* Access the Jones and Bartlett Publishers web site at http://www.jbpub.com/hwonline.

Choosing what's best for you.

Don't become a statistic; learn how to prevent STIs.

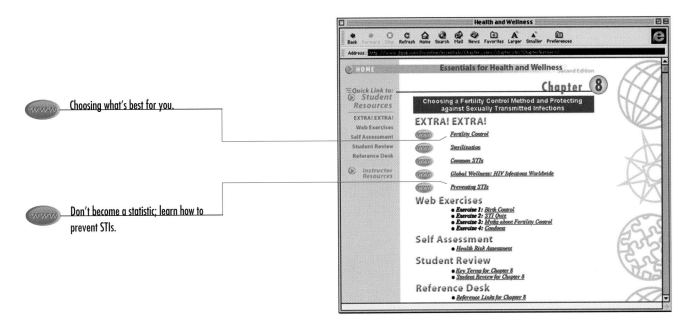

References

Centers for Disease Control and Prevention. (1997). Abortion surveillance: Preliminary analysis—United States, 1995. *Morbidity and Mortality Weekly Report, 46(48),* 1133–1135.

Centers for Disease Control and Prevention. (1997). *HIV/AIDS surveillance report,* Volume 9.

Fleming, D. T., et al. (1997). Herpes simplex virus type 2 in the United States, 1976–1994. *New England Journal of Medicine, 337,* 1105–1111.

Frisch, M., et al. (1997). Sexually transmitted infection as a cause of anal cancer. *New England Journal of Medicine, 337,* 1350–1358.

Goldberg, M. S. (1993, December). Choosing a contraceptive. *FDA Consumer,* 18–25.

Graves, K. L., & Hines, A. M. (1997). Ethnic differences in the association between behavior with a new partner. *AIDS Education and Prevention, 3,* 219–237.

Grodstein, F., & Rothman, K. J. (1994). Epidemiology of pelvic inflammatory disease. *Epidemiology, 5,* 234–242.

Hatcher, R. A., Trussell, J., Stewart, F., Cates, W., Stewart, G. K., Guest, F., & Kowal, D. (1998). *Contraceptive technology.* 17th ed. Media Ardent: New York.

Holmes, K. S. (1994). Human ecology and behavior in sexually transmitted bacterial infections. *Proceedings of the National Academy of Sciences, 91,* 2448–2455.

Kost, K., & Forrest, J. D. (1992). American women's sexual behavior and exposure to risk of sexually transmitted diseases. *Family Planning Perspectives, 24,* 244–246.

National Abortion Federation. (1997). What is medical abortion? Washington, DC.

Shah, K. V. (1997). Human papilloma viruses and anogenital warts. *New England Journal of Medicine, 337,* 1386–87.

Suggested Readings

Centers for Disease Control and Prevention. (1999). Trends in the HIV and AIDS epidemic. Atlanta: CDC. An up-to-date overview covering historical trends in AIDS incidence, trends in diagnoses, and implications for prevention.

Fackelmann, K. (1995). Staying alive: Scientists study people who outwit the AIDS virus. *Science News, 147,* 172–174. Five to 10% of HIV-infected persons are still healthy after 10 years; they appear to be genetically resistant to the effects of HIV infection.

Fraser, I., Tiitien, A., Affandi, B., Brache, V., Croxatto, H. B., Diaz, S., Ginsburg, J., Gu, S., Holma, P., Johansson, E., Meirik, O., Mishell D., Nash, H., Von Schoultz, B., & Sivin, I. (1998). Norplant consensus statement and background review. *Contraception, 57,* 1–9. The study analyzes the efficacy and safety of Norplant and discusses factors that influence the controversy behind this method of birth control.

Handsfield, H. H. (1997). A look at sexually transmitted diseases. *Postgraduate Medicine, 101,* 268–277. A highly readable account of STDs in human history.

Hatcher, R. A., Trussell, J., Stewart, F., Cates, W., Stewart, G. K., Guest, F., & Kowal, D. (1998). *Contraceptive technology,* 17th ed. Media Ardent: New York. A complete, practical guide for people who provide and use reproductive health services.

Nordenberg, T. (1998). Condoms—barriers to bad news. *FDA Consumer, 32*(2), 22–25. The article is an easy to understand and entertaining piece on the importance of using condoms during sexual encounters.

Marrs, R., Bloch, L. F., & Silverman, K. K. (1998). *Dr. Marr's fertility book.* NY: Dell Publishing. America's leading infertility expert tells you everything you need to know about getting pregnant.

Planned Parenthood Federation of America. (1998). *All about birth control: A complete guide.* NY: Three Rivers Press. A thorough, concise, and complete guide to all fertility control options available to women.

Revelle, M. (1995, April). Progress in blood supply safety. *FDA Consumer,* 21–24. Discusses the importance of a safe blood supply and the safeguards taken to prevent contaminated blood.

Royce, R. A. (1997). Sexual transmission of HIV. *New England Journal of Medicine, 336,* 1072–1078. Explains in detail how HIV is transmitted sexually and what contributes to the risk of infection. Surprising is the finding that HIV is transmitted in only about 1 per 1000 occasions of sexual intercourse in which one of the partners is HIV-positive.

Shilts, R. (1988). *And the Band Played On: Politics, People, and the AIDS Epidemic.* New York: Penguin Books. An account of the AIDS epidemic and how politics affected the lives of people. Also an excellent movie-on-video.

Tarantola, D. J. M., & Mann, J. M. (1996, October 15). Global expansion of HIV infection and AIDS. *Hospital Practice,* 63–79. Explains why HIV infection will continue to spread globally even if the rate of infection continues to decline in industrialized countries.

Making *Healthy Changes*

Humans are very social creatures, so it should come as no surprise that healthy relationships are good for health. People who are in healthy relationships (e.g., close intimate relationships, friendships, or members of supportive organizations and communities) are in better health, live longer, and are more satisfied with life. What factors contribute to a healthy relationship? Most people put trust and good communication at the top of the list. Self-acceptance and the willingness to accept and support others are important too. In the physical environment, you benefit personally when you manifest attitudes and behaviors that contribute to enhancing the overall environment because a healthy environment helps you be a healthy person. It's the same with the social environment. When your attitudes and behaviors contribute to the health of your relationships, those relationships are able to help you be healthy too.

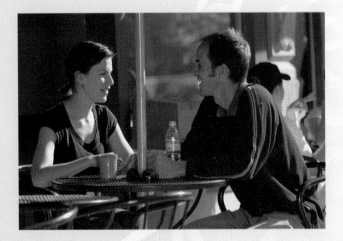

Emotional Wellness: Become an Effective Listener

It may seem peculiar, but experts in interpersonal communication agree that being a good listener is more important for healthy communication than being a good speaker. That's because by listening effectively, you can understand the speaker's thoughts and emotions, which both provides you with data about the speaker and tells the speaker that you are interested in what she or he has to say. Here's an example of not-so-effective listening:

Jim and Dee have been dating seriously for about six months. One day . . .

Jim says, "Wow. They just laid off my supervisor. All of us are worried that we're next."

Dee says, "Don't worry about it. You're a good employee. They'd never let you go."

"But if they do, I'm not sure what to do. All I see for my future is a blank movie screen."

"Maybe you shouldn't have turned down that teaching job. At least it was secure."

"But I didn't want to move that far away. And besides, teaching isn't really what I want."

"Maybe you should go to a career counselor. You're smart. You could do just about anything."

By this time Jim is probably muttering something like, "Oh, hell, what's the use?" A fight might even break out. Why? Because Dee is communicating to Jim that his anxiety is trivial, that he's a bad decision maker, and that he doesn't know how to run his life.

Dee is trying to be a good friend. But her attempts to help aren't working because she's not responding to Jim's feelings. Instead, she's controlling the conversation with advice, comments, and questions. She's trying to solve his problem when what he wants is to feel understood and supported.

This situation is extremely common. When someone shares a problem with us, we feel almost compelled to change the person's feelings, offer suggestions, point out mistakes—called constructive criticism—or minimize the severity of the situation. And when we're the source of the person's distress, we do all that and more: We offer excuses to defend ourselves, change the subject, withdraw from the conversation, or counter-attack, which moves the conversation onto the battlefield.

Being a good listener means being attentive, not only to what the person is saying, but more importantly, to what the person is feeling. When listening, think of yourself as a giant TV satellite dish. Your job is to take in as much data as you can: thoughts, feelings, body language. Resist the temptation to comment, fix, support, defend yourself, or attack. Just listen. And as you do, try to become the other person—to understand the reasons why she or he is feeling this way. Putting yourself in the other person's experience is called *empathy*.

Here is an exercise that can help you become an effective listener. Carry out Steps 1–4 with a close friend. Write a reaction to your experience in your journal by responding to the questions that follow.

Step One Ask your friend to tell you something that's important to her or him. The first time you do this, it's probably better to choose something that doesn't involve you personally or your relationship with the speaker so that you won't be tempted to react to what's said. Let the speaker talk for up to 5 minutes.

Step Two While the person is speaking, just listen, and notice any urges you have to stop paying attention or to interrupt with suggestions or comments. Notice where your attention goes, for example, if your mind drifts to other topics, or if you daydream. Notice whether you feel critical, or whether you have the urge to comment or advise.

Step Three When the speaker has finished, tell her or him what you experienced. Share with the speaker whether you were able to pay full attention to what was being said, whether you were bored, or whether your mind was busy with something else. If you're new at this, you'll probably notice that it's difficult simply to listen.

Step Four Do the exercise a second time with a different topic. This time, instead of telling the speaker your experience with listening, respond with a paraphrase of what was said, using an emotion word and a reason the speaker feels that emotion. "You seem *nervous* (emotion word) *about possibly not having a job in the future*" (reason for the emotion).

Once you've developed an awareness of how it feels to be an effective listener, with practice you'll become better at it, and those with whom you communicate—family, friends, lovers, and coworkers—will appreciate you greatly for it.

In your journal, respond to the following questions:

1. With whom did you carry out the listening exercise?
2. What topic did the speaker focus on in Step One?
3. What did you notice your mind doing while the speaker was talking (in Step One)?
4. What was the topic of the speaker's remarks in Step Four?
5. How well were you able to paraphrase (using an emotion word and summary) in Step Four? Write an example of your paraphrase.
6. What effect did this exercise have on your usual listening style?

Wise Consumer: Do Not Permit the Media to Determine Your Self-Image

Nearly everyone wants to be attractive, and many of us go to considerable lengths to attain our notions of personal attractiveness. After all, "looking good" makes us feel good about ourselves, and we believe that it increases our chances of finding romantic or sexual partners, and even getting a job.

Advertisers are masters at preying on our insecurities about our attractiveness. For example, many ads suggest that we are less attractive than we could be, and that by using the advertised product, our attractiveness and desirability will increase. Of course, this message is fundamental to advertising clothes, alcoholic beverages, and cosmetics, but it also appears in advertising for cars, travel, and even food.

A second way advertising preys on our fears of not being attractive is to show us images of models whose physical features are presented as perfect or ideal. Suggesting that we are physically imperfect because we look as we do is bad enough, but frequently the ads also suggest that because we do not look like the models in the ads, we are flawed as persons. This message is even more insidious when you consider that in real life, the models themselves rarely live up to their images.

Advertisers and media exist to make money; they are not in the business of promoting healthy persons and healthy relationships. Therefore, it is important not to accept any media message that you are flawed either physically or personally, or that you need their product.

Make a list of the cosmetics, health and beauty aids, or other products that you use to augment your physical appearance. After you've made your list, circle items that you bought because of an advertisement or because a friend recommended it.

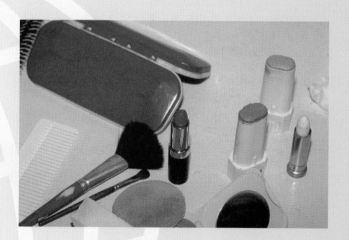

Then go over the list again and mark each item that you use on a regular basis and the reason for its use. Describe in your journal how the use of this product enhances your self-image and self-esteem.

Finally, go over the list one more time and cross out those items that you believe to be worthless or that you feel you do not really need. Describe in your journal the ways that you can improve your self-image or health without the use of advertised products.

Physical Activity: Couple's Walk-Talk

Many people complain that their lives are so busy that they don't have time to exercise and they don't have enough time for their personal relationships. Here's a two-for-the-price-of-one solution that may be the answer for you: the couple's walk-talk. Instead of taking the time to work out at a gym or in an exercise class by yourself, go for a run or take a walk with a special someone or close friend. Not only do you get your exercise, but you also create a time together for sharing feelings, dreams, and problems.

In your journal, keep a log of your walk-talks. Record what you talked about and notice any effects the activity has on feelings of togetherness and closeness in your relationship.

Managing Stress: Being Sexually Responsible

Sexually active college students probably never want to be involved in an unintentional pregnancy or test positive for a sexually transmitted disease, especially AIDS. Usually, college students focus on getting through school and not becoming parents. So an unintentional pregnancy, with the prospect of a massive and unanticipated life change, can be extremely distressing, even terrifying. Even the decision to get an abortion can be emotionally difficult. Acquiring AIDS, of course, may be one of the most distressing and terrifying experiences of all. Even acquiring a non-life-threatening STI is likely to produce a high degree of guilt and stress.

Studies show that almost all college students know the importance of using birth control and practicing safer sex. The same studies indicate, however, that knowledge of birth control and safer sex practices does not always translate into responsible sexual practices. While acknowledging that risks exist in general, students frequently deny that any undesired conse-

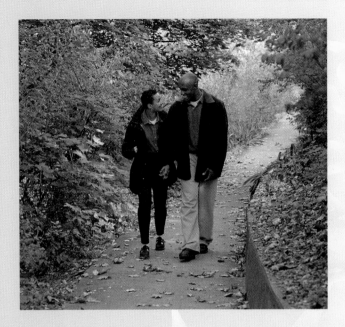

quences of sexual activity can happen to them personally, or they engage in sexual activity while intoxicated with drugs or alcohol and do not take precautions.

You can prevent a lot of stress in your life and the lives of your family and others by focusing your attention on being sexually responsible. To help you do that, imagine yourself being involved in an unintentional pregnancy or acquiring a genital herpes infection. In your journal, write how you would experience each situation.

For the unintentional pregnancy, imagine receiving the news that your pregnancy test is positive. How would you feel? How would you react? Imagine what you would say to your parents, or if you chose not to tell them, what would it be like for you to keep the secret? What would you do about the pregnancy? How do you feel about becoming a parent? Would you consider having an abortion? What effect would the pregnancy or parenthood have on your academic progress? How would the pregnancy affect your relationship with the other involved person? How would the pregnancy affect your future intimate relationships?

For the diagnosis of genital herpes, how would you feel about yourself? Your partner? How are you going to manage your future sexual relationships, knowing that herpes is a lifetime infection that can be transmitted to sexual partners?

Considering your reactions to these imaginary events in detail in your journal may help you to be sexually responsible in the future.

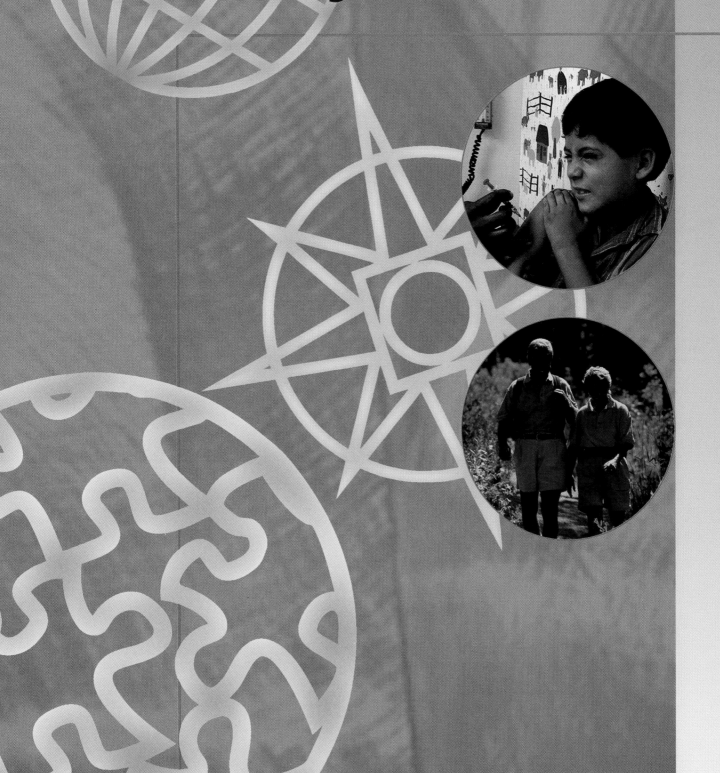

Part 4

Understanding and Preventing Disease

Learning Objectives

1. Define pathogen, communicable disease, vector, immunizations, opportunistic infections, nosocomial disease, immune system, antibodies, antigens, and autoimmune diseases.
2. Identify and explain how infectious diseases are prevented and treated.
3. Discuss the importance of antibiotics with regard to bacterial infections and the implications of antibiotic-resistant strains of bacteria.
4. Discuss how immunizations prevent infections.
5. Discuss the etiology, symptoms, and treatments for cold and flu.
6. Explain how antibodies battle infectious diseases.
7. Describe how unwanted activities of the immune system cause allergies.
8. Discuss organ transplants, blood transfusions, and the Rh factor.
9. Describe how HIV causes AIDS.

Exercises and Activities

WORKBOOK
Are You Current on All Your Vaccines?

Health and Wellness Online

 www.jbpub.com/hwonline

Wellness Guide: Are the Hamburgers Safe? Maybe Yes, Maybe No
Wellness Guide: A Cure for Asthma

Chapter 9

Reducing Infections and Building Immunity: Knowledge Encourages Prevention

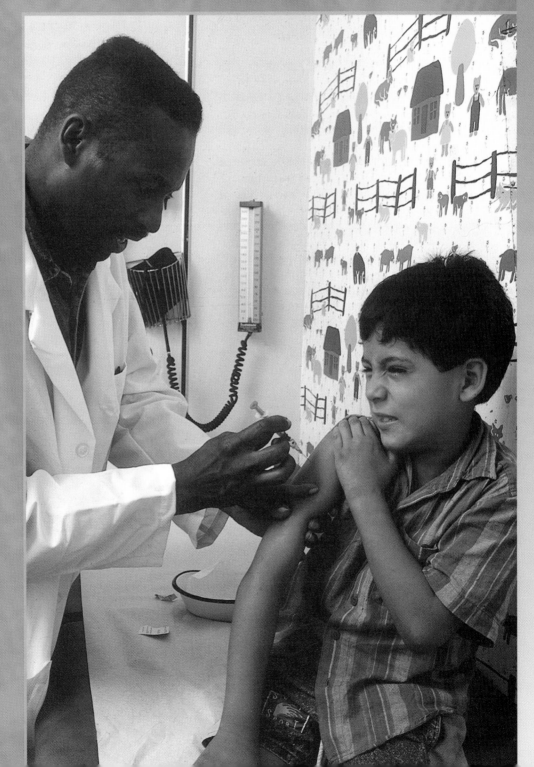

In past centuries, hundreds of millions of people died from infectious diseases caused by bacteria, viruses, protozoa, and other microorganisms. In this century, improvements in public sanitation, personal hygiene, nutrition, and immunizations have drastically reduced the amount of sickness and number of deaths from infectious diseases. However, infectious diseases such as malaria, tuberculosis, and cholera, still cause millions of deaths each year, primarily in poor, underdeveloped countries. Poverty and undernutrition create conditions that foster the spread and lethality of infectious diseases. Globally, infectious disease is still the single most common cause of death. In 1993, it was estimated that more than 16 million people died from infectious diseases caused by microorganisms (Fineberg and Wilson, 1996).

Bacterial contamination of beef, chicken, ice cream, and other foods has caused serious disease in the U.S. in recent years. And in many countries, thousands of people are infected every year by bacteria in their food that makes them seriously sick. Concern is growing in the U.S. over the safety of meat, dairy, and other foods (Tauxe, 1997).

A healthy body has a functionally active immune system that is able to cope with most infections. A nutritious diet, regular exercise, and low levels of stress are vital elements to maintaining a healthy immune system that can help ward off infections. However, even the healthiest person is exposed to microorganisms that may cause an infectious disease. We all have occasional colds, flu, or stomach upsets that are caused by viruses. Usually these infections are self-limiting, and we become well in a few days or weeks. Other infectious diseases such as pneumonia, tuberculosis, or "staph" infections are caused by bacteria that can be destroyed with antibiotics. However, there is growing concern over the upsurge in disease-causing bacteria that are resistant to many antibiotics.

Understanding how infectious microorganisms cause disease and how your immune system battles infections is essential for maintaining wellness and for recovering from an infectious disease.

Infectious Microorganisms

Not all microorganisms are harmful when they are present in or on the body. In fact, bacteria perform many essential functions in many parts of the body, but there are also areas of the body that must remain sterile (Table 9.1). If normally sterile areas of the body become infected by microorganisms, an infectious disease results. Any microorganism that infects the body and causes disease is called a **pathogen.**

TABLE 9.1   Bacteria in the Body
Some areas of the body harbor millions of bacteria, most of which are beneficial; other areas of the body are sterile.

Sterile Body Areas

Respiratory tract (below the vocal chords)

Sinuses and *middle ear*

Liver and *gall bladder*

Urinary tract above the urethra

Bones, joints, muscles, and *blood*

Cerebrospinal fluid (the brain and spinal column)

The *linings around the lungs* (pleura) and *abdominal cavity* (peritoneum)

Body Areas that are Colonized with Bacteria

Skin: Contains thousands of bacteria per square centimeter and some fungi. The microorganisms are beneficial or harmless unless the skin is damaged or a person is already sick.

Nasopharynx and oropharynx: May contain billions of bacteria per milliliter of fluid, including pathogenic bacteria that can cause pneumonia or influenza. These pathogens cause disease only in people whose immune systems are weak.

Esophagus and stomach: Thousands of bacteria are ingested with food. Most people have been infected with *Helicobacter pylori* but do not have any symptoms of ulcers.

Small intestine: Low concentration of bacteria; one of the more common ones is *Lactobacillus* species.

Large intestine: Billions of bacteria per milliliter of fluid are present; almost all anaerobic species (bacteria that only grow in the absence of oxygen). All fecal matter contains billions of bacteria.

Vagina: Contains millions of bacteria including *Lactobacillus* species and *Escherichia coli* as well as other anaerobic bacteria.

Recognizing Agents of Infectious Disease

A remarkable variety of microorganisms, including bacteria, viruses, protozoa, yeast, and small worms, can infect cells in the human body and cause disease and sickness (Figure 9.1). Viruses are not alive in the same sense that a bacterium is; all microorganisms except viruses are cells that can grow and reproduce on their own. Viruses only grow and reproduce after they infect a cell and usurp the cellular machinery to make more viruses. Some common human diseases caused by viruses are colds, flu, polio, hepatitis, chicken pox, mumps, measles, herpes and AIDS. Each of the viruses that cause these diseases is different and infects a specific tissue or organ in the body.

Other infectious diseases, such as pneumonia, tuberculosis, cholera, plague, typhoid fever, and gonorrhea, are caused by specific pathogenic bacteria. Often pathogenic bacteria and viruses cause disease only if the individual is already in a weakened state, particularly if the immune system is not functioning optimally.

If an infectious disease is shown to be caused by a specific microorganism, that cause is called its **etiology.** For example, tuberculosis usually is caused by a

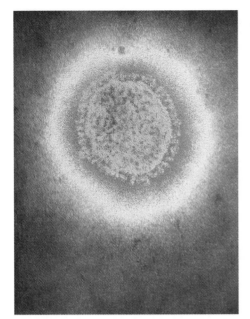
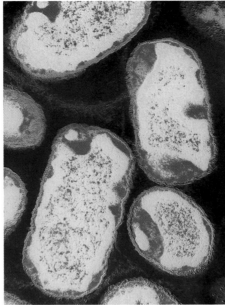

FIGURE 9.1   Infectious Organisms

Electron micrographs of (left) an influenza virus that causes flu and (right) *Salmonella* bacteria that cause food poisoning. Both the "flu" virus and the bacteria are easily passed from person to person and cause widespread epidemics.

specific bacterium called *Mycobacterium tuberculosis;* infectious mononucleosis is caused by the Epstein-Barr virus; and giardiasis (an infection of the small intestine) is caused by the protozoan *Giardia lambia.*

Infectious agents enter the body in a variety of ways. If the infectious organism is usually passed from person to person, the disease is called a **communicable disease.** Colds, measles, chicken pox, and gonorrhea are all communicable diseases. Infectious organisms also can be transferred to people from other animals, especially insects. In these instances the animal or insect is said to be the **vector,** or carrier, of the disease-causing microorganism. For example, **malaria** is usually caused by a microscopic protozoan called *Plasmodium falciparum.* When a person with malaria is bitten by a mosquito, blood (and the parasite) is taken up by the mosquito and injected into another person by a bite from the same mosquito. Thus, mosquitoes are the vectors for malaria. (Only a few species of mosquitoes carry the malarial parasite.)

Terms

pathogen: a disease-causing organism

etiology: specific cause of disease

communicable disease: an infectious disease that is usually transmitted from person to person

vector: the carrier of infectious organisms from animals to people or from person to person

malaria: a disease of red blood cells that produces fever, anemia, and death

Rabies is a disease of the nervous system caused by the rabies virus present in infected dogs, cats, bats, skunks, and other animals. The infected animals are the vectors for rabies, and the virus is transmitted in the saliva of the rabid animal.

While infectious diseases are usually ascribed to a specific etiologic agent as described above, in reality most infectious diseases do not have only one cause. Whether or not a person gets an infectious disease depends on a wide range of factors, including the competence of the immune system, nutritional status, the

> *It is more important to know what sort of patient has a disease than what sort of disease a patient has.*
>
> SIR WILLIAM OSLER, M.D.
> (1849–1919)

presence of other diseases, and environmental conditions (Figure 9.2). For example, many people are exposed to bacteria that can cause pneumonia. However, pneumonia usually develops in very old people whose immune systems are weak or in younger people who are susceptible to infections, such as AIDS patients. Some people are more resistant to infectious organisms than others because of genes that they inherited.

Resistance to infection also is increased by previous exposure to a similar virus; for example, a person generally is not infected by the same strain of cold virus in succession. Resistance to infection can be reduced by stress, poor nutrition, or infection by other viruses.

Tuberculosis (TB) is not simply caused by infection with the bacterium *Mycobacterium tuberculosis.* Robert Koch, a famous nineteenth-century microbiologist, called TB the "disease of poverty" because it was associated with squalor, overcrowding, poor nutrition,

FIGURE 9.2   Various internal and external factors determine if disease will result from infections by viruses, bacteria, and other kinds of infectious agents.

Internal

Age
Sex
Immunological competence
Previous infections
Hormonal status
Presence of other diseases
Nutritional status
Emotional stress level
Heredity

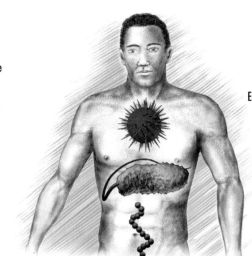

External

Infections in the community
Season of the year
Hygiene and sanitation
Drugs and medications
Environmental pollutants or toxins

and poor sanitation. Today many people have small tubercular lesions in their lungs, but have no symptoms of disease because they enjoy good nutrition, good living conditions, and are in good general health. However, in some urban areas where people live in squalor and poverty, TB is once again emerging as a communicable infectious disease.

In many areas of the globe, millions of people still die from infectious diseases (Table 9.2). Various kinds of worms (roundworm, pinworm, hookworm, and tapeworm) infect at least a billion people worldwide. Another 200 million people are debilitated by the waterborne parasite that causes the disease schistosomiasis.

TABLE 9.2   Estimated Deaths Worldwide from Infectious Diseases*

Cause of death	Estimated number
Acute respiratory infections	6,900,000
Diarrheal diseases	4,200,000
Tuberculosis	3,300,000
Malaria	1,000,000–2,000,000
Hepatitis	1,000,000–2,000,000
Measles	220,000
Meningitis, bacterial	200,000
Schistosomiasis (parasitic tropical disease)	200,000
Pertussis (whooping cough)	100,000
Amoebiasis (parasitic infection)	40,000–60,000
Hookworm (parasitic infection)	50,000–60,000
Rabies	35,000
Yellow fever (epidemic)	30,000
African trypanosomiasis (sleeping sickness)	20,000 or more

*Source: World Health Organization.

Malarial parasites still infect as many as 300 million people each year and cause at least a million deaths annually in Africa. Surveys show that about a billion children in Asia, Africa, and Latin America contract severe diarrhea caused by infectious organisms, and about 4 million children die from diarrhea each year in these areas. Many countries lack the resources to ensure safe water supplies, public sanitation, safe waste disposal, and adequate health care—factors that can control the spread of most infectious diseases.

Emerging Infectious Diseases

Several factors are contributing to the emergence of new infectious diseases in industrialized countries; some new infectious agents have the potential to cause serious illness and epidemics. Global travel by infected persons is a major factor in spreading viruses and bacteria.

People who move from remote villages in Africa, Asia, or other areas of the world to cities may carry infectious microorganisms with them that previously did not exist in the urban areas. Because of the close physical contact of people in cities, the infectious microorganisms may spread to persons who do not have any resistance to them. Many pathogens also can become established in insect, rodent, or other animal populations and then spread to other areas of the world. In past centuries, smallpox and measles wiped out millions of native North and South Americans when their countries were visited or invaded by Europeans who carried these infectious diseases with them.

Destruction of ecosystems and forest environments contributes to the spread of microorganisms. The building of giant dams, deforestation of large areas of land, poor water quality, and an increase in urbanization, which is occurring around the world, upset the balance of nature and encourage the spread of pathogens (Guenno, 1995).

Promiscuous human sexual activity, along with the increased use of injected drugs, around the world are largely responsible for AIDS and hepatitis B epidemics. Because so many factors contribute to the emergence of these infectious diseases, the diseases are likely to become more prevalent in the future (Morse, 1996). As with all areas of health, avoidance of high-risk behaviors can help protect you from contracting one of these diseases.

Fighting Infectious Diseases

Infectious diseases are fought in four ways: sanitation, treatment with antibiotics and other drugs, vaccinations, and healthful living. Stopping the spread of infectious organisms requires that they be destroyed in infected people, in the environment, or in both.

Scientific understanding of the causes of infectious diseases first began in the late nineteenth century with the research of the French scientist Louis Pasteur, who established the "germ" theory of disease by showing that microscopic organisms could cause infections and disease. Pasteur discovered that these microorganisms could be rendered harmless by heat or by treatment with antiseptic chemicals. Like many radically new scientific ideas, Pasteur's discoveries were ignored at first.

The use of antiseptic (sterile) techniques to reduce the number of infections and deaths after surgery was adopted slowly in the United States, despite the fact that a famous American physician, Joseph Lister, had successfully implemented Pasteur's advice in his hospital. (The antiseptic mouthwash Listerine is named in his honor.) Before antiseptic techniques were introduced in hospitals, surgery or giving childbirth in a hospital often led to death from subsequent infection.

Sanitation, sterile techniques, and public health programs were not actively implemented in the United States until the beginning of the twentieth century. Only then did the incidence of many infectious diseases, such as tuberculosis, plague, pneumonia, and diphtheria, begin to decline dramatically. Many medical historians argue that sanitation is the most significant medical advance of all time because it contributed to preventing millions of cases of infectious disease caused by contaminated water and food.

Understanding Antibiotics

In the late 1940s another highly effective tool was discovered for combatting infectious diseases caused by bacteria. The antibiotic **penicillin,** which is produced by a species of mold, was able to cure many kinds of bacterial infections. Today hundreds of antibiotic drugs

are available for treating infectious diseases caused by bacteria, yeast, worms, and other microorganisms, except for viruses. When antibiotics were first discovered they were greeted as wonder drugs capable of curing some of the most deadly infectious diseases, such as plague, tuberculosis, pneumonia, syphilis, and a slew of less serious diseases. Indeed, antibiotics have been exceptionally useful drugs over the past 50 years, but we are now witnessing a decline in their general effectiveness. One of the primary reasons is that many pathogenic bacteria have acquired new genes that make them resistant to one or several of the most common antibiotics (Gold and Moellering, 1996).

Antibiotics block essential biochemical reactions of microorganisms that infect the body, thereby preventing them from growing. The most useful antibiotics selectively interfere with the growth of bacteria without affecting the functions of body cells. Antibiotics kill both harmful and helpful bacteria in the body; however, once the harmful bacteria have been killed, the helpful bacteria quickly repopulate their normal sites.

> Life doesn't cease to be funny when people die anymore than it ceases to be serious when people laugh.
>
> GEORGE BERNARD SHAW, playwright

However, antibiotics do not destroy viruses because viruses are not living cells. Viruses infect and take over the cellular functions of body cells, thus ensuring their own growth and propagation. Finding a drug that will specifically kill a virus but not also kill body cells is very difficult.

Within a few years of the discovery of penicillin, penicillin-resistant bacteria began appearing in patients treated for bacterial infections. Bacteria also acquired resistance to later antibiotics, such as tetracycline, erythromycin, and chloramphenicol. Antibiotic resistance can be transferred among bacteria in nature in a small piece of genetic material (**DNA**) that carries antibiotic-resistance genes. Harmless bacteria of one species can transfer antibiotic-resistance genes to many other species of bacteria, including ones that cause disease. In this way bacteria that cause gonorrhea, pneumonia, tuberculosis and "staph" infections have become resistant to many previously effective antibiotics (Levy, 1998).

Terms

penicillin: an antibiotic produced by mold and capable of curing many bacterial infections

DNA (deoxyribonucleic acid): a chemical substance in chromosomes that carries genetic information

For example, vancomycin is the only effective antibiotic for treating deadly bacterial infections of the circulatory system and surgical wounds. Since 1988, vancomycin-resistant bacteria have been increasing in patients with these infections; consequently, some patients die because the antibiotic is no longer effective. The antibiotics rifampin and isoniazid had been very effective in treating TB, but now these drugs are sometimes ineffective because the TB bacteria have acquired multiple antibiotic resistance.

New antibiotics are constantly being developed, but nature is never far behind in the selection of resistant strains of bacteria. For example, millions of tons of antibiotics have been released into the environment as a result of their use in animal feed. The antibiotics in soil and water encourage the selection of resistant strains of bacteria that normally grow in soil and water. Only increased caution in the use of antibiotics will permit them to remain "wonder drugs" (Swartz, 1997).

How the Body Protects Itself

The best way to avoid infectious diseases caused by pathogenic microorganisms is to keep them out of the body. The skin and mucous membranes prevent the entry of most microorganisms into the body by functioning as physical barriers. That is why a wound often exposes the body to infection (Figure 9.3). The skin is mildly acidic and provides a poor habitat for most harmful microorganisms, although the skin is covered with beneficial bacteria.

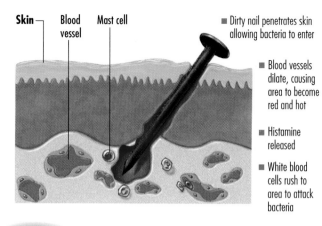

Skin — Blood vessel — Mast cell

- Dirty nail penetrates skin allowing bacteria to enter
- Blood vessels dilate, causing area to become red and hot
- Histamine released
- White blood cells rush to area to attack bacteria

FIGURE 9.3 **Inflammation Response** Penetration of the skin by any unsterile sharp object often produces an inflammation response, the normal response of the body to injury or infection.

The eyes, nose, throat, and breathing passages are protected by mucous membranes that continuously produce secretions that flush away harmful organisms and particles. Mucous membranes also secrete enzymes that can destroy toxic substances. The mouth, digestive system, and excretory organs also are protected by membranes that guard the internal organs.

Tears keep the surface of the eyes moist and serve to wash away foreign particles. Wax secreted from the ears protects the delicate hearing apparatus. The mucus coating of the respiratory tract is sticky and provides a trap for irritating particles and microorganisms in the air; microscopic hairs called **cilia** keep the mucus moving out of the bronchial tubes.

Wellness Guide

Sepsis Syndrome: A Cause of Death in Hospitals

We rightly regard our hospitals as places for emergency help, for surgery to repair broken and diseased body parts, and for help in healing when we become seriously ill. We don't usually regard admission to a hospital as being dangerous in its own right. However, approximately 1 out of every 50 patients admitted to a hospital will die of **sepsis syndrome** (also called septicemia or bacteremia). Sepsis syndrome refers to a bacterial infection of the blood that spreads infection throughout the body and often causes death from organ failure (Sands, 1997). Most often, the bacterial infection is acquired in the hospital as a result of some invasive test procedure.

Slightly more than half of the people who die from sepsis syndrome are in intensive care units (ICUs) and were admitted to the hospital in a critical condition, although most of them did not have the infection before admission. However, about one third of patients who die from sepsis syndrome are not in ICUs and did not have a blood infection on admission.

What causes sepsis syndrome? Any invasive procedure, from a simple injection to a catheterization, carries with it a certain risk of infection if the instrument inserted into the body is not sterile, if the wound is not cared for, or if the catheter is not replaced every few days. The rate of

sepsis syndrome in hospitals seems to be increasing with advances in medical technology and as the bacteria found in hospitals become increasingly resistant to antibiotics.

The message for any patient who is *not* admitted to a hospital in critical condition (e.g., after a heart attack) is to be sure that any recommended invasive procedure is absolutely necessary before giving consent. Also discuss the risk of infection for the recommended procedure in that hospital with your physician, because the frequency of hospital-acquired infections varies considerably among hospitals.

Managing Stress

Humor and Relaxation Are as Good as Anything for a Cold

Virtually everybody catches a cold sometime or other. Schoolchildren may contract as many as a dozen different colds a year. It is estimated that 100 million serious colds occur each year in the United States, causing 30 million days lost at school and work.

In 1914 a German scientist, W. Von Kause, first proposed that colds are caused by viruses. However, an actual cold virus (adenovirus R-167) wasn't isolated until 1953. Finally, in 1985, a detailed x-ray picture of a cold virus was obtained. Six major classes of cold viruses — rhinoviruses, coronaviruses, adenoviruses, myxoviruses, paramyxoviruses, and coxsackieviruses — have been identified. And within the rhinovirus class alone, more than 120 different strains have been observed. Scientists hope to find some common feature shared by the different cold viruses so that a single vaccine can

be developed, but this is still just a remote possibility.

Here is a brief history of research on the common cold. It shows what science can accomplish.

- **1930s:** Scientists announce that colds are contagious and are caught by shaking hands. Recommended treatment is aspirin, fluids, and rest.
- **1940s:** Scientists announce that taking hot baths followed by cold showers, eliminating wheat from the diet, and eating fruits and vegetables help develop immunity to colds.
- **1950s:** Scientists announce that a low-sugar, low-starch diet prevents colds. Bioflavenoids are the rage as cold remedies. Vitamin C is declared worthless. Development of a cold vaccine is predicted within 2 years.

- **1960s:** Scientists declare war on the common cold. They announce that a salt-free diet prevents colds. They also discover that more women than men catch colds.
- **1970s:** Linus Pauling, a Nobel prize winner, declares that massive doses of vitamin C prevent colds. The National Institutes of Health announce they have given up hope of finding a cure for the common cold.
- **1980s:** Fifty years after the first such announcement scientists announce that colds are spread by hand contact. They recommend aspirin, fluids, and rest if you catch a cold and not shaking hands with someone who has a cold.
- **1990s:** Gesundheit! Scientists recommend chicken soup.

Coughing and spitting are mechanisms that remove foreign material from the breathing passages. Sneezing and blowing the nose eliminate irritating particles that are inhaled.

Cells and enzymes in the blood quickly form clots that seal off any break in the skin, thereby preventing the entry of harmful substances and infectious organisms. If some bacteria do enter the wound before it is sealed off, other special cells that are part of the immune system attack and destroy the invaders.

If microorganisms or foreign particles penetrate the skin and enter the blood, they soon encounter specialized cells called **leukocytes,** the colorless white blood cells that can be distinguished from the red blood cells that transport oxygen. Only about 1 in 700 cells in the blood is a leukocyte, but their number can increase dramatically if an acute infection occurs. That is why blood is tested for the number of white blood cells when an infection is suspected.

Specialized white blood cells called **macrophages** are associated with specific organs and are vital to the body's internal defense mechanisms. Macrophages are able to engulf and digest foreign cells and particles that invade the body. Organ-specific macrophages protect the lungs, stomach, and other organs from damage by foreign substances.

Common Infectious Diseases

Some infectious diseases, such as AIDS and Lyme disease, have received more-than-average public attention and press coverage. Colds and flu are so common that almost everyone gets one or more infections each year. Infectious diseases, depending on their cause and consequences, present special public health problems and personal concerns for many people.

Colds and Flu

Most people especially children, contract several colds and flu every year. Both diseases are caused by viruses that infect cells of the respiratory tract. Colds are caused by more than 200 different species and strains

Terms

cilia: microscopic hairs in the lining of the bronchial tubes

sepsis syndrome: bacterial infection of the blood; may be fatal

leukocytes: white blood cells that fight infections

macrophages: specialized cells that destroy and eliminate foreign particles and microorganisms from the body

of viruses. A cold caused by one virus does not protect a person from catching a cold caused by a different one, which explains why colds can occur one after another or several times a year.

While cold symptoms may be quite discomfiting, colds generally do not result in long-term illness or death. Billions of dollars are spent by Americans every year on medications that are supposed to alleviate cold symptoms, such as sore throat, cough, congestion, runny nose, and pain. Physicians joke that a cold will go away in about a week with rest and medications or in about 7 days if nothing is done. It takes the immune system about a week to produce the specific proteins that inactivate the viruses and help tissues to heal.

Influenza, or flu, is caused by a different kind of virus than the ones that cause colds. Flu is a much more serious disease. The symptoms of flu are body aches, high fever, loss of appetite, and other complications that may result from the infection. Infections of the respiratory system by a flu virus can so weaken people that they contract pneumonia, a bacterial infection, and die.

There are many different strains of flu virus and new strains arise continually. Because flu is so debilitating and serious, vaccines are prepared each year. Scientists have to guess which flu strain will be the cause of the next epidemic, because it takes about a year to prepare and distribute the vaccine. In some years, flu vaccine is quite effective, but in others, it is not effective at all because it was prepared with the wrong strains of the virus. People with respiratory problems such as asthma, people with immune system deficiencies, or the elderly are advised to get a flu shot each year to help prevent infection.

Never catching a cold or flu is probably impossible in modern society. However, certain precautions can help reduce the risk. During seasons when colds and flu are present, try to stay away from crowds as much as possible. The viruses are easily transmitted in droplets from people who are coughing or sneezing. Being in a classroom, theater, bus, or any crowded place increases the risk of being infected. The viruses also are easily transmitted by bodily contact, such as shaking hands with someone with a cold who has recently wiped his or her nose or mouth. So it's a good idea to wash your hands frequently during cold and flu season.

Mononucleosis

Mononucleosis (also called mono) is an infectious disease common in young adults, especially those in college or living in crowded, unsanitary conditions. The disease is caused by infection by the Epstein-Barr virus (EBV), which is ubiquitous in human populations. About half of all children in the United States become infected with EBV by age 5; in most of these children, the infection goes unnoticed since it causes few or no symptoms. Once a person has been infected with EBV, it remains in the body for life without necessarily causing any disease symptoms. A number of other viruses also can become permanent residents in the body (Table 9.3).

Periodically, infected people shed the virus, primarily in secretions of the nose and mouth. The virus is very contagious and if saliva is shared between an infected and uninfected person, transmission of EBV occurs. This is why mononucleosis is described as the "kissing disease."

Infection by EBV as a child provides protection against infection as an adult because of the immunity that develops. However, infection by EBV as a young adult usually produces mononucleosis, a disease characterized by fatigue, fever, and swollen lymph nodes. There is no specific treatment for mononucleosis except rest, and most symptoms usually disappear within 2 weeks. Persons recovering from mononucleosis, however, should refrain from sports activities and weightlifting for at least 2 months because of the

---

TABLE 9.3   Viruses that Remain in the Body for Life After Infection

Virus	Symptoms	Spread by	Remains in
Herpes simplex I	Cold sores on lips or in mouth	Direct contact; most infectious when lesions are present	Nerve cells
Herpes simplex II	Painful blisters on genital organs	Direct contact; oral-genital sex can transmit type I or II to mouth or genital area	Nerve cells
Cytomegalovirus (CMV)	No symptoms in most children and adults; CMV can cause stillbirth and mental retardation in fetuses	Body fluids: blood, urine, saliva	White blood cells
Varicella zoster virus	Chicken pox in children; shingles in adults	Person to person	Nerve cells
Epstein-Barr virus (EBV)	Mononucleosis	Saliva (kissing)	Lymph glands
Human immunodeficiency virus (HIV)	From none to full symptoms of AIDS	Sexual intercourse (homosexual or heterosexual), blood transfusions, contaminated needles of injection drug users, mother-to-child transmission before or after birth	T-cells of the immune system and other body cells

risk of rupturing the spleen. In a very few cases (less than 1%), mononucleosis can precipitate more serious diseases. Once people have had mononucleosis, they are immune to subsequent infections by EBV.

Hepatitis

Serious infections of the liver can result from at least five different **hepatitis viruses.** Hepatitis A and hepatitis E are spread primarily by fecal-oral transmission and cause a relatively mild liver disease. Not washing the hands after going to the toilet and subsequently handling food is the primary route of transmitting these two viruses. If one person in a household has hepatitis A, others also are likely to get the infection. Symptoms may include jaundice (yellowing of the eyes), stomach pains, and diarrhea.

Infection by hepatitis B, hepatitis C, or hepatitis D causes persistent liver infection, chronic hepatitis, and eventually may lead to fatal liver cancer. About 16,000 persons die of hepatitis-associated liver cancer each year in the United States. Hepatitis C and a newly discovered hepatitis G are commonly acquired during a blood transfusion or by injected drug use, and the ensuing liver disease may go undetected for many years (Fackelmann, 1996).

Fortunately, effective vaccines are now available for both hepatitis A and hepatitis B (Lemon and Thomas, 1997). It is recommended that everyone, especially young children, be immunized with hepatitis B vaccine, because of the seriousness of the infection and the ensuing chronic liver disease. People at risk for hepatitis A infection, particularly those traveling to South America, Asia, or Africa where hepatitis A is prevalent, should also be vaccinated for hepatitis A.

Finally, there was the golfer in Ireland who came down with a case of nonviral hepatitis. It turned out that he licked his golf balls to clean them up before teeing off and was poisoned by a herbicide used on the golf course. The weed killers that he ingested each time he licked his ball damaged his liver to the point that he developed hepatitis. Weed killers (especially the amounts used on golf courses) can be toxic.

Hospital-Acquired Infections

We usually regard the hospital as a safe, sterile environment. Unfortunately, the modern hospital has become a place that sometimes endangers the health of patients, because it is a source of serious infectious diseases. About 5% of hospital patients in this country contract an infectious disease while hospitalized for an unrelated problem. These infections are called

Terms

mononucleosis: an infectious disease caused by the Epstein-Barr virus, common among college-age adults

hepatitis viruses: viruses that infect the liver

Wellness Guide

Are the Hamburgers Safe? Maybe Yes, Maybe No

The United States has an enviable record for the safety of its meat products, but bacteria are gaining ground. A particular strain of *Escherichia coli* bacteria (0157:H7), now found worldwide, causes serious outbreaks of disease when people eat food contaminated with it. In 1997, 25 million pounds of frozen hamburger were destroyed in the U.S. when a large meat processing plant was found to be contaminated with *E. coli* 0157:H7 (Morganthau, 1997). In 1996, more than 9,000 persons, most of whom were children, were infected with *E. coli* 0157:H7 in Japan.

The symptoms of infection by this pathogen include acute diarrhea and blood infections (Greenwald and Brandt, 1997). The bacteria release a toxin that causes the symptoms; killing the bacteria with antibiotics does not destroy the toxin which, once released, circulates in the blood. (Thoroughly cooking meat destroys both bacteria and toxins.)

The public health problem associated with *E. coli* 0157:H7 infection was recognized in the 1980s and has increased in magnitude ever since. The bacteria are usually found in beef products but occur in poultry, pork, lamb, and other meat and dairy products as well. The bacteria can also be passed from person to person. Some people have stopped eating meat, especially hamburgers, because of fear of infection. In 1998, TV talk-show personality Oprah Winfrey was acquitted by a jury in Texas on the charge of libeling the Texas meat industry. She had said on her TV show that she would not eat hamburgers again because of the risk of "mad cow" disease. The Texas meat industry claimed that they lost millions of dollars in beef sales because of her comment.

Sensitive tests for detecting bacterial contaminants in foods are being developed. Also, meat products may undergo some form of sterilization in the future (possible by gamma irradiation) to ensure that the meat is absolutely free of microbial contamination.

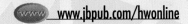 **www.jbpub.com/hwonline**

nosocomial diseases. Each year, approximately 7.5 million Americans undergo bladder catheterization in hospitals because they are immobilized. About a half million of these patients develop serious bacterial urinary tract infections, and some patients die from the hospital-acquired infections. Nosocomial diseases also prolong the patient's stay in the hospital and require extra treatment.

The two bacteria mainly responsible for nosocomial diseases are *Escherichia coli* and *Staphylococus aureus.* These bacteria normally are present in healthy individuals and usually do not cause disease. In hospital patients, however, similar, but different, strains of bacteria may invade other tissues and cause an infectious disease. Because hospitals use large quantities of antibiotics, bacteria that grow in hospitals are often resistant to the antibiotics. Thus, nosocomial diseases are difficult to treat.

The Immune System Battles Infections

The world teems with infectious viruses, bacteria, and other microorganisms that can cause disease if they invade the body. Most people stay well most of the time because the body contains a remarkable array of defense mechanisms that help keep disease-causing microorganisms out or that can destroy them if they invade the body. We only occasionally have an infectious disease because the **immune system** acts to protect the body from infectious organisms and foreign substances.

The immune system takes time to develop. At birth, a baby is protected from infectious diseases by antibodies that were present in the mother's blood and passed on to the newborn. **Antibodies** are proteins that recognize and inactivate viruses, bacteria, and harmful substances that can cause disease. Babies also receive antibodies in breast milk, which helps to protect them while their own immune systems mature during the first year or so of life.

Many factors can adversely affect the development and functioning of the immune system. Perhaps the most important factor is poor nutrition, especially early in life. Without a healthy diet, a child is extremely susceptible to infections that a weak immune system cannot fight. Inadequate nutrition and starvation are the principal reasons that children die in many undeveloped and impoverished countries of the world. Other factors that affect the development or functions of the immune system are hereditary disorders, viral infections, stress, and many drugs and chemicals, including alcohol and tobacco.

The Lymphatic System

The immune system, which is part of a larger and more complex system called the **lymphatic system,** has many organs and cells that must act in concert to protect people from infectious diseases (Figure 9.4). The lymphatic vessels contain fluid called lymph. At

Managing Stress

Chi—The Life Force

In the Western culture, there are several classifications of diseases: the two most predominant are infectious diseases and life-style diseases. In Chinese culture, diseases are grouped into one category: energy disease. Unlike Westerners, who view health as the absence of diseases and illness, the Chinese view health as an unrestricted current of subtle energy throughout the body.

According to the Chinese philosophy, there is a life force of subtle energy that surrounds and permeates us all. The Chinese people call this force "chi." To harmonize with the universe, to move in unison with this energy, to move as freely as running water, is to be at peace with the universe. This harmony promotes tranquillity and inner peace.

The study of mind-body-spirit medicine already indicates that stress management techniques strengthen our immune systems and inhibit the predisposition to infectious disease.

The following relaxation technique may help you to calm yourself and possibly strengthen your immune system.

Breathing Clouds

Breathing clouds is a meditation that serves as a cleansing process for the mind and body. To begin, close your eyes and focus all your attention on your breathing. Visualize the air you breathe as being clean, pure, and full of vitalizing energy. As you breathe in this clean, pure, air, visualize and feel air enter your nose (or mouth) and travel down your spine and circulate throughout your entire body. Now, as you exhale, visualize the air leaving your body carrying with it all the body's stress and frustrations in the form of a cloud of vapor. With each breath, allow the clean, pure air to clear your mind and rejuvenate your body. Repeat this breathing cycle for 5 to 10 minutes. As you repeat this cycle of breathing in pure air and breathing out polluted air filled with undesired feelings and toxins from the body, you should notice your body and mind becoming more relaxed and comfortable.

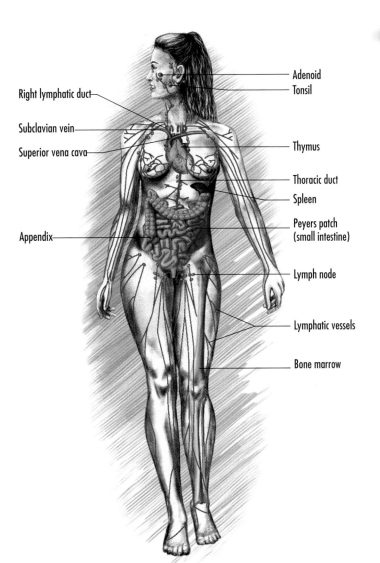

FIGURE 9.4   The Lymphatic System
Bone marrow, lymph nodes, and other organs of the immune system are shown. The lymphatic system performs many functions in protecting the body from infectious diseases.

Adenoid
Tonsil
Right lymphatic duct
Subclavian vein
Superior vena cava
Thymus
Thoracic duct
Spleen
Peyers patch (small intestine)
Appendix
Lymph node
Lymphatic vessels
Bone marrow

various intervals along the lymphatic vessels are nodules called **lymph nodes.** The "swollen glands" that people experience in the neck, under the arms, in the groin, or in other areas of the body are due to enlarged lymph nodes that are engaged in filtering out infectious organisms or foreign particles capable of causing disease. Thus, swollen and sore lymph nodes are a sign that the body is fighting an infection.

Bone marrow, tonsils, adenoids, spleen, and thymus all produce cells that allow the body to mount an immune response against infectious microorganisms. When bacteria or viruses infect the body, the immune system produces diverse kinds of white blood cells that function in different ways to destroy infectious organisms.

The foreign proteins on viruses, bacteria, and other infectious organisms are called **antigens** (*anti*body *gene*rators). Every person has a collection of cells circulating in the blood that can recognize any foreign protein on any infectious organism in the world that may be encountered during a person's lifetime.

A particular immune system cell can recognize a particular foreign antigen on a virus or bacterium and begin to make more B-cells just like itself. Eventually these B-cells (at this stage called plasma cells) synthesize vast amounts of one specific kind of antibody that

Terms

nosocomial diseases: an infectious disease contracted while in the hospital for an unrelated disease or problem

immune system: an interacting system of organs and cells that protect the body from infectious organisms and harmful substances

antibodies: proteins that recognize and inactivate viruses, bacteria, and other organisms and toxic substances that enter the body

lymphatic system: a system of vessels in the body that trap foreign organisms and particles; the immune system is part of the lymphatic system

lymph nodes: nodules spaced along the lymphatic vessels that trap infectious organisms or foreign particles

antigens: foreign proteins on infectious organisms that stimulate an antibody response

attaches to all of the infectious bacteria or viruses in the body. Once the antibodies have recognized and inactivated an invader, other white blood cells finish the job of destruction. To produce the correct antibodies in large amounts takes about a week after an infection, which is why other quicker-acting immune system defense mechanisms are also needed.

Immunizations

One of the great achievements of modern medicine has been the development of **immunizations** (vaccinations) to prevent many serious infectious diseases caused by bacteria and, more importantly, by viruses (Beardsley, 1995). Viral diseases (whooping cough, measles, mumps, and hepatitis) have been eliminated in the U.S. (smallpox, polio) or markedly reduced.

Vaccination is the administration, usually by injection (hence, the name "shot"), of substances called **vaccines.** When you are vaccinated, specific proteins from inactivated viruses, bacteria, or toxins are injected into the body. The body's immune system responds by producing antibodies (proteins) that can inactivate the infectious organisms. If you later encounter the active, disease-causing viruses, you are protected by the vaccination and cells that produce protective antibodies. For example, the crippling disease poliomyelitis has been eradicated in the United States as a result of the widespread use of the polio virus vaccine.

In general, vaccination is safe and effective in preventing a number of infectious diseases. Vaccinations are recommended for both children and adults, but vaccinations are crucial for young children (Figure 9.5). Other vaccinations are recommended only for people at risk of exposure to a certain disease. For example, travelers to a country where cholera, typhoid fever, or polio is prevalent should be vaccinated for these diseases.

A recent addition to the list of effective vaccines is one for the hepatitis B virus. About 300,000 cases of hepatitis B (HB) are diagnosed in the United States annually. HB is a serious viral disease that can lead to death from liver disease or liver cancer. Some people experience only mild symptoms after being infected, but others develop a chronic infection that gradually destroys the liver. Because HB causes such a serious disease, vaccination of infants with hepatitis B vaccine is strongly advised.

Understanding Allergies

Allergies are the immune system's response to foreign substances called **allergens** that the body thinks are harmful, but which usually are not. Pollens, molds,

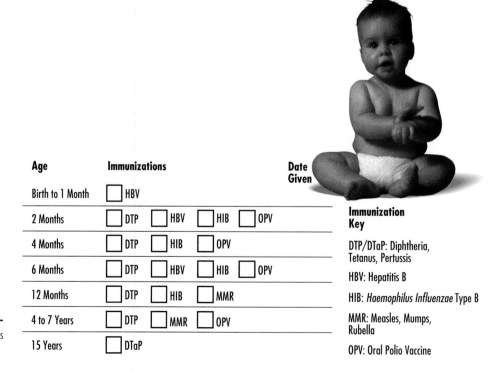

Age	Immunizations				Date Given
Birth to 1 Month	☐ HBV				
2 Months	☐ DTP	☐ HBV	☐ HIB	☐ OPV	
4 Months	☐ DTP	☐ HIB	☐ OPV		
6 Months	☐ DTP	☐ HBV	☐ HIB	☐ OPV	
12 Months	☐ DTP	☐ HIB	☐ MMR		
4 to 7 Years	☐ DTP	☐ MMR	☐ OPV		
15 Years	☐ DTaP				

Immunization Key

DTP/DTaP: Diphtheria, Tetanus, Pertussis

HBV: Hepatitis B

HIB: *Haemophilus Influenzae* Type B

MMR: Measles, Mumps, Rubella

OPV: Oral Polio Vaccine

FIGURE 9.5 **Recommended Immunizations for Children** Chickenpox immunization is recommended but optional.

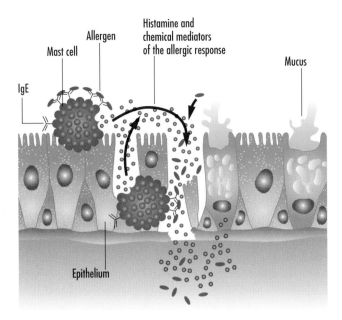

FIGURE 9.6 **Chemistry of an Allergic Response** An allergen (a substance from a plant, insect, or other organism) binds to antibody proteins (IgE) on mast cells. This triggers the release of histamines and other inflammatory substances that characterize the allergic response. These reactions occur mainly in the nose, lungs, skin, and digestive tract.

house dust, animal hair, foods, drugs, chemicals, and many other substances can act as allergens. The body responds by synthesizing a particular class of antibodies (immunoglobulin E, or IgE) that triggers the allergic reaction (Figure 9.6). No one knows why allergic responses evolved or what benefit they might have provided, but millions of people today can attest to the misery caused by allergic responses.

The allergic reaction is usually accompanied by the secretion of mucus and the release of **histamine,** an inflammatory chemical that is abundant in cells of the skin, respiratory passages, and digestive tract. That is why most allergic reactions are associated with the skin (eczema, hives, contact dermatitis), the respiratory passages (asthma, hay fever), and the digestive tract (swelling, vomiting, diarrhea).

Contact Dermatitis

Contact dermatitis affects millions of people because many of the things we touch or put on our skin can cause allergic reactions that manifest as rashes. Walking in the woods where poison ivy or poison oak grows can produce serious rashes in susceptible persons. Peeling a mango can cause people who are allergic to the skin of this fruit to break out in a rash; however, they usually can eat the flesh of the fruit without experiencing a reaction. As many as 17 million Americans may be allergic to natural rubber (latex) products.

Asthma

The incidence of asthma has been increasing in both adults and children in developed countries and has more than doubled in the U.S. in the past 20 years. The increase does not appear to be caused by air pollution (although that certainly exacerbates symptoms), and the reasons for the upsurge are still not clear.

While the symptoms of asthma vary from mild to very severe, deaths due to asthma are rare, although increasing. People no longer need to suffer from asthma and endure the fear of not being able to breathe. A range of effective medicines are now available that can control any asthmatic's symptoms, even the most serious. Short-acting bronchodilators that are inhaled at the onset of symptoms can provide immediate relief. For persistent asthma, short-term and long-term corticosteroid inhalers are available. With daily use, these can effectively suppress wheezing symptoms and breathing difficulties. Cromolyn inhalers also suppress symptoms in many people, and oral corticosteroids prevent asthma in the most severe cases.

Recently, a new class of drugs became available that blocks the actions of leukotrienes, chemicals produced in the body that cause muscles in the air passages to constrict. The goal of asthma treatment is to find the right medication at the lowest dose that leaves an asthmatic free of symptoms. And, of course, it is still important to eliminate from an asthmatic's environment as many allergens as possible to which the individual is sensitive.

Food Allergies

Food allergies, also called food intolerance, are allergic responses to a particular food. The reaction can be local (such as a stomach upset or swelling in the mouth) or it can involve the whole body. For example, an allergic reaction to a food or to an insect bite can cause

Terms

immunizations: vaccinations to prevent a variety of serious diseases caused by both bacteria and viruses

vaccines: inactivated bacteria or viruses that are injected or taken orally; the body responds by producing antibodies and cells that provide lasting immunity

allergens: foreign substances that trigger an allergic response by the immune system

histamine: a chemical released by cells in an allergic response; causes inflammation

contact dermatitis: an allergic reaction of the skin to something that is touched

food allergies: allergic responses to something that is eaten

Wellness Guide

A Cure for Asthma

One of the first successful treatments for an allergy dates from the sixteenth century. An Italian physician, Girolamo Gardano, was asked to come to Scotland to treat John Hamilton, Archbishop of St. Andrews, who suffered from asthma. After watching his patient for several days, Gardano asked the archbishop to give up his swan-feather pillows. This was almost heresy because only the upper classes were allowed to use such pillows. However, the archbishop did give them up and was cured.

Today avoidance of allergy-causing foods and environmental substances that cause allergic reactions is still the best therapy. In many patients with allergies, mental imagery, hypnosis, or suggestion are also effective in reducing or eliminating allergic reactions.

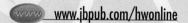 **www.jbpub.com/hwonline**

hives to break out all over the body. Food allergies are most common in children but can occur in anyone at any age.

When people are tested for food allergies, six substances account for 90 percent of the allergic reactions—eggs, peanuts, milk, fish, soy, and wheat. Severe allergic reactions produce **anaphylactic shock,** a systemic reaction that can quickly cause death. Anaphylactic shock can be brought on by an immediate, strong allergic reaction to food, a bee sting, or a drug.

Children are at particular risk of developing allergies to nuts, particularly peanuts. (Strictly speaking, the peanut is a legume, not a nut). Children tend to outgrow most of their childhood allergies, but this is not true for nut allergies. In addition to peanuts, many persons are allergic to Brazil nuts, almonds, hazelnuts, and walnuts. Because the reactions in nut allergies can be quite serious, including anaphylactic shock, most people with nut allergies have to be extremely careful about what foods they eat, since many manufactured products contain nuts.

Some allergists believe the increase in nut allergies is caused by feeding nuts to young children. Most nut allergies develop in children before age 7, a time when the immune system is still developing (Raloff, 1996). Not allowing children to eat nuts until they are older than 7 years might help reduce the incidence of nut allergies in the population.

Infants less than 1 year old can develop infant botulism from eating honey; therefore, infants should not be fed honey until their immune system can handle it, at about age 1.

About 20% of people report food intolerance of one sort or another at some time in their lives, yet studies show that the actual number of people who are physiologically sensitive to foods is more like 2% or less (Young et al., 1994). The discrepancy between what people report as an allergic reaction and what is demonstrated by allergy tests probably results from the power of suggestion. If someone reads or is told that many people are allergic to eggs, he or she may begin to experience an allergic reaction when eggs are eaten. Also, throwing up after eating a particular food can produce a subsequent aversion or allergic reaction to that food.

Food allergies (as well as other forms of allergy) should not be regarded as the result of imagination and, therefore, in some sense, "unreal." Whether the allergic reaction is brought on specifically by the interaction of an allergen with IgE antibodies or by a state of mind is largely irrelevant. In both instances, the physiological responses are real and need to be treated.

Autoimmune Diseases

The immune system must function without mistakes to distinguish "self" from "nonself" because any mistake that caused antibodies to attack the body's own cells could result in serious disease or death. Unfortunately, mistakes in the functioning of the immune system do occur and produce **autoimmune diseases** (Figure 9.7). Some inherited disorders, fortunately quite rare, can result in the loss of the immune system's ability to distinguish "self" from "nonself." Environmental factors, such as viral infections, nutri-

Terms

anaphylactic shock: a severe allergic reaction involving the whole body that can cause death

autoimmune diseases: mistakes in the functioning of the immune system that cause it to attack tissues in the body

lupus erythematosus: an autoimmune disease that mostly affects women

histocompatibility: the degree to which the antigens on cells of different persons are similar

HLA (human leukocyte antigens): antigens that are measured to determine the suitability of an organ for transplantation from donor to recipient

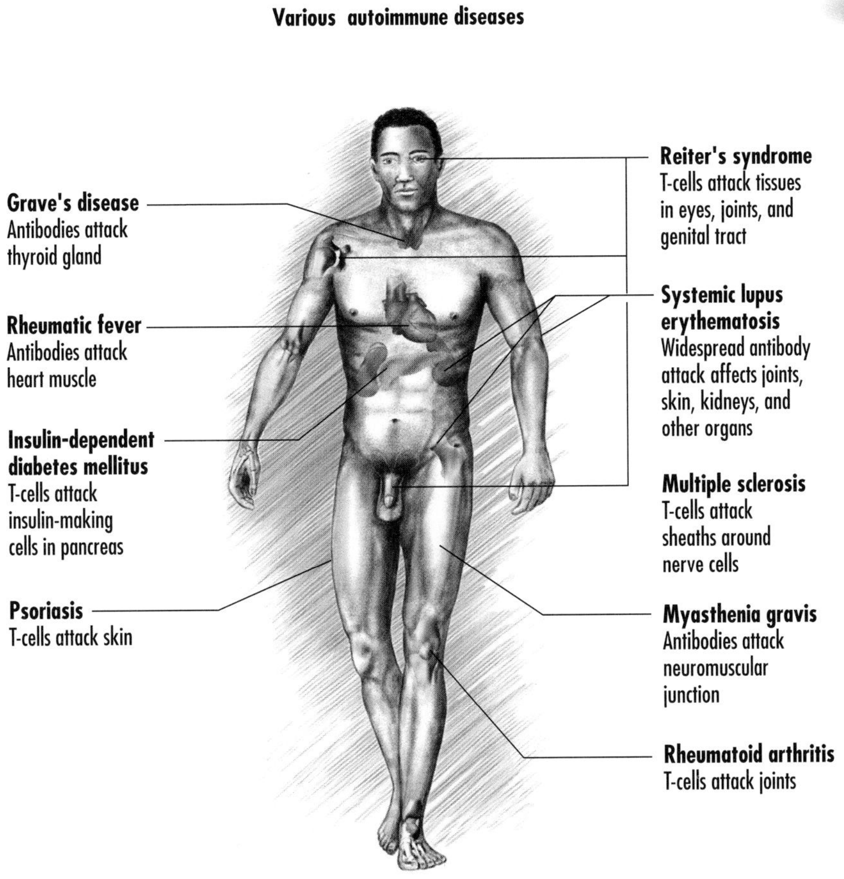

Various autoimmune diseases

Grave's disease
Antibodies attack
thyroid gland

Rheumatic fever
Antibodies attack
heart muscle

**Insulin-dependent
diabetes mellitus**
T-cells attack
insulin-making
cells in pancreas

Psoriasis
T-cells attack skin

Reiter's syndrome
T-cells attack tissues
in eyes, joints, and
genital tract

**Systemic lupus
erythematosis**
Widespread antibody
attack affects joints,
skin, kidneys, and
other organs

Multiple sclerosis
T-cells attack
sheaths around
nerve cells

Myasthenia gravis
Antibodies attack
neuromuscular
junction

Rheumatoid arthritis
T-cells attack joints

FIGURE 9.7   Autoimmune Diseases
These occur when the body's immune system goes awry and cells of the immune system begin attacking the body's own cells because they are mistakenly recognized as foreign.

tional problems, and other unknown agents may also cause the immune system to make mistakes that lead to autoimmune diseases.

Lupus erythematosus is an autoimmune disease that most frequently affects women between the ages of 18 to 35. In this disease, for reasons still unknown, antibodies are synthesized that attack the genetic information in cells (DNA), especially in cells of the blood vessels, skin, and kidneys. Many organs of the body are affected, and the symptoms—rashes, pain, and anemia—flare up and wane throughout life, which usually is shortened.

Arthritis is one of the most common chronic diseases; approximately 1 in 7 Americans has some form of arthritis. There are about 100 forms of arthritis and arthritis-related conditions, but the common denominator is pain and stiffness in joints throughout the body. The causes of arthritis vary widely, but many forms are the result of autoimmune disease in which the body's immune system mistakenly attacks cartilage and bone. Drugs can relieve many of the symptoms of arthritis, such as pain and inflammation, but the diseases themselves have no cure. Although drugs can help reduce the symptoms of autoimmune diseases, these diseases cannot be cured since they are caused by complex malfunctions of the immune system. Because the mind also affects the functions of

the immune system, many people who suffer from autoimmune diseases find relief in alternative therapies, mental relaxation techniques, and nutritional changes.

Organ Transplants

Like blood cells, all body cells have antigens on their surfaces that are different for everyone except identical twins. If tissue or organs from one person are grafted onto another, the immune system produces antibodies to the foreign cell antigens, causing destruction of the cells and rejection of the transplanted organ.

The more alike two persons are genetically, the more likely it is that the transplanted tissue will be accepted by the body. Identical twins are genetically identical; tissue transplants between identical twins have the greatest chance of success. To minimize the rejection of transplanted organs, the **histocompatibility** (similarity of cell surface antigens) between the donor and recipient is determined by immunological tests. Just as red blood cells have particular groups of strongly antigenic proteins on their cell surfaces, other cells in the body have antigenic proteins called **HLA (human leukocyte antigens)** that are crucial in determining whether a transplanted organ is accepted or rejected

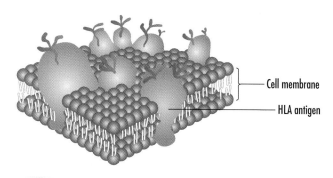

Cell membrane

HLA antigen

FIGURE 9.8   Antigens and the Immune System   A vast array of different HLA antigens are embedded in the outer membranes of cells, projecting beyond their surfaces. These antigens can be recognized by the body's immune cells and antibodies. Since every person's antigens are different, tissue transplanted from one person to another is usually rejected because the donor's HLA antigens are recognized as foreign and destroyed by the immune response of the recipient.

(Figure 9.8). The greater the similarity in HLA antigens between donor and recipient, the greater the chance that the tissue will be accepted and function normally in its new host. There are so many different HLA combinations that each person is immunologically unique.

Today, the transplantation of hearts, kidneys, livers, and other organs has become a relatively common procedure in many hospitals. However, organ transplants are extremely costly, complicated procedures and are not always successful, and more people are waiting for suitable organs than can be supplied.

The organ transplanted most often is the kidney. Since people have two kidneys, relatives sometimes donate one of their healthy kidneys to another close relative if their HLA genes are well matched. Brothers and sisters have one chance in four of inheriting the same HLA genes from their parents, which is why close relatives are examined first as possible donors.

The rejection of transplanted organs can be controlled to some degree with **immunosuppressive drugs** (corticosteroids, cyclosporine); however, treatment with these drugs lessens resistance to infections, and long-term immunosuppressive drug therapy results in increased susceptibility to cancer.

Blood Transfusions and Rh Factors

In the early part of the twentieth century, a blood transfusion often led to the patient's death. Because the patient's immune system recognized the donor's blood cells as being "foreign," it attacked them with antibodies. The antibodies caused clumps of blood cells to form in the veins and arteries, impeding the flow of blood and oxygen and causing death.

The two most important human red blood cell surface antigens are the ABO and Rh-positive/Rh-negative proteins. There are actually many other groups of antigens on red blood cells, but these two are by far the most important ones in evoking an immune response that can endanger health.

People with type O blood have neither A nor B antigens on their red blood cells and are **universal donors;** their blood cells will not stimulate an antibody response in the recipient, no matter what the blood type. People with type AB blood are **universal recipients** and accept blood from any of the four groups.

The Rh-positive antigen and the antibody that reacts against it cause problems primarily in pregnancy. A woman is Rh-negative if her red blood cells do not contain any of this antigen. If the red blood cells of a developing fetus have the Rh-positive antigen (inherited from the father) and if some of the fetus' red blood cells enter the mother's blood supply, production of anti-Rh antibodies can be stimulated by her immune system, which recognizes the fetal cells as foreign. This usually does not cause any difficulty during the first pregnancy and might even go unnoticed until the woman becomes pregnant again.

Now, if the second fetus is also Rh-positive, the Rh-positive antibodies (synthesized during the first pregnancy) in the mother's blood attack the developing infant's red blood cells, resulting in anemia, brain damage, or even death. Fortunately, doctors can manage this problem safely and effectively. At the time the first child is delivered, the mother is given an injection of anti-Rh antibodies that destroys any Rh-positive antibodies in her blood. In this way, any danger to the fetus during a subsequent pregnancy is avoided.

AIDS and HIV

The infectious disease that has received the most public and research attention since it was first detected in

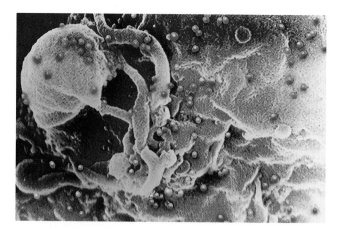

The AIDS virus as seen under the electron microscope. The red dots are presumed to be human immunodeficiency viruses being released from infected cells.

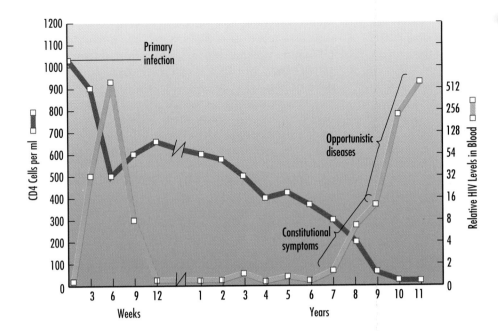

FIGURE 9.9 **HIV and the Immune System** After infection, the virus level rises sharply in the blood, but within 3 months is undetectable. However, the virus is usually multiplying slowly in lymph nodes. The infected CD4 T-cells gradually decrease in number over many years. At some point, the immune system is weakened so that the person becomes susceptible to any of dozens of infectious diseases. Although this figure shows a disease latency of 8 years, some HIV-positive individuals have had no symptoms for as long as 15 years.

the early 1980s is **AIDS (acquired immune deficiency syndrome)**. AIDS, like cancer, arthritis, or diabetes, is not a single disease. AIDS is defined by the Centers for Disease Control and Prevention (CDC) as consisting of more than two dozen specific diseases accompanied by a very low level of CD4 T-cells in the blood. A normal CD4 T-cell level in the blood is 800 to 1200 cells per milliliter.

HIV (human immunodeficiency virus), the cause of AIDS, is an unusual virus, because once it infects a cell it becomes a permanent resident of that cell. Proteins on the surface of the virus recognize receptors on the surface of CD4 T-cells, allowing the virus to inject its genetic information. The injected virus now is able to manufacture more viruses that can escape and infect other cells.

AIDS and the Immune System

Infection with HIV gradually weakens the body's immune system, exposing it to **opportunistic infections,** caused by any of a wide variety of microorganisms. AIDS patients become progressively weaker with each infection and eventually die. The course of HIV infection is unpredictable; some individuals progress to full-blown AIDS and die within months. Others have no symptoms even after 10 years or more of HIV infection (Figure 9.9).

About 1% of HIV-infected persons have remained healthy for as long as 15 years after they were infected, demonstrating that HIV infection does not inevitably lead to AIDS (at least within a certain timeframe) in everyone. Studies of these long-term survivors revealed that these lucky persons carry two copies of a rare gene (CCR5) that makes them

resistant to HIV infection. People who carry one copy of the rare gene along with a copy of the more common gene also survive longer than average with HIV infection. This important finding paves the way for scientists to devise drugs that can mimic the effect of the desirable gene in people who are not genetically resistant to HIV infection.

For the majority of HIV-infected patients, powerful drugs must be taken (more than 50 pills a day) to keep HIV in check and prevent progression to AIDS. Three classes of drugs that block HIV multiplication in infected individuals are available: reverse transcriptase inhibitors (AZT and 3TC), nonnucleoside reverse transcriptase inhibitors (Nevirapine, Delavirdine, and Loviride), and newly developed protease inhibitors (Saquinavir, Rotonavir, and Indinavir). These or other drugs must be taken daily to prevent HIV from infecting additional cells. Since all of these drugs are toxic,

Terms

immunosuppressive drugs: drugs to suppress the functions of the immune system (e.g., after organ transplants)

universal donor: a person whose blood is accepted by everyone during transfusion

universal recipient: a person whose blood type is compatible with anyone else's blood

AIDS (acquired immune deficiency syndrome): a syndrome of more than two dozen diseases caused by HIV

HIV (human immunodeficiency virus): the virus that causes AIDS

opportunistic infections: any infectious disease in a patient with a weakened immune system; often occurs in AIDS patients

there is a time limit as to how long they can be taken. Also, because of cost and other considerations, not all AIDS patients are receiving the most effective drug regimes (Cohen, 1997).

Although optimism for treating HIV infections has increased, a cure for AIDS is still a remote hope. Eventually, scientists hope to develop a vaccine for HIV infection; although many potential vaccines have been tested, none have proved effective as yet. In Asia and Africa, millions of people are still becoming infected with HIV; however, they have little hope of receiving the expensive and complicated treatments being developed in the U.S.

The AIDS Antibody Test

Upon infecting a person, HIV acts like all other viral infections by stimulating synthesis of antibodies capable of inactivating the virus. Detection of these antibodies is the basis of the **AIDS antibody test.** In reality, the test is an indirect measure of HIV infection; it does not measure whether a person has AIDS or will get AIDS.

The test is positive only after antibodies have reached a detectable level, which can take several weeks or even months after infection. In the interim, a person is highly infectious, but will show negative results on the AIDS antibody test. Thus, even a recent negative AIDS antibody test may not mean that a person is uninfected if they have been sexually active or use injected drugs.

Another problem with AIDS antibody tests is false-positive results that create unnecessary anxiety. A false-positive means that the test shows that the person has antibodies in his or her blood that resemble ones produced in response to HIV. In reality, the person is not infected and the test is in error. Infection by other viruses or bacteria whose antigens resemble those of HIV can lead to a false-positive result on the HIV antibody test. Any positive AIDS test result should be rechecked. The most accurate test for HIV infection is the **Western blot,** which tests for the presence of specific HIV proteins.

Preventing HIV Infection

Compared to other viral infections, such as ones that cause colds, flu, or hepatitis, HIV is not very infectious. The virus is *never* transmitted by casual contact between an infected person and uninfected persons. Never, in this context, means that no well-docu-

mented cases of HIV infection have been reported except as a result of sexual intercourse or the receipt of HIV-contaminated blood. HIV is not transmitted in saliva, spit, sweat, air, water, or other objects that have been used by an HIV-infected person.

You can protect yourself from HIV infection by understanding the facts about HIV and AIDS. HIV is transmitted only by sexual intercourse with an HIV-infected partner, by sharing blood-contaminated needles during use of illegal drugs, or by receiving HIV-contaminated blood in transfusions. With care, these are all situations that can be avoided.

Preventing Infections

Infections to some degree are unavoidable. However, the elements of healthy living that we have been emphasizing can both reduce the risk of contracting an infectious disease and also hasten recovery. Foremost is maintaining health by proper nutrition and a reasonable amount of exercise. These factors, as well as sufficient rest and sleep, increase the ability of the immune system to fight infectious organisms.

Vaccinations against certain infections can provide almost complete protection in most cases. Check your record of immunizations with your family physician and update any that have not been received on schedule or that you are not sure that you received as a child. Many infections, such as mumps or measles, that are usually mild in childhood, can be serious if acquired as an adult.

Stressful situations and emotional disturbances lower the body's defenses and make it more vulnerable to infectious microorganisms. Use common sense and stay away from people and situations that carry a high risk of infection. For example, do not travel to a country that is having a cholera epidemic. Do not expose yourself unnecessarily to people with colds, flu, hepatitis or other highly contagious diseases. With reasonable precautions many infectious diseases are preventable. And by maintaining good health, the body will quickly and completely recover from most infections when they do occur.

Terms

AIDS antibody test: detects antibodies in blood that are produced in response to infection by HIV

Western blot test: a test to determine the presence of specific HIV proteins; very accurate

Critical Thinking About Health

1. Describe one infectious disease you have had in the past few years (other than a cold). Discuss the following: (a) how you think you caught the disease, (b) what kind of microorganism caused it, (c) what the symptoms were, (d) how the disease was treated, and (e) any advice you were given on how to avoid contracting the disease in the future. Have you made any changes in your life-style to reduce the risk of contracting an infectious disease as a result of this experience?

2. What kind of infectious disease worries you the most: AIDS, hepatitis, tuberculosis, sexually transmitted diseases in general, or others? Explain your concerns over contracting this disease, including any circumstances in your life that might have given rise to your concerns. Describe all that you know about this particular disease and how your concerns have altered your life-style or behaviors.

3. Find out all that you can on food-borne infectious diseases. Describe the kinds of microorganisms in foods that cause disease and ways that people can protect themselves from becoming infected. Do you have any concerns about the foods that you eat? Can you reduce or eliminate these concerns by making changes in your diet?

4. A variety of mind-body exercises are effective in controlling the symptoms of allergies, asthma, arthritis, and other immune system diseases. Learn as much as you can about how the immune system works. Discuss how you think the mind affects the immune system and how it can affect symptoms of the diseases mentioned above. Have you had any personal experience in using your mind to change the symptoms of a disease that has its roots in some form of immune system malfunction?

Health in Review

- Infectious diseases are caused by a myriad of pathogenic organisms: viruses, bacteria, fungi, protozoa, and worms. Some pathogenic microorganisms are easily passed from one person to another and cause communicable diseases.
- Some infectious diseases are caused by a vector such as an insect or other animal that transmits the pathogenic microorganism to an uninfected person.
- Many pathogenic bacteria are becoming resistant to common antibiotics, making treatment of serious infectious diseases difficult.
- Antibiotics kill microorganisms but do not kill viruses, which are not alive in the sense that cells are.
- Infectious disease is fought in four ways: sanitation, antibiotics, vaccination, and healthful living.

- The skin and mucous membranes keep harmful substances from entering the body.
- The immune system produces cells that make antibodies, which are proteins that recognize any foreign substance or organism. Malfunctioning of the immune system causes autoimmune diseases and allergies.
- Transplantation of organs or blood requires that the donor and recipient be matched with respect to histocompatibility.
- AIDS results from infection by HIV, which destroys cells of the immune system. Immunodeficiency leads to opportunistic infections that eventually cause death.

Health and Wellness Online

The World Wide Web contains a wealth of information about health and wellness. By accessing the Internet using Web browser software, such as Netscape Navigator or Microsoft's Internet Explorer, you can gain a new perspective on many topics presented in *Essentials of Health and Wellness, Second Edition.* Access the Jones and Bartlett Publishers web site at http://www.jbpub.com/hwonline.

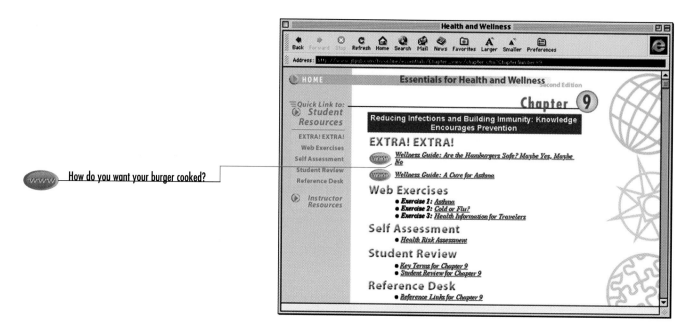

References

Beardsley, T. (1995, January). Better than a cure. *Scientific American,* 88–93.

Cohen, J. (1997). AIDS trials ethics questioned. *Science, 276,* 520–523.

Fackelmann, K. (1996, April 13). The hepatitis G enigma." *Science News,* 238–239.

Fineberg, H. V., & Wilson, M. E. (1996). Social vulnerability and death by infection. *New England Journal of Medicine, 334,* 359–360.

Gold, H. S., & Moellering, Jr, R. C. (1996). Antimicrobial drug resistance. *New England Journal of Medicine, 335,* 1445–1453.

Greenwald, D. A., & Brandt, L. J. (1997, April 15). Recognizing *E. coli* 0157:H7 infection. *Hospital Practice,* 123–140.

Guenno, B. L. (1995, October). Emerging viruses. *Scientific American,* 56–64.

Lederberg, J. (1996). Infectious diseases—A threat to global health and security. *Journal of the American Medical Association, 276,* 417–419.

Lemon, S. M., & Thomas, D. L. (1997). Vaccines to prevent viral hepatitis. *New England Journal of Medicine, 336,* 196–204.

Levy, S. R. (1998, March). The challenge of antibiotic resistance. *Scientific American,* 46–53.

Morganthau, T. (1997, September 1). *E. coli* alert. *Newsweek,* 26–32.

Morse, S. S. (1996, April 15). Patterns and predictability in emerging infections. *Hospital Practice,* 85–91.

Raloff, J. (1996). Family allergies? Keep the nuts away from baby. *Science News, 149,* 279.

Sands, K. E., et al. (1997). Epidemiology of sepsis syndrome in 8 academic medical centers. *Journal of the American Medical Association, 278,* 234–240.

Swartz, M. N. (1997). Use of antimicrobial agents and drug resistance. *New England Journal of Medicine, 337,* 491–492.

Tauxe, R. V. (1997). Emerging foodborne diseases: An evolving public health challenge. *Emerging Infectious Diseases, 3,* 425–434.

Young, E., et al. (1994). A population study of food intolerance. *Lancet, 343,* 1127–1130.

Suggested Readings

Guenno, B. L. (1995, October). Emerging viruses. *Scientific American,* 56–64. Explains the health danger of the many new viruses that are causing disease.

Morganthau, T. (1997, September 1). *E. coli* alert. *Newsweek,* 26–32. Discusses the bacteria that contaminate meat and other foods and how to protect yourself from infection.

Royce, R. A. (1997). Sexual transmission of HIV. *New England Journal of Medicine, 336,* 1072–1078. Explains in detail how HIV is transmitted sexually and what contributes to the risk of infection. Surprising finding: HIV is transmitted in only about 1 in 1000 occasions of sexual intercourse in which one of the partners is HIV-positive.

Smaglik, P. (1997). Proliferation of pills. *Science News, 151,* 310–311. Discusses the overuse of antibiotics by physicians and how this contributes to the development of antibiotic-resistant bacteria.

Learning Objectives

1. Define cardiovascular disease, infarction, coronary heart disease, stroke, and heart attack.
2. Explain the role atherosclerosis plays in heart disease.
3. Identify the major risk factors of heart disease that cannot be changed, major risk factors that can be changed, and other contributing factors.
4. List dietary supplements and foods that help maintain a healthy cardiovascular system.
5. Identify and describe the most important ways to prevent cancer.
6. Define the following terms: cancer, tumor, benign tumor, malignant tumor, metastasis, and xenoestrogen.
7. Describe the kinds of environmental agents that cause cancer.
8. Discuss how cigarette smoke and diet contribute to cancer.
9. Describe several coping mechanisms for someone with cancer.

Exercises and Activities

WORKBOOK
Testing for Risk of Heart Disease
Reduce Environmental Cancer Risks

Health and Wellness Online

 www.jbpub.com/hwonline

Understanding Cardiovascular Diseases
Diet and Cardiovascular Disease
Regulating Diet
Wellness Guide: Ways to Prevent Skin Cancer
Critical Thinking About Health

Chapter 10

Cardiovascular Diseases and Cancer: Risks and Prevention

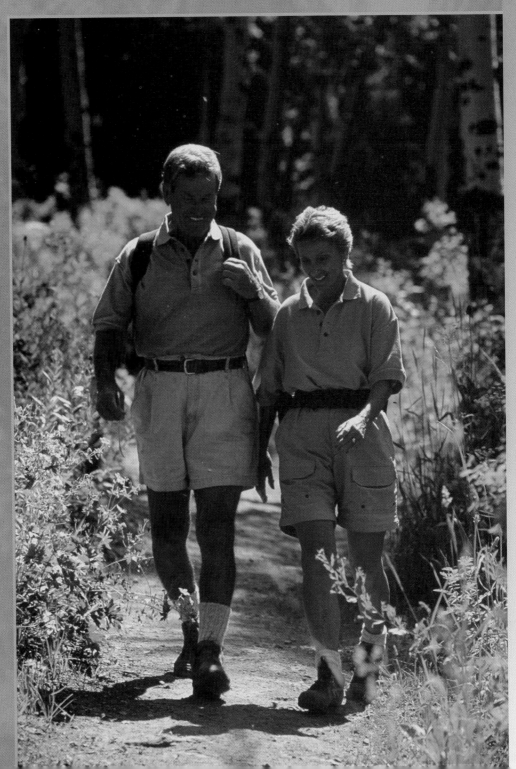

Cardiovascular disease and cancer share two important aspects. First, they are the number one and number two causes of death and disability year after year. Second, both are, to a large degree, *preventable* diseases in the majority of people who ultimately die from heart disease or cancer. Both

> *Have a heart that never*
> *hardens*
> *A temper that never tires*
> *A touch that never hurts.*
> CHARLES DICKENS

diseases usually make their appearance in older people, so most of us do not think about them while we are young (although we know that even young people may die from heart attacks or cancer).

Adopting a healthy life-style while young can dramatically reduce your risk of these diseases later in life: don't smoke; drink moderately; avoid drugs; eat lots more fresh fruits and vegetables and much less fat, salt, and sugar; exercise regularly; and know how to let go of stress and anxiety.

Terms

cardiovascular disease: any disease that causes damage to the heart or to arteries that carry blood to and from the heart

coronary arteries: two arteries arising from the aorta that supply blood to the heart muscle

heart attack: death of, or damage to, part of the heart muscle caused by an insufficient blood supply

infarction: death of heart cells resulting from a blocked blood supply

ischemia: an insufficient supply of blood to the heart

stroke: an insufficient supply of blood to the brain, resulting in loss of muscle function, loss of speech, or other symptoms

arteries: any one of a series of blood vessels that carry blood from the heart to all parts of the body

veins: blood vessels that return blood from tissues to the heart

capillaries: extremely small blood vessels that carry oxygenated blood to tissues

myocardium: muscular wall of the heart that contracts and relaxes

arteriosclerosis: hardening of the arteries

atherosclerosis: a disease process in which fatty deposits build up in the arteries and block the flow of blood

plaque: deposit of fatty substances in the inner lining of arteries

angina pectoris: medical term for chest pain caused by coronary heart disease; a condition in which the heart muscle doesn't receive enough blood, resulting in chest pain

angiocardiography: an x-ray examination of the coronary arteries and heart; produces a picture called an angiogram

arteriography (cardiac catheterization): visualization of blocked coronary arteries by injecting a dye and monitoring blood flow

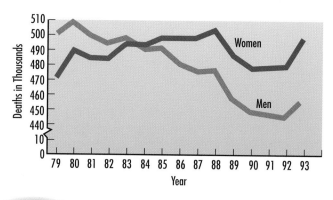

FIGURE 10.1   Mortality from Cardiovascular Disease in the U.S. (1979–1993)   Death from heart disease has been declining among men for about 20 years but has increased slightly among women.

Source: American Heart Association, Dallas, TX. Heart and Stroke Statistical Data, 1997.

Understanding Cardiovascular Diseases

Cardiovascular disease refers to any of a number of conditions that damage the heart or the arteries that carry blood to and from the heart. If the **coronary arteries** (the large blood vessels that carry blood to and from the heart) become diseased or blocked, a **heart attack** may result. If the cells of the heart do not receive a continual supply of blood and oxygen, the cells die, a condition known as an **infarction.** If the blood supply to the heart is only partially blocked, the process is known as **ischemia.**

More than 40% of all deaths each year in the United States result from cardiovascular diseases that lead to heart attacks and **strokes.** A stroke occurs when an insufficient supply of blood to brain cells causes them to die. While cardiovascular diseases tend to occur in the elderly, heart attacks can occur at any age, often without warning.

The rate of death from cardiovascular diseases among men has been declining steadily in the United States for over 20 years (Figure 10.1). Rates for women have not changed significantly over the same period. Certainly public awareness of the risk factors in cardiovascular disease has been a major contributor to the decline. Less fat and cholesterol in the diet, less cigarette smoking, and more exercising have all contributed to reducing deaths from cardiovascular disease. Like cancer, most heart disease is preventable and is caused primarily by unhealthy life-styles: poor diet, overweight, lack of exercise, and smoking.

The Heart and Blood Vessels

The circulatory system consists of the heart (the pump) and the various blood vessels. **Arteries** carry oxygenated blood from the heart to all organs and tissues in the body. **Veins** return blood to the heart after

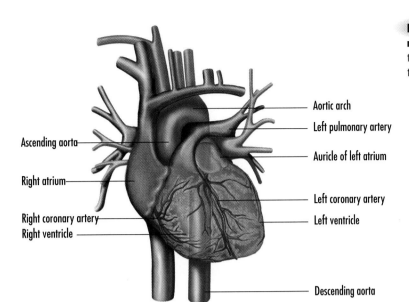

FIGURE 10.2 **Heart and Major Arteries** Oxygenated blood is pumped through the arteries (red) and oxygen-depleted blood is returned to the heart via the veins (blue).

Aortic arch

Left pulmonary artery

Auricle of left atrium

Ascending aorta

Right atrium

Left coronary artery

Right coronary artery

Left ventricle

Right ventricle

Descending aorta

oxygen and nutrients have been exchanged for carbon dioxide and waste products. **Capillaries** are tiny blood vessels that branch out from arteries and veins and circulate blood to all of the cells in the body. Blood vessels can be damaged by injury or by disease; this damage may obstruct the flow of blood carrying oxygen and nutrients.

The organ that keeps the blood circulating throughout the body is the heart, a highly specialized muscle about the size of an adult fist that pumps blood (Figure 10.2). The muscular wall of the heart is called the **myocardium.** If the blood supply to heart cells is blocked, cells begin to die and a heart attack results.

The heart contracts from 65 to 70 times a minute depending on the body's activity. The entire volume of blood in the body is recirculated almost once every minute. During an average lifetime of 70 years, the heart will pump between 30 to 40 million gallons of blood, and it will beat 2.5 billion times!

Atherosclerosis and Heart Disease

Arteriosclerosis, which literally means hardening of the arteries, includes all kinds of diseases that damage the arteries. However, the one form of arteriosclerosis that is of primary concern is **atherosclerosis.** This arterial disease begins with damage to cells of the heart's arteries and leads to the formation of a fibrous, fatty deposit called **plaque.** The arterial plaque slowly increases in size until eventually the amount of blood flowing through the artery is greatly reduced or completely blocked (Figure 10.3).

If the coronary arteries become partially blocked and the heart cells do not get enough oxygen, chest pain called **angina pectoris** results. The drug nitro-

glycerin dilates blood vessels and is used to relieve the pain of angina. If a coronary artery becomes completely blocked, the person usually has a heart attack.

Diagnosis of a Heart Attack

Each year in the United States more than a million people are admitted to hospitals because of possible heart attacks. Tests eventually rule out a heart attack in about 50% of those admitted. Chest pains that mimic those of a heart attack can be brought on by severe indigestion (heartburn), panic, and stress.

If a heart attack has occurred, the levels of certain proteins in the blood, such as creatine kinase, troponin, myoglobin, and myosin, begin to change. Tests are being developed that measure the levels of these proteins rapidly. This would allow physicians in emergency departments to quickly determine if a heart attack has occurred and to initiate appropriate treatment.

Repairing Blocked Arteries

When medical tests, such as an **angiocardiography**, a procedure for visualizing the flow of blood through the coronary arteries and chambers of the heart, confirm that one or several coronary arteries are blocked and that blood flow to the heart is restricted, additional tests or surgery are usually recommended.

A precise image of the flow of blood through the coronary arteries that supply blood to the heart is obtained by an invasive procedure called **arteriography** (also called cardiac catheterization). To visualize the blood flow, a thin tube is threaded from an artery in a leg or arm up into the coronary arteries. A dye is injected and high speed x-ray film records the flow of the dye in the arteries. Over a million cardiac

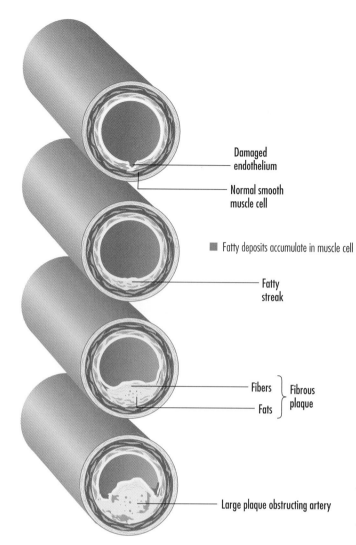

Damaged endothelium

Normal smooth muscle cell

■ Fatty deposits accumulate in muscle cell

Fatty streak

Fibers } Fibrous
Fats   } plaque

Large plaque obstructing artery

FIGURE 10.3   Development of an Atherosclerotic Lesion (Plaque) inside an Artery Plaque can eventually block blood flow, causing a heart attack or stroke. Many factors are suspected in the formation of a plaque, but none has been proven.

catheterizations are performed each year in the U.S. on patients with suspected partial blockage of their coronary arteries.

In **coronary bypass surgery,** the diseased segment of an artery is cut out and a segment of a healthy vein or artery is grafted onto the damaged artery to restore normal flow of blood to the heart. If one graft is made into a blocked artery, the surgery is called a single coronary bypass; if four grafts are made it is called a quadruple bypass.

An alternative surgical approach to opening a blocked artery is **percutaneous transluminal coronary angioplasty** (PTCA), or simply, angioplasty. In this procedure, a thin wire is threaded from the femoral artery in the thigh up to the point of blockage in a coronary artery. Another thin tube containing a deflated balloon is then slipped over the wire and threaded up to the area of the arterial plaque. The bal-

loon is inflated and pushes the plaque back into the wall of the artery, thereby opening it up.

Until recently, it was universally believed that atherosclerosis was a progressive and irreversible disease. However, an experiment with a small group of volunteers who had partial blockage of their arteries showed that this longstanding conviction is not necessarily correct. This study showed that over a period of 5 years, life-style changes could significantly reduce arterial blockage in over 70% of the experimental group (Ornish, 1998). While the life-style changes made by persons in the Ornish program are intense, the results show that behavioral changes (diet, exercise, meditation) can improve the biological health of coronary arteries. Also, people who stayed with the program had half the risk of a heart attack after 5 years as compared to a control group that did not make life-style changes (Ornish et al., 1998).

Stroke

Stroke is the third leading cause of death in the U.S., after coronary heart disease and cancer. As with the latter two diseases, stroke is, in most cases, a preventable disease (Bronner et al., 1995). High blood pressure is the most important risk factor and plays a role in at least 70% of all strokes.

Stroke is a form of cardiovascular disease that affects arteries supplying blood to the brain. If a brain artery becomes blocked or ruptures, brain cells die within minutes from lack of oxygen. Parts of the body that depend on these damaged or dead cells in the brain for functioning also are affected. Thus, a person who has a stroke can lose the ability to speak, become paralyzed in an arm or leg, or lose the use of one whole side of the body. The effects of strokes vary greatly, ranging from mild or unnoticed symptoms to sudden death.

The warning signs of a stroke are any of the following conditions that occur suddenly. Immediate medical attention is needed if any of the symptoms of stroke occur:

• Sudden weakness or numbness of the face, arm, or leg on one side of the body

• Sudden dimness or loss of vision, especially in one eye

T e r m s

coronary bypass surgery: surgery to improve blood supply to the heart muscle; most often performed when narrowed coronary arteries reduce the flow of oxygenated blood to the heart

percutaneous transluminal coronary angioplasty (PTCA): a procedure to open blocked arteries

Wellness Guide

Get a Second Opinion Before Undergoing Heart Surgery

High-tech surgical procedures, such as coronary bypass, angioplasty, and pacemaker implantation, have revolutionized the treatment of coronary heart disease (CHD). While these surgeries prevent some heart attacks and save lives, in many instances they are performed for heart conditions that do not warrant surgery. Many CHD problems such as angina (chest pain) can be controlled with medications.

In the 1950s, angina pain from partially blocked coronary arteries was relieved by an operation in which a chest artery was tied off in the hope that more blood would be supplied to the patient's heart. About 40% of the patients felt better following this operation. To determine whether the relief of angina pain was a placebo effect or actually resulted from the surgery, a number of mock operations were performed. (In the 1950s, informed consent was not mandatory in most hospitals.) Patients were given anesthesia, the chest was cut open, but nothing else was done to correct blood flow to the heart. Patients who underwent mock surgeries had just as much relief from angina as patients who had the chest artery tied off. As a result, this operation was abandoned.

In a similar fashion, coronary bypass operations may relieve angina as a result of the long period of rest and recuperation that patients undergo; life-style changes that people make also may contribute to their relief. A large part of the success of bypass surgery may be a placebo effect.

In 1999, a drug called vascular endothelial growth factor (VEGF) was developed to promote the growth of new blood vessels and to help prevent heart attacks in people with clogged arteries. The drug is injected directly into the coronary arteries. As with all clinical trials of new drugs, a placebo group of potential heart attack patients was given injections of an inert substance. Patients receiving the drug injections were able to walk 26 to 32 seconds longer on a treadmill test than they could previously. The placebo patients were able to walk 42 seconds longer! The drug company, not surprisingly, called the test a failure. But the researchers are wondering if the placebo patients actually grew new blood vessels simply because they were told that that was what the drug would do. Stay tuned.

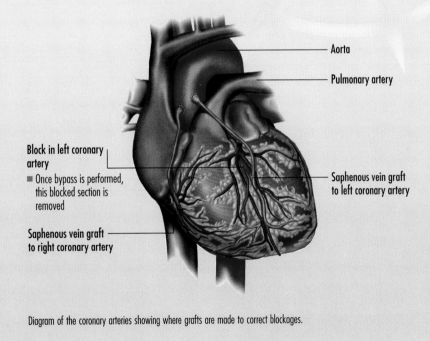

Aorta

Pulmonary artery

Block in left coronary artery
■ Once bypass is performed, this blocked section is removed

Saphenous vein graft to left coronary artery

Saphenous vein graft to right coronary artery

Diagram of the coronary arteries showing where grafts are made to correct blockages.

- Loss of speech, difficulty understanding speech, or trouble talking
- Sudden, severe headaches with no known cause
- Unexplained unsteadiness, dizziness, or sudden falls, especially with one of the other symptoms

The best way to prevent a stroke is to reduce the risk factors. There are five controllable risk factors for a stroke: (1) high blood pressure; (2) heart disease; (3) cigarette smoking; (4) transient ischemic attacks; and (5) high red blood cell count, which thickens the blood and facilitates formation of a clot. These risk factors can, for the most part, be controlled by life-style. Factors resulting from heredity or natural processes can't be changed. Risk factors for a stroke that cannot be changed include: 1) increasing age; 2) being male; 3) race; 4) diabetes mellitus; 5) prior stroke; and 6) heredity.

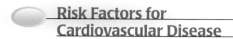

Risk Factors for Cardiovascular Disease

What starts the development of plaque in arteries and leads to cardiovascular disease, heart attacks, and strokes? Although no one really knows what causes arteries to become blocked by the buildup of plaques, a common bacterium, *Chlamydia pneumoniae,* may be involved. This bacterium, primarily known as a cause of sexually transmitted diseases, is frequently found in the plaques of patients with clogged arteries (Bachmaier et al., 1998). If bacterial infections are involved in coronary artery disease, it may be possible to develop a vaccine to prevent heart disease in the future. Arterial plaques are found in the hearts of healthy young people who die accidentally, suggesting that the disease process begins early in life in some individuals. Atherosclerosis is primarily a disease of modern, industrialized societies. Tribal people in New Guinea, !Kung tribes in Africa, and Eskimos in Greenland have a low incidence of cardiovascular disease. Tarahumara Indians in Mexico have virtually no heart disease or high blood pressure as long as they consume their native diet. However, when researchers switched a group of Tarahumara Indian volunteers to a typical American diet, they gained weight and had dramatic

TABLE 10.1   **Amount of Cholesterol in Various Foods**

Food	Cholesterol
Lard, 1 tablespoon	12 mg
Cream, 1 oz.	20 mg
Cottage cheese, 1/2 cup	24 mg
Ice cream, 1/2 cup	27 mg
Cheddar cheese, 1 oz.	28 mg
Whole milk, 1 cup	34 mg
Butter, 1 tablespoon	35 mg
Oysters, salmon, 3 oz.	40 mg
Clams, tuna, 3 oz.	55 mg
Beef, pork, lobster, chicken, turkey, 3 oz.	75 mg
Lamb, veal, crab, 3 oz.	85 mg
Shrimp, 3 oz.	130 mg
Beef heart, 3 oz.	230 mg
Egg, one yolk	250 mg
Liver, 3 oz.	370 mg
Kidney, 3 oz.	680 mg
Brains, 3 oz.	1,700 mg

The most common source of cholesterol in the diet is egg yolk. Only about half of the consumed cholesterol is absorbed. Additionally, the human liver itself synthesizes 1,000 to 1,500 mg of cholesterol a day.

increases in lipid and cholesterol levels in their blood (McMurry et al., 1991).

Some studies indicate that environmental chemicals and pollutants may damage cells in the lining of the blood vessels and initiate the formation of plaques. Thus, the same factors that trigger changes in cells that lead to cancer may also be risk factors in cardiovascular disease. In particular, cigarette smoking, high blood cholesterol levels, and high blood pressure are well documented risk factors that contribute to the development of both atherosclerosis and heart disease (Figure 10.4). Physical inactivity, stress, and high levels of glucose in the blood are additional factors that contribute to the risk of a heart attack once the blood supply to the heart has been restricted.

Cholesterol

Cholesterol is an essential component of body cells and is synthesized in the body as well as being obtained from food (Table 10.1). Cholesterol circulates in the blood mostly in the form of particles consisting of proteins, triglycerides (fats), and cholesterol. These particles are divided into two kinds. Called **high-density lipoproteins (HDL)** and **low-density lipoproteins (LDL),** their functions are different and, in some sense, are opposite to one another. Other kinds of cholesterol-carrying particles also are found in the blood, but these are ultimately converted into LDL particles.

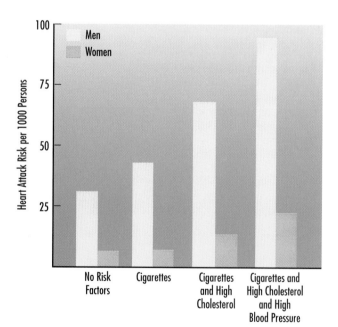

FIGURE 10.4   How Risk of Heart Attack Increases The graph shows how risk increases for a male or female, age 55, with the following risk factors: smoking 20 cigarettes per day, having a blood cholesterol level over 260 mg/dl, and having a systolic blood pressure over 150 mm Hg.

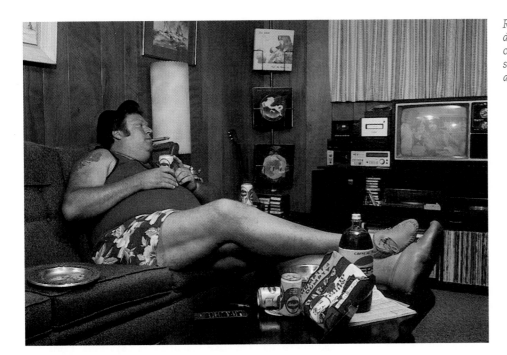

Risk factors for cardiovascular disease include being overweight, a sedentary life-style, smoking, and excessive alcohol consumption.

People differ markedly in their ability to process excess cholesterol, just as they differ in other traits. The most dramatic example of cholesterol metabolism is that of an 88-year-old man who had eaten twenty-five eggs a day for over fifteen years and yet had completely normal blood cholesterol levels (Kern, 1991).

At the other extreme are persons with a rare inherited disease called **familial hyperlipidemia (FH)**, which results in markedly elevated levels of cholesterol in the blood. People with this disease have two defective genes, one inherited from each unaffected parent. The normal forms of these genes are responsible for synthesizing LDL receptor proteins on liver cells that remove cholesterol from the blood. As a result of their defective genes, people with FH cannot synthesize these essential LDL receptor proteins. Cholesterol cannot be removed and processed in the liver, and it accumulates to exceptionally high levels in the blood. People with this disease usually have heart attacks at an early age. In a few cases, transplant of a normal liver has successfully reversed the effects of FH to a significant degree.

Measuring Cholesterol Levels Cholesterol and lipid levels in the blood are measured in various ways. Total cholesterol levels are measured in milligrams per deciliter (mg/dl) of blood. Generally, a cholesterol level below 200 mg/dl indicates relatively low risk of coronary heart disease (CHD); 240 mg/dl or higher doubles the risk of CHD. Blood cholesterol values between 200–239 mg/dl indicate moderate and increasing risk of CHD. However, the total cholesterol level may not be a reliable indicator of cardiovascular dis-

ease risk because the level of HDL in the blood is also important and can modify the risk inherent in high cholesterol levels.

Extensive research has shown a strong association between blood cholesterol levels and coronary heart disease; the higher the blood cholesterol level, the greater the risk of all forms of cardiovascular disease. However, many epidemiological studies show cholesterol levels are not always a reliable predictor of heart disease.

For example, the French enjoy a diet laden with eggs, meats, and fats. They have cholesterol levels that, on average, are much higher than those of Americans. Yet the French die of heart disease at less than half the rate observed in the United States (sometimes called the "French paradox"). Nobody can give a satisfactory explanation for the discrepancy; some heart experts attribute it to drinking wine with meals (which may reduce stress) and eating more vegetables (which may be protective in some way). Cholesterol level is a risk factor for cardiovascular disease, but the level at which it becomes a risk is still extremely controversial.

Terms

high-density lipoprotein (HDL): the carrier of cholesterol from tissues to the liver for removal from the circulation; carrier of "good" cholesterol

low-density lipoprotein (LDL): the carrier of "bad" cholesterol in blood

familial hyperlipidemia (FH): an inherited disease causing extremely high levels of cholesterol in the blood

High Blood Pressure

Medical surveys indicate that one in every four Americans suffers from **hypertension,** blood pressure that is above the range that is considered normal. About one-third of these individuals are unaware of their hypertension, which contributes to stroke and heart and kidney disease. The cause of high blood pressure in 90% to 95% of cases is unknown; the medical term for this is **essential hypertension.**

The remaining cases of high blood pressure are symptoms of a recognizable problem, such as a kidney abnormality, congenital defect of the aorta, or adrenal gland tumor. This type of high blood pressure is called **secondary hypertension.** Generally, when the cause of secondary hypertension is determined and corrected, blood pressure returns to normal.

High blood pressure may be caused by psychosocial factors, although the mechanisms by which these factors could cause it are not understood. For example, people with low income and poor education are at higher risk for high blood pressure. Being poor or jobless may generate stress and raise blood pressure.

Black and Hispanic Americans have a higher rate of high blood pressure than white Americans. The stress of being a member of a minority group may also increase the risk of high blood pressure and heart disease. Hypertension is a disease of modern societies; even today tribes in New Guinea or the forests of Brazil do not develop hypertension when they grow old.

High blood pressure is a major risk factor for heart attacks and stroke because blood vessels in the heart or brain are more likely to rupture under increased pressure. Hypertension is often called the "silent killer" because it is a disease without symptoms until something serious occurs. As many as 50 million Americans have high blood pressure, which can occur even in young children.

Each time the heart contracts, blood is pumped through the arteries and exerts pressure on the arterial walls (Figure 10.5). In fact, there are two pressures that are measured. The maximum pressure in the arteries occurs when the heart contracts (**systole**), pumping blood from the heart to the lungs and body. Between

---

Wellness Guide

Known Risk Factors for Heart Disease

Major Risk Factors That Cannot Be Changed

- **Heredity:** Both heart disease and atherosclerosis appear to be linked to heredity. If your parents have had heart disease, or if you are an African-American, your risk of heart disease is greater than that of the population at large.

- **Sex:** Men have a greater risk of heart disease than women early in life. However, after women reach menopause, their death rate from heart disease increases. Research indicates the potential reason for this is the decrease in estrogen after menopause.

- **Age:** The majority of people who die from heart attacks are age 65 or older.

Major Risk Factors That Can Be Changed

- **Smoking:** People who smoke are twice as likely to have a heart attack as those who do not smoke. Cigarette smoking is the greatest risk

factor for sudden cardiac death. Studies also indicate that chronic exposure to environmental tobacco smoke increases the risk of heart disease.

- **High blood cholesterol:** As your blood cholesterol level increases, so does your risk of coronary heart disease. A person's cholesterol level is affected by age, gender, heredity, and diet. With other risk factors such as high blood pressure and smoking, your risk of coronary heart disease increases even more.

- **High blood pressure (HBP):** High blood pressure is sometimes referred to as the "silent killer," because there are no specific symptoms or early warning signs. Eating properly, losing weight, exercising, and restricting sodium all will help reduce HBP. People with this factor should work with their doctor to control it.

- **Physical inactivity:** Physical inactivity is a risk factor for heart disease. Regular aerobic

exercise plays a significant role in preventing heart disease; even modest levels of low intensity physical activity are beneficial if done regularly over the long term.

Other Contributing Factors

- **Diabetes:** More than 80% of people with diabetes die of some form of heart disease or blood vessel disease.

- **Obesity:** If you are overweight, overfat, or obese, you are more likely than a person of normal weight to have heart disease, despite the fact you may not have any other risk factors.

- **Individual response to stress:** There is some evidence of a relationship between coronary heart disease and stress, behavior, habits, and socioeconomic status.

Source: Adapted from *Heart and Stroke Facts* (1999). (Dallas, TX.: American Heart Association).

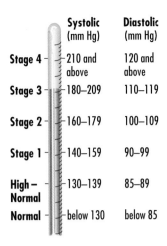

	Systolic (mm Hg)	Diastolic (mm Hg)
Stage 4	210 and above	120 and above
Stage 3	180–209	110–119
Stage 2	160–179	100–109
Stage 1	140–159	90–99
High Normal	130–139	85–89
Normal	below 130	below 85

FIGURE 10.5 **Stages of High Blood Pressure** According to current guidelines, normal blood pressure is 140/90 (systolic/diastolic) or below. High blood pressure (hypertension) is defined in four stages, the risk of heart disease being greater the higher the blood pressure. Weight loss, exercise, not smoking, and stress reduction are recommended ways to control hypertension at earlier stages; drugs may also be necessary at later stages.

contractions, the pressure falls (**diastole**) as blood flows from one chamber of the heart to another. Normal blood pressure is defined as a value less than 140/90 mm Hg (systole/diastole). Generally, the diastolic pressure is considered the more significant of the two with respect to health risk. A person with a diastolic pressure of 120 has double the risk of a heart attack or stroke compared to a person with a diastolic pressure of 90.

High blood pressure can be lowered by making certain changes in lifestyle. Obesity and excessive intake of calories are major risk factors that can be changed; increasing physical exercise also is required to reduce hypertension. Moderating salt and alcohol consumption also is beneficial. And ensuring that you are obtaining an adequate amount of potassium (eat more bananas) will also reduce blood pressure.

Blood pressure is the result of two forces. The first is created by the heart as it pumps blood into the arteries, the second created by the arterial blood vessels as they resist blood flow from the heart. Tiny receptors in the walls of the arteries respond to changes in blood pressure. If blood pressure rises, these receptors send signals to the nerves to relax the arteries and to slow down the heartbeat, thus returning blood pressure to normal levels. However, these regulatory mechanisms can be overcome by signals from the brain. Arteries can be constricted and blood pressure raised by thoughts and emotions. Fear, tension, anger, and anxiety activate the sympathetic nervous system, which sends signals to the arteries causing them to constrict. If one's life is overly stressful or full of anger and frustration, arteries may stay constricted and blood pressure remain elevated.

While drugs are the most expedient (and profitable) means of controlling hypertension, mental relaxation techniques are also effective. Many studies demonstrate that a variety of relaxation techniques are effective in lowering blood pressure in hypertensive patients. However, working with people to lower blood pressure through relaxation techniques is time-consuming and costly in a modern medical setting, so physicians prescribe antihypertensive drugs.

One of the lessons of history is that nothing is sometimes a good thing to do and often a clever thing to say.
WILL DURANT

Cigarettes and Cardiovascular Disease

Smoking cigarettes is another major risk factor contributing to the development of cardiovascular disease, heart attacks, and strokes. Smokers are at two to four times greater risk of dying from a heart attack than nonsmokers. The risk of heart disease from tobacco smoke extends to those who breathe secondhand smoke at work or at home (He et al., 1994). The more tobacco smoke a person is exposed to, the greater the risk of cardiovascular disease and a heart attack. Tobacco smoke is the most dangerous environmental pollutant known and is a major contributor to both heart disease and cancer.

Stopping smoking at any time can reverse many of the harmful physiological effects of tobacco on the cardiovascular system. After several years of not smoking, ex-smokers have about the same risk of cardiovascular disease as nonsmokers. One key to protecting your heart is not smoking and not living or working in a smoke-filled environment.

Diet and Cardiovascular Disease

As already mentioned, diet plays a major role in heart disease, especially as it contributes to being overweight and overfat and to elevated levels of cholesterol.

Terms

hypertension: high blood pressure

essential hypertension: high blood pressure that is not caused by any observable disease

secondary hypertension: high blood pressure caused by a recognizable disease

systole: the pressure in the arteries when the heart contracts (the higher number)

diastole: the pressure in the arteries when the heart relaxes (the lower number)

However, certain foods and vitamins in the diet seem to provide some protection from cardiovascular disease.

Vitamin E

While the oxygen gas that we breathe is essential to life, uncombined oxygen atoms in cells can react with many substances and cause damage. For example, consider what happens to iron that is exposed to the oxygen in air under moist conditions; it quickly rusts and disintegrates. Body tissues also can be destroyed by oxygen atoms. The body has many mechanisms for protecting cellular constituents from oxidation, among them the antioxidant action of vitamin C and vitamin E (Diaz et al., 1997).

Vitamin E acts as an antioxidant in blood and reduces the amount of oxidized LDL that is formed. When volunteers took vitamin E supplements (800 IU), their LDL particles were more resistant to oxidation. Also, a study of 2000 patients with CHD found that those who took 400 to 800 IU of vitamin E every day for 2 years had a 37% lower risk of heart disease compared to a group of men who did not take the vitamin supplement. (Rimm et al., 1993). A similar benefit from vitamin E was also reported for women.

B Vitamins

Other vitamins that protect against heart disease are three B vitamins, B_6, B_{12}, and folic acid (folate). As described above, high levels of the amino acid homocysteine are associated with atherosclerosis and heart disease. People with high levels of homocysteine in their blood also had low levels of the three B vitamins. On the other hand, people with low homocysteine levels had high levels of the B vitamins and were less likely to develop heart disease.

The key B vitamins can be obtained from food; however, many people do not obtain enough in their diets (Table 10.2). The evidence that B vitamins do, in fact, protect against heart disease is now strong enough that some health authorities recommend taking them in a daily multivitamin supplement.

Vitamin C

Like vitamin E, vitamin C is an antioxidant and can neutralize destructive oxygen atoms and other oxidizing substances called **free radicals** in the blood. These may damage the elastic tissues in arteries that allow blood vessels to expand and contract. If a blood vessel is damaged and cannot relax, blood pressure rises. Vitamin C prevents such damage from occurring by eliminating the free radical compounds in blood. Taking up to a gram of vitamin C supplement a day is safe; any that is not used is excreted in urine. However, taking megadoses of vitamin C (10 grams a day) can cause serious side effects, such as stomach irritation and kidney stones.

Calcium

Food profile studies indicate that half or more of all Americans of both sexes consume amounts of calcium that are less than the recommended amounts for bone development and health. Populations that are especially at risk are African Americans, pregnant women, obese persons, and elderly persons. Unless you consume foods that are high in calcium, such as milk and cheese, your daily calcium intake may be low.

Calcium deficiency is not only a risk factor for osteoporosis in women, it is also a significant risk factor for hypertension in persons of all ages (McCarron and Hatton, 1996). Calcium is readily obtained in the diet but levels can also be increased by taking calcium supplements, which cost much less and are much safer than antihypertensive medications.

Soy Products

Soybeans have been cultivated around the world for thousands of years; the Chinese name for soybean is *ta-tou*, which means "greater bean." Soy seems to boost the activity of LDL receptors in the liver, and thereby helps to remove cholesterol from the blood. Soy also seems to block oxidation of the LDL particles, which prevents them from sticking to the walls of arteries.

Studies in which people ate 1 to 2 ounces of soy daily showed that both cholesterol and LDL levels dropped about 10%. Other studies indicate that soy is especially effective among people with cholesterol levels above 240 mg/dL. Soy products are available in a multitude of products, such as soy sauce, soy milk, soft and firm tofu, and tofu burgers.

Fish Oils

Populations that consume large amounts of fish in their diets—Greenland Eskimos and Japanese islanders—have lower rates of CHD than others. Americans who consume fish regularly in their diets also

Vitamin	Foods
B_6	Meat, poultry, nuts, whole grain cereals, fish, green leafy vegetables
B_{12}	Meat, organ meats, eggs, dairy products, fish
Folic acid	Green leafy vegetables, fruits, liver, brewer's yeast, dried beans and peas, wheat germ

TABLE 10.2   Food Sources for B-Vitamins

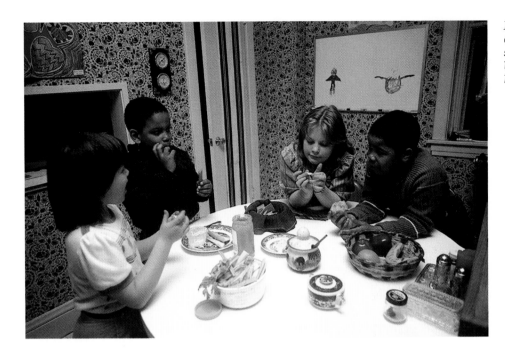

It's important to encourage children to eat heart-healthy snacks, so they won't have to break bad eating habits later in life.

have healthier hearts (Daviglus et al., 1997). The protective effects of dietary fish have been ascribed to fish oils, in particular to n-3-polyunsaturated oils. In some studies, supplements of fish oil have reduced levels of cholesterol and blood pressure.

One of the best studies demonstrating the beneficial effect of fish was carried out in Tanzania among Bantu villagers. One group of Bantu lived on the shores of a lake, and people consumed about a pound of fish a day. The other Bantu population lived in nearby hills and had a diet that consisted primarily of vegetables. The Bantu people who ate fish had high levels of n-3-polyunsaturated oils in their blood. They also had lower levels of cholesterol and lipoproteins (Pauletto et al., 1996). Sardines, salmon, and mackerel have high levels of n-3-polyunsaturated oils, but all fish have some.

Tea

Both green and black tea contain antioxidant chemicals that help block oxidation of LDL particles in the blood; herb teas do not contain antioxidants. Consuming green or black tea helps protect the coronary arteries in a manner similar to that of the C and E antioxidant vitamins. Asian people drink green tea daily, which may contribute to their reduced risk of CHD.

Aspirin

A commonly used drug can significantly reduce the risk of CHD and heart attacks. Aspirin helps to "thin" blood and also acts to combat inflammation, which increases the risk of a heart attack. Hundreds of studies have been carried out in which aspirin was given to both healthy people and to people who had had a

heart attack or stroke. In all studies, small amounts of aspirin (either a half tablet daily or a whole tablet taken every other day) reduced the risk of a heart attack.

It is now recommended that if you think you might be having a heart attack, first call 911 and then take a couple of aspirin, which will help prevent clotting. Whether healthy people who are at low risk of a heart attack should take aspirin on a regular basis is still an open question. As with vitamin supplements or drinking alcohol, each person must decide what is best for his or her health.

Alcohol

A large study of 275,000 middle-aged men showed that one or two drinks a day over 12 years reduced their risk of dying from a heart attack by about 20% in comparison to men who did not drink alcohol. However, more than two drinks a day *increases* the risk of a heart attack significantly. Women also experienced a benefit from a daily drink or two, but the small benefit to the heart is offset by a slight increased risk of cancer.

Although moderate alcohol drinking does have some health benefits, the issue of drinking is so controversial (and potentially harmful) that no recommendation can be made to drink because it may protect you from a heart attack. With the increased

Terms

free radicals: oxidizing substances in the body that can damage blood vessels and tissues

attention given to risk factors that cause cardiovascular disease, people are now armed with knowledge about reducing their chances of heart attacks and stroke. Cardiovascular disease can be prevented by adopting good health habits now!

Preventing Cancer

On the basis of recent statistics, one out of two men and one out of three women in the United States will develop some type of cancer during their lifetime. Despite the dismal statistics, the news about cancer is not all bad. Most cancers *are* preventable if people adopt healthy life-styles. Avoiding cigarette smoke and tobacco in *any* form is the most important action anyone can take to avoid cancer, especially lung and pancreatic cancers, which are most often incurable. Cigarette smoke is estimated to be the primary cause in the development of at least 30% of all cancers.

> *Statistics are like a bathing suit; what they reveal is interesting but what they conceal is significant.*
> ANONYMOUS

A healthy diet that includes low levels of animal fat and high levels of fresh fruits, vegetables, and grains will also markedly reduce the risk of cancer. Avoiding ultraviolet (UV) radiation in sunshine helps prevent skin cancer later in life. Finally, knowing what chemicals in the environment are cancer-causing can help you avoid dangerous substances. Overall, if

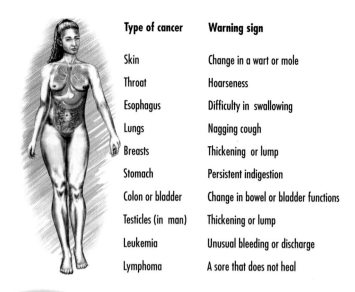

Type of cancer	Warning sign
Skin	Change in a wart or mole
Throat	Hoarseness
Esophagus	Difficulty in swallowing
Lungs	Nagging cough
Breasts	Thickening or lump
Stomach	Persistent indigestion
Colon or bladder	Change in bowel or bladder functions
Testicles (in man)	Thickening or lump
Leukemia	Unusual bleeding or discharge
Lymphoma	A sore that does not heal

FIGURE 10.6 **Some Warning Signs of Cancer** If any of these symptoms occur, see a physician promptly.

everything known about cancer prevention were practiced by everyone, up to two-thirds of *all* cancers could be prevented.

Another positive note is that about half of all cancer patients can be cured if their cancer is detected at an early stage before cancer cells have spread. Being "cured" of cancer means that a person's life expectancy is the same as for a person who never had cancer. It is important to have cancer screening tests as indicated for your age and risk group; tests for the

TABLE 10.3 **American Cancer Society Recommendations for the Early Detection of Cancer**

Test	Population Sex	Age	Frequency of testing
Sigmoidoscopy, preferably flexible	M & F	50 and over	Every 3–5 years
Fecal occult blood test	M & F	50 and over	Every year
Digital rectal exam	M & F	40 and over	Every year
Prostate exam*	M	50 and over	Every year
Pap test	F		All women who are, or who have been, sexually active, or have reached age 18, should have an annual Pap test and pelvic examination. After a woman has had three or more consecutive satisfactory normal annual examinations, the Pap test may be performed less frequently at the discretion of her physician.
Breast self-examination	F	20 and over	Every month
Breast clinical examination	F	20–40 Over 40	Every 3 years Every year
Mammography†	F	40–49 50 and over	Every 1–2 years Every year

*Annual digital rectal examination and prostate-specific antigen test should be performed on men 50 years and older. If either result is abnormal, further evaluation should be considered.

†Screening mammography should begin by age 40.

Source: Reprinted by the permission of the American Cancer Society.

early detection of breast, colon, prostate, and cervical cancers are recommended by the American Cancer Society (Table 10.3). You should also watch for early warning signs in functions of the body that may indicate that a cancer is developing (Figure 10.6).

Understanding Cancer

Incidence of Various Cancers

Cancers of the stomach, uterus, cervix, and testis and Hodgkin's disease have declined significantly in recent years. However, cancers of the lung, skin, liver, prostate, and kidney and non-Hodgkin's lymphoma have all increased in frequency. Overall, the mortality from cancer has remained virtually unchanged over the last generation.

The most serious increase has been the continuing rise in lung cancer in both men and women. Increases in lung cancer in men began to be noticed in the 1940s; in women, the increase did not become apparent until the 1960s. As everyone knows, the reason for the increase in lung cancer among both men and women is cigarette smoking. Women now die from lung cancer about half as often as men, and their rate of death is still increasing.

What Is Cancer?

The term *cancer* comes from the Latin word meaning crab. Cancer was characterized as a crablike disease by the Greek physician Hippocrates, who observed that cancers spread throughout the body, eventually cutting off life. Now **cancer** generally is defined as the unregulated growth of specific cells in the body. The word cancer actually refers to over 100 different diseases, but in all cases, certain body cells multiply in an abnormal, unregulated manner.

Normally, the growth and reproduction of every cell in the body are regulated; this regulation, in turn, determines the size and functions of tissues and organs. If a normal body cell begins to grow abnormally and reproduces too rapidly, a mass of abnormal cells eventually develops that is called a **tumor.** A tumor generally contains millions of genetically identical abnormal cells before it can be detected or felt.

If the cells of the tumor remain localized at the site of origin in the body and if they multiply relatively slowly, the tumor is said to be benign. **Benign tumors,** such as cysts, warts, moles, and polyps, do not spread to other parts of the body. Benign tumors usually can be removed surgically and generally are not a threat to life. In fact, benign tumors weighing several hundred pounds have been surgically removed from persons who then recovered fully. Benign tumors

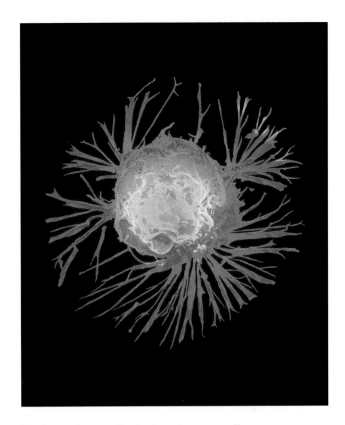

Electron micrograph of a breast cancer cell.

cannot regrow if all of the abnormal cells are removed by surgical excision of the tumor.

Malignant tumors are composed of cells that grow rapidly, have other abnormal properties that distinguish them from normal cells, and invade other normal tissues. In particular, malignant cells may have altered shapes and cell-surface characteristics that contribute to their rapid proliferation. Many malignant cells also have abnormal chromosomes or altered genes, and they manufacture abnormal proteins. The numerous altered properties of malignant cells enable a **pathologist,** who is a physician who specializes in the causes of diseases, to determine whether the cells removed from a tumor are abnormal and to what degree.

The cells of most malignant tumors also undergo **metastasis,** a process in which cells detach from the

Terms

cancer: unregulated growth of cells in the body

tumor: a mass of abnormal cells

benign tumor: a tumor whose cells do not spread to other parts of the body

malignant tumor: a tumor whose cells spread throughout the body

pathologist: a physician who specializes in the causes of diseases

metastasis: the process by which cancer cells spread throughout the body

FIGURE 10.7 *Four Major Categories of Cancers and Approximate Frequencies of Occurrence*

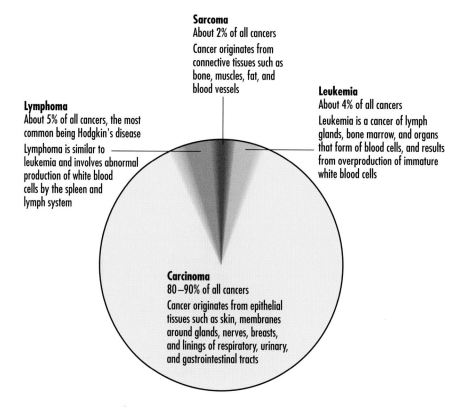

Sarcoma
About 2% of all cancers
Cancer originates from connective tissues such as bone, muscles, fat, and blood vessels

Leukemia
About 4% of all cancers
Leukemia is a cancer of lymph glands, bone marrow, and organs that form of blood cells, and results from overproduction of immature white blood cells

Lymphoma
About 5% of all cancers, the most common being Hodgkin's disease
Lymphoma is similar to leukemia and involves abnormal production of white blood cells by the spleen and lymph system

Carcinoma
80–90% of all cancers
Cancer originates from epithelial tissues such as skin, membranes around glands, nerves, breasts, and linings of respiratory, urinary, and gastrointestinal tracts

original tumor, enter the lymphatic system and bloodstream, and are carried to other organs. Once the malignant cells spread to other organs, they develop into new tumors that often grow more rapidly than cells in the original tumor. Metastases and the growth of new tumors in many organs of the body eventually disrupt a vital body function, which is the cause of death.

Cancers are medically classified according to the organ or kind of tissue in which the tumor originates. The four major categories of cancers are *carcinomas, sarcomas, leukemias,* and *lymphomas* (Figure 10.7). Within these major categories are numerous subgroups that generally describe the organ in which the cancer originates, such as adenocarcinoma of the stomach or oat cell carcinoma of the lung. About half of all human cancers originate in one of four organs: the lung, breast, prostate, or colon, which is why so much research is devoted to these particular forms.

Cancer does not develop all at once in a cell. Several changes must occur in the genetic information (i.e., DNA) carried in a single cell before it can become a cancer cell and multiply into a tumor. Cells change their abnormal growth properties one step at a time; each genetic change pushes the cell further along the spectrum of abnormal growth. Not all cells acquire the same genetic changes nor can anyone predict when the changes will occur. That explains to some extent why some cancers develop and grow rapidly and cause death in months; other cancers may grow so slowly that the person eventually dies from a cause other than cancer.

Once a tumor has been detected, cells can be removed from it in a procedure called a **biopsy;** the cells are then examined under the microscope by a pathologist. In stage I, cancer cells can be distinguished from normal cells. The cancer cells are still localized (usually referred to as cancer *in situ*) and surgical removal of the tumor usually results in a cure. In stage II, the cancer cells have begun to metastasize and may have migrated to nearby lymph nodes. That is why lymph nodes near the tumor are removed and examined during surgery to determine if cancer cells have spread. By stage III, the cancer cells have spread throughout the body, and tumors may have begun to grow in other organs. In stage IV, often a terminal stage, tumors are found throughout the body and usually are resistant to treatment.

Causes of Cancer

Most Cancers Are Not Inherited

Scientific studies indicate that 90% to 95% of all cancers, including breast, lung, stomach, colon, skin, or prostate, are *not* inherited from parents except in a few rare families in which members do inherit one or more cancer-susceptibility genes.

However, the genes in the chromosomes of any cell of your body, such as skin, lung, or stomach cells, can be chemically changed by environmental agents. These genetic changes in skin, lung, or stomach cells

TABLE 10.4   Environmental and Life-Style Risk Factors that Contribute to Cancer

Factor	Amount of risk	Types of cancer

Nutrition	About *half* of cancer deaths are caused by nutritional problems:
	    Excess calories
	    Excess fat consumption
	    Obesity
	Nutritional deficiencies, especially fiber and vitamin A
		Cancers of the colon, rectum, stomach, breast, and ovaries

Cigarettes and alcohol	About *one-third* of cancer deaths are caused by smoking cigarettes and excessive alcohol consumption	Cancers of the lung, pancreas, mouth, larynx, liver, esophagus, and bladder
Occupation	About 5% of cancer deaths are caused by substances in the workplace such as asbestos, benzene, and vinyl chloride	Cancers of the bladder, lung, stomach, blood, liver, bones, and skin
Radiation	About 3% of cancer deaths are caused by ionizing radiation, such as x-rays and ultraviolet light	Blood, skin
Other	Other cancer deaths result from heredity, chronic disease, drugs, and chemotherapy	Various cancers

may transform them into cancer cells. Thus, cancer is a genetic disease in that genes are changed in a person's body cells; however, it is *not* an inherited disease because defective genes were not passed on from parents in most cases.

Even if several close family members have died of cancer, it does not mean that cancer "runs in the family" and is an inherited disease. Currently, one out of every five deaths each year in the United States is due to cancer (American Cancer Society, 1999). If your parents and eight aunts or uncles died, probably two or three of them died of cancer simply by chance. If they all smoked cigarettes, it would not be surprising if more than three close relatives out of ten died of cancer.

Environmental Factors

The causes of cancer or, more correctly, the risk factors associated with the development of cancer are numerous and complex. It often is difficult to point to a single cause of a cancer, but certain environmental factors are strongly correlated with the occurrence of particular cancers. Two examples are the strong correlation between cigarette smoking and lung cancer and exposure to ultraviolet (UV) light and skin cancer. Even in these examples, not everyone who smokes heavily or stays in the sun day after day will get cancer.

Epidemiology is the branch of science that investigates the causes and frequencies of diseases in human populations. Many epidemiological studies show that as many as 80% to 90% of cancers are caused by exposure to environmental factors that are known to increase the risk of cancer (Table 10.4). For example, smoking cigarettes while young puts a person at 10 to 20 times higher risk of developing cancer later in life than persons who do not smoke. Eating fat-laden ham-

burgers and pizza frequently may be convenient, but it is ultimately unhealthy and may contribute to the development of certain cancers (Davis and Freeman, 1994). Because each of us can change our diets, stop smoking, and avoid other cancer-causing risks in the environment, preventing cancer is a realistic and attainable goal for most people.

Radiation and chemical carcinogens (cancer-causing chemicals) have been shown to increase the risk of cancer in both laboratory animals and people. Each of these agents increases the risk of cancer by producing chemical changes in genes that can cause cancer. If a cell undergoes one or more mutations in genes that regulate its growth, it may begin to multiply rapidly and develop into a tumor.

Ionizing Radiation

Ionizing radiation consists of x-rays, UV light, and radioactivity whose energy can damage cells and chromosomes. The high rate of leukemia among survivors of the Hiroshima and Nagasaki atomic bomb blasts in 1945 leaves no doubt that radioactivity increases the risk of cancer.

In the United States, among children born in southern Utah in the 1950s who were exposed to radioactive fallout from nearby atomic tests, leukemia deaths were two to three times greater than among

Terms

biopsy: removal of cells from a tumor for examination under a microscope

epidemiology: a branch of science that studies the causes and frequencies of diseases in human populations

ionizing radiation: radiation, such as x-rays, that can damage cells and cause cancer; also used to treat cancer

children born in southern Utah before and after the atomic tests. In a landmark legal decision in 1984, a federal court ruled that the U.S. government was negligent in conducting atomic bomb tests in southern Utah in the 1950s because they released radioactive material into the atmosphere. The court ruled that the families who were exposed to radioactivity as a result of these tests, and whose members died as a result of exposure to the radioactivity, were entitled to compensation.

Because any amount of ionizing radiation, however small, has the potential for causing damage to chromosomes and genes, one should minimize exposure to x-rays. For example, if you are healthy, periodic chest x-rays are unnecessary. Dental x-rays with each 6-month checkup also pose a cumulative risk. Some homes release radon, a radioactive gas present in some building materials. Long-term exposure to the invisible radon gas contributes to the risk of cancer.

The most common source of ionizing radiation is UV radiation in sunlight. Because children and young people tend to play in the sun, people acquire as much as 80% of their lifetime UV exposure by age 20.

Ultraviolet radiation in sunlight is characterized by two different wavelengths, called UVA and UVB. Until recently, it was thought that only UVB was dangerous, but now it appears that both forms of UV radiation are harmful. Reducing the time of exposure to intense sunlight and using sunscreen creams to protect exposed areas of the body reduce the risk of skin cancer.

Chemical Carcinogens

A **chemical carcinogen** is an environmental chemical that can interact with cells to initiate cancer, usually by chemically altering the chromosomes or genes in cells.

Many chemicals are now tested to determine their cancer-causing potential. Unfortunately, many thousands of chemical substances already in use have not been adequately tested. Of the thousands of chemical substances that have been tested, many have been found to be carcinogenic and should be avoided if at all possible. Carcinogens include cigarette smoke, pesticides, asbestos, heavy metals (lead, mercury, cadmium), benzene, and nitrosamines (Table 10.5).

Despite the long list of carcinogenic substances, some scientists and public health officials argue that tobacco is the only substance of consequence with respect to the numbers of cancers caused. While the argument has some basis, it is of small consolation to persons who acquire cancer from exposure, often without their knowledge, to carcinogenic substances in the environment or workplace.

In some industries, workers have cancers that almost never arise in the general population. For example, **mesothelioma** is a rare form of lung cancer that only occurs among persons exposed to asbestos fibers. Long-term exposure to the heavy metals beryllium and cadmium increases workers' risk of prostate cancer. Workers exposed to vinyl chloride, the starting material for polyvinyl chloride (PVC) pipes and other products, develop a rare form of liver cancer not found

TABLE 10.5   Examples of Occupational Cancers

Chemical/physical agent	Cancer type	Exposure of general population	Examples of workers frequently exposed or exposure sources
Arsenic	Lung, skin	Rare	Insecticide and herbicide sprayers; tanners; oil refinery workers
Asbestos	Mesothelioma, lung	Uncommon	Brake-lining, shipyard, insulation, and demolition workers
Benzene	Myelogenous leukemia	Common	Painters; distillers and petrochemical workers; dye users; furniture finishers; rubber workers
Diesel exhaust	Lung	Common	Railroad and bus-garage workers; truck operators; miners
Formaldehyde	Nose, nasopharynx	Rare	Hospital and laboratory workers; manufacture of wood products, paper, textiles, garments, and metal products
Man-made mineral fibers	Lung	Uncommon	Wall and pipe insulation; duct wrapping
Hair dyes	Bladder	Uncommon	Hairdressers and barbers (inadequate evidence for customers)
Ionizing radiation	Bone marrow, several others	Common	Nuclear materials; medicinal products and procedures
Mineral oils	Skin	Common	Metal machining
Nonarsenical pesticides	Lung	Common	Sprayers; agricultural workers
Painting materials	Lung	Uncommon	Professional painters
Polychlorinated biphenyls	Liver, skin	Uncommon	Heat-transfer and hydraulic fluids and lubricants; inks; adhesives; insecticides
Radon (alpha particles)	Lung	Uncommon	Mines; underground structures; homes
Soot	Skin	Uncommon	Chimney sweeps and cleaners; bricklayers; insulators; firefighters; heating-unit service workers

in the general public. Fortunately, with current occupational and safety regulations, these types of cancer occur infrequently.

The total number of cancers attributable to industrial chemicals is small compared to those caused by tobacco and diet, however, cancers caused by industrial chemicals are preventable or avoidable. Before you accept a job it might be wise to determine what chemicals you will be exposed to for long periods.

Do Xenoestrogens Cause Cancer?

Estrogens are hormones that regulate a variety of biological functions in women, including the growth and development of breast tissue. Many chemicals that we are exposed to in the environment mimic the action of normal estrogen to some degree; such chemicals are called **xenoestrogens** (literally, foreign estrogen). Exposure to xenoestrogens in the environment may cause breast cancer (Davis and Bradlow, 1995).

Substances that contain xenoestrogens include the pesticides DDT (now banned in the U.S., but still used elsewhere), methoxyclor, kepone, chlordane, atrazine, and endosulfan. Polychlorinated biphenyls (PCBs), which were used in electrical transformers for many years, also are xenoestrogens. Bisphenol-A, a component of polycarbonate plastics that are widely used, can leach into liquids when the plastic bottles are heated. Even the gasoline vapor inhaled at the pump can act as a xenoestrogen.

The effects of xenoestrogens can be tested on human cells grown in the laboratory. Normal estrogen binds to many cells and affects their growth. Xenoestrogens bind to the same cellular receptors as normal estrogen and exert some of the same effects on the growth of cells. The evidence that xenoestrogens can affect cell proliferation and reproductive organs is now well established.

Since 1976, when chlorinated pesticides were banned in Israel, and all pesticide residues eliminated from milk products, the incidence of breast cancer among Israeli women has been declining. Israel is the only industrialized country that has not experienced an increase in breast cancer in the past 20 years. These observations also lend support to the idea that xenoestrogens contribute to development of breast cancer.

It is impossible to avoid all exposure to xenoestrogens since they are everywhere in the environment. But certainly avoid unnecessary exposure. Also, eating broccoli, cabbage, and soy products may help counteract the effects of xenoestrogens. This advice comes from the observation that Asian women have much lower rates of breast cancer in comparison to white or black American women. Asian diets are richer in these vegetables, which may contain chemicals that block the biological activities of the xenoestrogens.

Common Cancers

Lung Cancer

Lung cancer causes more deaths among men and women than any other form of cancer. Smoking cigarettes is the primary cause of 80% to 90% of lung cancers; thus, it is almost a completely preventable disease if people would stop smoking tobacco. Most cases of lung cancer are detected only after considerable development and only after cancer cells have already spread to other parts of the body. In most forms of lung cancer, the abnormal cells are resistant to chemotherapy; however, one form of lung cancer called small-cell carcinoma often does respond to chemotherapy. Overall, the 5-year survival rate for people with a diagnosis of lung cancer is between 10% and 15%—not very good odds.

The rate of lung cancer in other nations is rising rapidly as more and more people take up cigarette smoking. China and other developing nations will have to cope with an epidemic of lung cancer early in the next century. The concerted effort in the U.S. to get people to stop smoking and to prevent access of young people to cigarettes is an attempt to reverse the epidemic of lung cancer in this country.

Breast Cancer

Both men and women can develop breast cancer, but it occurs very rarely among men. Although more women die from lung cancer than breast cancer, more than twice as many women had breast cancer as had lung cancer in 1997 in the U.S. Since 1940, the incidence of breast cancer among American women has more than doubled.

Increased weight, less exercise, and increased dietary fat have all been proposed as factors contributing to the increased rate of breast cancer. Other factors that increase the risk of breast cancer among women to varying degrees are:

- Mother who had breast cancer before age 60
- Onset of menarche before age 14
- First child born after age 30
- No biological children
- Menopause after age 55
- Benign breast disease

Terms

chemical carcinogen: a chemical that damages cells and causes cancer

mesothelioma: a form of lung cancer caused by asbestos

xenoestrogens: environmental chemicals that mimic the effects of natural estrogen

Wellness Guide

How to Examine Your Breasts

1. Lie down and put a pillow under your right shoulder. Place your right arm behind your head.

2. Use the finger pads of your three middle fingers on your left hand to feel for lumps or thickening. Your finger pads are the top third of each finger.

3. Press firmly enough to know how your breast feels. If you're not sure how hard to press, ask your health care provider. Or try to copy the way your health care provider uses the finger pads during a breast exam. Learn what your breast feels like most of the time. A firm ridge in the lower curve of each breast is normal.

4. Move around the breast in a set way. You can choose either the circle (a), the up and down line (b), or the wedge (c). Do it the same way every time. It will help you to make sure that you've gone over the entire breast area, and to remember how your breast feels.

5. Now examine your left breast using right hand finger pads.

6. If you find any changes, see your doctor right away.

Source: The American Cancer Society.

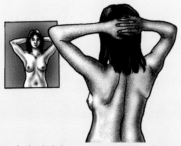

1. Under bright light, examine your breasts for any dimpling, puckering or change from the previous month.

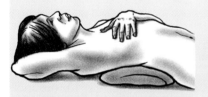

2. Lie down and put a pillow under your right shoulder. Place your right arm behind your head.

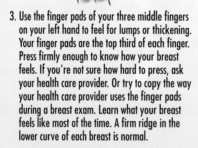

3. Use the finger pads of your three middle fingers on your left hand to feel for lumps or thickening. Your finger pads are the top third of each finger. Press firmly enough to know how your breast feels. If you're not sure how hard to press, ask your health care provider. Or try to copy the way your health care provider uses the finger pads during a breast exam. Learn what your breast feels like most of the time. A firm ridge in the lower curve of each breast is normal.

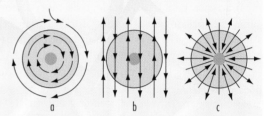

4. Move around the breast in a set way. You can choose either the circle (a), the up and down line (b), or the wedge (c). Do it the same way every time. It will help you to make sure that you've gone over the entire breast area, and to remember how your breast feels.

5. Now examine your left breast using right hand finger pads.

6. If you find any changes, see your doctor right away.

- Estrogen replacement therapy after age 55
- Consuming more than 3 ounces of alcohol a day
- Inheritance of BRCA1 or BRCA2 genes

However, all of the risk factors described above still account for only a small fraction of breast cancer cases.

The American Cancer Society still recommends **mammograms** every 1 to 2 years for women in their 40s and monthly breast self-exams beginning at age 20. However, even breast self-exams are controversial and may not help in early detection or reduced mortality from breast cancer. Preliminary results from 265,000 women participating in a breast self-exam study showed no benefits; equal numbers of women died of breast cancer irrespective of whether they performed a regular breast self-exam or not (Moon, 1997).

Testicular Cancer

The rate of testicular cancer among young men has been increasing but, as with breast cancer, the causes for the increase are unknown. It may be that exposure to xenoestrogens plays a role, but that has not been confirmed. Testicular cancer is still quite rare but usu-

Terms

mammogram: x-ray picture used to detect tumors in the breast

prostate-specific antigen: a blood test that detects a protein associated with abnormal growth of the prostate gland

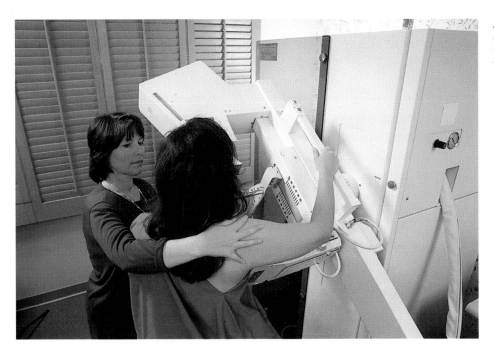

Mammograms can detect breast cancer at an early stage and improve chances for successful treatment.

ally can be cured if detected early. That is why it is recommended that young men perform a testicular self-exam regularly.

Prostate Cancer

Prostate cancer occurs primarily in men over age 65, although abnormal prostate cells can be detected at autopsy in young men who die from other causes. Generally, prostate cancers are very slow-growing and may never become life-threatening.

Early diagnosis of prostate cancer is facilitated by two tests. One is the finger rectal exam, in which a trained person can detect if the prostate is enlarged or otherwise feels abnormal. The **prostate-specific antigen (PSA)** test detects a protein in blood that is associ-

Wellness Guide

Inherited Genes for Breast Cancer: What to Do?

The genes BRCA1 and BRCA2 confer an inherited predisposition to development of breast and ovarian cancer. About 5% to 10% of all breast cancer cases is thought to be influenced by inheritance of these cancer susbeptibility genes. These genes do not cause breast cancer but they increase a woman's lifetime risk; some estimates of the increased risk are as high as 85% by age 70 (Burke et al., 1997). However, any estimated risks are really only educated guesses from studies of a few families whose female members have an exceptionally high rate of breast or ovarian cancer. Whether the risks calculated for these families can be extrapolated to other families is speculative. The increased risk, however great, is vitally important to each woman who has to make crucial health decisions.

Knowing that one is carrying a BRCA1 or BRCA2 gene (or other cancer suscpetibility genes) creates stress and problems for any woman (or couple) who choose to use the available tests for screening for these genes. Insurance coverage may be lost, job security may disappear, personal relations (including decisions on childbearing) are bound to be affected. And for the rest of her life, a woman will worry about the appearance of breast or some other cancer; such ongoing stress is bound to have a negative effect on health and on relationships.

For some women, knowing that they are at very high risk of developing breast cancer is sufficient cause for them to opt for prophylactic mastectomy; that is, they have their breasts removed while young to avoid the chance of breast cancer later in life.

Prophylactic oophorectomy is an option for women who are at high risk for ovarian cancer. Whether these procedures prolong life or whether the potential benefits offset the damage to the quality of life are still very controversial (Williams et. al., 1995).

Medical technology already can detect cancer susceptibility genes for breast cancer, ovarian cancer, and colon cancer. Tests for many more will become available in the near future. The only measure that people who have cancer susceptibility genes can take is to wait, worry, and watch for signs of a tumor. That is why many counselors and individuals believe that testing for these genes is a poor approach to healthy living. Promoting personal health is still the best approach to life, regardless of genetic makeup.

Wellness Guide

Ways to Prevent Skin Cancer

The number of people in the U.S. with various types of skin cancer, especially melanoma, has been increasing yearly. This need not be so, because skin cancers are among the most preventable of all cancers. The primary cause of most skin cancers is overexposure to sunlight, particularly its ultraviolet (UV) rays, which have enough energy to damage the DNA in skin cells and cause mutations. The best way to prevent skin cancer is to follow the **WAR** rule:

- **W**ear protective clothing.
- **A**void the sun between 10 AM to 3 PM.
- **R**egularly apply sunscreen with an SPF greater than 15 when outdoors, even on cloudy days. Sunscreen should be reapplied every 2 hours, and more often to replace what is washed from the body if swimming or exercising.

Protecting children from sunburn and overexposure is especially important since it is the lifetime exposure to UV that is associated with skin cancers in later life. By age 65, about one American in two has had some form of skin cancer. The ozone layer in earth's upper atmosphere filters out much of the sun's UV light; thinning of the ozone layer in recent years markedly increases the danger of overexposure to sunlight. Unless more people follow the **WAR** rule, the incidence of skin cancers is expected to continue to rise in the years ahead.

Wearing sunglasses that block at least 99% of all UV light is important for protecting eyes. Polarized lenses block glare but do not necessarily block UV unless the label says so. "Photochromic" lenses that darken in bright light also may not block UV light; always read the label. Over time, eye exposure to UV can cause cataracts.

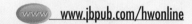 **www.jbpub.com/hwonline**

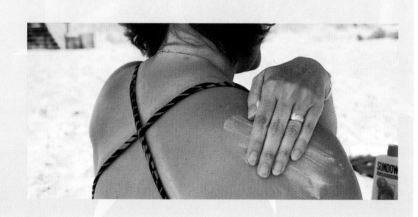

---

ated with abnormal growth of the prostate gland. A high PSA level may indicate prostate cancer, but also occurs with many other noncancerous conditions. Only additional tests can confirm the meaning of a high PSA level in blood.

An estimated 25 million men over age 50 have some detectible abnormal prostate cells; however, the majority never develop prostate cancer. And even among those who do, most eventually die from causes other than prostate cancer. Thus, the first question is whether it is worth screening for prostate cancer, and second, whether slow-growing prostate cancers should even be treated (Collins and Barry, 1996).

In 1996, a U.S. Preventive Services Task Force recommended *against* any routine screening for prostate cancer, including the digital exam, the PSA test, and ultrasound scan (Kuritzky, 1996). These medical experts concluded that screening would not reduce mortality from prostate cancer and would lead to treatments that would adversely affect the health and lives of many men. One form of treatment for prostate cancer, radical prostatectomy, usually causes urinary, sexual, and bowel dysfunction and makes life generally miserable.

As with breast cancer and colon cancer, a susceptibility gene for prostate cancer (HPC1) has been identified. When screening tests for this gene become available, men will have to decide whether or not they want to know if they carry a gene that puts them at higher-than-average risk for prostate cancer.

Skin Cancer

Skin cancers are on the rise everywhere, but they are especially prevalent in regions of the world exposed to intense sunlight. **Melanoma,** a malignant form of skin cancer, is now the most common cancer in women aged 25 to 29 and the second most common in women aged 30 to 34. Overall, melanoma is the fifth most frequent cancer diagnosed among Americans.

Exposure to sunlight is the primary cause of all forms of skin cancer. The exposure to sunlight that most of us receive as children largely determines the

Terms

melanoma: a particularly dangerous form of skin cancer

risk of skin cancer later in life. Two factors contribute to the dramatic rise in the rate of skin cancers. First, in the last generation or two we have become a nation of sun bathers and sun worshipers. Tans are associated with health, vigor, and beauty. Second, the continuing depletion of the ozone layer (see chapter 16) has resulted in more UV radiation reaching the earth's surface; it is the UV radiation in sunlight that causes mutations in skin cells that may lead to cancer. To reduce the risk of skin cancer, you must reduce your exposure to sunlight (Fackelman, 1998).

To protect yourself from melanoma remember these "ABCD" rules when examining moles on your body for any changes. If you suspect anything, consult a physician immediately.

- **A**ssymetry—one half of a mole looks different from the other half.
- **B**order irregular—the edges of a mole are ragged or indistinct.
- **C**olor—the pigmentation in the mole is uneven.
- **D**iameter—any mole that is larger than the diameter of a pencil or that has increased in size.

Colon Cancer

Colon cancer is rarely diagnosed in persons under age 40 but begins to appear more frequently in persons over age 50. The primary screening tests for colon cancer are occult blood tests and flexible sigmoidoscopy. In the occult blood test, stool samples are analyzed for the presence of blood, which may be a sign of colon cancer. In sigmoidoscopy, a flexible instrument is inserted via the rectum into the lower part of the colon to allow the physician to visually examine the lining of the colon. If any abnormal tissue is observed, a complete examination of the colon (colonoscopy) is recommended.

Neither screening test for colon cancer is completely accurate; therefore, a positive sign from either test usually is an indication for further tests. As with screening tests for breast and prostate cancers, the tests for colon cancer also are controversial; they are costly and entail some medical risks. Moreover, the polyps that are detected often never develop into cancer, so patients may be subjected to unnecessary surgical procedures.

Certain inherited genes are known to increase a person's risk for colon cancer. Persons from families known to be at high risk can be genetically tested to see if they have inherited a colon cancer susceptibility gene. They may benefit from the genetic information by more frequent examination of their colon, but they also must be willing to accept the lifelong stress that comes with knowing that they are at high risk for colon cancer.

www Regulating Diet

Many epidemiological studies show that the risk of certain cancers is influenced by diet. For example, stomach cancer is very common in Japan but uncommon among white Americans in Hawaii.

> *Faith. You can do little with it and nothing without it.*
> SAMUEL BUTLER

TABLE 10.6   Dietary Recommendations to Help Prevent Cancer
About 50% of all cancers are thought to derive from nutritional deficiencies.

Substance or food	Effect on cancer risk	Advice
Fiber	Helps decrease colon and rectal cancer	Obtain fiber from vegetables, fruits, whole grains
Cruciferous vegetables (broccoli, cauliflower, brussels sprouts)	Phytochemicals in these vegetables may detoxify cancer-causing chemicals	Eat more; raw or undercooked is best
Allium vegetables (onion, garlic, chives)	Sulfur-containing chemicals in allium vegetables may help prevent cancer	Eat more
Beta-carotene (15 mg), vitamin E (400 IU), and selenium (50 mcg)	A daily supplement reduced cancer (mainly stomach and esophagus) in a large Chinese population	Use supplements in moderation; selenium in high doses is toxic
Folic acid	Deficiency in this vitamin increases genetic damage that may contribute to cancer	Supplement if diet is deficient
Green tea	Reduced esophageal cancer in Chinese population	Most tea drunk in U.S. is black tea; try green tea
Shitake mushrooms	Extracts of shitake mushrooms reduced tumors in laboratory animals; also reduces blood cholesterol	Add to diet
Vitamins C and E	Boost immune system and may help prevent cancer	Supplement diet if desired

TABLE 10.7 Foods That Contain Cancer-Preventing Substances
Chemical compounds such as carotenoids, flavonoids, saponins, indoles, and phytochemicals inhibit the growth of cancer cells in laboratory experiments. Eat at least three different colors of fruits and vegetables daily.

Vegetables			
Cruciferous	*Pigmented*	*Green, leafy*	*Fruits*
Broccoli	Acorn squash	Chard	Apricot
Bok choy	Beets	Collard greens	Cantaloupe
Brussels sprouts	Carrot	Green tea	Grapefruit
Cabbage	Pumpkin	Kale	Grapes
Cauliflower	Red pepper	Kohlrabi	Guava
Turnips	Sweet potato	Lettuce	Mango
	Tomato	Okra	Orange
		Spinach	Papaya
			Peach
			Plum
			Watermelon

Japanese-Americans in Hawaii have stomach cancer rates that are almost as low as the white American population. Excessive consumption of smoked and pickled foods may contribute to the higher rates of stomach cancer in Japan.

Despite the scientific uncertainty over what specific foods increase the risk of cancer, certain dietary choices may help in preventing cancer (Table 10.6). Most of these dietary recommendations also help boost the immune system, which is the body's main defense against foreign cells (see chapter 9). B vitamins, vitamin C, vitamin E, folic acid, and carotenoids have been shown to boost the immune system and, as a consequence, may also help destroy cancer cells. These vitamins and substances can be taken as supplements, but also are readily available in fresh fruits and vegetables (Table 10.7).

Over the years, vitamin C has received much attention both as a preventive agent and as a cure for cancer when taken in extremely high doses. Some cancer patients who received megadoses of vitamin C have survived longer than expected, but other studies involving vitamin C and cancer have shown no positive therapeutic effect.

Our ancestors foraged for their food. They collected and ate seeds, roots, fruits, vegetables, and occasionally meat. Refined sugar, salt, and animal fats were scarce or nonexistent. Meat, milk, and cheese were certainly a rarity in the ancestral diet. Thus, the diet we consume today, filled with excess sugar, salt, fat, and meat, may be incompatible with the body chemistry we have inherited from our ancestors. The modern diet, heavy with processed foods, may result in the accumulation of toxic chemicals or an insufficient amount of some essential nutrients found in fresh fruits and vegetables.

Cancer Treatments

The three medical treatments for cancer are surgery, **radiation therapy,** and **chemotherapy.** Surgical removal of all or as much of a tumor as possible is considered the best treatment for cancer, particularly if the tumor is small and cells have not spread throughout the body. If even a few cancer cells remain, however, they may grow into new tumors, which is the reason that surgery, such as mastectomy, often removes a great deal of tissue in addition to the tumor.

If there is evidence that tumor cells have spread, or if some of the tumor could not be removed surgically, then radiation or chemotherapy, or both, are used to kill the remaining cancer cells. X-rays or other forms of high-energy radiation can destroy cancer cells as can the powerful drugs used in chemotherapy. Because radiation therapy and chemotherapy destroy normal cells as well as cancer cells, only limited amounts of each treatment can be administered.

Despite improvements in surgical techniques and development of new chemotherapeutic drugs, cancer treatments today are not noticeably more successful than they were in the past, a fact that is reflected in the more or less unchanged death rates for most cancers. Because of the limited success of current cancer therapies, new approaches are being tested.

An analysis of cancer mortality over the past 40 years in the U.S. led to the following conclusion:

> The best of modern medicine has much to offer to virtually every patient with cancer, for palliation if not always for cure, and every patient should have access to the earliest possible diagnosis and the best possible treatment. The problem is the lack of substantial improvement over what treatment

Terms

radiation therapy: use of high-energy radiation, such as x-rays, to kill cancer cells and treat some forms of cancer

chemotherapy: use of toxic chemicals to kill cancer cells and treat some forms of cancer

could already accomplish some decades ago. A national commitment to the prevention of cancer, largely replacing reliance on hopes for universal cures, is now the way to go (Bailar and Gornik, 1997).

Cancer patients often become desperate and depressed about their condition, the pain of treatments, and the prospect of death. In this state, some patients turn to unconventional therapies and promises of "miracle" cures (Table 10.8). Many cancer patients turn to alternative therapies in hope of a cure when conventional medicine has nothing to offer. Although unconventional therapies may be helpful or at least produce more peace of mind, patients and their families need to be wary of practitioners who make unfounded claims for unlicensed drugs and unproven therapies. Things that are "too good to be true" usually are.

Coping with a Diagnosis of Cancer

A diagnosis of cancer raises serious problems for the patient and for family and friends. Often the patient enters a state of disbelief or shock. The family has to cope with new problems. The patient must face surgery or other treatment. Along with treatment, the patient usually must deal with fear of death, anger at the disease, loss of income, changes in living habits, and, above all, the uncertainty of the outcome, which may last for months or years. These are some of the reasons why coping with cancer can be difficult. Stress and emotional upset can depress the normal functions of the immune system. There also is evidence that hostile feelings, resentment, deeply

felt personal loss, and feelings of hopelessness may be important factors in cancer development and lowering of disease resistance.

> *Prediction is very hard, especially when it's about the future.*
>
> YOGI BERRA,
> former catcher,
> New York Yankees

The coping strategies for dealing with the emotional distress resulting from cancer, AIDS, and other serious diseases are similar. They all depend on using the mind in positive ways. The effectiveness of any therapy and the ability to cope with a life-threatening illness depend on focusing the mind on ways to enhance the healing process. Meditation and relaxation techniques are important in reducing stress. Learning how to use visual imagery can help with the effectiveness of treatments. Along with mental relaxation techniques, the mind can focus on images and suggestions that may help the immune system fight and destroy cancer cells.

A dramatic illustration of the power of belief in altering the course of cancer is the case of Mr. Wright, a patient in the 1950s. At that time, a drug called krebiozen was touted by some as a "miracle drug" that could cure cancer. Mr. Wright, who had terminal lymphosarcoma, was given a life expectancy of two weeks by his physician. However, Mr. Wright had enormous faith in the miracle drug and insisted that he be treated with it. After a single injection, his doctor noted that "the tumor masses had melted like snowballs on a hot stove, and in only these few days, they were half their original size" (Klopfer, 1957).

Mr. Wright was symptom-free for 2 months until he read in the newspaper that krebiozen was worthless in treating cancer, whereupon he relapsed and was readmitted to the hospital. With nothing to lose, his doctor assured him that a fresh, double-strength injection of krebiozen would cure him. In actuality, Mr. Wright received an injection of salt water. Once again he was symptom-free for 2 months. Then headlines again proclaimed "nationwide tests show krebiozen to be a worthless drug in treatment of cancer." Mr. Wright relapsed and died in 2 days.

Coping with cancer requires courage and conviction. A cancer patient must not give up hope, despite what the statistics predict or what physicians say about the prognosis. The patient must believe that a cure is possible and work toward that end. For many people, coping with cancer is a transforming experience and gives renewed meaning to life.

The most important thing to remember about cancer is that most cancers *are* preventable. Abstain from using any tobacco and follow a diet rich in fresh fruits and vegetables. Also avoid excess exposure to sunlight and to chemicals that are known to be carcinogenic.

TABLE 10.8	**Unproven Cancer Therapies**

Many cancer patients who are desperate or who have exhausted all medical treatments turn to unconventional therapies for which benefits are scientifically unproven.

Therapy	Rationale
Metabolic therapy	Toxins and wastes in the body cause cancer. Treatments remove cellular poisons and detoxify the body.
Herbal remedies	Herbs have natural, sacred, curative properties not known to science.
Megavitamins	High doses of vitamins kill cancer cells and rejuvenate the body.
Diet therapy	Special diets (grape, macrobiotic, shark cartilage) restore balance to the body and cure the cancer.
Electronic devices	Electrical or magnetic energy harmonizes the life forces and kills the cancer cells.
Immunotherapy	Treatments stimulate or restore immune system functions, which will then be able to destroy cancer cells. (Immunotherapies are being tested by scientists but are a long way from clinical use.)

Managing Stress

The Art of Visualization

The new field of psychoneuroimmunology has provided some amazing insights into the mind-body-spirit connection. For example, several people with terminal cancer so severe that no medical treatment was suggested began to work with alternative methods of healing. To the surprise of many, their tumors went into remission. What was their secret? When these people were studied to find what they did to initiate their own healing process, one common theme emerged: a change in attitude. As director of Biofeedback Research at the Menninger Clinic in Topeka, Kansas, Dr. Patricia Norris has documented several cases where mental imagery and visualization were used successfully to complement traditional medical treatment. Dr. Norris cites eight specific characteristics which help to make mental imagery and visualization effective as a healing tool, specifically with regard to cancer:

1. **Make the visualization personal.** The images must be self-generated. Images that are created by the practitioner and not the patient appear to be ineffective.

2. **Make the imagery "egosyntonic."** Egosyntonic means that the image must fit the values and ideals of that person. If, for example, the individual is pacifistic, then combative or warlike imagery will undermine the effectiveness of this type of treatment.

3. **Make the imagery positive.** Negative imagery reinforces negative thoughts, which are

not conductive to healing. As an example, Norris notes that sharks, as a healing image, are not a good idea.

4. **Take an active role in the imagery.** Rather than imagining watching the imagery on a movie screen, you must feel the sensations of your images in the first person. You must have a sense that what you are seeing is happening inside your body, not "out there somewhere."

5. **Make the image anatomically correct and accurate.** Knowing exactly what body region and physiological system is in a disease state will dictate the type of imagery used. Consequently, you need to know whether to access the central nervous system or the immune system. Norris states that more than one image can be used in the healing process.

6. **Be constant, use dialogue.** Constancy means to be regular in generating your imagery. Norris suggests three 15-minute sessions per day, with intermittent shorter sessions throughout the day. When you feel pain, your body is communicating to you. She suggests making pain your friend. In the dialogue style of self-talk, she suggests thanking the pain for making you aware of the problem so that you may be able to fix it. Finally, she suggests "destroying" a tumor with its permission. Respond with love. Make peace with your body.

7. **Create a blueprint.** The concept of the blueprint is a strategy. A blueprint visualization is like time lapse photography where a flower (symbolizing a tumor) is shown to bloom within seconds, and then closes up again and fades away. An example would be to see the construction of a building, starting from the hole in the earth to opening day, where you are cutting the ribbon at the front entrance.

8. **Include the treatment in the imagery.** Norris has found that patients who use mental imagery with chemotherapy treatment and radiation do better than those who "fight" these medical procedures. She notes that it helps to have benevolent feelings versus ambivalent feelings toward the treatment. She suggests one mentally "welcome the treatment into the body." Consider the treatment as a guest in your house. Based on her patient research, she offers these examples:

(a) *Chemotherapy*—a gold-colored fluid that healthy cells, acting as a bucket brigade, pass along to the cancer cells, who in turn drink up the chemotherapy

(b) *Radiation treatment*—a stream of silver energy aimed at the cancerous tumor(s). Ask the white blood cells to move away or to shield themselves and act like mirrors to reflect the radiation toward the cancer cells, then watch the cancer cells die.

Critical Thinking About Health

1. Black Americans as a group have higher blood pressure, on average, than White Americans. Various hypotheses have been advanced to explain the differences in blood pressure between the races, including genetic differences, social factors, economic factors, diet, and behavioral differences. Find out all that you can on racial differences in blood pressure (your local branch of the American Heart Association is a good place to start for information). Then write a report giving your views as to why the blood pressure discrepancy exists among races and ethnic groups in our society.

2. Make a list of all the factors discussed in this chapter that increase the risk of cardiovascular disease, heart attacks, and stroke. How many of

the risk factors do you have? Among the risk factors that can be changed, discuss how you would go about reducing them in your life to improve your cardiovascular health now and for the future.

3. Make a list of all the factors you can think of that increase the risk of developing cancer. Order the items in your list from highest risk to lowest in your judgment. Are any of the risk factors relevant to your life? If so, describe how you could modify your life-style or behaviors to reduce the risk of developing cancer.

4. The "war against cancer" is fought by physicians and scientists in two fundamentally different ways. On the one hand, medical research tries to discover better treatments for all forms of cancer. On the other hand, epidemiologists and other researchers believe that we need to shift the scientific emphasis from seeking cures to prevention, since we understand many of the environmental factors that cause cancer. Reducing exposure to risk factors could prevent as many as half of all human cancers. In your judgment, which of these positions is correct; or do you believe both positions are equally valid? Develop facts and arguments that substantiate your views and write a report of your conclusions.

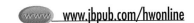 **www.jbpub.com/hwonline**

Health in Review

- Damage to the heart or arteries is called cardiovascular disease, which is the leading cause of death in the United States.
- Major risk factors of heart disease that can be changed are: cigarette or tobacco use, high blood cholesterol, high blood pressure, physical inactivity, and poor diet.
- Vitamins E, C, B_6, and B_{12}, and folic acid all help protect against heart disease.
- Calcium, soy products, fish oils, and green tea also help keep the heart healthy.
- Heart disease is caused by modern life-styles and can be prevented. Making changes in your diet, smoking, and exercise behaviors while you are young can help keep the heart and arteries healthy throughout life.
- Cancer refers to a number of different diseases, all of which share the common property of abnormal, unregulated cell growth in the body.
- Dietary factors and environmental agents, such as smoking and sunlight, act on the genetic material in cells to cause chemical changes that may initiate a tumor, which is a mass of abnormal cells.
- If everything known about cancer prevention were practiced, up to two-thirds of cancers would not occur; thus cancer is largely a preventable disease.
- Recovery from cancer depends on good nutrition, positive attitudes, healing mental images, and medical treatment appropriate for the particular cancer. A healthy, active immune system also is an essential component in cancer prevention and recovery.
- Cigarette smoking is responsible for about one-third of all cancers.
- Dietary deficiencies or excesses are responsible for about one-half of all cancers.
- Significantly reducing cancer requires major changes in peoples' life-styles, including more attention to a healthy diet, elimination of tobacco use, limiting alcohol consumption, and reducing exposure to intense sunlight and chemical carcinogens.

Health and Wellness Online

The World Wide Web contains a wealth of information about health and wellness. By accessing the Internet using Web browser software, such as Netscape Navigator or Microsoft's Internet Explorer, you can gain a new perspective on many topics presented in *Essentials of Health and Wellness, Second Edition.* Access the Jones and Bartlett Publishers web site at http://www.jbpub.com/hwonline.

Your heart will hold a grudge.

Working on that perfect tan?

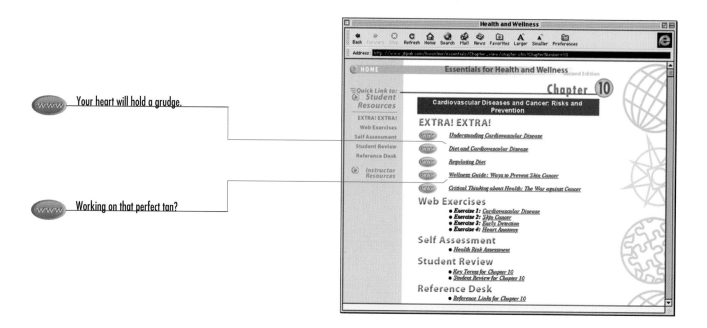

References

American Cancer Society. (1999). *Cancer Facts and Figures, 1999.*

Bachmaier, K., et al. (1998). Chlamydia infections and heart disease linked through antigenic mimicry. *Science, 283,* 1335–1338.

Bailar, J. C., & Gornik, H. L. (1997). Cancer undefeated. *New England Journal of Medicine, 336,* 1569–1574.

Bronner, L. L., et al. (1996). Primary prevention of stroke. *New England Journal of Medicine, 333,* 1392–1400.

Burke, W., et al. (1997). Recommendations for follow-up care of individuals with an inherited predisposition to cancer. *Journal of the American Medical Association, 277,* 997–1003.

Collins, M. M., & Barry, M. J. (1996). Controversies in prostate cancer screening. *Journal of the American Medical Association, 276,* 1976–1967.

Davis, D. L., & Bradlow, H. L. (1995, October). Can environmental estrogens cause breast cancer? *Scientific American,* 166–173.

Daviglus, M. L., et al. (1997). Fish consumption and the 30-year risk of fatal myocardial infarction. *New England Journal of Medicine, 336,* 1946–1052.

Diaz, M. N., et al. (1997). Antioxidants and atherosclerotic heart disease. *New England Journal of Medicine, 337,* 408–415.

Fackelman, K. (1998). Melanoma madness: The scientific flap over sunscreens and cancer. *Science News, 153,* 360–363.

He, Y., Lam, T. H., & Li, L. S. (1994). Passive smoking at work a risk factor for coronary heart disease in chinese women who never have smoked. *British Medical Journal, 308,* 6925.

Heart and stroke facts, 1996. Dallas, Tex.: The American Heart Association Publications.

Heart and stroke facts, statistical supplement. (1999). Dallas, Tex.: The American Heart Association Publications.

Kern, F. (1991). Normal plasma cholesterol in an 88-year-old man who eats 25 eggs per day. *New England Journal of Medicine, 324,* 13.

Klopfer, B. (1957). Psychological variables in human cancer. *Journal of Prospective Techniques, 21,* 331–340.

Kuritzky, L. (1996, June 15). PSA: To screen or not to screen. *Hospital Practice,* 145–146.

Marmot, M. (1994). The cholesterol papers. *British Medical Journal, 308,* 6925.

McCarron, D. A., & Hatton, D. (1996). Dietary calcium and lower blood pressure. *Journal of the American Medical Association, 275,* 1128–1129.

McMurry, M. P., Cerqueira, M. T., Connor, S. L., & Connor, W. E. (1991). Changes in lipid and lipoprotein levels and body weight in Tarahumara Indians after consumption of an affluent diet. *New England Journal of Medicine, 325.*

Moon, M. A. (1997, May 1). Breast self-exams have yet to show benefit. *Internal Medicine News,* 38.

Ornish, D., et al. (1998). Intensive lifestyle changes for reversal of coronary heart disease. *Journal of the American Medical Association, 280,* 2001–2007.

Pauletto, P., et al. (1996). Blood pressure and atherogenic lipoprotein profiles of fish-diet and vegetarian villagers in Tanzania: The Lugalawa study. *Lancet, 348,* 784–788.

Stephens, N. G., et al. (1996). Randomized controlled trial of vitamin E in patients with coronary disease. *Lancet, 347,* 781–790.

Verschuren, W. M., et al. (1996). Serum total cholesterol and long-term coronary heart disease mortality in different cultures. *Journal of the American Medical Association, 274,* 131–136.

Suggested Readings

American Cancer Society. *Cancer facts and figures.* Published yearly by the American Cancer Society and available at any branch of the society. Contains the latest statistics on all forms of cancer.

American Heart Association (AHA). *Heart and stroke facts, 1999.* Published yearly and obtainable from any AHA office. Contains the latest information on cardiovascular diseases, treatments, and statistical data.

Cooper, R. S., Rotimi, C. N., & Ward, R. (1999, February). The puzzle of hypertension in African-Americans. *Scientific American,* 56–63. Explores the question of whether the marked differences in high blood pressure between Black and White Americans is due to biological differences, social and economic differences, or a combination of both.

Cowley, G. (1998, November 30). Cancer and diet. *Newsweek,* 60–66. A good discussion of foods that may increase cancer risk and fruits and vegetables that help prevent cancer.

Cowley, G. (1997, August 11). The heart attackers. *Newsweek,* 54–59. The latest findings on what causes heart disease.

Groopman, J. (1998, October 26). Dr. Fair's tumor. *The New Yorker,* 78–106. Examines what happened to a famous physician when he learned that he had advanced colon cancer.

Hogan, P. J. (1996). *Texas heart institute heart owner's handbook.* New York: Wiley. Outlines a step-by-step program to improve and protect the health of your heart.

Lerner, M. (1994). *Choices in healing: Integrating the best of conventional and complementary approaches to cancer.* Cambridge, Mass.: MIT Press. Discusses both conventional and alternative treatments for cancer.

Pickering, T. (1996). *Good news about high blood pressure.* New York: Simon and Schuster. Explains the risk factors for hypertension and how to control hypertension without drugs, if possible.

Winawer, S. J., & Shike, M. (1996). *Cancer free: The comprehensive cancer prevention program.* New York: Touchstone. Describes a five-part program for healthy persons that will help them prevent cancer.

Making Healthy Changes

The key to remaining healthy most of the time in a world that teems with infectious microorganisms ready to invade your body and trigger illness is having a healthy immune system. As with all of the body's systems (circulatory system, nervous system, digestive system), the immune system consists of many different organs, cells, and biological signals, which coordinate the immune system's attack on microorganisms that penetrate the body and initiate an infection. The immune system also plays a key role in destroying cancer cells that arise in the body. Keeping your immune system operating at optimum levels requires a healthy diet, regular exercise, and a positive mental state.

It is relatively easy to understand how diet and exercise would affect the immune system's functions (as well as lowering the risk of heart disease and cancer), since the body's chemistry depends on what foods we eat and how active we are. It is less easy to understand how the mind affects the immune system (and other body systems), but many studies show that it does. We will help you to understand how powerful your mind is in affecting your physiology (digestion, breathing, blood pressure, and so forth) by describing an experience that everyone is familiar with—going to the movies.

The Movie Experience

By examining what happens when you go to a movie, you will begin to understand how easily your mind can be manipulated so that your physiology is changed—often in ways that are damaging to your health. The first step in the movie experience is deciding what kind of movie you want to see—action, comedy, horror, melodrama. You go to the theater and pay for a ticket, an action that commits you to the experience (and virtually guarantees that you will not walk out even if the movie is awful). Then you enter the movie theater and sit down with a hundred or more other people. The theater goes dark, and after the previews, the movie begins.

If the film is well done and you become engrossed in the story, you forget that you are in a movie theater. You do not worry about schoolwork, babysitters, what you have to do tomorrow, or anything except what is happening on the screen. That is why movies (and other kinds of entertainment) are called "diver-sions," because they divert your thoughts from what you were thinking that day or when you entered the theater.

Have you ever cried while watching a movie? Of course. Almost everyone has. Think about this unusual behavior for a moment. Crying is a complex physiological response to what the mind is thinking and feeling. And yet, when you cry at a movie you are crying at something totally imaginary. You are watching light images being projected onto a screen, and you respond by becoming sad or angry or upset. You may find your hands become sweaty or your stomach knots up even though nothing "real" is happening.

Even though nothing "real" occurs on the movie screen, our minds interpret what we see as "real" and respond with strong emotional and physiological changes, most of which are not healthy. In the words of one critic, "Horror films scare you, melodrama makes you cry, and porn arouses you." Each of these reactions involves complex physiological changes resulting from imaginary thoughts and feelings.

Movie images also can create lasting harm, especially in the minds of young children, who are easily frightened by things that they do not understand. Children interpret what they see and hear in a very literal sense. If a person is made up to look like a monster, the child sees a monster and does not comprehend that it is only a person dressed up. The mind records and remembers all frightening experiences, because that is how it is able to protect itself (and you) from a similar frightening situation in the future.

To protect yourself from the stress, decreased immune system functions, and physiological harm that come from frightening images, you can decide not to expose your mind to movies full of bloodshed or horror. You may elect not to watch the news (invariably full of scenes of destruction and brutality) on TV or to read certain stories in the newspapers. Each person must decide how affected he or she is by "unreal" images or by information that is upsetting.

Stress Management: Examining Fears Produced by Watching Movies

To begin to examine some of the fears that your mind may have recorded over the years, describe in your journal any movies or images that you remember that were particularly frightening or upsetting. What were the images that upset you? What were your feelings while you were watching those images? Do you remember any changes that took place in your body as a result of being frightened or upset at a movie? Do you recall becoming ill in any way shortly after watching the frightening movie?

Next time you go to a movie that affects you emotionally, describe in your journal what your feelings were and how you felt afterward. Note in your journal if your sleep or appetite or behaviors were affected in any way.

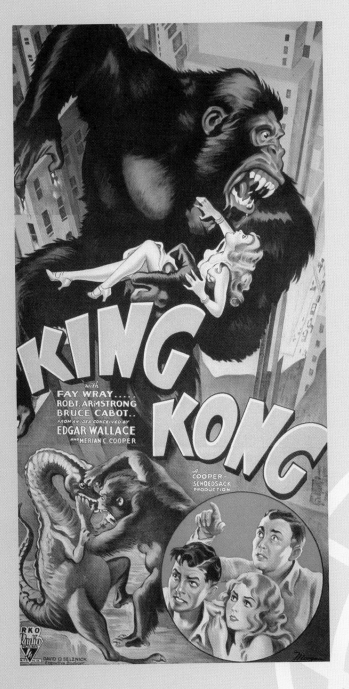

Safe Haven Update

If you have continued to do this exercise and have become comfortable using it in times of stress, note whether your experience is different after you have seen a powerful or disturbing movie. Sometimes when the mind is quiet, it feels safe to bring to your awareness fears and uncomfortable feelings that normally would not be conscious.

Describe in your journal how your "safe haven" may have become harder to reach after you have become upset or anxious as a result of watching a movie or TV program.

Improving Your Diet: Adding Antioxidants

All animals require oxygen to generate chemical energy and to stay alive. (Some bacteria and organisms deep in the ocean do not need oxygen to stay alive.) In the body's cells, oxygen is converted by a series of chemical reactions into water. However, along the way different, highly reactive forms of oxygen are produced that can damage and destroy tissues. To counteract this the body uses *antioxidants*, substances that neutralize the harmful forms of oxygen generated in cells.

The primary nutrients that function as antioxidants and which are available as supplements are vitamin C, vitamin E, carotenoids, coenzyme Q, and selenium. Although these nutrients are in fruits and vegetables, the amounts most people ingest usually are less than needed for optimal health. Antioxidants have been shown to reduce the risks of cardiovascular disease, cancer, and some of the unhealthy effects of aging.

The amount of antioxidant supplements a person might choose to take on a daily basis is a matter of personal choice, but here are some guidelines.

Nutrient	Daily amounts
Vitamin C	1–5 milligrams
Vitamin E*	400–800 IU
Mixed carotenoids	10,000–25,000 IU
Coenzyme Q	50–100 milligrams
Selenium	50–200 micrograms

*Vitamin E (chemically known as tocopherol) comes in d and l forms and occurs naturally in foods in eight different chemical structures. It is suggested that you supplement with 400 IU of the d-alpha form and about 400 IU of the other naturally occuring chemical forms.

After thinking about the benefits of taking antioxidant supplements, investigate where they can be purchased and compare prices and amounts. Try to obtain more information about antioxidants from different sources.

Discuss in your journal what you have discovered about antioxidants and health and whether you have decided to supplement your diet with one or all of the antioxidants listed.

Physical Activity: Walking More

Discuss in your journal how consistent you have been in walking every day (assuming you are not otherwise physically active). Is walking something that you now enjoy or is it a chore? Consider increasing the intensity of your walk by walking a longer distance, walking faster, or both. As your body adjusts to regular physical activity, you should find it easier to do more. If you enjoy bicycling or in-line roller skating, you could add these activities to your physical regime by biking or skating one day and walking the next.

Improving the Diet: Choosing Healthy Cooking Oils

Most of us are familiar with butter and margarine but we are less knowledgeable about the nutritional value of cooking oils. Butter and margarine are less healthy than vegetable oils because butter and margarine contain "saturated" fats (which keeps them solid at room temperature. Vegetable oils are "unsaturated," which is why they are liquid at room temperature). Oils can

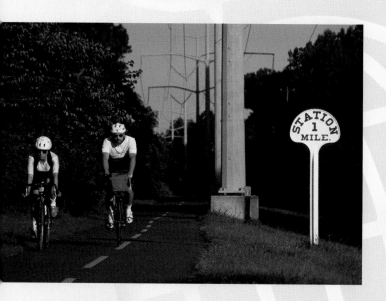

be extracted from all kinds of vegetables and nuts: corn, safflower, soy, canola, olive, almond, macadamia nut, grape seed, and so forth. Each oil contains different forms of fats (cholesterol is not present in any vegetable or nut), some of which are considered better for health than others. In general, canola oil and olive oil are regarded as the best choices for cooking and other uses. Small amounts of these "healthy" oils can be substituted in many instances where you would use butter, margarine, mayonnaise, or lard.

Describe in your journal any changes that you make in your diet by reducing your use of butter and margarine. Remember that pastries usually contain large amounts of fats.

Stress Management: Breathing Exercises

Breathing is the only major body function that we control both voluntarily and involuntarily. Most of the time we breathe without thinking about it. However, we hold our breath when startled or increase it when lifting a weight or exercising. Many breathe shallowly, which does not fully empty or expand the lungs. Correct breathing has been shown to improve blood pressure, digestive problems, heart arrhythmias, blood circulation, sleep problems, and anxiety. Breathing properly is probably the best (and most inexpensive) stress reduction technique known.

Many people have learned how to improve their breathing through the practice of yoga. A major component of yoga is working with *prana*, which means breath or spirit. (In many languages, the words for breath and spirit are the same.) Training yourself to breathe properly can make a major contribution to your health and energy.

Suggestions for improving your breathing include:

1. Begin by observing how you breathe. Sit or lie in a comfortable position and simply watch how you are breathing. Just paying attention to each breath will quiet your mind, reduce tension, and gradually cause your breathing to become slower and more regular.

2. Practice taking slow, deep breaths whenever you have a chance. This can be done while driving, sitting in class, or waiting in line at the store. The more you practice paying attention to breathing, the more benefits you will notice. Paying attention to breathing is calming and increases energy by increasing the supply of oxygen to tissues and the removal of waste products.

3. Learn to breathe with your abdominal muscles. You should feel your stomach move in and out

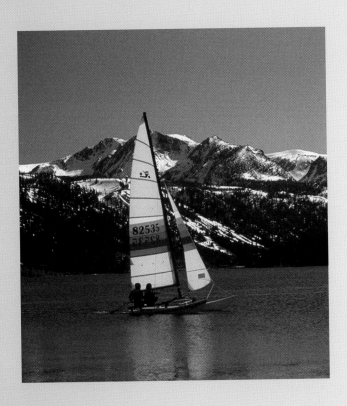

with each deep breath. Notice if the air is entering through one or both nostrils. Often we use only one nostril and sometimes switch unconsciously to using the other nostril. You might want to practice closing off one nostril with finger pressure and notice the difference in breathing with each nostril.

4. Pay attention to the exhalation. Try to exhale as much air as possible with each breath. You may notice that your exhalation is much shorter than your inhalation. Try to adjust your breathing so that the cycle of exhalation is longer than the inhalation. A good way to improve exhalation is to purse your lips and exhale completely and slowly through your mouth. This helps you to prolong the exhalation and empty your lungs as completely as possible.

After you have been practicing deep breathing for a while, discuss in your journal any changes in your body that you notice or how you feel mentally. Do you feel more alert or energetic? Are you calmer more of the time? How many times a day do you practice deep breathing?

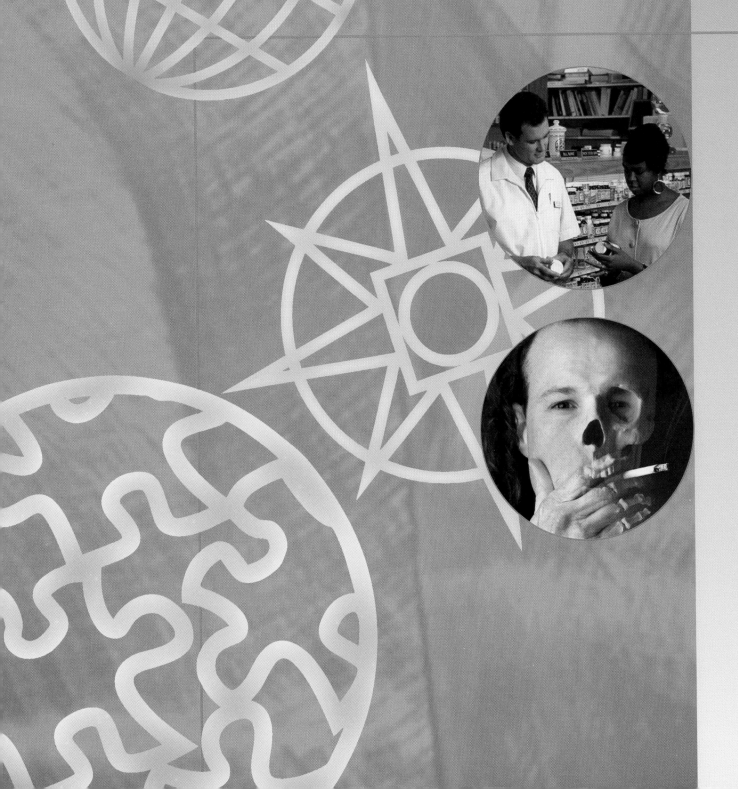

Part 5

Explaining Drug Use and Abuse

Exercises and Activities

WORKBOOK
The Drugs You Take
Be a Knowledgeable Consumer

Health and Wellness Online

 www.jbpub.com/hwonline

The Overmedicating of Americans
Consequences of Drug Use
Wellness Guide: Risk Factors for Addiction

Chapter 11

Using Drugs Responsibly

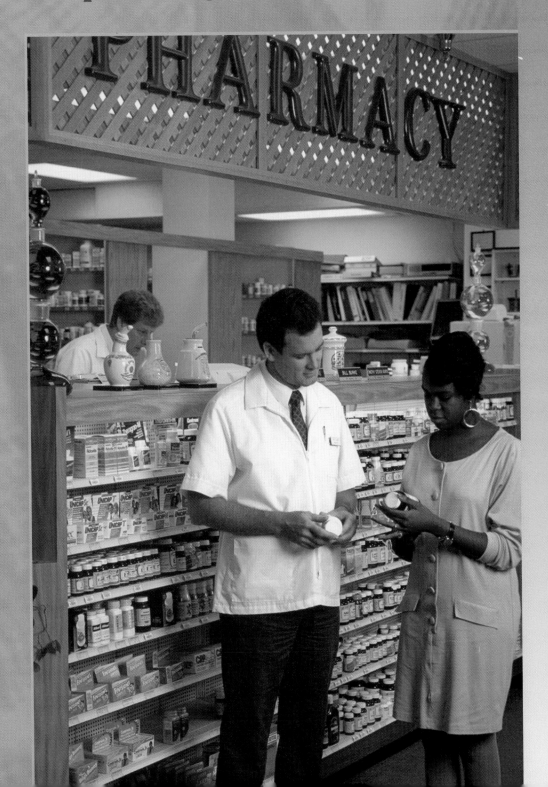

For thousands of years, people have been ingesting substances to heal themselves, change consciousness, produce sleep, drive out evil spirits, and promote tribal and family harmony. For most of that time, such substances were obtained by chewing the leaves of a particular plant, brewing a tea from a plant's bark or roots, or mixing a potion made up of plant and animal materials, as the three witches in Shakespeare's *Macbeth* did when they concocted "eye of newt and toe of frog, wool of bat and tongue of dog." Today, some healing substances are still obtained by ingesting plant and animal tissues or their extracts directly, whereas others are single, chemically pure substances that are manufactured by modern chemical and biological technologies.

No matter how they are obtained, many substances are of enormous value in relieving pain, preventing disease, and facilitating healing. However, indiscriminate or inappropriate use and overuse of drugs also are major problems in our society. For example, in 1997, the combination of phentermine and fenfluramine ("phen/fen"), taken by millions of people to control body weight, was found to cause heart valve damage, and the drugs were banned. Overuse of antibiotics has led to the creation of antibiotic-resistant organisms, against which no antibiotic drugs are effective (see chapter 9). Alcohol and the use of other drugs are associated with a greater risk of homicide and suicide (Rivara et al., 1997). And everyone has heard of the "war on drugs," which is concerned with the social and legal problems associated with the use of cocaine, heroin, and other illegal substances.

> It ain't what we know that gives us trouble. It's what we know that ain't so that gives us trouble.
>
> WILL ROGERS

The use of drugs in our society has become so commonplace and accepted that many people automatically turn to drugs to solve their physical, mental, and emotional problems, failing to understand the dangers and health hazards. When people have symptoms of headache, backache, fatigue, stomach upset, colds, or allergies, many believe that taking drugs is the *only* source of relief. Although many medicines are extremely valuable, reliance on drugs to solve life's problems opens the way for chemical dependency. Many people do not consider the possible consequences of drug use, which often have a negative impact on well-being.

What Is a Drug?

A **drug** is a single chemical substance in a medicine that alters the structure or function of some of the body's biological processes. The alteration can start, stop, speed up, or slow down a process, depending on the specific drug and its effect. A **medicine** is a drug (or combination of drugs) that is intended to: (a) prevent illness, as vaccines do; (b) cure disease, as antibiotics do; (c) aid healing, as ulcer medications do; or (d) suppress symptoms, as pain relievers do. Not all drugs—for example, alcohol and nicotine—are medicines.

Drugs are usually classified according to the particular biological process they affect rather than by their chemical properties. For example, all substances that increase urine production, regardless of their chemical structure, are called **diuretics;** those that reduce pain are **analgesics;** and those that produce nervous system excitation are **stimulants.**

How Drugs Work

Many drugs act by interacting with specific cells in the body that carry **receptors,** usually proteins with which the drugs interact; a drug-receptor interaction is akin to the way a key fits into a lock (Figure 11.1). When a drug binds to a receptor, it affects the biological process or processes of cells and organs. Frequently, a drug may chemically resemble a natural body component, such as a hormone or a neurotransmitter, which interacts with the receptor as part of normal functioning. The drug, acting like a counterfeit key, binds to the receptor in place of the natural substance, and thereby alters physiology.

For example, many antibiotics cure bacterial infections by binding to receptors in bacteria and blocking their reproduction. Many chemotherapeutic drugs used in cancer treatment also work by blocking cell reproduction; in this instance, the reproduction of the body's cancer cells are the target (see chapter 10). The

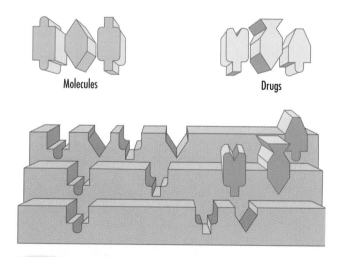

FIGURE 11.1   Bindings of Drugs to Cellular Receptor Sites   The molecular structures of many drugs are similar to molecules normally produced in the body. The drugs compete for receptor sites on cells and alter the physiological functioning of organs and tissues.

Common side effects with drugs of abuse

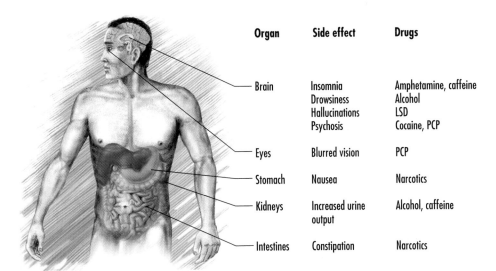

Organ	Side effect	Drugs
Brain	Insomnia	Amphetamine, caffeine
	Drowsiness	Alcohol
	Hallucinations	LSD
	Psychosis	Cocaine, PCP
Eyes	Blurred vision	PCP
Stomach	Nausea	Narcotics
Kidneys	Increased urine output	Alcohol, caffeine
Intestines	Constipation	Narcotics

FIGURE 11.2   Common Side Effects with Drugs of Abuse   Almost every organ or system in the body can be unintentionally altered by the effects of substances of abuse.

Source: G. Hanson and P. J. Venturelli, *Drugs and Society,* 4th ed. (Boston: Jones and Bartlett, 1995), p. 103.

aim of chemotherapy is to destroy the cancer cells, which tend to reproduce rapidly, while affecting normal, healthy cells to a lesser degree, allowing them to recover.

Side Effects of Medication

Even though a drug may be intended to have a single effect, it often has more than one, because it binds to a variety of receptors in or on different cells. Unintended drug actions are called **side effects** (Figure 11.2), which may be minor or severe. Some side effects include allergic reactions (**drug hypersensitivity**); harm to developing embryos and fetuses (**teratogen**); or physical dependence.

Drug side effects can be quite dangerous. One study estimated that, each year in the U.S., drug side effects are responsible for injury and illness in over 2 million hospitalized patients (Lazarou et al., 1998). Furthermore, drug side effects are responsible for the deaths of 100,000 hospitalized patients per year, making them the sixth leading cause of death in the U.S. These adverse drug reactions are caused by the unintended effects of the drugs and not to errors in prescribing or dosing, drug abuse, or accidental poisoning. This means that in the present climate of heavy drug advertising, it is necessary for good health to remember and respect that drugs are potent biological agents with both benefits and potentially fatal drawbacks.

In addition to side effects, a drug also may be harmful if the drug-taker has a condition that is aggravated by that drug. A medical reason for not taking a drug is called a **contraindication.** For example, a history of blood vessel disease is a contraindication for taking birth control pills. The need to screen for contraindications is one reason why many medicines are available only by prescription.

Medical practitioners should be knowledgeable about the side effects and contraindications of drugs, but sometimes these are overlooked. About one-third of hospital stays are needlessly extended because inappropriate medications are administered or managed improperly by medical staff. Consumers of medications should learn as much as they can about the intended use and side effects of their drugs, and they should ask their medical providers to explain the rationale for the medications prescribed for them.

Routes of Administration

Drugs can be taken by mouth, inhalation, or injection into the muscles, under the skin (from which they diffuse into surrounding tissues and blood) or directly into the bloodstream. Drugs also can be absorbed

Terms

drug: a single chemical substance in a medicine that alters one or more of the body's biological functions

medicine: drugs used to prevent, treat, or cure illness; aid healing; or suppress symptoms

diuretics: drugs that increase urine production

analgesics: drugs that relieve pain

stimulants: drugs that produce nervous system excitement; including cocaine, caffeine, and amphetamines

receptor: protein on the surface or inside a cell to which a drug or natural substance can bind and thereby affect cell function

side effects: unintended and often harmful actions of a drug

drug hypersensitivity: an allergic reaction to a drug

teratogen: a drug that affects the development of a fetus, causing birth defects

contraindication: any medical reason for not taking a particular drug

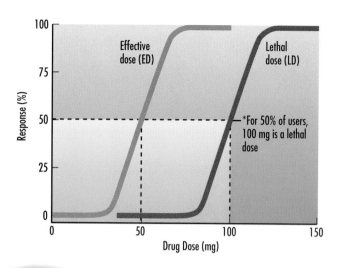

FIGURE 11.3   Method for Calculating a Drug's Therapeutic Index (LD-50/ED-50)   The LD-50 is the drug dose that causes lethality in 50% of the users (100 mg in figure). In this example, the therapeutic index is 2 (100/50 = 2). The greater the therapeutic index, the safer the drug.

Source: G. Hanson and P. J. Venturelli, *Drugs and Society,* 4th Ed. (Boston: Jones and Bartlett, 1995), p. 106.

through the skin and the mucous membranes of the nose, eyes, vagina, and anus. Regardless of the route of entry, most drugs remain active in the body for a relatively short time, often only a few hours.

Once in the body, drugs are degraded or destroyed by the liver and the lungs. Drugs are also filtered by the kidneys and eliminated from the body in urine. Drugs such as inhalatory anesthetics or nitrous oxide are eliminated in expired air.

Effectiveness of Drugs

The **dose** of a drug is the amount that is administered or taken. The effectiveness of a particular dose of a drug is influenced by a person's body size, how rapidly the drug breaks down and is eliminated, and sometimes, by the presence of other drugs and foods recently consumed (Table 11.1). A drug's effectiveness also depends on the person's expectations of the drug's efficacy (placebo effect) (see chapter 2) and the person's mental state. For example, when stressed or anxious,

many people require higher doses of analgesics to relieve pain than when they are relaxed. Most drugs have a narrow range of effectiveness, i.e., doses that produce intended results. In excess, many drugs are toxic and some are lethal (Figure 11.3). If the dose is too low, insufficient therapeutic effect may result.

The effects of a drug or medicine are often determined scientifically by performing double-blind clinical trials, which involve administering the drug and a look-and-taste-alike placebo to matched groups of patients. Neither the people administering the drug nor the patients know who is receiving the drug and who is receiving the placebo (thus the expression **double-blind**). Only after the trial is the code revealed that tells which patients received the drug. What is most remarkable about many of these drug trials is not that drugs show a therapeutic effect, but that placebos often come very close to giving the same relief or results as do the drugs.

In 1984, ibuprofen was introduced into the over-the-counter (OTC) market. Because aspirin and acetaminophen compounds commanded over 90% of the pain-reliever market, manufacturers of ibuprofen advertised heavily in medical journals to get physicians to recommend or prescribe the new drug. One advertisement showed that, after 4 hours, Nuprin, the trade name for an ibuprofen drug, relieved headaches about 8% more effectively than acetaminophen (Figure 11.4). From a holistic health perspective, however, the more significant result is that 40% of headache sufferers got the same relief with a placebo. Thus, 4 out of 10 headache sufferers found relief simply by believing that they had taken a pain-relief medicine.

An even more remarkable placebo effect is shown by the ability of balding men to stimulate hair growth simply by believing that they are using a hair-stimulating drug called Rogaine. The Upjohn Company, manufacturer of Rogaine, advertises extensively in the most prestigious medical journals and on TV. In these ads, the company emphasizes the effectiveness of Rogaine compared to a placebo solution applied to the scalp. Rogaine produces minimal to moderate growth

TABLE 11.1   Drug and Food Interactions That Should Be Avoided

If you take	Avoid	Because
Erythromycin or penicillin-type antibiotics	Acidic foods; pickles, tomatoes, vinegar, colas	These antibiotics are destroyed by stomach acids
Tetracycline-type antibiotics	Calcium-rich foods: milk, cheese, yogurt, pizza, almonds	Calcium blocks the action of tetracycline
Antihypertensives (to lower blood pressure)	Natural licorice (artificial is OK)	A chemical in natural licorice causes salt and water retention
Anticoagulants (to thin blood)	Vitamin K: green leafy vegetables, beef liver, vegetable oils	Vitamin K promotes blood clotting
Antidepressants (monoamine oxidase inhibitors)	Tyramine-rich foods: colas, chocolate, cheese, coffee, wine, avocados	Tyramine elevates blood pressure
Diuretics	Monosodium glutamate (MSG)	MSG and diuretics both increase water elimination
Thyroid drugs	Cabbage, brussels sprouts, soybeans, cauliflower	Chemicals in these vegetables depress thyroid hormone production

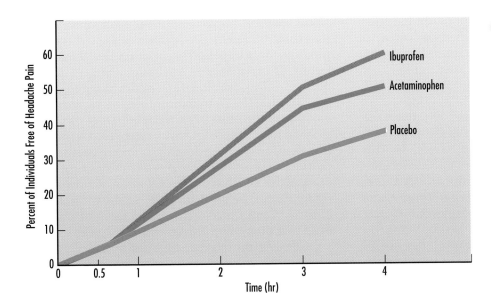

FIGURE 11.4   A Study of the Effectiveness of Ibuprofen versus Acetaminophen in Relieving Headaches   Note that 40% of headache sufferers get relief with no drug at all.

of new hair in 33% of patients receiving the drug. However, a placebo containing no active ingredient produces minimal to moderate hair growth in 20% of patients. While this fact is ignored by the advertising, it means that one out of five men who have pattern baldness (an inherited trait) can stimulate new hair growth simply because they believe they are using a drug. How the mind changes physiology to accomplish this is unknown. The point, however, is never to underestimate the power of your mind to act like a drug and help you to heal an injury or illness.

The Overmedicating of Americans

Americans consume an enormous quantity of drugs. In the United States, about two billion drug prescriptions are filled each year at an annual cost of $100 billion. In addition, there are about 100,000 different kinds of nonprescription, or **over-the-counter (OTC) drugs,** purchased, for which Americans pay $12 billion a year. Millions of people ingest herbal extracts and teas for their purported medicinal value, and millions more take vitamins, not as nutritional supplements, but as medicine. Indeed, when Americans are sick, four times out of five times they self-treat with OTC drugs and so-called alternative medicines rather than visit a medical doctor.

More than one-fourth of the legal drugs sold in the U.S. are **psychoactive,** i.e., they alter thoughts, feelings, and sensations. Psychoactive drugs include tranquilizers, sleeping pills, and mood modifiers. About 100 million Americans use alcohol regularly, another 53 million smoke cigarettes or chew tobacco for the stimulant effects of nicotine, and more than one-third of adult Americans ingest caffeine daily for its stimulatory effects. In addition, about 12 million Americans

regularly use illegal drugs (e.g., marijuana, cocaine, LSD, heroin) for the drug experience, to fit in socially, to self-medicate, or to ward off the misery of not taking a drug to which one is addicted.

As a group, older persons tend to take the most drugs, usually because they have a variety of chronic medical complaints. Two-thirds of those over age 65 take one drug per day; one-fourth of people over age 65 take three or more drugs per day (Williams, 1997). It is not uncommon for some older people to take 10 or more different medications daily, which may have been prescribed by different physicians at different times. Occasionally these drugs interact with each other to cause additional problems. That's why it's important for older people and their families and caretakers to keep a list of all medications and their doses and to inquire of health providers about possible harmful drug interactions.

In American society, the belief that drugs are legitimate and desirable solutions to life problems is pervasive. One example of the power of this belief can be found in the approval and use of troglitazone, a drug used in the treatment of non–insulin dependent diabetes, also referred to as type II, or adult-onset, diabetes. In 1997, research showed that troglitazone could cause fatal liver damage, which prompted the government in Great Britain to ban the drug's use. In

Terms

dose: amount of drug that is administered

double-blind: when neither the person receiving the drug nor the person administering the drug know whether it is a placebo or the real drug

over-the-counter (OTC) drugs: drugs that do not require a prescription

psychoactive: any substance that primarily alters mood, perception, and other brain functions

the U.S., however, the FDA chose not to ban the drug, insisting that its benefits outweighed its potential harm and that doctors could reduce the risk by monitoring patients who use the drug for early signs of liver damage. Critics of this decision argued that the risk posed by troglitazone was unnecessary since other anti-diabetes medications were safe, effective, and cost one-tenth as much. Proponents of the drug, consisting primarily of the manufacturer, several diabetes experts, and several large health care provider organizations, countered by arguing that diabetes is an extremely prevalent disease and difficult to control, and so any medication that could help is needed, even if there is a risk.

A basic premise of the debate over the use of troglitazone is whether the best way to treat non–insulin dependent diabetes is through medications, which overlooks the fact that the disease often is associated with overweight and responds to weight loss. The fact that the debate centers on drugs, instead of prevention and adopting a wellness life-style, emphasizes how drug-focused our culture is. However, health care providers that support the approval of troglitazone know that it is very difficult for people with diabetes to lose weight and maintain a healthy diet.

The Role of Drug Company Advertising

Through advertising to both consumers and health care providers, drug companies encourage drug-taking. Because most drug sales come from prescription medications, the heaviest drug company advertising is directed toward physicians. Drug companies spend thousands of dollars per year per physician trying to persuade them to prescribe the drugs that they manufacture. Drug companies send sales representatives to doctors' offices, hospitals, and health maintenance organizations (HMOs) to inform them of the company's products and to leave free samples. Drug companies sponsor seminars and courses often accompanied by free lunches or vacations to update health care providers on the diagnosis and treatment of particular diseases (for which the company manufactures a drug). And drug companies deluge physicians with pharmaceutical "junk" mail; one doctor received over 500 pounds of drug company junk mail in 1 year.

Consider this ad that appeared in a medical journal in 1997: A middle-aged man sits at a table in a restaurant on which there's a bowl of chili, a plate of fried food, and a bottle of hot sauce. The man's face signals discomfort and his right hand is placed on his obviously upset stomach. The headline in the ad says "OH, MY GERD," referring to the man's recurring problem with heartburn (called "**gastroe**sophageal **re**flux **d**isease" in medical language). The ad, of course, is for a drug that relieves the symptoms of heartburn. No mention is made of the possibility that avoiding foods that cause this man to be so miserable (the ones on the table before him) is another way for him to feel better.

Pharmaceutical companies spend $3 billion each year promoting their products. The Food and Drug Administration (FDA) regulates advertising and requires that print media ads carry information about effectiveness, side effects, precautions, contraindications,

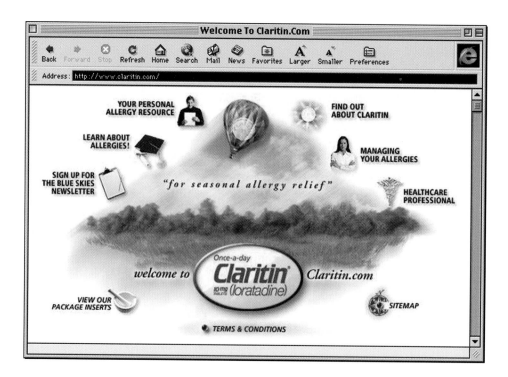

Many pharmaceutical companies market prescription drugs directly to the public through television, radio, and magazine advertising as well as using the World Wide Web to provide information on the drug and the illness it treats.

and potential reactions. The FDA also requires that these ads include "adequate directions for use." The regulations for print media ads surpass the regulations for TV and Internet advertisements, which say little about effectiveness, side effects, precautions, contraindications, and potential reactions.

Consumers are affected by advertising for prescription medications. This is why budgets for drug ads in newspapers, popular magazines, and TV are increasing. Consumer advertising jumped from $345 million in 1995 to over $1 billion in 1997. Such advertising is designed to encourage consumers to demand certain drugs from their health providers in the belief that the drugs they see in advertisements are the best, while generic and lesser known drugs are inferior. This creates pressure on health care providers to prescribe certain drugs when they may not wish to, because they fear that patients will complain to supervisors or find a more cooperative provider.

About half of doctor visits are for nonmedical or mental health problems that manifest as fatigue, lethargy, gastrointestinal upset, aches and pains, and sleeplessness. Often patients expect health care providers to prescribe a medicine, and just as often, health care providers feel obligated to offer some remedy, even if a medically legitimate one does not exist. The answer to this dilemma is provided by pharmaceutical companies that manufacture and advertise mood-altering drugs. If a person is anxious, drug ads suggest offering a tranquilizer; for depression, an antidepressant; for sleep problems, a sedative or hypnotic.

In some cases, the tranquilizer or sleeping pill may help temporarily. Sometimes people become so depressed or upset over a life situation that they cannot muster the clear thinking and action necessary to deal with the problem. In such instances, a sleeping medication, tranquilizer, or antidepressant may help achieve a calmer psychological state in which appropriate action can be taken. Unfortunately, too many people and their doctors mistakenly assume that the drug itself will solve the problem; whereas, it may, instead, substitute for proper help and treatment.

Many physicians recognize this problem. They would prefer to deal only with physically ill people—the patients whose problems they were educated to treat. But many patients resist the suggestion that they do not have a disease for which there is a diagnosis and insist that they receive a drug; this is a serious form of drug abuse. As people become more informed and aware of the undesirable consequences of taking drugs and how infrequently drugs are really necessary, they will elect to cope with stress and anxiety in ways that do not involve drugs.

Being healthy means, among other things, being responsible for the drugs you use. You do not have to resort to "chemical coping" for emotional problems.

You can resist being pushed into "pill popping" by drug company advertising. Seeking alternatives to prescription or over-the-counter drug use may be the most healthful action you can take.

Consequences of Drug Use

The human body is capable of tolerating and eliminating small quantities of virtually any substance or drug with no permanent harmful effects. However, it may be harmful to ingest large doses or to use a drug often even in small quantities. Generally, using any drug to the point where health is adversely affected or the ability to function in society is impaired can be defined as **drug abuse.**

Drug abuse refers not to the type or amount of a drug taken but to whether or not the person taking the drug is personally or socially impaired. If a drug is used to mask anxiety or facilitate undesirable behaviors, it is being abused. If a drug is used continually to combat the effects of stress, it is being abused. If pleasure is experienced only when a drug is taken, the drug is being abused. If a person cannot control the use of a drug, it is being abused.

> *If I called the wrong number, why did you answer the phone?*
> JAMES THURBER

Most of the commonly abused drugs are psychoactive substances that affect thoughts, perceptions, feelings, and moods; in other words, they change consciousness (Table 11.2). Consciousness is the state of being aware of one's mental processes. Each of us has a "normal" state of consciousness, although many people would have difficulty describing what they mean by "normal." However, everyone knows when his or her state of consciousness deviates from normal—for example, when drunk, extremely angry, sad, or depressed. A high fever can alter consciousness even to the point of hallucinations.

There are numerous activities not generally regarded as consciousness-altering that produce changes in consciousness comparable in many respects to those produced by psychoactive drugs. Long-distance runners may experience a change of consciousness that is described as a "runners' high"; dancing can produce psychic "highs" and even ecstatic states of consciousness, which is the goal of the whirling dervishes

Terms

drug abuse: persistent or excessive use of a drug without medical or health reasons

TABLE 11.2   Classifications of Drugs That Affect the Central Nervous System

Drug classification	Common or trade name	Medical uses	Effects of average dose	Physical dependence	Tolerance develops
Narcotics	Codeine Demerol Heroin Methadone Morphine Opium Percodan	Analgesic (pain relief)	Blocks or eases pain; may cause drowsiness and euphoria; some users experience nausea or itching sensations	Marked	Yes
Analgesics	Darvon Talwin	Pain relief	May produce anxiety and hallucinations	Marked	Yes
Sedatives	Amytal Nembutal Phenobarbital Seconal Doriden Quaalude Halcion	Sedation, tension relief	Relaxation, sleep; decreases alertness and muscle coordination	Marked	Yes
Minor tranquilizers	Dalmane Equanil/Miltown Librium Valium Xanax	Anxiety relief, muscle tension	Mild sedation; increased sense of well-being; may cause drowsiness and dizziness	Marked	No
Major tranquilizers (phenothiazines)	Mellaril Thorazine Prolixin	Control psychosis	Heavy sedation, anxiety relief; may cause confusion, muscle rigidity, convulsions	None	No
Alcohol	Beer Wine Liquor	None	Relaxation; loss of inhibition; mood swings; decreased alertness and coordination	Marked	Yes
Inhalants	Amyl nitrite Butyl nitrite Nitrous oxide	Muscle relaxant, anesthetic	Relaxation, euphoria; causes dizziness, headache, drowsiness	None	?
Stimulants	Benzedrine Biphetamine Desoxyn Dexedrine Methedrine Preludin Ritalin	Weight control, narcolepsy; fatigue and hyperactivity in children	Increased alertness and mood elevation; less fatigue and increased concentration; may cause insomnia, anxiety, headache, chills, and rise in blood pressure; organic brain damage after prolonged use	Mild to none	Yes
Cocaine	Cocaine hydrochloride	Local anesthetic, pain relief	Effects similar to stimulants	Marked	No
Cannabis	Marijuana Hashish	Relief of glaucoma, asthma, nausea accompanying chemotherapy	Relaxation, euphoria, altered perception; may cause confusion, panic, hallucinations	None	No
Hallucinogens	LSD PCP Mescaline Peyote Psilocybin	None	Altered perceptions, visual and sensory distortion; mood swings	None	Yes
Nicotine	(In tobacco)	None	Altered heart rate; tremors; excitation	Yes	Yes

who practice particular forms of Sufi dancing. Fasting can produce profound changes in consciousness, which is why prolonged fasts are often part of religious training. Many "thrill" activities, such as riding on roller coasters, shooting the rapids on river rafts, or bungee-jumping, change consciousness and presumably are enjoyed for that reason. Put into this perspec-

tive, ingesting psyhoactive drugs is only one of many ways people use to change consciousness.

Taking psychoactive drugs to alter consciousness is particularly dangerous because the cognitive, emotional, and behavioral processes that the drugs alter are required for harmonious adaptation to one's environment. Drugs that induce pleasant emotions can give a false sense of benefit. Drugs that block uncomfortable emotions (e.g., sadness, fear, pain) can impair useful defenses (Messe and Berridge, 1997). Furthermore, regular use of psychoactive drugs can alter the biology of the brain to the point that drug-using becomes a goal in itself, irrespective of any desire to alter thoughts and emotions (Koob and Le Moal, 1997).

Addiction

One of the many dangers of drug abuse is **addiction,** which is a progressive, chronic, primary disease that is characterized by (Leshner, 1997):

- Compulsion: An overwhelming preoccupation, desire, or drive to use a psychoactive drug, which can include obsessive thinking about a drug and drug-seeking and drug-hording behavior
- Loss of control: The inability to control use of a drug or loss of control over one's behavior because of taking a drug (e.g., impulsive actions, verbal or physical violence, impulsive sexual behavior)
- Continued drug use despite adverse consequences: The tendency not to stop drug use in the face of arrest, job loss, family breakdown, and health problems
- Distortions in normal thinking: Not admitting that problems are the result of drug-taking (denial)

Addiction is chronic and progressive: It tends to get worse over time, not better. Family members who wait for an addicted family member to "get better" generally are severely disappointed. Addiction is classified as a primary disease because, from a medical point of view, addiction has certain characteristics and treatments regardless of the substance to which a person is addicted.

Physical Dependence

Addiction is often associated with **physical dependence** (also called tissue dependence), which is biological adaptation to long-term exposure to a drug. First-time or infrequent use of a psychoactive drug causes intoxication because the drug upsets the biological balance in the brain. With continued use of a psychoactive drug, actual physical changes take place in brain tissues to adapt to the continual presence of the drug (Figure 11.5).

Both legal and illegal drugs can cause physical dependence. The legality of a drug is more a function of social, political, and economic considerations than the drug's toxicity or pharmacology (Kleber, 1994). From a personal and community health standpoint, alcohol causes far more harm than all other drugs combined, yet it is legal (Angell and Kassirer, 1994).

The legal status of drugs changes with social customs and people's beliefs. In the 1920s and 1930s, al-

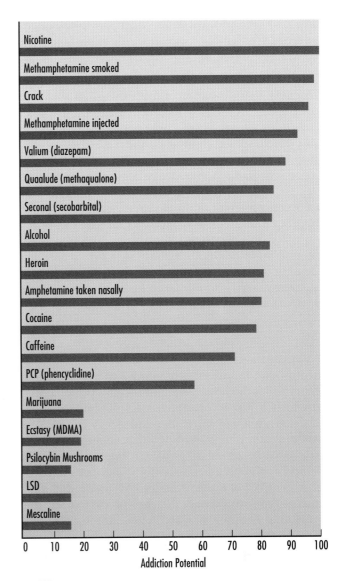

FIGURE 11.5   Health experts' ratings of how easy it is to become addicted and how difficult it is to stop using the following drugs, with 100 being the highest addiction potential. Note that both legal and illegal drugs can be highly addictive.

Source: Hanson and Venturelli, *Drugs and Society,* 5th ed. (Boston: Jones and Bartlett, 1998), p 95.

cohol was illegal in the United States but marijuana was legal. During the early twentieth century, opium, morphine, and cocaine were openly advertised and sold in the form of tonics and cough syrups. Coca-Cola, concocted by a Georgia pharmacist in 1886, was sold as both a remedy and an enjoyable drink. "Coke"

Terms

addiction: physical and psychological dependence on a drug, substance, or behavior

physical dependence: a physiological state that depends on the continuous presence of a drug; absence of the drug may cause discomfort, nervousness, headaches, and sweating (withdrawal symptoms) and sometimes death

contained cocaine until 1906, when the cocaine was replaced by caffeine.

Tolerance

Tolerance is an adaptation of the body to a drug so that larger doses are needed to produce the same effect. Thus, the longer one uses a drug, the more of that drug must be consumed to produce the desired effect. Because not all parts of the body become tolerant to a drug to the same degree, these higher doses may be dangerous. For example, a heroin or barbiturate user can become tolerant to the psychological effects of the drug, but the user's respiratory center in the brain, which controls breathing, does not. If the person takes a high dose of heroin or barbiturate to overcome the tolerance to the drug's psychological effects, the brain's respiratory center may cease to function as a result of the overdose, and the person may stop breathing.

Withdrawal

A consequence of physical dependence is the experience of withdrawal (or abstinence syndrome), which occurs when the body adapts to the absence of a drug on which it has become physically dependent. Withdrawal is often uncomfortable, and it may be fatal. For example, someone physically dependent on heroin may experience anxiety, pain, sweating, muscle cramps, frightening hallucinations, and fatal seizures when deprived of the drug. Indeed, for those who have experienced withdrawal, the fear of experiencing it again may become a greater motivator to continue drug use than the effects of the drug itself.

With many drugs, **withdrawal symptoms** are the opposite of the drug's primary effects. In general, withdrawal from central nervous system depressants, such as alcohol, opiates, tranquilizers, and sedatives, leads

to symptoms such as hyperexcitedness, anxiousness, irritability, and susceptibility to seizures. Withdrawal from stimulants, such as cocaine, amphetamines, and caffeine, on the other hand, can produce sleepiness, depression, and loss of consciousness.

Psychological Dependence

Besides physical dependence, drugs can create **habituation** (also called **psychological dependence**), which does not involve changes in cells and organs, but is manifested as an intense craving for the drug. Habituation becomes injurious when a person becomes so consumed by the need for the desired drugged state that all of that person's energy is siphoned into compulsive drug-seeking behavior. Physically addicting drugs like heroin, alcohol, and nicotine often produce habituation. As a consequence of compulsive drug-seeking behavior, relationships, jobs, and families may be destroyed.

Stimulants

Stimulants are substances that increase the activity of the central nervous system. These drugs include cocaine, amphetamine, amphetamine-like drugs, and caffeine. Their main effects are an increase in mental arousal and physical energy and production of a state of euphoria, which is why they are referred to as "uppers." Stimulants also can cause restlessness, talkativeness, and difficulty sleeping. Long-term use of stimulants tends to produce physical and psychological dependence.

Cocaine

Cocaine is obtained from the leaves of the coca shrub, *Erythroxylum coca*, a plant indigenous to the Andes. For thousands of years, inhabitants of Peru, Bolivia, and Colombia have chewed coca leaves to obtain a moderate stimulant effect intended to overcome fatigue. After the Spanish conquest of the Inca empire in the sixteenth century, coca leaves were introduced to Europe and later to North America. In the late nineteenth century, Angelo Mariani, a Corsican, received a medal from the pope for manufacturing an extract of coca leaves that "freed the body of fatigue, lifted the spirits, and induced a sense of well-being." In the United States in the 1880s, Atlanta pharmacist J. C. Pemberton mixed extracts of coca leaves and kola nuts to produce Coca-Cola, claimed at the time to be not only refreshing but also "exhilarating, invigorating, and a cure for all nervous afflictions." Today, of course, Coke no longer contains cocaine, although cocaine-free extracts of coca leaves are still used for flavoring. Sigmund Freud extolled the use of cocaine as a mood elevator, a possible antidote to depression, and a treatment for morphine addiction. However, witnessing a friend's severe and terrifying psychotic reaction to cocaine tempered Freud's enthusiasm for the drug.

As an illegal recreational drug, cocaine is most commonly taken into the body by sniffing ("snorting") it as a white powder, injecting it directly into the bloodstream (an obvious risk factor for AIDS), or smoking "free base" or "crack" cocaine. Each of these methods rapidly produces euphoria, a sense of power and clarity of thought, and increased physical vigor. The drug's effects last from minutes to an hour, depending on dose and the route of administration into the body. After the initial "high," users tend to experience a letdown ("crash") and an intense craving for more of the drug.

Cocaine increases heart rate and blood pressure. Continued use of the drug can result in appetite and weight loss, malnutrition, sleep disturbance, and altered thought and mood patterns. Frequent cocaine sniffing can inflame the nasal passages and cause permanent damage to the nasal septum. An overdose can cause seizures or death. Pregnant women who ingest cocaine risk giving birth to cocaine-addicted babies, who may be permanently handicapped or even die in infancy.

Cocaine does produce tolerance, physical dependence, and withdrawal. The potential for psychological dependence is great, probably the greatest among all psychoactive drugs. Some people develop such a strong craving for the drug that their lives are consumed by their cocaine habit.

Amphetamines

Amphetamines are manufactured chemicals that stimulate the central nervous system. The most common amphetamine substances are dextroamphetamine, methamphetamine, dextromethamphetamine, and amphetamine itself. Amphetamines are usually taken orally but they can also be injected ("mainlined") and smoked. The effects of an oral dose usually last several hours. Slang terms for amphetamines include dexies, footballs, orange, bennies, peaches, meth, speed, and ice.

Although amphetamines may be used medically to treat narcolepsy and attention-deficit hyperactivity disorder, they are principally used (illegally) to produce feelings of euphoria, increased energy, and greater self-confidence; an increased ability to concentrate; increased motor and speech activity; a perception of improved physical performance; and weight loss. Besides being used by those wishing to experience an amphetamine high, these drugs are frequently abused by people who fight sleep, such as students cramming for exams, entertainers, and truck drivers.

Excessive amphetamine use can cause headaches, irritability, dizziness, insomnia, panic, confusion, and delirium. The user often experiences a "crash," which occurs when the stimulants wear off, during which he or she usually is very depressed and tired and sleeps for long periods.

Prolonged use of amphetamines can lead to tolerance, especially for the euphoric effects and for appetite suppression. Amphetamines can cause mild physical dependence, and create a psychological dependence and a particular pattern of use called the "yo-yo," which is a cycle of amphetamine use for the stimulatory effect followed by use of a depressant in order to sleep, followed by more amphetamines the next day to get going. Chronic use can cause an amphetamine psychosis, consisting of auditory and visual hallucinations, delusions, and mood swings.

A particularly dangerous form of amphetamine is "ice"—a smoked form of pure methamphetamine hydrochloride. The inhaled drug reaches the brain almost immediately, producing a high that can last for several hours. Because the drug can be so easily inhaled, the potential for compulsive use, tolerance, and abuse is also very great. This amphetamine is manufactured at clandestine laboratories; the purity of the drug varies considerably from one laboratory to another, which adds to the risks of abusing it.

Methylenedioxymethamphetamine, an amphetamine called "Ecstasy," "Adam," "XTC," "X", "E," MDMA, or MDM, has become popular in recent years. Users of this drug experience hallucinogenic effects and euphoria, become more verbal, and find it easier to express feelings. A few psychiatrists have used the drug as part of therapy to relieve patients' anxieties and help them gain emotional insights. However, the drug is illegal and potentially dangerous. It alters the natural balance of neurotransmitters, particularly serotonin, in the brain and may permanently damage brain cells (Schwartz and Miller, 1997).

Caffeine

Caffeine is a natural stimulant found in a variety of plants used in coffee, tea, chocolate, and soft drinks (Table 11.3). These beverages and foods are an integral part of American eating habits and may be enjoyed partly for their psychoactive properties.

The effects of caffeine are familiar to most people. They include decreased drowsiness and fatigue (especially when performing tedious or boring tasks), faster and clearer flow of thought, and increased capacity for sustained performance (for example, typists work faster with fewer errors). In higher doses, caffeine produces nervousness, restlessness, tremors, and insomnia and it may have a negative effect on performance of complex tasks. In very high doses (10 grams, or 60

Wellness Guide

Risk Factors for Addiction

Risk factor	Leading to this effect
Biologically Based Factors (e.g., genetic, neurological, biochemical)	
• A less subjective feeling of intoxication	• More use to achieve intoxication (warning signs of abuse absent)
• Easier development of tolerance; liver enzymes adapt to increased use	• Easier to reach the addictive level
• Lack of resilience or fragility of higher (cerebral) brain functions	• Easy deterioration of cerebral functioning, impaired judgment, and social deterioration
• Difficulty in screening out unwanted or bothersome outside stimuli (low stimulus barrier)	• Feeling overwhelmed or stressed
• Tendency to amplify outside or internal stimuli (stimulus augmentation)	• Feeling attacked or panicked; need to avoid emotion
• Attention deficit hyperactivity disorder and other learning disabilities	• Failure, low self-esteem, or isolation
• Biologically based mood disorders (depression and bipolar disorders)	• Need to self-medicate against loss of control or the pain of depression; inability to calm down when manic or to sleep when agitated
Psychosocial and Developmental "Personality" Factors	
• Low self-esteem	• Need to blot out pain, gravitate to outsider groups
• Depression rooted in learned helplessness and passivity	• Need to blot out pain; use of a stimulant as an anti-depressant
• Conflicts	• Anxiety and guilt
• Repressed and unresolved grief and rage	• Chronic depression, anxiety, or pain
• Post-traumatic stress syndrome (as in veterans and abuse victims)	• Nightmares or panic attacks
Social and Cultural Environment	
• Availability of drugs	• Easy, frequent use
• Chemical-abusing parental model	• Sanction; no conflict over use
• Abusive, neglectful parents; other dysfunctional family patterns	• Pervasive sense of abandonment, distrust, and pain; difficulty in maintaining attachments
• Group norms favoring heavy use and abuse	• Reinforced, hidden abusive behavior that can progress without interference
• Misperception of peer norms	• Belief that most people use or favor use or think it's "cool" to use
• Severe or chronic stressors, as from noise, poverty, racism, or occupational stress	• Need to alleviate or escape from stress via chemical means
• "Alienation" factors: isolation, emptiness	• Painful sense of aloneness, normlessness, rootlessness, boredom, monotony, or hopelessness
• Difficult migration or acculturation with social disorganization, gender or generation gaps, or loss of role	• Stress without buffering support system

Source: Hanson and Venturelli, *Drugs and Society*, 5th ed. (Boston: Jones and Bartlett, 1998).

www.jbpub.com/hwonline

cups of coffee), it can produce convulsions, which can be fatal.

In the past, caffeine was prescribed for a variety of complaints, but it is rarely used medically any more.

TABLE 11.3   Caffeine Content of Beverages and Chocolate

Beverage	Caffeine content (mg)	Amount
Brewed coffee	90–125	5 oz.
Instant coffee	14–93	5 oz.
Decaffeinated coffee	1–6	5 oz.
Tea	30–70	5 oz.
Cocoa	5	5 oz.
Coca-Cola	45	12 oz.
Pepsi-Cola	30	12 oz.
Chocolate bar	22	1 oz.

Source: Hanson and Venturelli, *Drugs and Society*, 5th ed. (Boston: Jones and Bartlett, 1998), p. 278.

However, it is still a key ingredient in over a thousand over-the-counter drugs. For example, many "energizers" and "stay-awake" products are pure caffeine. Pain relievers, cough medicines, and cold remedies contain caffeine to counteract the drowsiness produced by other ingredients in these medications. Caffeine is also put into weight control and menstrual pain products because it increases urine output and water loss.

Psychological dependence may result from chronic use of caffeine, and tolerance to the stimulant effect may gradually develop. Mild withdrawal symptoms, such as headache, irritability, restlessness, and lethargy, may occur when caffeine use is stopped.

Depressants

Depressants comprise a vast number of drugs whose common effects include a reduced level of arousal, motor activity, and awareness of the environment and

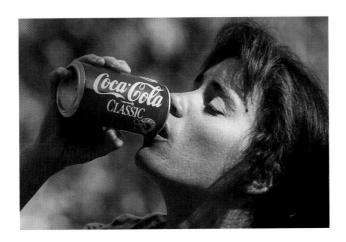

Most Americans consume more soft drinks than glasses of water. This can mean a significant daily intake of caffeine.

increased drowsiness and sedation. The depressants include alcohol (see chapter 12), and drugs that affect sleep, sedatives, hypnotics, and opiates. A number of other drugs, such as antihistamines and some medications used in the treatment of high blood pressure or heart disease may also act as depressants. In low doses, depressants produce a mild state of euphoria, reduce inhibitions, or induce a feeling of relaxation. In high doses, they may impair mood, speech, and motor coordination.

Depressants are dangerous. All carry the potential for physical and psychological dependency, tolerance, unpleasant withdrawal symptoms, and toxicity from continual use or overuse. Acute overdoses may produce coma, respiratory or cardiovascular collapse, and even death. Aggravating the potential for lethal overdose are the synergistic actions of depressants. That is, when taken together, two or more different depressants can produce a much stronger effect than the sum of both drugs. The most common synergistic effect occurs when people drink alcohol while taking depressant medications, such as barbiturates or tranquilizers.

Sedative and Hypnotic Drugs

A **sedative** is a drug that promotes mental calmness and reduces anxiety. A **hypnotic** is a drug that promotes sleep or drowsiness. Because of their potential for inducing dependence, almost all sedatives and hypnotics are highly regulated and are available only by prescription. Nevertheless, sedative-hypnotics are among the most widely used drugs in the U.S.

The most common sedative-hypnotics are drugs called benzodiazepines, more popularly known as **tranquilizers.** Medically, these drugs are used to relieve anxiety, promote relaxation, induce sleep, alleviate muscle spasm and lower back pain, treat convulsive disorders, and lessen the discomfort of alcohol and opiate withdrawal. Benzodiazepines are most

helpful when used on a short-term basis (a few weeks) as an adjunct to psychotherapy or medical therapy. Long-term use (more than 4 months) increases the risk of both dependence and of not confronting and overcoming issues and symptoms for which the benzodiazepines were originally prescribed.

Rohypnol (flunitrazepam) is a benzodiazepine with the nicknames "Ropies," "Roofies," and "Rope." The drug is illegal in the United States, but it is legal in some other countries, from which it is smuggled into the U.S. Rohypnol has been dubbed "the date-rape drug" for its purported effect of reducing a woman's level of consciousness and, therefore, her resistance to sexual assault. Several victims of sexual assault have apparently been intoxicated with the drug—in some instances because it was given to them without their knowledge or consent—before the attack.

Barbiturates are sedative-hypnotic drugs that include barbituric acid and its derivatives: amobarbital (Amytal), pentobarbital (Nembutal), phenobarbital (Luminal), secobarbital (Seconal), and Tuinal (50% amobarbital plus 50% secobarbital). Because they are less safe than benzodiazepines, barbiturates tend not to be prescribed for medical conditions that call for sedative-hypnotic drug therapy.

Opiates

The **opiates** are a group of chemically related drugs that depress the central nervous system. These substances cause physical dependence, habituation, and tolerance and produce serious withdrawal symptoms. Opiates are derived from the opium poppy, *Papaver somniferum*, extracts of which have been used for thousands of years in a variety of cultures to produce euphoria, to relieve pain, and to treat various diseases.

Medically, opiates are used for pain relief, cough suppression, and treatment of diarrhea. They can be taken by mouth, injection, snorting, and smoking. Heroin is converted to morphine in the body, and the morphine is eventually excreted in urine, saliva, sweat, and the breast milk of lactating women (which means that nursing infants can become addicted). Be-

Terms

sedatives: CNS depressants used to relieve anxiety, fear, and apprehension

hypnotics: CNS depressants used to induce drowsiness and encourage sleep

tranquilizers: central nervous system depressants that relax the body and calm anxiety

opiates: CNS depressants derived from the opium poppy

cause morphine crosses the placenta, a developing fetus may become addicted even before birth and may experience withdrawal symptoms after it is born.

Opiates are commonly abused substances, taken for their pain-relieving and psychoactive effects. The psychological sensations produced by opiates include feelings of warmth and belonging, relaxation, and mellowness. Regular use of opiates can produce tolerance to the psychological effects, constipation, loss of appetite, depression, loss of interest in sex, constriction of the pupil of the eye, disruption of the menstrual cycle, and drowsiness. Very large doses or prolonged use can be fatal because of respiratory failure.

Marijuana

Marijuana is another name for the plant *Cannabis sativa*, which grows in temperate climates all over the world. Species of this plant have been cultivated for thousands of years as a source of hemp fiber used to make clothing and rope or for a substance that, when ingested, produces euphoria, a sense of relaxation, mood elevation, and altered perceptions of space and time.

The principal psychoactive ingredient in marijuana is a chemical called *delta-9-tetrahydrocannabinol* (THC). This substance is found in the plant's leaves, buds, seeds, and resins. THC can be ingested by smoking the dried and crushed flowers and leaves or by eating food that has been prepared with marijuana as a minor ingredient.

Hashish (a resin generally smoked in a special pipe) is a highly potent derivative of marijuana obtained from the sticky resin found on the flowers and leaves of marijuana plants. *Ganja,* another derivative of marijuana, consists of the dried tops of female plants. *Bhang* (called "ditch weed") is made from parts of the plant that contain lesser amounts of THC. *Sinsemilla* (from the Spanish word "without seeds") is a potent form of marijuana derived exclusively from female plants. All male plants are removed from the plot to prevent seed formation and to allow more of the female plant's energy to be directed into the growth and formation of psychoactive compounds.

Besides its intended psychoactive effects, marijuana ingestion may evoke confusion, anxiety, panic, hallucinations, and paranoia. Speech and short-term memory may be impaired, which may be interpreted as humorous changes in one's normal mental state. However, because perception, motor coordination, and reaction time are also impaired, driving a car or operating other machines while intoxicated with THC is unsafe. Marijuana use may also aggravate an existing mental health problem or negative mood.

Some of the possible health dangers of long-term marijuana use include the risk of bronchitis caused by marijuana smoke, increased heart rate and blood pressure, and possibly a slight depression of immune system functions. Long-term use of highly potent marijuana may produce tolerance and a mild physical dependence. Marijuana smoke, like tobacco smoke, contains carcinogens (see chapter 10). Research has not yet ascertained whether long-term use contributes to a syndrome of lack of motivation and reduced productivity (*amotivational syndrome*). Contrary to what was once popular belief, marijuana does not turn users into crazed murderers and rapists nor does it cause genetic damage.

Marijuana has been shown to be effective in treating glaucoma (by reducing ocular fluid pressure) and in relieving the nausea and vomiting that often accompany cancer chemotherapy and AIDS treatments. Several states have passed referenda or legislation permitting the medical use of marijuana; however, federal laws (which take precedence over state laws) still prohibit its use for any medical condition. Despite the U.S. government's view, considerable evidence supports marijuana's effectiveness in treating a number of serious medical conditions (Grinspoon and Bakalar, 1997).

Hallucinogens

The **hallucinogens** comprise a variety of chemical substances derived from as many as 100 kinds of plants as well as by chemical synthesis in the laboratory (Table 11.4). Despite their chemical differences, hallucinogens share the ability to alter perception, thought, mood, sensation, and experience. The similarity of their effects to psychotic hallucinatory experience is one reason they are called hallucinogens, but in many respects the psychedelic drug experience is not the same as a psychotic hallucination. Psychotic hallucinations are generally auditory and frightening, and the hallucinator believes them to be real. Drug-induced

---

T e r m s

marijuana: a psychoactive substance present in the dried leaves, stems, flowers, and seeds of plants of the genus *Cannabis*

hashish: the sticky resin of the *Cannabis* plant

hallucinogens: psychoactive substances that alter sensory processing in the brain; produce visual or auditory sensations that are not real (i.e., that are hallucinatory)

LSD: a powerful hallucinogenic chemical; ingestion alters brain chemistry and produces a variety of hallucinogenic and behavioral effects

phencyclidine (PCP): drug that, depending on the route of administration and dose, can be a stimulant, depressant, or hallucinogen; originally developed as an animal anesthetic

inhalants: vaporous substances that, when inhaled, produce alcohol-like intoxication

TABLE 11.4 **Substances Considered to Be Hallucinogenic or Psychedelic**

Substance or active ingredient	Common name
D-lysergic acid diethylamide	LSD
Trimethoxyphenylethylamine	Mescaline (peyote)
2,5-Dimethoxy-4-methyl-amphetamine	STP
Dimethyltryptamine	DMT
Diethyltryptamine	DET
Tetrahydrocannabinol (cannabis)	Marijuana
Phencyclidine	PCP
Psilocybin	Mushrooms

hallucinations tend to be visual, usually are enjoyable, and the individual is aware that the experience is unusual and is not part of his or her normal state of consciousness.

Hallucinogens are most often ingested orally, either by eating the plant itself or by ingesting powder containing the active chemical. Normally, a hallucinogenic drug begins to take effect in 45 to 60 minutes. The first effects are physical: sweating, nausea, increased body temperature, and pupil dilation. These symptoms eventually subside, and the psychological effects become manifest within an hour or two of ingestion. Depending on the particular substance and the amount ingested, the "trip" lasts anywhere from 1 to 24 hours. Perhaps the most commonly used hallucinogen is **LSD** (D-lysergic acid diethylamide), commonly called "acid."

A common feature of the hallucinogenic experience is the suspension of the normal psychic mechanisms that integrate the self with the environment. The distortion of self-environment interactions makes the user extremely open to conditions in the surroundings. For this reason, experience in any particular drug episode is highly influenced, for better or worse, by the environmental setting in which the trip takes place and by the "psychic set"—the expectations and attitudes—of the user.

Phencyclidine (PCP)

Phencyclidine, also known as **PCP,** angel dust, hog, crystal, and killer weed, was developed originally for medical use as an animal anesthetic. But because of the drug's many adverse effects, it was removed from legal sale and became an illegal recreational drug. In the 1960s, phencyclidine was called the PeaCePill—a serious misnomer in view of the drug's effects.

The effects of PCP are variable: depending on the dose and the route of administration, it can be a stimulant, a depressant, or a hallucinogen. Some of the intended effects are heightened sensitivity to external stimuli, mood elevation, relaxation, and a sense of omnipotence. Some of the common unintended effects are paranoia, confusion, restlessness, disorientation, feelings of depersonalization, and violent or bizarre behavior. In high doses, the drug can cause coma, interruption of breathing, and psychosis.

Many admissions to psychiatric emergency rooms are for PCP intoxication. The drug impairs perception and muscular control, and users are prone to accidents such as falling from heights, drowning, walking in front of moving vehicles, and collisions while driving under the influence of the drug. PCP does not induce tolerance or physical dependence, but because it is eliminated slowly from the body, chronic users may experience the drug's effects for an extended period.

The effects of PCP are unpredictable and frequently unpleasant, if not terrifying and life-threatening. PCP produces more unwanted and dangerous symptoms of drug intoxication than

> *I do not take drugs. I am drugs.*
>
> SALVADOR DALI

any other psychoactive substance. Drug dealers often surreptitiously mix PCP with marijuana or cocaine or sell PCP while claiming it to be LSD, DMT, or some other drug. Because PCP is relatively easy to manufacture, it is one of the more readily available and dangerous of the illegal recreational drugs.

Inhalants

Inhalants are a wide variety of chemical substances that vaporize readily and when inhaled produce various kinds of depressant effects similar to those of alcohol. Like alcohol, inhalants are depressants of the central nervous system. Generally, their intended effect is loss of inhibition and a sense of euphoria and excitement. Unintended effects include dizziness, amnesia, inability to concentrate, confusion, impaired judgment, hallucinations, and acute psychosis.

Inhalants commonly used for recreational purposes include:

1. Commercial chemicals, such as model airplane glue, nail polish remover, paint thinner, and gasoline, and substances such as acetone, toluene, naphtha, hexane, and cyclohexane.
2. Aerosols—found in aerosol spray products.
3. Anesthetics, such as amyl nitrite, nitrous oxide ("laughing gas"), diethyl ether, and chloroform.

Because they are vaporous, these substances enter the body rapidly. The fumes are usually inhaled from plastic bags. The intoxicant effects are often felt within minutes, and the high lasts less than an hour. Regular users tend to be preteens and others without the money to buy other drugs. Some adults use amyl nitrite ("poppers") during sexual relations, believing that the drug enhances the sexual experience. Some medical personnel are frequent users of nitrous oxide or "laughing gas" because it is easily available.

The inhalant chemicals do not produce tolerance or withdrawal, nor do they induce physical dependence. However, they are dangerous. In addition to any harm resulting from uncontrolled behavior (such as driving while intoxicated), these chemicals damage the kidneys, liver, and lungs and can upset normal rhythmic heartbeat. Some users have suffocated while inhaling the fumes from plastic bags, and the potential for explosion is always present.

Anabolic Steroids

Characteristics and Use

Anabolic steroids are synthetic derivatives of the male hormone testosterone. The full name is androgenic (i.e., promoting masculine characteristics) anabolic (i.e., building) steroids (i.e., the class of drugs). These derivatives of testosterone promote the growth of skeletal muscle and increase lean body muscle. Anabolic steroids were first abused by elite athletes seeking to improve performance. Today, athletes and nonathletes use steroids to enhance performance and also to change physical appearance. A national survey revealed (National Institute on Drug Abuse, 1993):

- 2.1% of high school seniors had used anabolic steroids at least once in their lifetimes.
- 1.7% of both 8th and 10th graders had used anabolic steroids at least once, and 1.1% had used them within the past year.
- Males accounted for more users of anabolic steroids than females.
- Over 90% of those surveyed disapprove of people who use steroids.
- 15.1% of 8th graders, 25% of 10th graders, and 51.7% of twelfth graders believed it would be fairly or very easy for them to get steroids.

Steroids are taken orally or injected. Athletes and other abusers use them typically in cycles of weeks or months, rather than continuously, in patterns called cycling. Cycling involves taking multiple doses of steroids over a specified period, stopping for a while, and starting again. In addition, users frequently combine several different types of steroids to maximize their effectiveness while minimizing negative side effects, a process known as stacking.

Health Hazards

Anabolic steroids produce increased lean muscle mass, strength, and ability to train longer and harder; but the long-term effects of high-dose steroid use are largely unknown. Many, but not all, of the hazards of short-term use are reversible. Side effects of anabolic steroid use include liver tumors, jaundice, fluid retention, high blood pressure, severe acne, and trembling. Shrinking of the testicles, reduced sperm count, infertility, baldness, and development of breasts have been observed in males. In females, growth of facial hair, changes or cessation of menstrual cycle, enlargement of the clitoris, and deepened voice are among the side effects.

Reducing Drug Use

Almost everyone takes drugs of one kind or another at one time or another. People take drugs to relieve headaches, heartburn, tension, cramps, fatigue, and anxiety. Drugs are used to get to sleep and to stay awake. They are used for body problems and emotional problems. When used appropriately, drugs can play a vital role in the treatment and prevention of disease.

However, as a society we are overmedicated and overly dependent on drugs. The healthiest approach is to be as free of drugs as possible. Wellness is not achieved by taking drugs. No drug should ever be taken casually, whether prescribed, over-the-counter, or offered in a social setting. Each person should learn when drugs are necessary to maintain or restore health and when the benefits of the drug outweigh the risks.

All drugs are dangerous, and illegal recreational drugs are especially so, since you cannot be sure of either the quality or the strength. The use of most recreational drugs is illegal, and if caught, users and sellers are prosecuted as criminals. Still, many people in American society, especially young people, experiment with one or more illegal drugs. Experimenting with drugs is just that: you are taking a chance of getting caught, or getting high and causing an accident, or getting the wrong dose and dying.

Critical Thinking About Health

1. The graph below shows the results of a test of a new drug. Four groups of patients were involved. Group 1 received placebo; Group 2, 20 mg of the drug; Group 3, 40 mg; and Group 4, 80 mg.
    a. Do the data support the hypothesis that the drug is effective? Why or why not?
    b. What percentage of people get well without the drug? What's a likely explanation?
    c. What's the maximum percentage of people that can be expected to get well from taking the drug?
    d. If 80 mg produces the desired effect in the largest number of people, why didn't the experimenters report the effects of 100 mg?

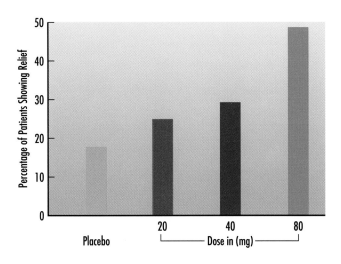

2. Bob Kozlo came home from work early one day. Upon hearing his dad's car pull up in the driveway, Jamie, Bob's 16-year-old son, quickly disposed of the joint he and his friend Max were sharing. Mr. Kozlo, who as a teenager also had experimented with marijuana, smelled the telltale odor and knew immediately what Jamie and Max had been up to.
    a. Should Mr. Kozlo ignore this situation or take some kind of action, and if so, what should he do?
    b. Should he tell Max's parents?
    c. What is your opinion of teenagers experimenting with marijuana or any other drugs, including alcohol and tobacco?
3. Why are some drugs illegal? What characteristics distinguish a legal drug from an illegal one? If you had unlimited power and resources, what would you do to solve the illegal drug problem in the U.S.?
4. In what ways has substance use and abuse touched your life?

Health in Review

*   People have been ingesting drugs throughout recorded history for a variety of reasons, including curing illness and facilitating social interaction.
*   A drug is a chemical substance capable of producing a change in physiology. Most drugs react by binding to receptor sites in or on cells, which alters biological activity.
*   Legal or illegal, medical or nonmedical, drug use in the United States is widespread. Drug use is encouraged by extensive advertising by the pharmaceutical, alcohol, and tobacco industries.
*   Drug abuse is the overuse of a drug, often to the point of loss of control. Many drugs of abuse are psychoactive, meaning that they alter thoughts, feelings, and perceptions. Many psychoactive drugs cause physical dependence; some cause psychological dependence.
*   Tolerance is the adaptation of the body to repeated drug use so that ever increasing doses of the drug are required to produce an effect.
*   The most commonly used psychoactive drugs in the United States include stimulants (cocaine, amphetamine, caffeine); depressants (sedatives, tranquilizers, hypnotics); opiates; marijuana; hallucinogens; PCP; and inhalants.

Health and Wellness Online

The World Wide Web contains a wealth of information about health and wellness. By accessing the Internet using Web browser software, such as Netscape Navigator or Microsoft's Internet Explorer, you can gain a new perspective on many topics presented in *Essentials of Health and Wellness, Second Edition.* Access the Jones and Bartlett Publishers web site at http://www.jbpub.com/hwonline.

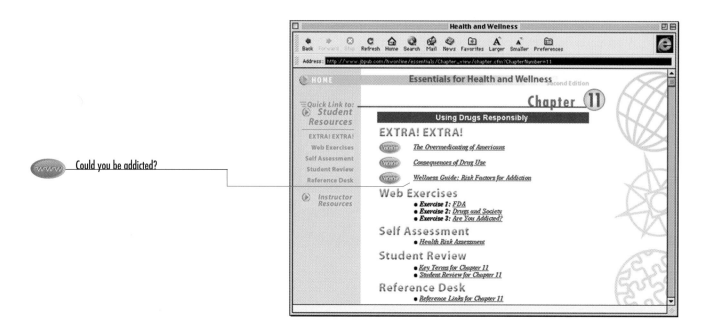

References

Grinspoon, L., & Bakalar, J. B. (1997). *Marijuana, the forbidden medicine.* New York: Yale University Press.

Hanson, G., & Venturelli, P. J. (1998). *Drugs and society.* (4th ed.). Boston: Jones and Bartlett Publishers.

Koob, G. F., & Le Moal, M. (1997). Drug abuse: Hedonic homeostatic dysregulation. *Science, 278,* 52–58.

Lazarou, J., Pomeranz, B. H., & Corey, P. N. (1998). Incidence of adverse drug reactions in hospitalized patients. *Journal of the American Medical Association, 279,* 1200–1205.

Leshner, A. I. (1997). Drug abuse and addiction treatment research. *Archives of General Psychiatry, 54,* 691–694.

Meese, R. M., & Berridge, K. C. (1997). Psychoactive drug use in evolutionary perspective. *Science, 278,* 63–66.

Rivara, F. P., et al. (1997). Alcohol and illicit drug abuse and the risk of violent death in the home. *Journal of the American Medical Association, 278,* 569–575

Schwartz, R. H., & Miller, N. S. (1997). MDMA (ecstasy) and the rave: A review. *Pediatrics, 100,* 705–508.

Williams, R. D. (1997, April). Medication and older adults. *FDA Consumer,* 17–21.

Viviano, F. (1998, May 14). In land of champagne and croissants, pills are king: French lead world in use of medications. *San Francisco Chronicle,* p. 1.

Suggested Readings

Baum, D. (1997). *Smoke and mirrors: The war on drugs and the politics of failure.* Boston: Little, Brown. A retrospective look at the war on drugs and an interpretation of why it has failed.

Blendon, R. J., & Young, J. T. (1998). The public and the war on illicit drugs. *Journal of the American Medical Association, 279,* 827–832. This article presents a review of 47 national surveys regarding American public opinion of the social, political, and law enforcement policy regarding illicit drugs.

DuPont, R. L., & Voth, E. A. (1996). Drug legalization, harm reduction, and drug policy. *Annals of Internal Medicine, 123,* 461–465. A review of U.S. drug policy options.

Graedon, J., & Graedon, T. (1997). *Deadly drug interactions.* New York: St. Martin's Griffin. Explains how most commonly used drugs interact with foods, other drugs, vitamin and mineral supplements, herbs, and alcohol.

Koob, G. F. (1998). Drug abuse and alcoholism overview. *Advances in Pharmacology, 42,* 969–977. A thorough explanation of research to date on the biological and psychosocial factors that contribute to substance abuse.

MacCoun, R., & Reuter, P. (1997). Interpreting Dutch cannabis policy: Reasoning by analogy in the legalization debate. *Science, 278,* 47–52. An analysis of how the depenalization and *de facto* legalization of marijuana in Holland can guide American policy.

Moore, Thomas J. (1998). *Prescription for disaster: The hidden dangers in your medicine cabinet.* New York: Simon and Schuster. An analysis of the dangers of prescription drugs.

The new era of lifestyle drugs. (1998, May 11). *Business Week,* 92–97. Discusses the social and economic implications of the use of drugs to enhance a person's life rather than to cure a serious illness.

Winder, H. (1997). *The complete guide to prescription and non-prescription drugs.* (15th ed.). NY: Perigee. A complete encyclopedia for the average person.

Learning Objectives

1. Describe the hazards of cigarette smoking.
2. Describe the hazards of smokeless tobacco use.
3. Identify and explain the physiological effects of tobacco.
4. Discuss the short-term and long-term health-related and social consequences of tobacco use.
5. Discuss the effects of smoke on nonsmokers, and the implications for both smokers and nonsmokers.
6. Identify advertising themes targeted at young men and women.
7. Explain why some people smoke.
8. Identify ways to quit smoking.
9. Discuss the prevalence of drinking, types of drinking, reasons for drinking, and attitudes toward drinking among college students.
10. Explain the effects of alcohol on the body.
11. Describe how alcohol is absorbed into the body and how this absorption relates to blood alcohol concentration.
12. Discuss the effects of alcohol on behavior, including sexual behavior.
13. Describe the long-term effects of alcohol overconsumption.
14. Define alcohol abuse, alcohol addiction, and alcoholism.
15. Explain the phases of alcoholism.
16. Describe how alcohol affects one's significant others and the help that is available for both the family and the alcoholic.

Exercises and Activities

WORKBOOK

Why Do You Smoke?
Do You Have a Drinking Problem?

Health and Wellness Online

 www.jbpub.com/hwonline

Tobacco Use
Global Wellness: Beyond the Clouds—
  Tobacco Smoking in China
Youth and Tobacco Advertising
Drinking on Campus
Alcohol Abuse and Alcoholism

Chapter 12

Eliminating Tobacco Use and Alcohol Abuse

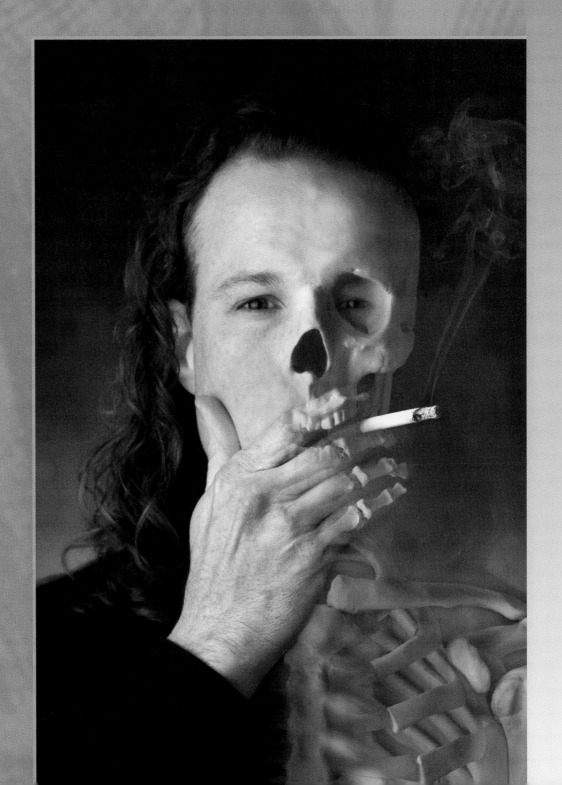

"Warning: The Surgeon General Has Determined That Cigarette Smoking Is Dangerous to Your Health." This message and other warnings from government officials and medical experts have reached just about everyone. The 1988 U.S. Surgeon General's Report on Nicotine Addiction concluded that cigarettes and other forms of tobacco, such as cigars, pipe tobacco, and chewing tobacco, are addictive and that nicotine is the drug in tobacco that causes addiction. In addition, the report determined that smoking was a major cause of stroke and the third leading cause of death in the United States. Despite this warning, about 62 million Americans aged 12 and older (29%) are currently cigarette smokers, making nicotine the most heavily used addictive drug in the United States. In 1995, approximately 47 million adults in the United States were current smokers (American Cancer Society, 1999). However, trends over the past three decades show adult smoking rates dropping (Figure 12.1). Each year, smoking kills more people than AIDS, alcohol, drug abuse, automobile accidents, murder, suicides, and fires combined!

> *Things are more like they are now than they have ever been before.*
> DWIGHT D. EISENHOWER

Tobacco Use

The health costs of smoking are staggering. Each year about 430,700 Americans die as a result of smoking; this adds up to nearly one in five deaths in the United States annually. Another 10 million have diseases caused by smoking. Cigarette smoking causes 30% of all human cancers, including about 87% of lung cancers. Government officials estimate that cigarette smoking costs the nation more than $100 billion in health care costs and lost productivity annually (American Cancer Society, 1999). Despite the fact that smokers die younger than the average American, over the course of their lives, current and former smokers add an estimated $501 billion in excess health care costs. On average, each cigarette pack sold costs Americans more than $3.90 in smoking-related expenses (American Cancer Society, 1999).

Tobacco is the single most preventable cause of death in our society (Figure 12.2). Since the release in 1964 of the first Surgeon General's report on smoking and health, the scientific knowledge about the health consequences of tobacco use has greatly increased. It is now well documented that smoking can cause chronic lung disease, coronary artery disease, and stroke, as well as cancer of the lungs, larynx, esophagus, mouth, and bladder. In addition, smoking is known to contribute to cancer of the cervix, pancreas, and kidney. The World Health Organization estimates that more than 3 million people die worldwide each year as a result of smoking.

Trends in Tobacco Use Among Youth

Adolescence (ages 10 through 18) is the crucial life stage for preventing tobacco use and its consequences, because this is when onset, regular use, and dependence begin. Each day, more than 3,000 young Americans begin to smoke. Among persons who had tried a cigarette, 88% had done so by age 18; among persons who had smoked daily, 71% had done so by age 18 (Elders, Perry, Erickson, & Giovino, 1994).

Tobacco use among teenagers rose by nearly one-third during the nineties, with an alarming increase

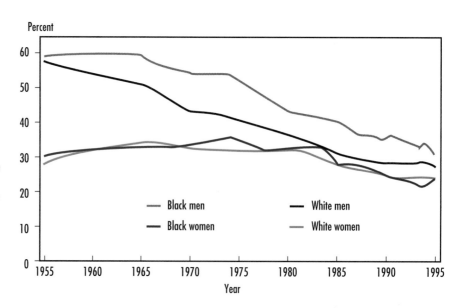

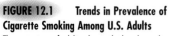

FIGURE 12.1   **Trends in Prevalence of Cigarette Smoking Among U.S. Adults**
The percentage of adults who smoke has dropped substantially in the United States over the past three decades. A greater percentage of men were smokers, and that group has experienced the largest drop in smoking prevalence. During the 1990s, adult smoking rates overall have changed little.

Note: In 1992 there was a change in smoker definition, which increased estimates by 0.9%.

Sources: Current Population Survey (Census Bureau, 1955) and National Health Interview Survey (National Center for Health Statistics, 1965–1995).

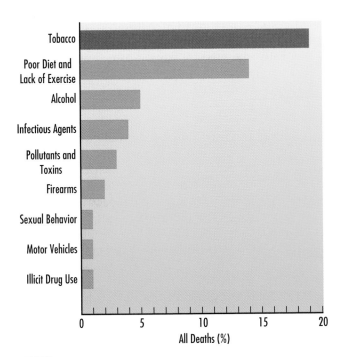

FIGURE 12.2   Actual Causes of Death in the United States, 1990

Source: McGinnis, J.M., & Foege, W.H. (1993). Actual causes of death in the United States. *Journal of the American Medical Association, 270,* 2207–2212.

among African-American youths. The 1995 Youth Risk Behavior Survey (YRBS) found that high school students were more likely to be current smokers in 1995 (34.8%) than in 1993 (30.5%) and 1991 (27.5%) (Everett, Husten, Warren, Crossett & Sharp, 1998). From 1991 to 1997 the rates of cigarette use rose among high school students from 27.5% to 36.4%. In 1997, the prevalence of current cigarette smoking was greater among white students (39.7%) than among

Hispanic (34.0%) or black (22.7%) students (Centers for Disease Control and Prevention, 1998a). The 1997 YRBS found that the consistent decline in smoking once seen among African-American youths reversed sharply, increasing from 12.6% to 22.7% between 1991 and 1997 (Centers for Disease Control and Prevention, 1998b).

In 1995, the Centers for Disease and Control and Prevention (1997) surveyed over 4,500 college students throughout the United States regarding six health-risk behaviors including tobacco use (Figure 12.3). Almost three fourths (74.8%) of college students had ever tried cigarette smoking. Students 25 or over (83.1%) were more likely than students 18–24 years of age (70.0%) to have ever tried cigarettes. Among college students who smoked cigarettes during the 30 days prior to the survey, 34% smoked more than 11 cigarettes per day; students over 25 years of age (54.1%) were more likely than students aged 18–24 (22.6%) to smoke more than 11 cigarettes per day. Among college students who were current cigarette smokers, over two-thirds (67.7%) had tried to quit smoking.

The Harvard School of Public Health College Alcohol Study examined the changes in cigarette smoking among college students between 1993 and 1997 (Wechsler, Rigotti, Gledhill-Hoyt, & Lee, 1998). The survey measured self-reports of cigarette smoking in the past 30 days and in the past year, age at first cigarette, and number of attempts to quit. One hundred and sixteen nationally represented colleges were selected, for a total of 15,103 and 14,251 randomly selected students in 1993 and 1997, respectively. Results indicate an increase in the prevalence of current cigarette smoking across gender, ethnicity, and year in school. Eleven per-

Global Wellness

Beyond the Clouds—Tobacco Smoking in China

Smoking prevalence among adults has remained relatively unchanged since 1990 in the United States, and smoking prevalence among youth has remained static since 1985. On a global scale, the picture is very different. In developing countries, data suggests that cigarette smoking is rising by 3% per year, and estimated total number of deaths attributable to smoking worldwide will increase to 12 million by the year 2050 (Bartecchi, MacKenzie, & Schrier, 1995).

China is the world's largest tobacco-producing country and has the most smokers, over 300 million

(Hing Lam, He, Sun Li, Shou Li, Fang He, & Qing Liang, 1997). Smoking in China has increased rapidly during the past few decades, but it is only in the early stage of an epidemic. Studies indicate that today Chinese men and women initiate smoking 3 years earlier than they did in the early 1980s and that the average number of cigarettes smoked by both men and women has increased as well.

China has been proactive with regard to tobacco use prevention by establishing the Chinese Association on Smoking and Health in 1990, and in 1995, banning all cigarette advertising in print and

electronic media. In some major cities, smoking has been banned in public places. China was also the first country to ban smoking on all domestic air flights.

Tobacco use prevention and control efforts have been intensified in China, as they take on the challenge of an ever-increasing population (predicted to rise from 1.25 billion to 1.513 billion by 2025), made up of people who may or may not take up the habit of cigarette smoking.

www **www.jbpub.com/hwonline**

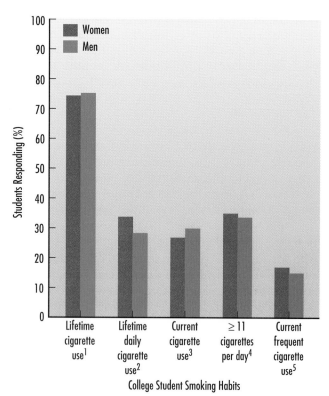

1 Ever tried cigarette smoking, even 1 or 2 puffs.
2 Ever smoked ≥ 1 cigarette every day for 30 days.
3 Smoked cigarettes on ≥ 1 of the 30 days preceding the survey.
4 Among those who had smoked cigarettes on ≥ 1 of the 30 days preceding the survey.
5 Smoked cigarettes on ≥ 20 of the 30 days preceding the survey.

FIGURE 12.3   Tobacco Use: National College Health Risk Behavior Survey—United States, 1997

Source: Centers for Disease Control and Prevention. (1997). Youth Risk Behavior Surveillance: National College Health Risk Behavior Survey—United States, 1995. *CDC Surveillance Summaries, 46*(55–6), 1–64.

cent of the college smokers had their first cigarette at or after age 19 and 28% began to smoke regularly at or after age 19. At least half of the current smokers tried quitting during the previous year, and 18% had made five or more attempts to quit smoking.

What Is Tobacco?

Processing tobacco for consumption involves harvesting the tobacco leaves and curing them by any one of several drying methods. The cured tobacco leaves are shredded, and various types of leaves are blended into commer-

cially desirable mixtures. Often flavorings and colorings are added, as well as chemicals that facilitate even burning. Finally, the mixture is used to manufacture cigarettes, pipe tobacco, and chewing tobacco, or is wrapped in specially cured tobacco leaves to make cigars.

The most familiar chemical constituent of tobacco is **nicotine,** but when tobacco is burned, approximately 4,000 other chemical substances are released and carried in the smoke. These chemicals include acetone, acrolein, carbon monoxide, methanol, ammonia, nitrous dioxide, hydrogen sulfide, traces of various mineral elements, traces of radioactive elements, acids, insecticides, and other substances. Besides these chemical compounds, tobacco smoke also contains countless microscopic particles that contribute to the yellowish brown residue of tobacco smoke known as **tar,** a documented cause of lung cancer.

The Food, Drug, and Cosmetic Act defines a drug or device as an article "intended to affect the structure or any function of the body." The FDA states that the nicotine in cigarettes and smokeless tobacco causes and sustains addiction and causes other mood-altering effects, including tranquilization and stimulation.

Not only is tobacco harmful in itself, nicotine also acts as a "gateway" drug (Hackbarth & Schnopp-Wyatt, 1997) that can introduce young people to the use of alcohol, marijuana, and hard drugs. Cigarette smokers were about three times more likely than nonsmokers to have drunk alcohol, eight times more likely to have used marijuana, and twenty-two times more likely to have used cocaine.

Physiological Effects of Tobacco

Most of the physiological effects of tobacco smoking are attributable to the pharmacological effects of nicotine. The most prominent effects include increased heart rate, increased release of adrenaline, and a direct stimulatory effect on the brain, which combine to produce the mild "rush" cigarette smokers may experience when they light up. It also lowers skin temperature and reduces blood flow in the legs and feet. Nicotine is also responsible for the nausea and vomiting experienced by most beginning smokers. Addiction to nicotine is probably responsible for perpetuating a smoker's habit. Nicotine addiction has been determined to be as powerful as addiction to heroin and cocaine.

Some harmful cardiovascular effects of cigarette smoking probably result from nicotine and carbon monoxide, which are believed to contribute to the development of heart and blood vessel disease. A host of other harmful chemicals contribute to the development of cancer and diseases of the respiratory tract. Among these chemicals are benzoapyrene, aza-arenes, N-nitrosamines, and radioactive polonium. Polonium

Terms

nicotine: an addicting chemical in tobacco that produces rapid pulse, increased alertness, and a variety of other physiological effects

tar: the yellowish brown residue of tobacco smoke

chewing tobacco: a form of shredded smokeless tobacco; chewed or placed in mouth between lower lip and gum

snuff: a form of smokeless tobacco; made from powdered or finely cut leaves

moist snuff: a form of snuff made from air- and fire-cured tobacco leaves; most hazardous form of smokeless tobacco

is a product of the breakdown of radioactive lead, a natural constituent of soil. Radioactive particles in the soil become deposited on sticky tobacco leaf hairs and eventually become part of tobacco smoke. Radon, a radioactive gas, is also present in tobacco smoke inhaled both by the smoker and nonsmoker via second-hand smoke. These radioactive substances can become trapped in tiny air sacs in the lungs, where they induce cancerous changes in lung tissue.

Smokeless Tobacco

Smokeless tobacco is available in two main forms: **chewing tobacco** and **snuff.** Chewing tobacco is processed into three different forms: loose leaf, firm/moist plug, and twist/rope chewing tobacco. A portion of chewing tobacco is either chewed or placed in the mouth and held in place between the lower lip and gum. Snuff is made from powdered or finely cut tobacco leaves and is available in two forms, dry and moist. In many European countries dry snuff is inhaled through the nose. However, in the United States a pinch of snuff is placed in the mouth and held in place between the cheek and gum, referred to as "snuff dipping." Dipping snuff is highly addictive and exposes the body to levels of nicotine equal to those of cigarettes. **Moist snuff** is made from air- and fire-cured tobacco leaves that are processed into fine particles, flavored, and packaged in moist form in round, flat containers. Moist snuff is considered the most hazardous form of smokeless tobacco because of the methods used in processing it.

Prevalence of Smokeless Tobacco Use

Chewing tobacco has been replaced by moist snuff as the most hazardous form of tobacco. The Centers for Disease Control and Prevention's 1997 Youth Risk Behavior Survey reported the overall prevalence of current smokeless tobacco use was 9.3% (CDC, 1998b). The prevalence of current smokeless tobacco use was higher among male students than female students, and among white students than among black and Hispanic students. Nationwide, about 7% of men aged 18 to 24 reported smokeless tobacco use in 1994 (National Center for Health Statistics, 1996). The National College Health Risk Behavior Survey found 5.4% of college students had used smokeless tobacco during the 30 days prior to the survey (CDC, 1997). Male students and students aged 18–24 were more likely than female and students 25 years and older to report current smokeless tobacco use, respectively.

Advertisers have intentionally promoted smokeless tobacco to athletes as being a healthy alternative to smoking—this is a myth! Smokeless tobacco is not healthier than smoking; but despite this fact advertisers continue to spend hundreds of millions of dollars annually targeting young athletes. The Federal Trade Commission (1997) reported to Congress that more than $127 million was spent on advertising and promotion of smokeless tobacco products in 1995; an increase of $7.7 million from 1993. The report noted increases in spending for magazine advertising, public entertainment, coupons, and value added promotions, such as "buy one get one free." In 1986, the U.S. Surgeon General concluded that the use of smokeless tobacco "is not a safe substitute for smoking cigarettes. It can cause cancer and a number of non-cancerous oral conditions and can lead to nicotine addiction and dependence."

> *Cigarettes are the only legal product that when used as intended cause death.*
>
> LOUIS W. SULLIVAN, former Secretary of Health and Human Services

Health and Social Consequences

Smokeless tobacco, or spit tobacco, as it is now called, is not a safe alternative to smoking. Smokeless tobacco mixes with saliva, and the nicotine and other chemicals are absorbed into the bloodstream. Tobacco in this form leads to nicotine addiction just as cigarette smoking does. Smokeless tobacco causes various kinds of oral cancer. It also causes other less serious diseases of the mouth, such as hard white patches on the gums (leukoplakia) and inflammatory lesions of the gum (gingivitis).

The risk of developing oral cancers—cancers of the throat, larynx, mouth, and esophagus—is much greater among smokeless tobacco users than nonusers. Incidence is more than twice as high in men as in women and is greatest in men over age 40 (American Cancer Society, 1999). It is projected that 29,800 new cases of oral cancer will be diagnosed in 1999 and that an estimated 8,100 people will die from oral cancer.

Smokeless tobacco has also been linked to other health problems. Taste-enhancing sugars and sweeteners found in loose chewing tobacco may lead to tooth decay. Abrasive ingredients found in tobacco cause receding gums in areas where the tobacco is held for long periods between the teeth and lower lip or the teeth and the cheek. Tobacco users often experience halitosis or a loss of taste and smell.

Social consequences for using smokeless tobacco include yellow and brown stains on the teeth, clothing, and automobile; the tobacco may cling to teeth, lips, tongue, and clothing. Spitting tobacco juice poses problems for users; thus some have learned to swallow the juice, which can contribute to stomach disorders.

Reducing Smokeless Tobacco Use

The health risks of smokeless tobacco have become increasingly apparent, and various steps have been taken to alert the public to this problem. Federal legislation has been enacted to help combat smokeless tobacco use.

In 1986, the Comprehensive Smokeless Tobacco Health Education Act was passed. This bill banned all smokeless tobacco ads on television and radio, and mandated that health hazard warnings be placed on all tobacco packages. However, advertisements in print media and at car races and rodeos have increased the use of smokeless tobacco among young people.

Cigars

Americans consume only 4.6 billion cigars annually, compared with 470 billion cigarettes. Cigar packages are not required to say anything about health hazards, and cigar smokers generally don't inhale, making the health dangers appear negligible. Despite the fact that we really don't know how many deaths are attributable to cigars, we do know that tobacco smoke is a carcinogen, whether it comes in the form of a cigarette or a cigar, and that there is no safe level of exposure to a carcinogen.

There appears to be a trend toward cigar use, because it is becoming more popular among celebrities and is considered a status symbol by some. Cigar bars and nightclubs and restaurants promoting new cigar smoking sections are seen with increasing frequency. And it is not only men—women are smoking cigars as well. Since 1993, cigar use in the United States has increased almost 50% (American Cancer Society, 1998a).

A recent study examined the prevalence of cigar use in 22 North American communities between 1989 and 1993 as part of the National Cancer Institute's Community Intervention Trial for Smoking Cessation (COMMIT) (Hyland, Cummings, Shopland, & Lynn, 1998). Their data indicated that regular cigar use increased 133% from 1989 to 1993. "Regular" was defined as "at least three or four times per week." Based on this study and others, there appears to be a resurgence of cigar use.

Cigar smokers are not as likely to develop lung cancer or have a stroke as cigarette smokers. However, cancers of the mouth, larynx, and esophagus are all associated with cigar smoking, and these risks are amplified if alcohol is drunk while smoking. Also keep in mind that the abrasive particles in the cigar's outer wrapping can erode teeth and that the 23 poisons and 43 carcinogens in its smoke can affect bystanders as well as smokers. Cigar smokers may spend up to an hour smoking one cigar; this one cigar may contain as much tobacco as a pack of cigarettes (Henningfield, Hariharan, & Kozlowski, 1996).

Cigars contain as much nicotine as several cigarettes. Although many cigar smokers do not inhale, they are still at risk for nicotine addiction because the nicotine is absorbed through the lining of the mouth.

Cigars fall under fewer federal regulations than do cigarettes and smokeless tobacco. In 1996, the Food and Drug Administration (FDA) regulated cigarettes and smokeless tobacco products as drugs. However, cigars were not included. There are also no required health warnings on cigars as there are for cigarettes and smokeless tobacco. Unlike cigarettes and smokeless tobacco, cigars are not banned from being advertised on television, radio, or any form of electronic communication. Finally, regardless of the price of the cigar, the highest federal tax on a cigar is only 3 cents.

Smoking and Disease

Almost from the beginning of tobacco use in Europe and America, people have been concerned about the possible harmful effects of smoking. Several articles in the medical literature of the eighteenth and nineteenth centuries claimed tobacco smoking as a cause of cancer of the lip, tongue, and lung. Modern research on the health consequences of cigarette smoking has provided overwhelming evidence that, among smokers as a group, the incidence of certain diseases is greater, sometimes much greater, than among nonsmokers. Smoking has been established as a factor in the development of coronary artery disease; lung cancer; bronchitis; emphysema; cancer of the larynx, lip, and oral cavity; cancer of the bladder and stomach; duodenal ulcer; and allergies.

Overwhelming data demonstrate that the death rate from cancer, heart disease, and respiratory diseases is higher among cigarette smokers than among

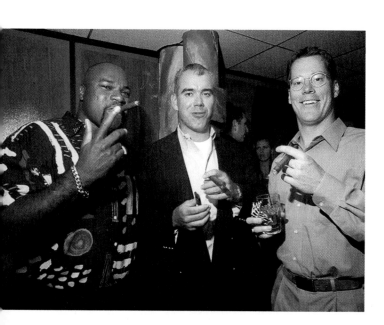

Cigar bars have become very popular in recent years.

nonsmokers. In fact, smoking decreases a person's life expectancy by an average of 7 years. Smokers between the ages of 35 and 70 have death rates three times higher than those who have never smoked.

Short-Term Health Effects of Tobacco Use

Tobacco use jeopardizes health and well-being, causing many short-term health problems. The body weight of babies of smoking women average six ounces less at birth than babies of nonsmoking women. A direct relation can be shown statistically between smoking during pregnancy and spontaneous abortions, stillbirths, death among newborns, and sudden infant death syndrome (SIDS). Research shows that the risk of SIDS triples for babies of mothers who smoke during pregnancy; two-thirds of SIDS deaths among babies of women who smoked during pregnancy can be attributed to smoking. A father who smokes a pack a day risks having his baby's weight reduced by over four ounces at birth as a result of second-hand smoking effects. Aligne and Stoddard (1997) estimate that approximately 46,000 low birth weight births and 2,800 perinatal deaths per year are caused by maternal smoking, leading to almost $5 billion in direct medical and loss-of-life costs.

Some serious short-term health outcomes of tobacco associated with pregnancy and infant health include intrauterine growth retardation, lower infant birth weight, and infant mortality (Marcus, Giovino, Pierce, & Harel, 1993; McGinnis & Foege, 1993). Other short-term health consequences of cigarette smoking occur in the respiratory and cardiovascular systems. Smokers exhibit higher rates of cough, sputum production, shortness of breath and nausea, and lower levels of physical fitness than do their nonsmoking counterparts (Marcus, Giovino, Pierce, & Harel; Davis et al., 1997). Smoking also diminishes the ability to smell and taste.

Long-Term Health Effects of Tobacco Use

Smoking kills more people than AIDS, poor diet and sedentary life-styles, car accidents, alcohol, homicides, illegal drugs, suicides, and fires combined (McGinnis & Foege, 1993). It contributes substantially to deaths from cancer (especially cancers of the lung, esophagus, oral cavity, pancreas, kidney, and bladder), cardiovascular disease (i.e., coronary disease, stroke, and high blood pressure), lung disease (i.e., chronic obstructive pulmonary disease and pneumonia), burns, and problems in infancy caused by low birth weight.

The health risks of cigarette smoking can be eliminated only by quitting. For those who continue to smoke, some reduction in cancer risk may occur from a switch to lower tar and nicotine cigarettes, if the smoker does not increase the number of cigarettes smoked or inhale more deeply to compensate for the lower tar and nicotine. The National Cancer Institute indicates that research has shown that there is no such thing as a "safe" cigarette.

Lung Cancer

Lung cancer is responsible for more deaths among men and women than any other type of cancer. Each year approximately 178,000 persons receive a diagnosis of lung cancer and about 160,000 people die of this disease, accounting for 28% of all cancers (American Cancer Society, 1999). The number of men dying of lung cancer has increased steadily since 1940. While the rate of increase among men is beginning to decline because fewer men are smoking cigarettes, the rate of increase among women is rising because more women have been smoking during the last three decades. Thirty-year trends in cancer death rates show an increase for both men and women. In 1987, for the first time in U.S. history, lung cancer passed breast cancer as the leading cancer-related cause of death in women.

A full biological explanation of how smoking causes lung cancer (and contributes to cancer at other sites) is not yet available. There are 43 known **carcinogens** found in tobacco smoke that are thought to cause the cellular changes leading to cancer.

Not all lung cancer deaths are attributable to cigarette smoking. The data suggest that about 80% of lung cancer deaths are related to smoking; the other 20% are likely caused by a variety of environmental factors, including air pollution (some studies indicate that twice as many city dwellers die of lung cancer as do people who live in rural areas); airborne substances encountered in work environments, such as particles of chromate, iron, radon, or asbestos, and breathing **sidestream smoke (passive smoking)** at home or at the worksite.

Heart Disease

Smoking cigarettes increases the risk of heart disease, which is America's number one killer. Almost 180,000 Americans die each year from cardiovascular disease caused by smoking. Smoking, high blood pressure, high blood cholesterol, and lack of exercise are all risk factors for heart disease, but smoking alone doubles the risk of heart disease. Also, comparing smokers and nonsmokers who have had heart attacks, smokers are more likely than nonsmokers to have another.

> We do not see things as they are. We see things as we are.
>
> TALMUD

Terms

carcinogens: any substances that can cause cancer in people and other animals

sidestream smoke (passive smoking): smoke released into the environment directly from lighted cigarette tips

It is not completely understood how cigarette smoking increases the risk of heart disease; however, researchers are beginning to understand the process better. Smoking can increase tension in the heart muscle walls, speed up the rate of muscular contraction, and increase the heart rate. As the heart's workload increases, so does the need for oxygen and other nutrients. Smoking also reduces the amount of high-density lipoprotein (HDL) cholesterol (i.e., the "good" cholesterol), facilitating plaque formation and blood clotting.

Bronchitis and Emphysema

Bronchitis and **emphysema** are respiratory diseases sometimes classified with asthma as **chronic obstructive pulmonary diseases (COPD).** Each of these diseases is associated with breathing difficulty caused by obstruction or destruction of some part of the respiratory system. Often persons suffer from more than one of these conditions at the same time. About 81,000 people die each year from COPD; cigarette smoking is responsible for the majority of these deaths.

Bronchitis is an inflammatory condition of the upper part of the respiratory tract, principally the **trachea,** which is part of the larger bronchial airways. Bronchitis is characterized by excessive production of mucus by cells that line the airways, which causes the major symptoms of bronchitis—such as a continual cough (smoker's cough) and the production of large amounts of sputum. Some affected people also experience shortness of breath, particularly during exertion.

Unquestionably, smoking is a factor in the development of chronic bronchitis; however, air pollution, passive smoke, and breathing hazardous chemicals and asbestos particles also contribute to developing the disease. Apparently, excessive production of mucus by the glands of the bronchi is a reaction to irritation caused by cigarette smoke and other air pollutants.

Fortunately, the pathology that produces the symptoms of bronchitis can be almost completely reversed by quitting smoking, reducing exposure to polluted air, or both. However, many people "live with" their persistent cough for many years and are not concerned with the message their body is giving them. If the disease is left to run its course, sufferers increase their vulnerability to other respiratory illnesses, and the airways may become irreversibly damaged.

Smoking is the primary cause of emphysema, which results from the destruction of the tiny air sacs deep in the lungs called **alveoli** (Figure 12.4). Each lung contains millions of alveoli; across their thin membranes the function of breathing is accomplished—the exchange of the respiratory gases, oxygen and carbon dioxide.

Emphysema is a disabling condition in which the walls of the air sacs in the lungs lose their elasticity and are gradually destroyed. The lungs' ability to obtain oxygen and remove carbon dioxide is impaired, requiring the heart to work harder, which results in the heart becoming enlarged. Emphysema involves a slow, irreversible process of alveolar destruction; as the disease progresses, affected people have greater and greater trouble breathing.

Tobacco Smoke's Effects on Nonsmokers

Nonsmokers who are exposed to tobacco smoke run a health risk. People who work or live in environments heavily laden with tobacco smoke inhale the same smoke-borne substances as do smokers. In fact, about two-thirds of the smoke from a burning cigarette enters the environment.

FIGURE 12.4   Respiratory System
Provides oxygen and removes carbon dioxide. Oxygen enters and carbon dioxide leaves via tiny air sacs in the lungs called alveoli. The rest of the respiratory system facilitates gas exchange in the alveoli.

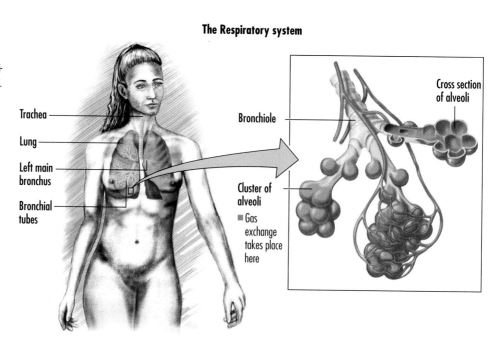

The Respiratory system

Trachea
Lung
Left main bronchus
Bronchial tubes

Bronchiole
Cluster of alveoli
■ Gas exchange takes place here
Cross section of alveoli

In 1993, the Environmental Protection Agency (EPA) declared secondhand smoke, or environmental tobacco smoke (ETS), as a human carcinogen. Annually, almost 3,000 nonsmoking adults die of lung cancer as a result of environmental tobacco smoke (American Cancer Society, 1999). Secondhand smoke contains over 4,000 chemical compounds, including four that are known human carcinogens (benzene, 2-naphthylamine, 4-aminobiphenyl, and polonium-210), and another 10 chemicals that are classified by the EPA as probable human carcinogens.

A nonsmoker in a smoke-filled room can inhale in one hour the equivalent of a cigarette's worth of nicotine, carbon monoxide, and carcinogenic substances. Also, many people are allergic to tobacco smoke, which can produce eye irritation, headache, cough, nasal congestion, and asthma. Nonsmokers forced to inhale tobacco smoke for long periods, such as workers in enclosed smoke-filled workplaces, can suffer impaired lung function equivalent to that of smokers who inhale while smoking 10 cigarettes a day. A recent study of bartenders in California before and after the smoking prohibition revealed that the establishment of smoke-free bars and taverns was associated with a rapid improvement of respiratory health (Eisner, Smith, & Blanc, 1998).

Passive cigarette smoking can also affect children. According to reports from the EPA, children of smokers have increased rates of bronchitis, pneumonia, chronic cough, missed school days, and hospital admissions. Maternal cigarette smoking has been shown to hinder the development of the lungs of the fetus and to impair respiratory function, which may predispose these children to respiratory illnesses later in life. Smoking during pregnancy also impairs a child's body stature, cognitive development and learning ability and predisposes them to later cigarette use.

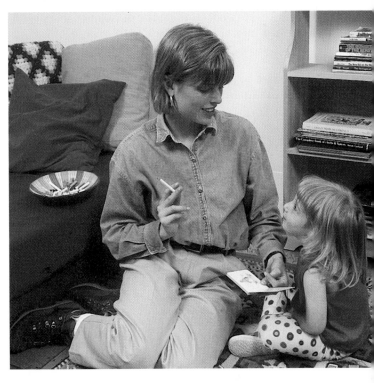

Children who live in homes where adults smoke have more respiratory problems than children who are raised in smoke-free environments.

Predicting Smoking Behavior

Personal Factors

Experimentation, usually through taking a few puffs on a cigarette smoked by an older sibling, friend, or parent, often marks the beginning of the smoking initiation process. Regular cigarette smoking probably reflects dependency on nicotine (Marcus et al., 1993). Most young smokers are addicted to nicotine and report that they want to quit but cannot; they experience relapse rates and withdrawal symptoms similar to those reported by adults.

Peer influence (friends who smoke) and family influence (siblings and parents who smoke) may be predictors of future smoking behavior. Pressure exerted by peers or siblings in a social situation appears to be the most common final pathway to smoking initiation and usually involves a member of the same sex (Williams & Wynder, 1993). If peers respond favorably to this image, smoking becomes a habit and is likely to continue.

Feelings of invincibility may be a factor in predicting smoking behavior. People are aware of the dangers associated with smoking and nicotine addiction, yet they do not believe that these dangers apply to them.

Tobacco use has repeatedly been shown to be related to poor academic achievement; 21% of below-average students are heavy smokers compared with 7% of above-average students (Elders et al., 1994).

Environmental Factors

Environmental factors associated with smoking are easy access to cigarettes and pervasive tobacco adver-

Terms

bronchitis: inflammation of the bronchi of the lungs as a result of irritation; often accompanied by a chronic cough

emphysema: a progressive degeneration of the lung alveoli, causing breathing and oxygen assimilation to become more and more difficult

chronic obstructive pulmonary diseases (COPD): diseases that restrict the ability of the body to obtain oxygen through the respiratory structures (bronchi and lungs); including asthma, bronchitis, and emphysema

trachea: upper part of respiratory tract

alveoli: tiny air sacs in the lungs that exchange oxygen and carbon dioxide

tising. These two factors are the most amenable to public policy interventions (Hackbarth et al., 1997). Cigarettes can be purchased from vending machines and self-service displays and from retailers who do not enforce their legal responsibilities and therefore sell cigarettes to minors. Cigarettes also may be received free by distribution in public places or through the mail.

Genetic Factors

Until recently, there have been few studies that showed a genetic basis for cigarette smoking. A recent study reported the first evidence that the dopamine transporter (SLC6A3) genotype is associated with smoking risk, age at smoking initiation, and ability to quit smoking (Lerman et al., 1999). Plomin (1998) states that a "better understanding of genetic, neuropharmacologic, and environmental determinants can lead to the development of improved prevention and treatment strategies tailored to the needs of individual smokers."

Youth and Tobacco Advertising

Cigarettes are one of the most heavily advertised products in America (Hackbarth & Schnopp-Wyatt, 1997). Tobacco companies spend approximately $6 billion a year in advertising. To combat declining sales, U.S. tobacco companies target women, teenagers, and non–Caucasian males in the U.S. Young people are a strategically important market for the tobacco industry, because they constitute the chief source of new consumers. These young people are "replacement smokers" who take the place of adult smokers who either quit smoking or die from a smoking-related disease. About 85% of adolescent smokers prefer either Marlboro, Newport, or Camel, the three most heavily advertised cigarette brands. The Surgeon General has concluded that cigarette advertising appears to capitalize on the disparity between an ideal and actual self-image and suggests that smoking may close that gap.

Tobacco companies use several themes that only attract the attention of children. For example, "Joe Camel," the cartoon camel used to advertise Camel cigarettes, is as familiar to children aged 6 as Mickey Mouse's silhouette. Ninety-one percent of 6-year-olds recognized Joe Camel and linked him with his product; the same recognition level was found for the Disney icon. The tobacco industry purposely targets young people in its advertising to encourage them to begin smoking and eventually become addicted. Many young adults who began smoking as teens say they want to quit the habit but find it difficult because of the addictive properties of nicotine.

There are several advertising themes aimed at young boys that tap into their insecurities and needs for acceptance. For example, advertising aimed at young boys is sensitive to feelings of lack of independence and control; thus, the campaign for the brand Marlboro, which uses "Marlboro Man," who is strong, rugged, and independent, is successful. Other marketing ploys emphasize acceptance by peers, risk taking, excitement, and the ability to do well in individual, rather than team, sports. Advertising portrays healthy, active young males engaging in risky activities that are likely to appeal to teens (Hackbarth et al., 1997).

Marketing aimed at young girls centers around four themes: women's liberation, glamour, health, and thinness. For example, a long-running Virginia Slims campaign has shown smoking as a mark of freedom and equality with men, implying that sophisticated, liberated women smoke. Another ad portrayed young women in glamorous clothes and hairstyles. These women are portrayed as being popular with both sexes and having fun with others. The health theme can be seen in promotions of women's cigarettes that are filtered, low in tar, low in nicotine, and flavored with menthol. The most successful advertising theme in luring and keeping young girls as smokers is the implication that cigarette smoking will make a girl become thin and desirable; hence, the cigarettes are long and slender. It is reasonable to conclude that a belief in the psychological benefits of smoking, derived from advertising, precedes and contributes to the adoption of smoking.

Why People Smoke

Most people begin to smoke in their teen years, emulating parents, others who smoke, or cigarette ad models. Teenagers also smoke to attain acceptance in their peer group. About half of those who experiment with smoking continue the habit into adulthood. There must be some very compelling reasons that people continue to smoke despite the unpleasant taste, the initial adverse physiological reactions to smoke and nicotine, and the knowledge—now widespread—that tobacco smoke causes cancer and other life-threatening diseases.

According to the American Cancer Society, the motivations of smokers fall into six general categories:

- **Stimulation.** Some people experience a psychological lift from smoking. They say that smoking helps them to wake up in the morning and organize their energies. They often report that smoking increases their intellectual capacities.

- **Handling.** Some people enjoy the mere handling of cigarettes and smoking paraphernalia, such as lighters.

- **Pleasurable relaxation.** Some smokers say they smoke simply because they like it. Smoking brings them true pleasure and relaxation and is often practiced to enhance other pleasurable sensations, such as the taste of food and alcoholic beverages. However, smoking actually dulls the tastebuds.

- **Reducing negative feelings (crutch).** Approximately one-third of smokers say they smoke because it temporarily helps them deal with stress, anger, fear, anxiety, or pressure.
- **Craving.** Some people crave cigarettes and have no other explanation for their habit except that they have a frequent need to smoke, regardless of the tension-relieving effects that smoking might bring.
- **Habit.** Some smokers light up only because of habit. They no longer receive much physical or psychological gratification from smoking; often they smoke without being aware of whether or not they really want the cigarette.

The question that still eludes a definitive answer is: What distinguishes people who smoke from those who do not? The list of suggested answers includes a biological susceptibility to dependence on nicotine; a variety of personal, sociological, and environmental traits; and a need to deal with stress. There may be as many reasons as there are smokers. Whatever the case, people smoke by choice. In the final analysis, smoking, like any other habitual, health-threatening behavior, is a personal matter. In the case of smoking, the choice can ultimately be—and often is—fatal.

Quitting Smoking

Each year about 17 million people try to quit for at least a day during the American Cancer Society's Great American Smoke Out. Of these quitters, more than 4 million still aren't smoking after 3 months. About 90% of those who have tried to quit have done

---

Wellness Guide

Quit Smoking Tips

Over 40 million Americans have made the decision to quit smoking. Each one had to make the same decision you're thinking about now. Smoking cigarettes is an expensive and destructive habit—it's time to stop. You've probably heard of all the reasons why you should quit, so we won't dwell on them here. However, you should reflect on the benefits of quitting. When you quit smoking, the body starts to repair itself almost immediately, unless damage has been done that cannot be reversed. Familiar symptoms like shortness of breath, sinus troubles, and persistent cough start to disappear.

Preparing to Quit

1. Ask yourself three key questions:
   How much do I smoke?
   Why do I smoke?
   What will be my most difficult hurdle in quitting?
2. If you're feeling ambivalent about quitting, ask yourself which you want most—to smoke or to stop. (Remember, you don't have to get rid of the desire to smoke before stopping.)
3. Choose a method of quitting. Cold turkey is the most successful, but a gradual approach is fine.
4. Set a final quit date.

Ways to Cut Down Your Smoking Day by Day

Note: Do not allow this gradual approach to become a way of procrastinating, rather than quitting.

1. Decide to cut down by a certain number of cigarettes per day, and increase your reduction by that number each succeeding day; *or* postpone the first cigarette of the day by an hour and extend that time daily.
2. Make it hard to get and smoke a cigarette. Wrap up the package and put elastic bands around it. Smoke with your left hand if you usually smoke with your right.
3. Change to a brand you don't like. Buy only one pack at a time.
4. If you always have a smoke with your coffee, switch to tea, juice, or soda.
5. Do something for your body. Get back into shape. Exercise is great for relaxation.
6. Call up your friends and tell them you're going to quit. (Choose to tell the friends who will offer only positive reinforcement.)
7. If you quit for one day, you can quit for another. Try it.

8. Save all the money you would have spent on cigarettes and buy yourself something. You deserve it.
9. If you break down and have a cigarette, don't give up. Some people take several tries before they make it. Just don't have a second cigarette.

On the Day You Quit

1. Throw away all cigarettes and matches. Hide lighters and ashtrays.
2. Visit the dentist and have your teeth cleaned to get rid of the tobacco stains. Notice how nice they look, and resolve to keep them that way.
3. Make a list of things you'd like to buy yourself or someone else. Estimate the cost in terms of packs of cigarettes, and put the money aside to buy these presents.
4. Keep very busy on the big day. Go to the movies, exercise, take long walks, or go bike riding.
5. Buy yourself a treat or do something special to celebrate.

Source: American Cancer Society. (1998). *Quitting smoking.*

so on their own by either stopping "cold turkey" or using other methods.

In 1994, an estimated 69% of current smokers reported that they wanted to quit smoking completely. Quit attempts, i.e., abstaining from smoking for at least 1 day during the preceding 12 months, were made by about 46% of current everyday smokers.

> *I do not think that the measure of a civilization is how tall its buildings of concrete are, but rather how well its people have learned to relate to their environment and fellow man.*
>
> SUN BEAR,
> Chippewa tribe

People stop smoking for a variety of reasons: to reduce the risk of early death from heart or lung disease; to enjoy, once again, the unpolluted taste of food; to please non-smoking loved ones; to eliminate the ever-present ashes and smell of cigarette smoke from their homes; and to fulfill a simple commitment to personal health. Frequently, a positive change in other aspects of life leads to cessation of smoking. For example, many people who take up meditation, t'ai chi ch'uan, jogging, or other physical activity automatically stop smoking. They simply lose the desire to smoke.

It is never too late to quit. The sooner smokers quit, the more they can reduce their chances of getting cancer and other diseases. Within 20 minutes of smoking the last cigarette, the body begins a series of regenerating changes. After 20 minutes, blood pressure drops to normal. After 48 hours, nerve endings start regrowing and the ability to smell and taste is enhanced. In 1 to 9 months, coughing, sinus congestion, fatigue, and shortness of breath decrease and cilia regrow in the lungs. After 5 years, the lung cancer death rate decreases by almost half. After 15 years, the risk of coronary heart disease is that of a nonsmoker and the risk of dying from lung cancer is only slightly higher than that of a nonsmoker. The extent to which these risks are reduced depends on the total amount the person smoked, the age the person started smoking, and the amount of inhalation.

Managing Stress

Progressive Muscular Relaxation

Of all the relaxation techniques known to help people quit smoking, progressive muscular relaxation (PMR) seems to be the most effective. PMR is a technique for learning how to relax muscles made tense by stressors confronted in a normal day. Muscle tension is the number one symptom of stress. Learning to relax your muscles helps promote the relaxation response. In turn, feeling relaxed helps negate some of the most obvious symptoms of stress, and may, in fact, also help you quit smoking.

People who do smoke may tell you that they do so to relieve stress and tension. Perhaps you are one of these people. Although smoking may seem to calm your nerves, the chemicals in cigarette smoke actually keep the body's nervous system in a heightened state of stress. In an effort to kick the habit, smokers often adopt another, healthier behavior in place of smoking to deal with stress, in this case PMR. Here is how they do it:

When feelings of stress and tension begin to surface, give yourself some positive feedback by saying to yourself *"I have the ability to control my stress levels without any outside help."* Next, do a quick body scan to determine if any one area is more tense than others, like your facial muscles, your neck and shoulders, or your stomach area. Then, before you light up try the following:

1. Squeeze the muscles of your eyes and forehead really tight, as if you were squinting as hard as you can. Hold this position for about 5 to 10 seconds and then let go by relaxing those same muscles around your face. Feel the difference between the levels of tension and relaxation. Think to yourself: The muscles of my face and eyes feel calm and relaxed.

2. Tense the muscles of your jaws as hard as you can, like you are biting on something really hard. Hold this position for about 5 to 10 seconds and then let go by relaxing the muscles of the jaws. Feel the difference between the levels of tension and relaxation. Think to yourself: The muscles of my jaws feel calm and relaxed.

3. Contract the muscles of your neck and shoulders really hard. Hold this position for about 5 to 10 seconds and then let go by completely relaxing the neck and shoulder muscles. Feel the difference between the levels of tension and relaxation. Think to yourself: The muscles of my neck and shoulders feel calm and relaxed.

4. Make a fist with both hands and tighten them both really hard. Hold this tension level for about 5 to 10 seconds and then let go by relaxing your hands completely, opening and spreading the fingers wide. Feel the difference between the levels of tension and relaxation. Think to yourself: The muscles of my hands and forearms feel calm and relaxed.

5. Tense the muscles of your stomach area as hard as you can. Hold this position for about 5 to 10 seconds and then let go by relaxing the muscles and organs in your abdominal area as much as you can. Feel the difference between the levels of tension and relaxation. Think to yourself: My stomach area feels calm and relaxed.

It may take a few tries with this technique to both reduce levels of stress and tension and rid your desire for a smoke, but with time you may find this to be just the technique to stop the smoking habit.

Types of Nicotine Substitutes

The nicotine patch, gum, or nasal spray are also known as nicotine replacement therapy or nicotine substitutes. All three are medicines that provide nicotine without the other harmful effects. Nicotine replacement delivers nicotine to the bloodstream more slowly than smoking. However, there are several advantages for people trying to quit:

- Nicotine replacement is a cleaner form of nicotine. It avoids the thousands of poisons that are found in burning tobacco.
- Nicotine replacement delivers a lower dose of nicotine.
- Nicotine replacement reduces withdrawal symptoms, allowing the smoker to focus on the psychological aspects of quitting (American Cancer Society, 1998b).

Using Alcohol Responsibly

Alcohol abuse is one of the most significant health-related drug problems in the United States and in many other countries. Although cocaine and other illegal drugs receive much more attention from governments and the news media, these drugs affect far fewer people and cause far fewer health problems than alcohol. Each year, over 100,000 deaths are alcohol-related, many resulting from automobile fatalities, and alcohol abuse is responsible for approximately $120 billion in health and social costs. Excessive alcohol use is also associated with thousands of divorces, perhaps as many as 80% of the incidents of family violence, and millions of hours of school and job absenteeism. In addition, alcohol abuse is linked to a long list of diseases and disorders.

Alcohol use has long been a part of social events, such as parties, dinners, weddings, ball games, and picnics. The liquor industry encourages alcohol use by advertising in newspapers and magazines, and on radio and television. No direct link between advertising alcoholic products and alcohol abuse has been established. However, public health authorities and organizations such as the American Medical Association are concerned that advertising that associates drinking with athletic prowess, material wealth, social prestige, and sex encourages irresponsible drinking behavior. Breweries and liquor distributors are especially active on college campuses, spending millions of dollars each year on advertising in campus newspapers and promoting their products by sponsoring "pub nights," giving away items with product logos, and underwriting some of the costs of college athletic events.

Alcohol's positive public image makes many people doubt that they need to learn about alcohol use and abuse. Most people who drink believe that they can "hold their liquor" and that alcoholic beverages, especially beer, are no more harmful to health than soft drinks. As with so many other aspects of health, for most people responsible and moderate alcohol consumption is more desirable than overzealous adherence to a single course of action. Everyone can benefit from knowing more about the effects of alcohol.

Drinking on Campus

In 1997, two university students died from alcohol poisoning from ingesting massive quantities of alcohol as part of fraternity initiation ceremonies. In its coverage of these tragic occurrences, the national media reminded Americans (once again—since this kind of tragedy happens periodically) that drinking is as much a part of going to college as is going to class. Indeed, American college students spend more money on alcoholic beverages each year than they do on textbooks and soft drinks combined (Cohen, 1997).

In 1995, the Centers for Disease Control and Prevention (1997) surveyed over 4,500 college students throughout the United States regarding six health-risk behaviors, including alcohol use. Over two-thirds of the college students had had at least one drink of alcohol on at least one occasion during the preceding 30 days; more than one-third had had five or more drinks of alcohol. During the 30 days preceding the survey, more than one-third (35.1%) of the college students had ridden with a driver who had been drinking, and more than one-fourth (27.4%) had driven a vehicle after drinking. Almost half of the college students reported having received information on responsible alcohol use while in college.

Whereas it is true that many students drink to excess and that, by virtue of being underage, they drink illegally, it is wrong to assume that college campuses are taverns in disguise. On the contrary, college students are only a bit more likely to drink alcohol than their age peers who are not attending college (Gfroerer et al, 1997).

Although the majority of college students drink responsibly (or not at all), some engage in drinking behaviors that are dangerous. About 10% of students are **heavy drinkers,** which means that they consume 14 or more drinks per week—a degree of alcohol consumption that risks the drinker's health and the safety of

Terms

heavy drinkers: people who drink more than 14 alcoholic drinks a week

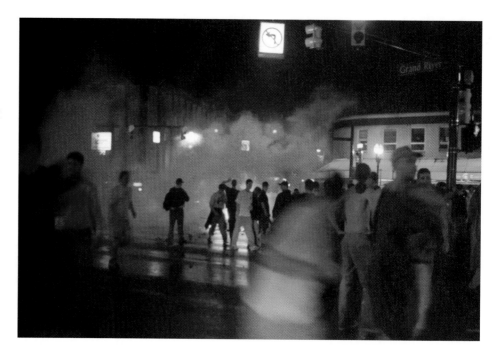

A student protest against a ban on alcohol use during tailgate parties turned into a 3000-person riot at Michigan State University in May 1998. Protesters built bonfires, threw bottles and stopped traffic throughout the night. Police used tear gas to disperse the crowd.

others in the community. Some students engage in **binge drinking,** which is defined as ingesting five or more drinks on one occasion. About 44% of students report binge drinking once in a while; however, 19% of students binge drink regularly (Wechsler et al., 1997). Frequent binge drinking is associated with a number of alcohol-related problems. For example, compared with non–binge drinkers, binge drinkers are much more likely:

- Not to use protection when engaging in sex
- To engage in unplanned sexual activity
- To get into trouble with campus police
- To damage property
- To get injured
- To engage in dangerous driving behaviors
- To disturb, insult, quarrel with, or assault others
- To require care from others while being sick from drunkenness

In general, the cultural attitude of the campus regarding alcohol use has a tremendous influence on student drinking behavior. A campus culture that encourages legal and responsible alcohol use and discourages underage drinking, binge drinking, and alcohol-induced anti-social behavior promotes responsible behavior among the students (Haines & Spear, 1996). The opposite is true for a campus that has few or no student alcohol-use policies and at which students perceive that just about anything goes with regard to alcohol use. College students who drink heavily tend to view campus attitudes toward drinking as liberal (Baer, Stacy, & Larimer, 1991). Students with the most enthusiastic attitudes toward drinking are typically the heaviest drinkers.

To reduce the degree of heavy and binge drinking, college campuses are changing the campus climate around alcohol use. Irresponsible drinking is not viewed as a rite of membership in campus organizations (e.g., clubs, athletic teams, fraternities, sororities), as an acceptable way to lessen social anxiety in party or other social situations, as the definition of partying, as an acceptable means to deal with academic stress, or as a rite of passage to adulthood and independence from parental control.

How Alcohol Affects the Body

Composition of Alcoholic Beverages

The alcohol in beverages is a chemical called **ethyl alcohol (ethanol).** The amount of ethanol in a commercial alcoholic product usually is listed on the product label (beer is the exception). The amount of alcohol in beer and wine is usually given as the percentage of the total volume. Beer, for example, is generally about 4% alcohol, although some beers contain more or less (so-called light beers have nearly the same alcohol content as regular beers). Wine is about 12% alcohol. The amount of alcohol in distilled liquors (e.g., scotch, vodka, bourbon, tequila, rum) is given in terms of **proof,** a number that represents twice the percentage of alcohol in the product. Thus, an 80-proof whiskey is 40% alcohol; 100-proof vodka is 50% alcohol.

Most standard portions of alcoholic drinks contain about one-half ounce of ethanol. For example, a 12-ounce can of beer that is 4% alcohol contains 0.48 ounce of alcohol. The same amount of alcohol is contained in a 4-ounce glass of wine. The alcohol content of a cocktail mixed with one shot (1 ounce) of a 100-proof bourbon is 0.5 ounce. So, a can of beer, a glass of wine, and a highball contain approximately the same amount of alcohol.

How Alcohol Is Absorbed, Excreted, and Metabolized

After alcohol is ingested, it is readily absorbed into the body through the gastrointestinal tract. About 20% of ingested alcohol is absorbed by the stomach and the rest by the small intestine. The alcohol is then carried through the bloodstream to all the body's tissues and organs. Although not strictly a food (it contains no protein, vitamins, or minerals), alcohol does contain calories—in fact, 7 calories per gram (almost twice as many calories per gram as sugar).

Several factors affect the rate at which alcohol is absorbed into the body tissues. For example, food in the stomach—especially fatty foods or proteins—slows the absorption of alcohol. Nonalcoholic substances in beer, wine, and cocktails can also slow absorption of alcohol. The presence of carbon dioxide in beverages, such as champagne, sparkling wines, beer, and carbonated mixed drinks, increases the rate of alcohol absorption. That is why people feel intoxicated more quickly when drinking champagne or beer, especially on an empty stomach. The higher the alcohol content in a drink, the faster it is absorbed.

The concentration of alcohol in the blood is called the **blood alcohol content (BAC),** which is measured in grams of alcohol per deciliter of blood. A simple way to estimate BAC is to assume that ingesting one standard drink per hour (one beer, one glass of wine, one mixed drink), which contains approximately one-half ounce of ethyl alcohol, produces a BAC of 0.02 in a 150-pound male. Thus, the BAC of an average-sized man who drinks five beers during the first hour at a party will be 0.10; this level of alcohol in the blood violates the drinking-and-driving laws of most states. This shorthand method of approximating BAC changes depending on a person's body size, body composition (e.g., muscle, fat), and sex. All other things being equal, the BAC of a large person is less than that of a smaller person because the alcohol is diluted more in the large person's tissues. Women tend to have a higher BAC from the same number of drinks as men because they generally weigh less than men, have proportionately more body fat (which does not absorb alcohol as readily as muscle and other tissues), have sex hormones that tend to increase alcohol absorption and decrease its elimination, and tend to absorb more alcohol from the stomach.

Alcohol is eliminated from the body in two ways. About 10% is excreted unchanged through sweat, urine, or breath (hence the use of breath analyzers to test for drinking). The portion of alcohol that is not excreted (about 90%) is broken down primarily by the liver (metabolized), ultimately winding up as carbon dioxide and water. The liver detoxifies alcohol at a rate of about one-half ounce per hour; there is no way to speed up the process. Sobering-up remedies, such as drinking a lot of coffee, taking a cold shower, or engaging in vigorous exercise, do not accelerate the rate at which the liver removes alcohol from the body.

> *Outside of a dog, a book is man's best friend. Inside of a dog, it's too dark to read.*
> GROUCHO MARX

The Hangover

An occasional consequence of drinking alcohol is a **hangover,** which may involve stomach upset, headache, fatigue, weakness, shakiness, irritability, and sometimes vomiting after drinking too much. The frequency and severity of hangovers vary. The particular factors in alcohol that cause a hangover are unknown, but several causes have been suggested:

- When alcohol is present in the body, normal liver functions may slow in order to break down the alcohol. This slowdown may reduce the amount of sugar the liver releases into the blood, resulting in temporary hypoglycemia and its resultant fatigue, irritability, and headache.
- Alcohol may inhibit REM sleep, resulting in fatigue, irritability, and trouble concentrating.
- **Congeners,** which are chemical substances in an alcoholic beverage or the breakdown products produced in the liver may cause a hangover.
- **Acetaldehyde,** a toxic substance produced when the liver breaks down alcohol, may be responsible for hangover symptoms.

The best way to deal with a hangover is to sleep, to drink juice to replace lost body fluid and blood sugar (alcohol increases urine output), and perhaps to

Terms

binge drinking: ingesting five or more drinks on one occasion

ethyl alcohol (ethanol): the consumable type of alcohol that is the psychoactive ingredient in alcoholic beverages; often called grain alcohol

proof: a number assigned to an alcoholic product that is twice the percentage of alcohol in that product

blood alcohol content (BAC): the amount of alcohol in the blood

hangover: unpleasant physical sensations resulting from excessive alcohol consumption

congeners: flavorings, colorings, and other chemicals present in alcoholic beverages

acetaldehyde: a toxic substance produced when the liver breaks alcohol down

take an analgesic for a headache. Ingesting more alcohol will only prolong the hangover symptoms.

The Effects of Alcohol on Behavior

Pharmacologically, alcohol acts as a central nervous system depressant, which means that it slows certain functions in some parts of the brain. In moderate amounts, alcohol may affect the parts of the brain that control judgment and inhibitions, which is why many people have a drink or two at a party to help "loosen up" or to become less shy and more able to interact freely with others. While some people may talk or laugh more than usual, others may become boisterous, argumentative, irritable, or depressed.

The behavioral effects of alcohol depend on the BAC (Table 12.1). At a BAC of 0.02, the "loosening-up" effects of alcohol become manifest. At a BAC of 0.10, the depressant effects of the drug become pronounced, the person may become sleepy, and motor coordination is affected. Speech may become slurred and postural instability may become noticeable.

Alcohol's effects on motor skills, judgment, and reaction times make driving after drinking extremely dangerous. Even after just one or two drinks, although an individual may not be legally drunk, reaction time, perception, and judgment are impaired. Approximately 40% of the nearly 40,000 highway fatalities each year involve people who are intoxicated. Highway accidents are among the 10 leading causes of death in the United States. One-third of male college students and nearly one-fourth of female college students report driving after having consumed alcohol (Douglas et al., 1997).

Each year there are over 120 million episodes of alcohol-impaired driving in the United States (Liu et al., 1997). Men in the 21 to 34 age group have the highest frequency of alcohol-impaired driving; men in the 18 to 20 age group have the second-highest frequency, despite the fact that all states prohibit drinking for persons under age 21. By contrast, the rate of alcohol-impaired driving among women in the same age groups is one-fourth that of their male peers. The frequency of alcohol-impaired driving declines as people become middle-aged.

Besides impaired driving, alcohol consumption contributes to arguments, fights, jeopardized relationships, employee absenteeism, school failure, and lost jobs. According to the National Institute on Drug Abuse, 30% of all drinkers aged 18 to 25 reported that they had become "aggressive" while drinking; 19% had been in "heated arguments"; and 11% had been absent from school or work as a result of drinking. More than three-fourths of incidents of domestic violence are alcohol-related (Brookoff et al., 1997).

Sexual Behavior

The effects of alcohol on sexual desire and performance vary from person to person, and depend on the BAC. In some individuals, small amounts of alcohol may dispel uncomfortable feelings about sex and may facilitate sexual arousal. Higher amounts of alcohol (a BAC of 0.10 or more) may cause problems for males, such as getting and maintaining an erection or ejaculating, and for females, such as inadequate vaginal lubrication and difficulty reaching orgasm. Even at moderate BACs, some individuals are too intoxicated to effectively give and receive sexual pleasure.

Alcohol consumption may contribute to a variety of undesired consequences of sexual behavior. While intoxicated, people can forget to use a birth control method or simply ignore the practice altogether and thus become unintentionally pregnant. Not using condoms or having sex with a stranger increases the risk of transmission of STIs and AIDS. Alcohol can blur one's judgment and can lead to unintended sexual experiences.

Acquaintance rape has been linked to alcohol consumption on college campuses (see chapter 13). A sexual assault study revealed that 26% of men who acknowledged committing sexual assault on a date reported being intoxicated; 29% reported being slightly intoxi-

---

TABLE 12.1   Behavioral Effects of Alcohol in a 150-Pound Male

Number of drinks	Ounces of alcohol	BAC* (g/dl)	Approximate time for removal	Effects
1 beer, glass of wine, or mixed drink	½	0.02	1 hour	Feeling relaxed or "loosened up"
2½ beers, glasses of wine, or mixed drinks	1¼	0.05	2½ hours	Feeling "high"; decrease in inhibitions; increase in confidence; judgment impaired
5 beers, glasses of wine, or mixed drinks	2½	0.10	5 hours	Memory impaired; muscular coordination reduced; slurred speech; euphoric or sad feelings
10 beers, glasses of wine, or mixed drinks	5	0.20	10 hours	Slowed reflexes; erratic changes in feelings
15 beers, glasses of wine, or mixed drinks	7½	0.30	15–16 hours	Stuporous, complete loss of coordination; little sensation
20 beers, glasses of wine, or mixed drinks	10	0.40	20 hours	May become comatose; breathing may cease
25–30 beers, glasses of wine, or mixed drinks	15–20	0.50	26 hours	Fatal amount for most people

*BAC, blood alcohol content.

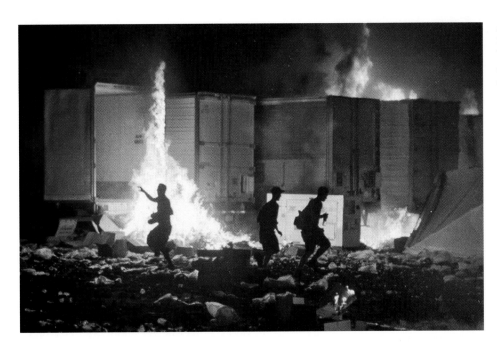

A number of factors contributed to the riot that concluded Woodstock '99, among them alcohol and drug use by concertgoers over the 3-day event.

cated. In this same study, 21% of the women who were victims of sexual aggression on a date reported being intoxicated; 32% were slightly intoxicated. A woman's alcohol consumption may prevent her from realizing that her friendly behavior is being perceived as seductive; men may be inclined to perceive friendly cues from a woman as a sign of sexual interest.

Other Effects of Alcohol

Alcohol can impair the functioning of body organs other than the brain. Alcohol can irritate the organs of the gastrointestinal (GI) tract—the esophagus, stomach, intestine, pancreas, and liver—causing upset or irritability, nausea, vomiting, or diarrhea. Alcohol can

also dilate arteries and cause bloodshot eyes. Dilation of arteries in the arms, legs, and skin can cause a drop in blood pressure and decrease body heat, explaining why people occasionally feel flushed when they drink. Giving people alcohol to "warm them up" actually produces the opposite physiological effect.

Alcohol should not be ingested simultaneously with other central nervous system depressants such as tranquilizers, sedatives, and antihistamines, which are found in cold medicines. In many instances, the depressant effects of alcohol and the other drug interact so that the combined effects of the two drugs is greater than the simple additive effects of either drug taken separately. Seemingly reasonable amounts of alcohol taken with another depressant drug can dangerously suppress brain function and respiration (Table 12.2).

Long-Term Effects

Long-term heavy drinking can affect the immune, endocrine, and reproductive functions and can cause neurological problems, including dementia, blackouts, seizures, hallucinations, and peripheral neuropathy. Various cancers associated with heavy drinking include cancers of the lip, oral cavity, pharynx, larynx, esophagus, stomach, colon, rectum, tongue, lung, pancreas, and liver. Long-term heavy drinking can also increase the risk of chronic gastritis, hepatitis, hypertension, cirrhosis of the liver, and coronary heart disease.

Chronic alcoholic men may become "feminized," with breast enlargement and female body hair patterns. Chronic alcoholic women may experience menstrual disturbances, loss of secondary sex characteristics, and infertility. Women who drink heavily experience more gynecological problems and have surgery more often than women who do not.

TABLE 12.2   Alcohol and Drugs That Don't Mix
Alcohol should NOT be consumed when taking drugs such as these.

Drug	Dangerous interaction
Acetaminophen (Tylenol, Anacin-3)	Moderate use plus alcohol can cause liver damage.
Aspirin (Anacin, Excedrin)	Heavy use plus alcohol can cause bleeding of stomach wall and GI tract.
Antihistamines (Chlor-Trimeton, Benadryl)	Drowsiness and loss of coordination increased by alcohol.
Tranquilizers, sedatives (Valium, Dalmane, Miltown)	Alcohol increases their effects.
Painkillers (codeine, Percodan, morphine)	Alcohol increases sedation and reduces ability to concentrate.
Barbiturates (Amytal, Seconal, phenobarbital)	Potentially FATAL. NEVER use with alcohol.

Fetal Alcohol Syndrome

Alcohol can harm the health of anyone, man or woman, young or old. Even a fetus can be damaged by alcohol. Over the last 10 years, evidence has accumulated showing that numerous kinds of birth defects and mental retardation may result from ingestion of alcohol by pregnant women—a condition known as **fetal alcohol syndrome.** Fetal alcohol syndrome is estimated to be the third leading cause of birth defects and mental retardation among newborns. Since the harmful effects on the fetus are believed to occur during the first few weeks or months of prenatal development, a time during which much of the nervous system is being formed, women should refrain from drinking if they are trying to become pregnant or if they suspect they are pregnant. Studies have also shown that the level of alcohol in the fetus' blood may be ten times greater than the BAC of the mother. This explains why even a couple of drinks early in pregnancy can endanger normal fetal development.

 ## Alcohol Abuse and Alcoholism

Alcohol abuse is the principal drug problem in the United States. Approximately 12 million Americans of different ages, religions, races, educational backgrounds, and socioeconomic status have problems with alcohol. Over 3 million American teenagers between ages 14 and 17 have a drinking problem. More than a third of all suicides involve alcohol. Approximately 6 million adults have personal and health problems associated with alcohol that are severe enough to warrant the label **alcoholic** and be said to have **alcoholism.** These people are unable to control their drinking; some are physically dependent on alcohol and may experience withdrawal symptoms, including **delirium tremens**

> *I don't even know what street Canada is on.*
>
> AL CAPONE

(DTs), characterized by hallucinations and uncontrollable shaking, when deprived of alcohol.

Problem drinking can cause numerous negative consequences. Job and school performance can be impaired, family relationships and friendships can be destroyed, and drunk driving may cause financial problems, injuries, legal problems and fatalities. Because alcohol supplies calories, alcoholics are rarely hungry. They may have vitamin deficiency syndromes, which result in loss of muscular coordination and mental confusion.

The cause or causes of problem drinking and alcoholism are unknown, although hypotheses abound. Before the advent of modern psychology and medicine, alcohol abuse was thought to be a manifestation of immorality and irreligiousness. Some people still hold that view, but many professionals (and problem drinkers) interpret alcohol abuse as a behavioral disorder or a medical disease. For example, some people may drink in order to feel better about themselves or to try to cope with life's adversities. Instead, they may add a drinking problem to their other problems.

Some evidence indicates that, at least for some people, alcoholism may have a biological basis, either because people metabolize alcohol differently or because their brains respond differently to alcohol. Some experts resist considering alcohol abuse a disease be-

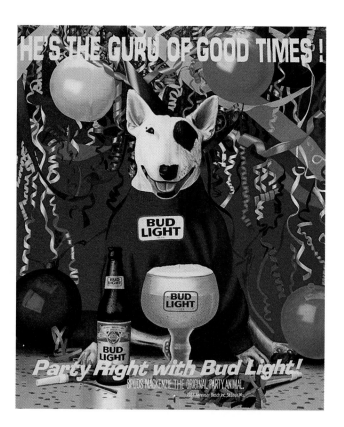

Alcohol advertisements, like cigarette ads, emphasize the connections among drinking, sex, and fun.

Terms

fetal alcohol syndrome: birth defects and mental retardation caused by ingestion of alcohol during pregnancy

alcohol abuse: frequent, continued use of alcohol; binge drinking

alcoholic: a person dependent on alcohol

alcoholism: loss of control over drinking alcohol

delirium tremens (DTs): hallucinations and uncontrollable shaking sometimes caused by withdrawal of alcohol in alcohol-dependent individuals

blackout: failure to recall normal or abnormal behavior or events that occurred while drinking

bender: several days of binge drinking

cause doing so may remove the sense of personal and social responsibility for problem drinking. Others argue that calling alcohol abuse a "disease" fosters successful treatment because it removes the stigma, lessens guilt, and offers a supervised and presumably scientifically based plan for treatment.

The Phases of Alcoholism

Alcoholism usually develops from a prealcoholic stage of needing to drink to relieve tensions and anxieties. The prealcoholic phase may last for years, during which tolerance to alcohol gradually develops. Progression to a state of alcoholism is characterized by three phases:

- **The warning phase.** In this first stage of alcoholism, problem drinkers increase tolerance for alcohol and become more preoccupied with drinking. For example, when invited to a party they may ask what alcoholic beverages will be served rather than who is going to be there. In this stage problem drinkers may sneak drinks often and may deny that they are drinking too much. **Blackouts** may also occur. Blackouts are periods in which others observe the drinker as behaving normally or abnormally, but the drinker has no recall of events that happened while drinking.

- **The crucial phase.** This phase of alcoholism is characterized by loss of control over how much alcohol is consumed. The person may not drink every day, but cannot control the amount of alcohol consumed once drinking has begun. In this stage, the problem drinker may rationalize drinking behavior and actually believe that there are good reasons for heavy drinking. Alcoholics may still carry out responsibilities (e.g., housework, job, schoolwork) for some time, and they may employ a series of strategies to keep the family from rejecting them, including promises to stop drinking. Often alcoholics' extrav-

agant measures to prove they do not have a drinking problem appear successful, but eventually they begin drinking heavily again. At this point the problem with alcohol is sometimes blamed on the kind of drinks preferred or on the usual place of drinking; as a result, problem drinkers may change to a different form of alcoholic beverage or to a different place in which to drink.

- **The chronic phase.** In this phase, the alcoholic is dependent on the drug, and drinking behavior consumes all aspects of life. Friends and family have resigned themselves to the problem and may be angry or ignore the alcoholic. At this stage of alcoholism the person may miss work or school occasionally. The health consequences of alcohol abuse may intensify and the person may need medical attention and even hospitalization. When physical addiction to alcohol occurs, continual drinking is needed to prevent withdrawal symptoms. Drinking for days at a time (a **bender**) may take place. The great majority of alcoholics do not wind up on "skid row," but instead struggle with their problem within their families and communities.

The Effects of Alcoholism on the Family

Alcoholism can severely disrupt marital and family relationships. One family member's drinking problem can put stress on all the other members, causing them mental and emotional suffering and sometimes financial hardship. Alcoholism is costly to many people, not just the alcoholic.

Close relatives of a problem drinker can experience a variety of emotions, ranging from joy and relief when the problem drinker stops drinking for a time to feelings of failure and depression when the problem drinker begins drinking again. In between the highs and lows, family members can feel anger, shame, guilt, pity, and constant anxiety. They may try to cope

---

Wellness Guide

Warning Signs of Problem Drinking or Alcoholism

1. Gulping drinks.
2. Drinking to modify uncomfortable feelings.
3. Personality or behavioral changes after drinking.
4. Getting drunk frequently.
5. Experiencing "blackouts"—not being able to remember what happened while drinking.
6. Frequent accidents or illness as a result of drinking.
7. Priming—preparing yourself with alcohol before a social gathering at which alcohol is going to be served.
8. Not wanting to talk about the negative consequences of drinking (avoidance).
9. Focusing social situations around alcohol.
10. Sneaking drinks or clandestine drinking.
11. Preoccupation with alcohol.

with the situation in different ways. Some may try to assume responsibility for the problem; others may be designated as scapegoats and blamed for it, while some family members blame others (i.e., other family members, other people) for the drinker's problem. Some may withdraw in silence while others try to maintain their sense of humor. These behaviors are all defense mechanisms against the family's psychological pain.

Like the problem drinker, family members may deny the problem, try to rationalize it, isolate themselves from friends and relatives, and, in some cases, actually feel responsible for the other's drinking problem. This **enabling,** or protection process, keeps the alcoholic from feeling responsible for his or her drinking—which is part of the paradox experienced by families of alcoholics. In their attempts to protect the alcoholic, family members may unwittingly contribute to the drinking problem; they may try to protect the alcoholic from serious social consequences of excessive drinking, for instance, making excuses for absenteeism from work or school.

Family members of alcoholics may attend Alanon, an organization that helps spouses, families, and friends of alcoholics. Alateen is a similar organization that helps children of alcoholics. Alanon and Alateen help family members understand how alcoholism has affected their lives and help them to explore the family relationships that contribute to the alcohol problem. Family therapy (with or without the problem drinker's participation) may help a family find ways to cope with the problem and regain harmony in their family life.

Children of Alcoholics

The National Clearinghouse for Alcohol and Drug Information estimates that there are 26.8 million children of alcoholics (COAs) in the United States, 11 million of whom are under the age of 18. Adult children of alcoholics (ACOAs) and COAs grew up in families in which one or both parents had a drinking problem. As children, many of these individuals experienced neglect, emotional deprivation, an unstable family environment, and sometimes violence and abuse. As a result, they may have developed ways of thinking and behaving that impair personal and relationship harmony in adulthood. Children of alcoholics are at a high risk of becoming alcoholics themselves.

To numb the emotional pain stemming from parental alcoholism, many ACOAs learn as children to block from their awareness the truth of their situation—both the fact of a parent's alcoholism and also the emotional pain resulting from it. This tendency is referred to as **denial.** The consequences of denial by the ACOA go beyond issues of parental alcoholism to become a generalized way of approaching life. As adults, many ACOAs are constricted in their capacities to see the world as it really is and also to experience emotional fulfillment.

Denial gives many ACOAs a negative self-image and a tendency to be hypercritical of themselves. Rather than face the painful truth, many ACOAs, when children, believed themselves to be the cause of their parent's erratic, violent behavior. Indeed, sometimes the troubled parents reinforced this assumption by blaming their children for their problems. The children not only come to believe themselves to be "bad," but they also tend to believe they are responsible for everyone else's emotions. Thus, they become very other-focused, a behavior called **codependency.**

Another consequence of growing up in an alcoholic family is the tendency to try to control situations and other people. Because family life was unstable and painful, many ACOAs come to believe that their interpersonal environment is likely at any moment to become emotionally painful, violent, or disruptive. Thus, ACOAs tend to be constantly anxious and hypervigilant for signs of danger. To minimize the threat (experienced as criticism, abandonment, or abuse), ACOAs tend to be compliant and agreeable and actively try to please. Believing that others cannot be trusted and that the world must be made safe, ACOAs also try to be totally self-reliant and in control of their lives.

Denial, a negative self-image, the tendency to take responsibility for others, the need to control oneself and the environment, and other characteristics help an ACOA survive childhood in an alcoholic family. Unfortunately, in adulthood these same "survival" mechanisms limit the opportunity to grow and develop unique individual qualities and to experience healthy interpersonal relationships. Fortunately, these self-limiting beliefs and behaviors can be changed through counseling, 12-step programs, such as Codependents Anonymous, and various spiritual practices.

Seeking Help: Treatment Options

The situation of problem drinkers and alcoholics is serious but not hopeless. Recovery is possible if the person is strongly motivated to stop drinking. Moreover, as in other aspects of health, "an ounce of prevention is worth a pound of cure."

Sometimes the motivation to stop drinking comes in the form of a threat—a drinking-related legal problem or illness, severe disruption of family life, the loss of a job. The motivation to stop drinking can also come from the person's own resolve to stop his or her self-destructive behavior and to stop feeling helpless, hopeless, and confused.

Wellness Guide

Some Characteristics of Adult Children of Alcoholics

- Guessing at what normal behavior is and having a higher tolerance for abusive behavior
- Tendency to perceive things as all good or bad ("all-or-none" thinking)
- Feeling different and cut-off from other people
- Mercilessly self-critical
- Fearful of losing control of one's feelings and behaviors

- Trying to control others
- Resisting and overreacting to change
- Constantly seeking approval and affirmation
- Lack of awareness of emotions
- Fearful of expressing one's true thoughts and feelings
- Being overly responsible for others' feelings

- A tendency toward compulsive behavior: overeating, drug or alcohol abuse, workaholism
- A tendency to be a "rescuer" or "victim" in interpersonal relationships
- Difficulty relaxing, letting go, and having fun

Alcoholics Anonymous (AA), the worldwide non-profit self-help organization, has assisted many people to get on the road back to wellness and enjoyment of life. AA bases its program on total sobriety, anonymity, and a step-by-step program of recovery. The environment at AA meetings is relaxing, caring, and open. Members share their experiences, strengths, and hopes with each other, with the goal of helping new and old members identify and learn more about their own problems with alcohol. Practical tips on how to remain sober are shared, and telephone numbers are exchanged so that a member can contact another member if stressful situations arise that previously led to drinking.

Alcoholics Anonymous emphasizes that sobriety is a state of mind, which means that recovering from a drinking problem involves changing values, attitudes, and life-styles. The AA program helps problem drinkers honestly examine their feelings, recognize their limitations, and accept responsibility for past wrongs. For problem drinkers, remaining sober is an ongoing process, which involves finding new ways to satisfy emotional, spiritual, and social needs.

Besides AA, problem drinkers can receive help from individual and group psychotherapy. Many therapists are trained specifically to help problem drinkers and their families recover. Also, certain medicines may help. Disulfuram ("Antabuse") causes uncomfortable physical and mental feelings when alcohol is ingested. Naltrexone ("ReVia") can help reduce the craving for alcohol.

Responsible Drinking

Each person has the option of drinking or abstaining from alcohol. Each of you has the responsibility for determining the occasions for drinking and the amounts of alcohol that you consume. If you are one of the millions of people who already enjoy drinking, here are some guidelines to remember:

- Make sure that alcohol use improves your social interactions and does not harm or destroy them.
- Drink slowly and avoid mixing alcohol with other drugs.
- Be sure that using alcohol enhances your general sense of well-being and does not make either you or other persons feel disgusted with your actions.
- If you plan to drink, decide beforehand that you will not drive and designate someone who will not drink to be the driver.

In addition to being responsible for your own drinking habits, you can also help others to drink responsibly. Respect the wishes of the person who chooses to abstain from drinking and don't push drinks on people at parties. If you are giving a party, be sure to provide alternatives to alcohol. You may also offer places to sleep for those who have been drinking and should not drive home. Remember to eat when you drink and to provide food at your parties.

There is no evidence to indicate that total abstinence from alcohol is necessary for health and wellness. On the other hand, there is a great deal of evidence showing that excessive alcohol use can destroy personal health and family relationships, can cause traffic deaths and suicides, and can produce birth defects in newborns. We believe that you can significantly improve your health and happiness by developing responsible drinking habits while you are young and maintaining moderate drinking habits throughout life.

Terms

enabling: denial of, or excuses for, the excessive drinking by an alcoholic to whom one is close

denial: refusal to admit you (or someone else) have a drinking problem

codependency: a relationship pattern in which the nonaddicted family members identify with the alcoholic

Critical Thinking About Health

1. Smoking takes a toll on everyone—those who smoke and those who do not. Government officials estimate that cigarette smoking costs the nation about $100 billion a year in health care costs and lost productivity. These costs are borne equally by nonsmokers and smokers.
   a. Should nonsmokers pay for the health care expenses of people who smoke? Why or why not?
   b. Should cigarettes be taxed by the government to cover their full cost to society, which could lessen tobacco consumption, put tobacco growers out of business, and drastically reduce tobacco companies' profits?

2. Purchase a popular magazine and count the number of cigarette ads in that issue. Review each ad and respond to the following questions:
   a. Who is the ad targeting? (e.g., women, men, young, old)
   b. How is the ad appealing to its target audience? (e.g., sex, friends)
   c. Besides the warning label (which is required by law) does the ad mention any negative side effects of smoking?
   d. What does the ad imply will happen if you smoke their brand of cigarette?

3. Visit or call your local health department and ask them for a list of restaurants in your community that are smoke-free.
   a. What percentage of your community's eating establishments are smoke-free?
   b. What can you do to promote smoke-free eating establishments within your community?
   c. Should all public places—indoor and outdoor—be smoke-free?

4. After about a month it was clear that inviting Chris to be their roommate had been a brilliant move. With a 3.9-plus GPA, Chris was a fountain of help with every subject from history to chemistry. Getting into law school was a forgone conclusion. The real question was how to get Chris on "Jeopardy!"

   When mid-term exams rolled around, the roommates noticed that Chris was coming home every day with a 12-pack of beer—six cans would disappear before dinner and the rest disappeared as the night's studying progressed. Although Chris showed no signs of impairment from ingesting this quantity of alcohol, the roommates were concerned.
   a. What concerns might the roommates have? If you were Chris' roommate, would you be concerned?

   b. Given Chris' obvious success in school and the fact that Chris shows no outward sign of impairment, would you agree or disagree that Chris has a problem with alcohol?
   c. Do you think Chris' roommates should try to change Chris' drinking behavior, or is it none of their business?

5. Every summer, State U. invites the parents of incoming students to "Parents' Day," a chance to visit the campus and talk to faculty, students, and administrators. Last summer, Dr. Meredith, one of the university's newest faculty members, gladly volunteered to give a "sample lecture" on paleontology to the parents and to chat with them at the luncheon in the Faculty Dining Room.

   A father of an incoming female student engaged Dr. Meredith in conversation about his daughter's likely experiences living in the college dormitory and swimming on the swim team.

   "My daughter's never been away from home before," said the father. "I want to be sure she'll be OK."

   Dr. Meredith silently gulped hard, for he knew that the dormitories had the reputation for massive illegal drinking during the first month or two of the school year, and that the swim coach would drink beer with the team members after swim meets.
   a. Does the father have anything to be concerned about?
   b. Should Dr. Meredith tell the father about alcohol use at the college?
   c. To avoid having to encounter another parent with similar concerns, Dr. Meredith vowed never again to help out at Parents' Day. What else could Dr. Meredith do to avoid such unpleasant experiences? Remember that Dr. Meredith is new at the university and without tenure.
   d. What is the campus climate toward tolerating alcohol use among students on your campus?

6. A college needs an electronic scoreboard for its football stadium, and a beer company is willing to buy it in exchange for exclusive advertising rights on the scoreboard and in the football game programs. The college president is against this deal, arguing that it promotes drinking on campus. However, the athletic director and the president of the alumni association favor it, arguing that it's vital to have the new scoreboard and besides, "beer and college always have gone together and always will, and there's nothing wrong with it."

a. Do you favor or object to the scoreboard deal?

b. Do you agree or disagree with the college president about the fact that advertising promotes drinking?

c. Do you agree or disagree with the athletic director and alumni president that beer and college always have and always will go together?

Health in Review

- No public health message is disseminated as widely as that on every package of cigarettes and in every cigarette advertisement: "Warning: The Surgeon General Has Determined That Cigarette Smoking Is Dangerous to Your Health."

- Despite the overwhelming evidence that cigarette smoking is associated with higher death rates from cancer, heart disease, and respiratory diseases, approximately 62 million Americans smoke. Smoking also is associated with a higher risk of emphysema and bronchitis.

- Users of smokeless tobacco also have increased health risks, particularly for lip and oral cancer.

- Besides smokers, nonsmokers who breathe smoke-laden air also have greater risk for lung cancer and other respiratory diseases. Children are harmed by breathing parents' cigarette smoke. Children of women who smoke during pregnancy tend to weigh less at birth (a health risk) and have developmental problems during childhood.

- Despite nicotine's capacity to cause physical dependence, the main reason people smoke is ultimately the desire to do so. For some, that desire results from the stimulation they receive from smoking; for others, smoking is a means to increase pleasure or to decrease stress.

- Smoking is a matter of personal choice: people can stop smoking if they choose. Many stop-smoking programs are available to assist a motivated quitter. Success relies on the smoker's resolve to quit and on replacing the smoking habit with personally rewarding behaviors.

- Alcohol abuse is the major drug problem in the United States. Consumption of alcohol is responsible for almost half of all highway fatalities and for numerous social, family, and health problems.

- Alcoholic beverages contain ethyl alcohol, which is produced by the action of yeast on sugar (fermentation) in grains and the juices of berries and fruits. Beer and wine are direct products of fermentation; "hard" liquor, such as whiskey, vodka, rum, and brandy, is made from distilled fermented liquids. Most standard portions of alcoholic beverages contain one-half ounce of ethyl alcohol.

- Social and normative influences on drinking behavior are evident in specific drinking patterns among college students. Drinking on campus increases the risk of violence, including sexual assault.

- Alcohol enters the bloodstream within minutes after ingestion. The physical and behavioral effects of alcohol depend on the blood alcohol content (BAC). A BAC of 0.02 produces a "loosening up" effect. A BAC of 0.10 seriously impairs motor coordination and judgment; in most states it is illegal to drive with a BAC of 0.10.

- Frequent and constant use of alcohol can lead to physical dependence and tolerance for the drug (alcoholism). Alcoholism develops in stages, starting with the inability to control drinking and advancing to complete physical dependence.

- Alcoholics may encounter severe health problems and their personal lives, family relationships, and friendships may be disrupted. Millions of children who grew up in families where one or both parents were alcoholics experience, as adults, personal problems, which stem from their childhoods.

- Organizations, such as Alcoholics Anonymous, and individual or group psychotherapy can help people recover from problem drinking and alcoholism. Alcohol abuse can be prevented by taking responsibility for one's drinking behavior.

Health and Wellness Online

The World Wide Web contains a wealth of information about health and wellness. By accessing the Internet using Web browser software, such as Netscape Navigator or Microsoft's Internet Explorer, you can gain a new perspective on many topics presented in *Essentials of Health and Wellness, Second Edition.* Access the Jones and Bartlett Publishers web site at http://www.jbpub.com/hwonline.

Can legislation make a difference?

A tale of two students.

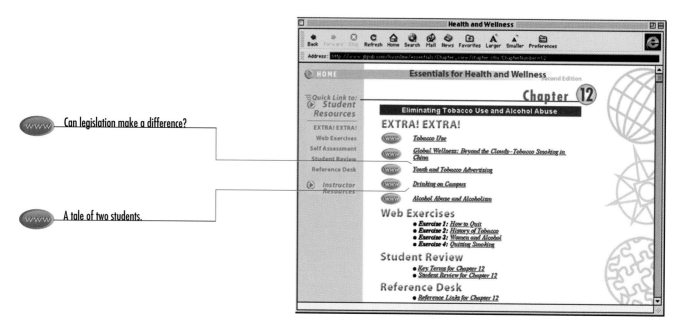

References

Aligne, C. A., & Stoddard, J. J. (1997). Tobacco and children: An economic evaluation of the medical effects of parental smoking. *Archives of Pediatric and Adolescent Medicine, 151,* 648–653.

American Cancer Society. (1998a). *Cigar smoking and cancer.* Atlanta: American Cancer Society.

American Cancer Society. (1998b). *Quitting smoking and cancer.* Atlanta: American Cancer Society.

American Cancer Society. (1999). *Cancer facts and figures.* Atlanta: American Cancer Society.

Baer, J. S., Stacy, A., & Larimer, M. (1991). Biases in the perception of drinking norms among college students. *Journal of Studies of Alcohol, 52* (6), 580–586.

Bartecchi, C. E., MacKenzie, T. D., & Schrier, R. W. (1995). The global tobacco epidemic. *Scientific American,* May, 44–51.

Brookoff, D., et al. (1997). Characteristics of participants in domestic violence. *Journal of the American Medical Association, 277,* 1369–1373.

Centers for Disease Control and Prevention. (1996). Tobacco use and usual source of cigarettes among high school students—United States, 1995. *Morbidity and Mortality Weekly Report, 45*(20), 413–418.

Centers for Disease Control and Prevention. (1997). Youth Risk Behavior Surveillance: National College Health Risk Behavior Survey—United States, 1995. *CDC Surveillance Summaries, 46*(SS-6), 1–64.

Centers for Disease Control and Prevention. (1998a). Tobacco use among high school students—United States, 1997. *Morbidity and Mortality Weekly Report, 47,* 229–233.

Centers for Disease Control and Prevention. (1998b). Youth Risk Behavior Survey—United States, 1997. *CDC Surveillance Summaries, 47*(SS-3), 1–97.

Cohen, A. (1997, September 8). The endless binge. *Time Magazine,* 54–56.

Douglas, K. A., et al. (1997). Results from the 1995 national college health risk behavior survey. *Journal of American College Health, 46,* 55–64.

Davis, T., Arnold, C., Nandy, I., Bocchini, J., Gottlieb, A., George, R., & Berkel, H. (1997). Tobacco use among male high school athletes. *Journal of Adolescent Health, 21,* 97–101.

Eisner, M. D., Smith, A. K., Blanc, P. D. (1998). Bartenders' respiratory health after establishment of smoke-free bars and taverns. *Journal of the American Medical Association, 280,* 1909–1914.

Elders, J., Perry, C., Erickson, M., & Giovino, G. (1994). The report of the Surgeon General: Preventing tobacco use among young people. *American Journal of Public Health, 84*(4), 543–547.

Everett, S. A., Husten, C. G., Warren, C. W., Crossett, L., & Sharp, D. (1998). Trends in tobacco use among high school students in the United States, 1991–1995. *Journal of School Health, 68*(4), 137–140.

Federal Trade Commission. (1997). *1997 smokeless tobacco report.* Federal Trade Commission: Washington, D.C.

Gfroerer, J. C., Greenblatt, M. S., & Wright, D. A. (1997). Substance use in the U.S. college-age population. *American Journal of Public Health, 87,* 62–65.

Hackbarth, D., & Schnopp-Wyatt, D. (1997). Tobacco advertising restrictions as primary prevention for childhood nicotine addiction. *Journal of Addictions Nursing, 9*(3), 112–117.

Haines, S., & Spear, S. F. (1996). Changing the perception of the norm: A strategy to decrease binge drinking among college students. *Journal of American College Health, 45,* 134–140.

Henningfield, J. E., Hariharan, M., & Kozlowski, L. T. (1996). Nicotine content and health risks of cigars. *Journal of American Medical Association, 276*(23), 1857–1858.

Hing Lam, T., He, Y., Sun Li, L., Shou Li, L., Fang He, S., & Qing Liang, B. (1997). Mortality attributable to cigarette smoking in China. *Journal of American Medical Association, 278*(18), 1505–1508.

Hyland, A., Cummings, K. M., Shopland, D. R., & Lynn, W. R. (1998). Prevalence of cigar use in 22 North American communities: 1989 and 1993. *American Journal of Public Health, 88*(7), 1086–1089.

Lerman, C., Audrain, J., Main, D., Boyd, N. R., Caporaso, N. E., Bowman, E. D., Lockshin, B., & Shields, P. G. (1999). Evidence suggesting the role of specific genetic factors in cigarette smoking. *Health Psychology, 18*(1), 14–20.

Liu, S., et al. (1997). Prevalence of alcohol-impaired driving. *Journal of the American Medical Association, 277,* 122–125.

Mackay, J. (1997). Beyond the clouds—Tobacco smoking in China. *Journal of the American Medical Association, 278*(18), 1531–1532.

Marcus, S., Giovino, G., Pierce, J., & Harel, Y. (1993). Measuring tobacco use among adolescents. *Public Health Reports, 108*(1), 20–24.

McCormick, J., & Kalb, C. (1998, June 15). Dying for a drink. *Newsweek,* 30–34.

McGinnis, M., & Foege, W. (1993). Actual causes of death in the United States. *Journal of American Medical Association, 270*(18), 2207–2212.

National Center for Health Statistics. (1996). *Healthy people 2000 review, 1995–96.* Hyattsville, MD: Public Health Service.

Plomin, R. (1998). Using DNA in health psychology. *Health Psychology, 17,* 343–350.

Thun, M. J., et al. (1997). Alcohol consumption and mortality among middle-aged and elderly U.S. adults. *New England Journal of Medicine, 337,* 1705–1714.

Wechsler, H., Davenport, A., Dowdall, G., Moeykens, B., and Castillo, S. (1994). Health and behavioral consequences of binge drinking in college. *Journal of the American Medical Association, 272,* 1672–1677.

Wechsler, H., Davenport, A. E., Dowdall, G. W., Grossman, S. J., & Zanakos, S. I. (1997). Binge drinking, tobacco, and illicit drug use and involvement in college athletics. *Journal of American College Health, 45,* 195–203

Wechsler, H., Rigotti, N. A., Gledhill-Hoyt, J., & Lee, H. (1998). Increased levels of cigarette use among college students: A cause for national concern. *Journal of the American Medical Association, 280,* 1673–1678.

Williams, C., & Wynder, E. (1993). A child health report card: 1992. *Preventive Medicine, 22* (4), 604–628.

Suggested Readings

An, L. C., O'Malley, P. M., Schulenberg, J. E., Bachman, J. G., Johnston, L. D. (1999). Changes at the high end of risk in cigarette smoking among U.S. high school seniors, 1976–1995. *American Journal of Public Health, 89*(5), 699–705.

Argentine FRICAS Investigators, Ciruzzi, M., Pramparo, P., Esteban, O., Rozlosnik, J., Tartaglione, J., Abecasis, B., Cesar, J., De Rosa, J., Paterno, C., & Schargrodsky, H. (1998). Case-control study of passive smoking at home and risk of acute myocardial infarction. *Journal of the American College of Cardiology, 31*(4), 797–803.

Ashworth, M., & Gerada, C. (1997). ABC of mental health. Addiction and dependence II: Alcohol. *British Medical Journal, 315,* 358–360. This article explains alcohol addiction.

Chaloupka, F. J., & Wechsler, H. (1997, June). Price, tobacco control policies, and smoking among young adults. *Journal of Health Economics, 16*(3), 359–373. Analysis of anti-smoking policies and the effects of smoking among young adults.

Hyland, A., Cummings, K. M., Shopland, D. R., & Lynn, W. R. (1998). Prevalence of cigar use in 22 North American communities: 1989 and 1993. *American Journal of Public Health, 88*(7), 1086–1089. Examines the prevalence and characteristics of cigar use.

O'Brien, C. P. (1997). A range of research-based pharmacotherapies for addiction. *Science, 278*, 66–70. This article reviews modern pharmacological approaches to the treatment of addiction, including alcoholism.

O'Connor, P. G., & Schottenfeld, R. S. (1998). Patients with alcohol problems. *New England Journal of Medicine, 338*, 592–602. This article reviews patterns of alcohol use in the United States, and the health consequences and medical treatment of alcohol abuse.

O'Malley, P. M., & Johnston, L. D. (1999). Drinking and driving among U.S. high school seniors, 1984–1997. *American Journal of Public Health, 89*(5), 678–684.

Rorabaugh, W. J. (1991, Fall). Alcohol in America. *Organization of American Historians Magazine of History.* In 1830, Americans drank three times the quantity of alcohol they do today. Article gives a history of alcohol use and abuse.

Sabol, S. Z., Nelson, M. L., Fisher, C., Gunzerath, L., Brody, C. L., Hu, S., Sirota, L. A., Greenberg, B. D., Lucas, F. R., Benjamin, J., Murphy, D. L., Marcus, S. E., & Hamer, D. H. (1999). A genetic association for cigarette smoking behavior. *Health Psychology, 18*(1), 7–13.

Making Healthy Changes

Let's face it—our society believes in taking drugs. Not just prescription and over-the-counter medicines, but substances of all kinds, including herbals, teas, elixirs, and a variety of "recreational" drugs (both legal and illegal) that alter thoughts and feelings, including tobacco (nicotine) and alcohol.

Three factors contribute to excessive use of drugs: (1) advertising and other promotions by manufacturers and distributors of drugs; (2) consumer demand for drug solutions to their problems; and (3) doctors who want to help patients in some way and, hence, prescribe medications to please rather than to cure.

Drugs and medicines have a place in society. It is important, however, to be aware of one's attitudes about drugs to be sure that they are used responsibly and wisely and not because of advertising, peer pressure, or to solve personal problems.

Wise Consumer: Becoming More Critical of Drug Advertising

Drug companies have long focused their advertising for prescription drugs on doctors, since they are the ones who write prescriptions for medications. Now, however, consumers are just as likely to be the targets of prescription drug advertising, called "Direct to Consumer Advertising." In such advertising, celebrities may be used to pitch a certain drug, or the ads may focus on people's suffering with symptoms that the drug can alleviate, or the ads may feed into people's fears of a heart attack, cancer, or crippling arthritis.

As a result of these ads, consumers often pressure their doctors to prescribe the advertised drugs, which may not be the wisest course because advertised drugs tend to be new and lack a history of safe or effective use. Also, over-the-counter drug ads can be misleading; they may overstate a drug's benefits and not clearly indicate its risks. Furthermore, new drugs often cost much more than older drugs that may be just as—or even more—effective.

In your journal, set aside some pages for a "Drug Ad Log." Every time you see a drug ad in a magazine, newspaper, or on TV that catches your interest, make an entry in your journal:

1. Describe how the advertiser uses images and words to convince you to use the drug. In what ways does the ad try to convince you to buy the product?

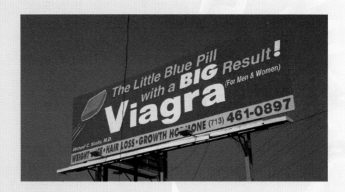

2. Would you be tempted to use the drug if you had the condition for which it is recommended?
3. How would you determine if the drug is safe and effective?
4. Would you rely solely on your doctor's recommendation? Instead of demanding a certain drug from your doctor just because you saw it on TV, use the Internet to find out about the drug (don't search the manufacturer's Web site), and ask your doctor what her or his evaluation of the drug is and whether other patients have used it.

A good source of unbiased information about drugs is the monthly newsletter "Worst Pills, Best Pills" (www.citizen.org/hrg).

Stress Management: Alternatives to Binge Drinking

Studies show that a large percentage of college students binge drink, meaning that they consume five or more alcohol-containing drinks in one session. Students binge drink for two major reasons: to relieve academic stress and to reduce social anxiety.

Preparing for exams and writing papers can be intense, highly stressful experiences. And when they are over, it's natural to want to reward oneself for simply "surviving" and to "blow off" the accumulated tension. At many colleges, binge drinking, whether in one's dorm, apartment, or at a party, is a socially acceptable way to recover from academic stress.

Students also binge drink to lessen their nervousness in party situations. Large amounts of alcohol can numb the anxiety of being at a party, especially if you don't know many of the guests or if you imagine that others are judging your behavior. Also, alcohol can lessen the mental conflict when your personal values are not in accordance with behaviors considered acceptable by others at the party, for example, behaving rudely, destroying property, or engaging in sexual activity with a stranger.

There are many healthy ways to relieve academic stress and social anxiety without binge drinking. In your journal, describe ways of reducing academic stress and social anxiety that might work for you and that do not involve drinking.

Emotional Wellness: Getting Rid of "Smoker's Mind"

Despite the warnings printed on every package of cigarettes and extensive public education efforts about the dangers of cigarette smoking, 25 percent of Americans still smoke cigarettes. These people have "smoker's mind"; tobacco has captured their minds as well as their bodies. Not only are they physically dependent on nicotine, but also they are in denial of the reality of the consequences of their actions. Research shows that the majority of heavy smokers do not perceive themselves at risk for heart disease and cancer.

Another example of "smoker's mind" is identification with film actors who smoke cigarettes in their roles on screen. Even though 25 percent of Americans smoke cigarettes, 57 percent of leading characters in the most popular films smoke—on average, about once every 3 to 5 minutes. Films tend to present smokers as successful, sophisticated, attractive, and vigorously healthy (the greatest lie of all).

If you do smoke, describe in your journal your personal reasons for smoking. Discuss whether you really *believe* smoking damages your health. Discuss the reasons you continue to smoke. If you are convinced that smoking is destructive to health, what efforts can you make to stop smoking?

Wise Consumer: Don't Send Your Money Up in Smoke

A smoking habit costs a pack-a-day smoker more than $1000 a year for cigarettes. If that thousand dollars a year were invested in a mutual fund at an annual 8 percent compounded rate of return, it would yield:

After 5 years $7,335
After 10 years . . . $16,645
After 30 years . . . $123,345

By the time an ex-smoker reaches retirement age, he or she would be wealthy instead of facing death from heart disease, emphysema, or lung cancer!

Physical Activity Update: Exercising More

If your walking has been going well and you are feeling up to it, you may want to consider becoming more active. In addition to walking, you may want to begin to jog or run to increase aerobic fitness. Or you may want to take up a sport with friends, such as tennis or golf. However, if you decide to become more active, be sure that you are physically ready to take on more exercise without the risk of injury. The goal of exercise is to have fun and to feel good—not to compete to the point of exhaustion or injury. Describe in your journal the progress you have made over the past few months in increasing physical activity. Have you increased the kind, duration, or frequency of exercise?

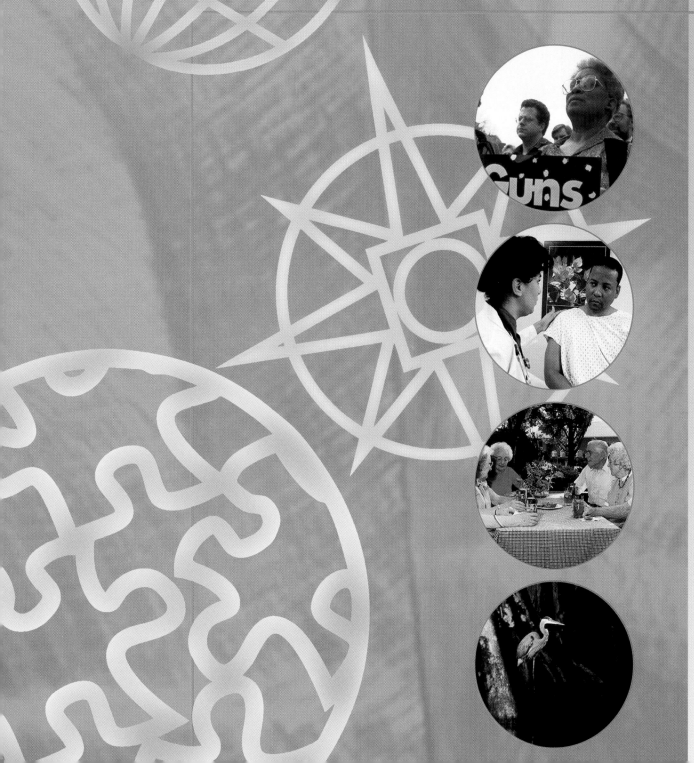

Part 6

Making Healthy Choices

Learning Objectives

1. Describe the different kinds of interpersonal violence.
2. Explain ways that violence affects health.
3. Discuss the symptoms and long-term effects of post-traumatic stress disorder.
4. Describe the different forms of child abuse and why the incidence is different in different cultures.
5. Define sexual assault, forcible rape, and acquaintance rape.
6. Discuss the reasons that underlie forcible rape and acquaintance rape.
7. Define elder abuse and the factors that contribute to it.
8. Discuss the ways in which firearm abuse affects the health of individuals and disrupts society.
9. Define safety, accidents, and unintentional injuries.
10. Describe various strategies to prevent unintentional injuries.
11. Use the epidemiological triad to identify unintentional injury risk factors.
12. Describe the Haddon matrix and explain why it was developed.
13. Discuss various ways to prevent motor vehicle crashes, motorcycle accidents, bicycle accidents, and pedestrian accidents.
14. Describe various strategies to improve home safety.

Exercises and Activities

WORKBOOK
Crime Prevention Tips
Prevention of Intentional Injury

Health and Wellness Online

 www.jbpub.com/hwonline

Interpersonal Violence
Managing Stress: "Road Rage" on the Rise
Sexual Assault
Firearm Violence
Unintentional Injuries and Accidents
Motor Vehicle Safety

Chapter 13

Enhancing Personal Safety

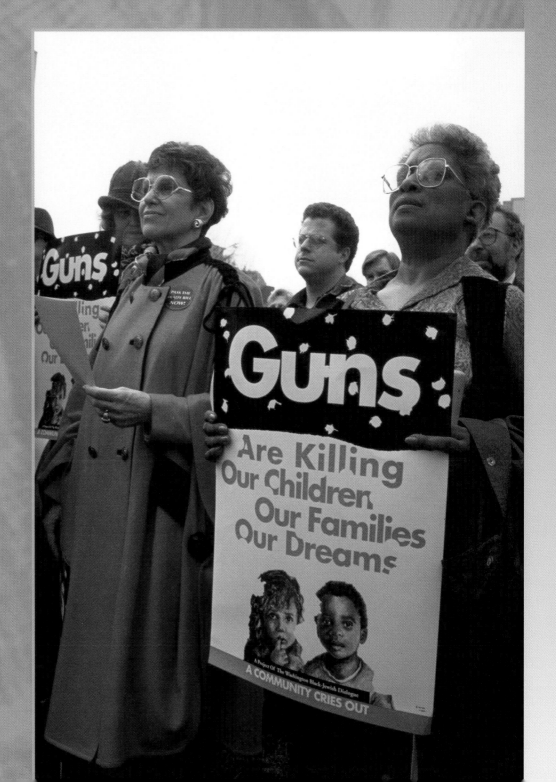

Violence is an integral part of the animal kingdom, as the expression "eat or be eaten" implies. Predator animals practice offensive violence, while their victims practice defensive violence. Animals invariably engage in these kinds of violent behavior to gain access to food and water and to reproduce. Human beings, however, are far ahead of all other animal species in the degree and occasions for practicing violence. In peace, as well as in war, people attack, injure, and kill other people for a multitude of reasons.

Violence is a physical or verbal behavior in which the aim is to harm, injure, or destroy someone or something. Human beings are unique in understanding the future possibility of injury and death and so will fight for many reasons, including being threatened by loss of personal freedom. People also have many intangible things to fear—fear of being hungry, fear of being poor, fear of being attacked, and fear of being unwanted or unloved are examples. All of these fears can provoke violent behavior.

Some people use violence as a means of gaining power over others. In its simplest form, power is the ability to satisfy one's needs. Power and its accompanying violence manifest in society in a variety of ways—as rape, domestic violence, physical and sexual child abuse, elder abuse, homicide, suicide, terrorist attacks, gang fights, and wars between nations.

More than 20,000 persons die in the U.S. every year from homicide, and over 2 million persons are injured in violent attacks. Homicide is the second leading cause of death among persons aged 15 to 24, and suicide is the third in the same age group. The consequences of violence in society are broken families, battered women, maimed and handicapped children, and countless unnecessary injuries and deaths.

To repair the effects of violence on the minds and bodies of people is expensive, difficult, and often unsuccessful. The *only* solution to violent human behavior, as with other serious diseases, is prevention (Gellert, 1997). While some people believe that violence in human societies is inevitable, many others do not and choose to live nonviolent lives.

Interpersonal Violence

Historically, violence in the family was ignored for centuries both in the United States and in other developed countries. Until the 1960s, most people considered family violence a rare event. Since then, awareness of interpersonal violence as a major health problem has increased partly as a result of required reporting of suspected cases of domestic violence and child abuse by hospitals, physicians, and police departments and partly to increased research (Kantor and Jasinski, 1998). In the 1990s, publicity about child abuse, sexual abuse, spousal abuse (primarily by men), and elder abuse has greatly increased public awareness.

The killings of Nicole Brown Simpson and Ronald Goldman focused public attention on interpersonal violence as never before in the 1990s. (Gelles, 1997). The three most widely quoted "facts" about interpersonal violence by commentators of the trial of O. J. Simpson, the alleged killer, were:

- More women are treated in hospital emergency rooms for battering injuries each year in the U.S. than for muggings, rapes, and traffic accidents combined.
- Interpersonal violence has killed more women in the past 5 years in the U.S. than the total number of Americans killed in Vietnam.
- Battering during pregnancy is the leading cause of birth defects and infant mortality.

The FBI estimates that a woman is beaten by her husband or boyfriend every 15 seconds in this country. Clearly, interpersonal violence is out of control. Recognizing that domestic violence is as serious a health problem as communicable diseases, the federal government has declared October as National Domestic Violence Month. During this month, extra efforts are made to increase public awareness and to educate people on how to prevent and avoid violence in the family.

Domestic Violence

Women who experience battering by a partner or rape have medical problems and may also suffer from anxiety, depression, chronic pelvic pain, gastrointestinal upset, substance abuse, obesity, or headaches. Assaulted women may also develop symptoms of **post-traumatic stress disorder (PTSD)** and its variants which are battered women's syndrome or rape trauma syndrome. Many long-term health consequences of battering, rape, and sexual abuse are associated with PTSD. For example, traumatized individuals tend to be more susceptible to arousal by stimuli that makes it difficult for them to differentiate normal aches, pains, and sensations from signals of disease, leading

Terms

violence: a physical or verbal behavior, in which the aim is to harm, injure, or destroy someone or something

post-traumatic stress disorder (PTSD): reactions after an event that is outside the range of usual human experience and would be distressing to almost anyone

to increased incidence of seeking help from health professionals. Also, emotional tension and guardedness can produce painful muscle tension and skeletal misalignment. Chronic anxiety can lead to gastrointestinal upsets. Alcohol, nicotine, and other drugs may be used to block out memories of abuse and to alleviate uncomfortable emotions and physical sensations that accompany memories of the assault or abuse.

Recovering from the trauma of relationship violence requires patience and support. Victims are encouraged to seek psychological counseling from professionals who specialize in helping victims of relationship violence and to join support groups of other assaulted individuals. Support can hasten healing and recovery and help restore the trust that is shattered by assault. Support groups can also provide a place to stay if the victim needs to escape the abuser, or the group can offer companionship if the victim is afraid to be alone.

Symptoms of PTSD include:

- Re-experiencing the traumatic event(s) via recurrent intrusive images, thoughts, dreams of the trauma, and "flashbacks"—having a sense of reliving the trauma, including re-experiencing the disturbing accompanying emotions.

- Intense reactions to things that symbolize the traumatic experience. For example, in recovering from a rape, victims may intensely fear being in locales that resemble the scene of the assault.

- Some may experience nausea when thinking of the rape, and some may have difficulties with sexual relations.

- Being unable to recall the trauma (denial), or being able to "make the mind go somewhere else" to avoid the pain associated with the memory of the trauma (dissociation). They may feel detached or estranged.

- Manipulation of others and the environment as a way to keep things calm and under control. They may become compliant as a way to avoid real or imagined abuse.

- Persistent arousal symptoms, such as difficulty falling or staying asleep, being edgy, jumpy, irritable, and sometimes irrationally angry. Victims may have difficulty concentrating, be hypervigilant to their surroundings, and have an exaggerated startle response.

Causes of Domestic Violence

There is no single cause of domestic violence, but contributing factors include:

- A high level of conflict and stress in the family

- Male dominance and the view that women and children are men's property
- Cultural norms that permit family violence
- Displays of violence on TV and other media
- Being raised in a violent family
- Alcohol and drug abuse
- Victim-blaming ("people get what they deserve")
- Denying the existence of physical violence or sexual abuse

Ways to prevent domestic violence include providing shelters, safe houses, and other protective environments for abused women; reducing contributing social and economic factors (unemployment, poverty, and racism); holding the abusers accountable for their actions; training law enforcement and health care professionals to recognize and intervene in cases of domestic violence; training everyone in nonviolent conflict resolution; and reducing the amount of violent imagery on TV, in films, and in popular music.

> *For a while we pondered whether to take a vacation or get a divorce. We decided that a trip to Bermuda is over in 2 weeks, but a divorce is something you always have.*
>
> WOODY ALLEN

Domestic violence not only affects adults who are in an abusive relationship; children who share the abusive environment also suffer (Table 13.1). Resolution of conflicts between parents or partners is essential to the long-term health of children. And children who grow up in physically or sexually abusive environments are much more likely to find themselves in abusive relationships as adults.

TABLE 13.1 **Symptoms of Parental Violence in Children**
Children who are exposed to parental violence are subject to a variety of symptoms.

Behavioral symptoms			
Aggression	Tantrums	Immaturity	Delinquency
Emotional symptoms			
Anxiety and depression	Low self-esteem	Anger	Withdrawal
Cognitive symptoms			
Poor performance in school	Poor language skills		
Physical symptoms			
Eating disorders	Poor motor skills	Sleep problems	Retarded growth
Psychosomatic disorders			

Managing Stress

Coping with Anger

Anger. The word itself brings to mind images of pounding fists, yelling, and violent behavior. But anger is as natural a human emotion as love. Anger is a survival emotion; it's the fight component of the fight or flight response. We use anger to communicate our feelings, from impatience to rage. We employ anger to communicate boundaries and defend values. Although feeling angry is within the normal limits of human emotions, anger is often mismanaged and misdirected. Unfortunately, we have been socialized to suppress our feelings of anger. As a result, it either tears us apart from the inside or promotes intermittent eruptions of verbal or physical violence, which can be seen played out in local and national headlines. In most cases, we do not deal with our anger wisely.

Research reveals four very distinct ways in which people mismanage their anger. They include:

1. **Somatizers:** People who never show any signs of anger and internalize their feelings until eventually there is major bodily damage (i.e., temporomandibular joint syndrome, colitis, migraine headaches).

2. **Exploders:** Individuals who erupt like a volcano and spread their temper like hot lava, destroying anyone and anything in their path with either verbal or physical abuse. This type of mismanaged anger style is what makes the news headlines.

3. **Self-Punishers:** People who neither repress their anger nor explode, but rather deny themselves a proper outlet of anger because of feelings of guilt. Examples of their behavior include excessive sleeping, eating, and shopping.

4. **Underhanders:** Individuals who sabotage or seek revenge against someone through barely socially acceptable behavior (e.g., sarcasm, tardiness, not returning phone calls).

When anger is mismanaged and left unresolved it becomes a control issue, if not a control drama.

Here are some ways to deal with anger sensibly or creatively:

1. Take "time-out" from the situation, followed by a "time-in" to resolve the issue.

2. Communicate your feelings diplomatically.

3. Think of the consequences of your anger.

4. Plan several options to a situation.

5. Lower personal expectations.

6. Most important, learn to forgive—"make past anger pass."

Although anger is an emotion we all experience and should recognize when it arises, it is crucial to manage anger. Sometimes just writing down what frustrates you can be the beginning of the resolution process. Above all, make a habit of resolving your angry feelings once they arise. Learn to let go of your feelings of anger before they become toxic to your mind, body, and spirit.

Child Abuse

Children have been abused for centuries in all cultures and countries. The widely accepted definition of **child abuse,** which applies to all cultures is: "Child abuse is the portion of harm to children that results from human action that is proscribed, proximate, and preventable" (Finkelhor and Korbin, 1988). In plain English, child abuse is any human action that causes injury to children and is preventable.

About 16 million American children are taken to hospital emergency rooms each year for treatment of injuries caused by child abuse (Peterson and Gable, 1998). Several hundred thousand of these children require hospitalization, and at least 30,000 of them suffer permanent disabilities. Child abuse assumes several forms, all of which invariably lead to serious harm (Garbarino and Eckenrode, 1997).

Physical Abuse   When intentional force of any kind that results in injury is used on a child, the child has suffered physical abuse. Injuries can also result from accidents, which are not the result of physical abuse. For example, a child may fall and be bruised while running during play. This is understood by the child to be an accident and may lead to more careful behavior. It may also be something the child is proud of and can be "brave" about.

However, physical force that is used to discipline or control a child or adolescent can cause serious physical and psychological injury. Often a parent is venting anger over some other issue that is irrelevant to the child's behavior; the child is the unwitting victim of the anger and knows that the punishment is unjust. The younger the child, the more likely a serious injury will result from the use of physical force. Shaking a baby repeatedly to get it to stop crying, or for any other reason, can cause death.

Emotional Abuse   Psychological abuse can cause severe emotional distress and can produce illness and violent behavior that may lead to suicide or homicide. Being screamed at repeatedly, and told that one is worthless, stupid, or defective can permanently damage psychological and social development.

Sexual Abuse   This is another form of maltreatment of children. Sexual contact between adults and children is forbidden by both cultural taboos and by crim-

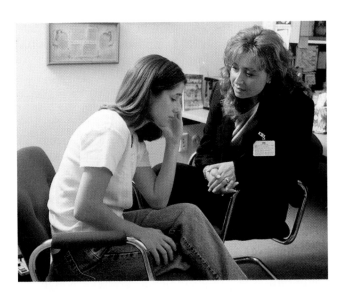

Being able to tell an understanding person what happened helps.

inal law. Although it is difficult to determine with accuracy the prevalence of child sexual abuse in this country, some surveys find that as many as 15% of women and 6% of men have experienced sexual abuse as children (Swenson and Hanson, 1998). Because this subject is not one that most people are willing to discuss, the prevalence of child sexual abuse may be higher than reported. Sexual abuse of children may result in depression, anxiety, and general dysfunction later in their lives.

Neglect   This is probably the most common form of maltreatment of children. Neglect includes failure to provide a child with adequate nourishment, proper clothing, prescribed medications, or to oversee a child's hygiene. Neglected children are left to their own devices for long periods without adult supervision, and many neglected children engage in self-destructive behaviors.

While it is true that males are the usual perpetrators of violence on children, especially female children, mothers also abuse their children both physically and sexually. Women who inflict serious injury on their children are often mentally ill and may suffer from dissociative identity disorder, formerly known as multiple personality disorder (Mitchell and Morse, 1998).

Child abuse affects children not only physically (e.g., broken bones, burns, or even death), but emotionally as well (e.g., they may become abusive themselves, suicidal, or withdrawn). Effects are both short- and long-term and invariably devastating to all victims. As the abused child reaches age 10 and older and becomes more independent, he or she may feel in a hopeless situation and may run away from home. The consequences for many runaways are dismal: teenage prostitution, illicit drug and alcohol use, higher rates of juvenile crimes, and higher school dropout rates. Child abuse is costly to society and directly or indirectly affects everyone.

Social Aspects of Child Abuse

Because many cases of child abuse go unreported, reliable data are difficult to obtain; also, abusers and the abused usually do not offer information freely. As a result, much information on child abuse has been incorrect or misleading (Allen and Epperson, 1993).

As more women enter the work force, more males assume greater responsibility for child care. For whatever reasons, males tend to abuse their children at a higher rate than females. However, no unique factors have been found that distinguish male abusers of children from female abusers. Male children are abused more frequently and seen by parents as more deserving of harsh treatment than female children. Male children even blame themselves more than female children do for their own maltreatment.

Two-thirds of all abused children are between the ages of 5 and 17. Younger children are abused more frequently because they lack both physical strength to resist child abuse and knowledge about what is normal and abnormal behavior. Infants are attacked less frequently than older children by abusive parents, but are at greater risk of death than older children, especially when shaken. As children pass the age of 15, they are more likely to be abused by peers than by family members.

Children with physical or mental handicaps such as blindness, deafness, mental retardation, or cerebral palsy are at a greater risk for child abuse than others. It is unclear if the physical handicap itself provokes the abuse or if stress created by caring for such a child is the underlying cause of the abuse. Children who are temperamental, impulsive, aggressive, depressed, or hyperactive are also at a higher risk for being abused. These behaviors create parental stress that may contribute to child abuse.

Cultural Aspects of Child Abuse

Different cultural beliefs play a role in the risk of child abuse. Latino men tend to regard themselves as *macho* (masculine), which may be used to justify

---

Terms

child abuse: physical or mental injury, sexual abuse or exploitation, maltreatment, or neglect of a child by a person who is responsible for the child's welfare; circumstances in which a child's health or welfare is harmed or threatened

abusive behavior towards their families and children. Their society accepts macho behavior as the social norm, although as Latino families become acculturated to the value system of middle-class Americans, child abuse declines. *Machismo* (the need for males to appear powerful) is observed in all ethnic groups and child abuse occurs among all socioeconomic classes.

Lack of knowledge and skills about child care may predispose parents to child abuse, possibly because of frustration and stress created by the needs of a child and its apparent lack of cooperation. Males who are primary care givers usually have received little or no training regarding child care.

The same holds true for adolescent mothers and mothers with low levels of education, for example, high school dropouts. They, too, lack the knowledge and skills necessary for adequate child care. This lack places them in a stressful situation in which abuse is more likely to occur. These mothers feel they have no one to turn to for help, and they may not even know where to obtain help. In frustration, they abuse their children.

If the family lives in an unsafe neighborhood, family members may feel afraid to venture out to seek help for their problems. This fear results in even more isolation and may exacerbate family conflicts and abuse. If the family lives in an area of limited public transportation or owns no car, these factors also contribute to the risk of child abuse. Contributing reasons for child abuse seem to be social isolation, lack of friends, dangerous neighborhoods, or lack of access to transportation (Finkelhor and Dziuba-Leatherman, 1994).

Child Abuse Prevention

There are child abuse prevention programs that can help parents reduce the stress that is a risk factor in child abuse. These programs emphasize educating parents on how to care for their children and how to avoid abuse. Different stress reduction programs have been developed for adolescent mothers, young parents, fathers who have never been in charge of child care before, working mothers, single parents, step parents, and siblings who are in charge of child care. Stress management programs are particularly important in communities where unemployment rates are high.

Conflict resolution programs can also help prevent child abuse. If people are able to manage conflict without using physical force, the risk of child abuse is lower. Both anger mediation programs and conflict resolution programs have been shown to help lower rates of child abuse. Training in life and social skills for all individuals involved with child abuse is recommended. Training in parenting skills for both males and females of all ages is also strongly suggested. This training also educates them about resources for assistance.

Managing Stress

"Road Rage" on the Rise

A report by the American Automobile Association in 1997 observed that "motorists . . . are increasingly being shot, stabbed, beaten, and run over for inane reasons." The reasons that provoke rage among today's drivers include being cut off by a car pulling into your lane, aggressive tailgating, headlight flashing, and verbal abuse (Adler, 1997).

All of us have been irritated at one time or another while driving; most of us also have driven in a manner that was irritating to another driver. There is something about getting behind the wheel of a two-ton automobile that seems to raise the level of aggression in many people and causes them to ignore the safety of others. It is no coincidence that sport utility vehicles, large vans, and pickup trucks are called "suburban assault vehicles."

Whenever you get into a car to drive somewhere, remind yourself that being courteous (even if the other driver is not) can save your life. Play a relaxing tape while driving. Your goal should be to get where you are going as safely as possible and without incident. Your health and survival depend on it. Do not let yourself become a victim of "road rage."

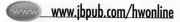 **www.jbpub.com/hwonline**

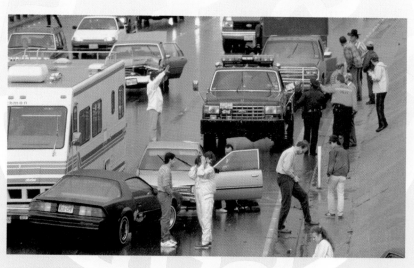

Wellness Guide

How to Prevent Date Rape

Be wary of a relationship that is operating along classic stereotypes of dominant male and submissive, passive female. The dominance in ordinary activities may extend to the sexual arena.

Be wary when a date tries to control behavior or pressure others in any way.

Be explicit with communication. Don't say "no" in a way that could be interpreted in any way as a "maybe" or "yes."

Avoid ambiguous messages with both verbal and nonverbal behavior. Saying "no" and permitting heavy petting implies confusion or ambiguity.

First dates with an unknown companion may be safer in a group.

Avoid remote or isolated spots where help is not available.

Source: L. L. Alexander and J. H. LaRosa. *New Dimensions in Women's Health* (Boston: Jones and Bartlett, 1994).

Sexual Assault

Rape, incest, attempted rape, and unwanted sexual touching are called **sexual assault.** There has been a significant increase recently in public recognition of sexual crimes against women, including intense media scrutiny of rape issues in high profile rape trials. The legal definition of **forcible rape** varies from state to state. However, rape is generally viewed as penetration by force or threat of force of a body orifice, including the mouth, rectum, or vagina. Penetration includes the use of objects or other body parts, such as fingers. Forced sexual activity can occur between men and women, men and men, women and women, and married and unmarried people. Regardless of the identity of the victims and perpetrators, sexual assault is a criminal activity; it is not sex and has nothing to do with sex. Sexual assault is an act of power, an attempt to humiliate a victim. Whether the term is sexual assault or forcible rape, the end result is physical violence to the victim.

Some men try to deny the fact of sexual assault with statements such as "women enjoy being raped," "she asked for it," and "I didn't think she meant no." These kinds of statements are heard repeatedly; however, the facts of sexual assault are plain (Donat and D'Emilio, 1998):

- Sexual assault is an act of power and control—*not* an act of sex or passion.
- Most sexual assaults go unreported.
- Most sexual assaults do not occur on impulse or in remote areas.
- In 80% of all sexual assaults, according to some estimates, the assailant was a casual acquaintance, friend, or relative of the victim.
- Sexual assailants come from *all* socioeconomic and ethnic backgrounds.
- Rapists are not sexually deprived people.
- Women do not secretly want to be raped.
- Forced intimacy in a dating situation is sexual assault.

Acquaintance Rape

Acquaintance rape, or date rape, occurs when a person known to the victim uses force to coerce the victim into having sex. Warsaw (1988) reports that 84% of all sexual assaults are committed by an acquaintance of the victim, 57% of all sexual assaults occur during a date, and 60% of men raped by other men knew their attacker. Acquaintance rape carries the same legal penalties as sexual assault committed by a stranger.

Women of high school and college age are the most vulnerable to acquaintance rape. A survey of 6,000 students from 32 colleges found that one in six female students had been a victim of rape or attempted rape within the preceding year, and one of fifteen male students reported committing sexual assaults within the preceding year (Koss and Harvey, 1991).

Since 1990, more than 100,000 forcible rapes have been reported each year in the U.S. This number is probably low, because many rapes are not reported by the victim. In 1960, only about 15,000 forcible rapes were reported, a statistic that provides a sad record of how much this form of violence has increased in one generation (Dobrin, Wiersema, Loftin, and McDowall, 1996).

Cultural views on sexual relationships between men and women play a significant role in acquaintance rape. Many young women who are victims of attacks that meet the legal definition of rape do not know that what happened to them was sexual assault. Victims may believe that a sexual assault can only be committed by a stranger or they may blame themselves for the act. A rapist may not realize that the victim's refusal

Terms

sexual assault: violent actions that include rape, incest, attempted rape, and unwanted sexual touching

forcible rape: sexual assault using force or threat of force and involving sexual penetration of the victim's vagina, mouth, or rectum

acquaintance rape: (also known as "date rape") sexual assault occurring when the victim and the rapist are known to each other and may have previously interacted in some socially appropriate manner

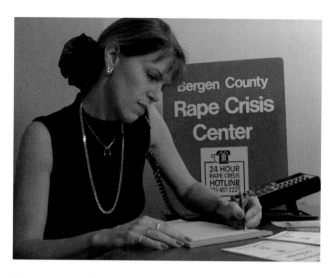

Many communities have crisis centers for rape victims.

really means NO. Aggressive males mistakenly believe that when women say no, men should insist.

In a survey conducted by *Ms.* magazine, 84% of men whose actions came under the legal definition of sexual assault believed they had not committed sexual assault. This reinforces the myth that women really do not mean NO when they say no. Another study found that 43% of college-aged men admitted using coercion to have sex, including ignoring a woman's protest, using physical aggression, and forcing intercourse. Fifteen percent of the same group acknowledged they had committed acquaintance rape, and 11% admitted using physical restraint to force a woman to have sex (Rapaport and Posey, 1991).

Consequences of Acquaintance Rape

Victims of acquaintance rape often suffer serious, long-term psychological effects. Compared with victims of stranger rapes, acquaintance rape victims often blame themselves for what happened. They often have difficulty trusting people in later relationships. It may take acquaintance rape victims longer to recover, particularly if the rape involved physical violence. Acquaintance rape victims are less likely than other rape

victims to seek crisis services, tell someone, report the incident to the police, or seek counseling. Family and friends may not provide the same support for acquaintance rape victims as they might offer victims of stranger rape. If victims tell friends or family, the severity of the attack may be minimized or the victim may be blamed for the sexual assault.

Family members and significant others have also been victimized when someone they know, love, and care for has been sexually assaulted. Significant others may also have expressed or controlled reactions that indicate a state of shock from the incident. Some common feelings felt by the sexual assault victim's family members and significant others are listed in Table 13.2.

Victims usually have two types of behavioral reactions, expressed or controlled. Those who express their feelings usually manifest fear, anger, and anxiety. They may display these emotions through crying, tension, nervousness, restlessness, and hysteria. Those who control their feelings may appear calm or quiet, but either reaction indicates that the victim is in a state of shock (Table 13.3). Expressed or controlled feelings may occur at any time and often come and go more than once after the incident. Acknowledging or recognizing these feelings are a normal part of the healing process.

What to Do after a Sexual Assault

A person who has been sexually assaulted is advised to do the following:

- Contact a rape-crisis hotline.
- DO NOT shower, bathe, douche, change or destroy clothing, or straighten up the area where the sexual assault occurred (if indoors), because these actions would destroy important evidence.
- Go to the nearest hospital emergency room.
- Notify the police.
- Seek professional counseling.

Each person's reaction to being sexually assaulted is different and it is natural that each victim's pain and needs are unique. All victims of sexual assault should seek counseling from someone they trust.

TABLE 13.2   Reactions and Feelings of Significant Others of Sexual Assault Victims

Anger	Concern	Guilt	Embarrassment	Vulnerability
• At assailant for committing crime • At system for letting "those kinds of people" run the streets • At survivor for engaging in "risky behavior"	• For the survivor's well-being and safety • About how the relationship between survivor and significant other will change • For the survivor's rights	• For not having prevented assault ("I should have been with them" OR "I should have given them a ride home") • For not having been there to protect survivor	• Worry about gossip (myth and stigma hold strong effect) • Embarrassed for survivor	• Realization that it can happen to them as well • Intensely heightened awareness of environment

Source: Adapted with permission from Illinois Coalition Against Sexual Assault, Springfield, Ill.: 1993.

TABLE 13.3   Feelings Reported by Sexual Assault Victims

Fear of rapist	*Embarrassment*	*Shame*	*Guilt*	*Anxiety*
• Fear of death • Fear of rapist	• Embarrassed to discuss details • Embarrassed about their bodies	• Destruction of self-esteem, self-worth, self-respect • Ashamed at having the medical exam • Ashamed at having to perform a sexual act in order to stay alive	• Feelings of shame and of having provoked the rape • Feeling of blame for the assault	• Shaking • Nightmares • Difficulty sleeping or sleeping all the time • Constantly reminds self what "should or shouldn't have" been done
Stupidity	*Vulnerability*	*Concern for rapist*	*Anger*	*Loss of control*
• Feels stupid for engaging in risk-taking behavior(s) • Feels stupid for being too trusting	• General fear of people • Paranoid feelings • Intensely heightened awareness of environment	• Will the rapist get psychiatric help? • What will happen to offender if rape is reported?	• Toward assailant • Toward self • Toward men and women in general, especially if they resemble assailant	• Small decisions seem monumental • Unsure about self or actions

Source: Adapted from *Illinois Coalition Against Sexual Assault*, Springfield, Ill.: 1993.

Elder Abuse

We are an aging society, and with increasing frequency adult children are required to care for disabled or demented elderly parents and grandparents. It is only within the last generation that the problem of elder abuse has been recognized and documented. Studies now indicate that over 1 million elderly persons are victims of abuse each year in the U.S. (Quinn and Tomita, 1997). In addition to abuse by their adult children, elderly persons also are abused frequently by their spouses. The magnitude of elder abuse in the U.S. is now only slightly less than that of child abuse.

Elder abuse is defined as the physical, sexual, or emotional maltreatment or financial exploitation of an adult, age 60 or older. The abuse or neglect may be by any caregiver—spouse, child, relative, or friend—and occurs in a domestic setting. Self-neglect is also included in the definition, because almost half of the cases of elder abuse involve self-neglect.

Self-neglect may result from physical or mental disability of the elder person. He or she may not be able to obtain essential food, clothing, shelter, or medical care. Quite often the financial affairs of a neglected elder person are in disarray. Despite increased public attention to the problems of elder abuse, much maltreatment of elders still remains hidden to a large extent.

A variety of abusive methods are used by caregivers in the domestic setting to control the elder persons under their care. These include screaming and yelling (the most frequent form of abuse), physical restraint, forced feeding or medicating, blows and slaps, and threats to send the person to a nursing home.

However, the abuse is not all one way. Elder persons who are disabled or immobilized also use abusive methods to control their caregivers. Elder persons scream and yell, pout and withdraw, refuse food and medication, cry or become emotional, throw objects, and threaten to call the police. As with other forms of abuse, the reasons for the abusive behaviors by both persons in the relationship are many. Alcohol plays a role in many situations, and emotional illness contributes, as does mental impairment, on the part of one or both parties.

The reason why much elder abuse remains hidden or undocumented is that many elderly people are concerned about the family's privacy and fear public exposure and embarrassment. The victim also may feel shame at having raised the child who has now become abusive. If the child is stealing money, the elderly parent may fear that the child will be sent to jail if the abuse is reported (Quinn and Tomita, 1997). And, despite the abusive treatment, the elder person may feel that the situation is preferable to being sent to a nursing home. Elder abuse will become an ever greater problem during the next century, as more and more people live to be age 80 or older and as the number of people with dementia increases (see chapter 15).

Firearm Violence

Year after year, the use of pistols, rifles, and other firearms causes thousands of deaths in the United States, both accidental and deliberate. In 1987, almost 33,000 deaths were caused by firearms—about half of these were suicides, about 13,000 were homicides, and the rest were unintentional accidents or involved

Terms

elder abuse: physical, sexual, or emotional maltreatment or financial exploitation of an adult age 60 or older

shootings by police officers. Every year more than 60,000 injuries result from firearms. Numerous studies come to the same conclusion; ready availability of firearms in the United States is associated with an increased risk of suicide and homicide (Kellerman et al., 1992).

> The streets are safe in Philadelphia. It's only the people who make them unsafe.
>
> FRANK RIZZO

Americans have a longstanding love-hate relationship with firearms, and many people believe strongly in the constitutionally guaranteed right to carry and use firearms. Their views are defended with money and lobbying by the National Rifle Association (NRA), which works to prevent passage of laws limiting or regulating the purchase and use of guns by civilians. The NRA is opposed by physicians, health organizations, and law enforcement agencies including the Federal Bureau of Investigation (FBI), which supports stricter gun control laws.

The Brady Handgun Violence Prevention Act, or Brady Law, which took 7 years to pass in Congress, was signed into law on November 30, 1993, and went into effect on February 28, 1994. The Brady law imposed a 5-day waiting period for the purchase of handguns and required local police agencies to determine if the prospective buyer had a criminal record. The law affected 32 states when it was first implemented. Several of these states subsequently passed laws requiring background checks on handgun purchasers, which exempted the states from the Brady law.

On November 30, 1998, the provision requiring the five-day waiting period expired. It was replaced by a mandatory, computerized National Instant Check System (NICS), which provides the information for criminal background checks on all firearm purchasers, not just those buying handguns. Most background checks and firearm sales conducted under this system are completed within minutes. The impact of this change in the federal law varies from state to state.

Twenty-five states use the NICS system for all background checks conducted at the time of purchase: Arkansas, Delaware, Idaho, Kansas, Kentucky, Louisiana, Maine, Massachusetts, Minnesota, Mississippi, Missouri, Montana, New Hampshire, New Mexico, New York, North Dakota, Ohio, Oklahoma, Rhode Island, South Dakota, Texas, West Virginia, and Wyoming. Fifteen states use their state-based system for the permit background check when purchasing a handgun: Arizona, California, Colorado, Connecticut, Florida, Georgia, Hawaii, Illinois, Nevada, New Jersey, South Carolina, Tennessee, Utah, Vermont, and Virginia. Some states still have waiting periods to obtain a permit to purchase a handgun. These waiting periods range from 2 to 30 days.

Violence and the use of firearms in the United States has become one of society's most pressing concerns. Juveniles under 21 now account for about one-quarter of all arrests for the possession or use of a gun. Black American youths are three times more likely to be arrested for a gun violation than are white American youths, and about half of all homicide victims are black Americans. Most homicides are not racially motivated, however, because 94% of victims are killed by members of their own race and 83% of white American murder victims are killed by other whites.

The majority of homicides involve juveniles, many of whom are in gangs and involved in selling and using illegal drugs. While law enforcement can be increased in some ways, laws cannot solve the problems of violence and murder. Solutions to the social problems that underlie the violence must come from parents, clergy, teachers, and the youths involved.

Youth Gangs

Youth gangs exist in nearly every major city in the U.S. Recent surveys indicate that more than 200,000 adolescents and young adults are members of almost 4,000 gangs. Previously, gangs were primarily focused in major cities, such as Los Angeles, Chicago, and New York, but they have since spread to most large cities in the midwest, northwest, south, and southwest. The sale of drugs has been a key factor in the movement of gangs to more and more cities. In most cities with gangs, it is not only poor areas that are affected, but gang activities have spread to traditionally safe suburbs and to schools.

A number of factors contribute to a teenager or young adult deciding to join a gang: poverty, failure at school, substance abuse, dysfunctional family life, and

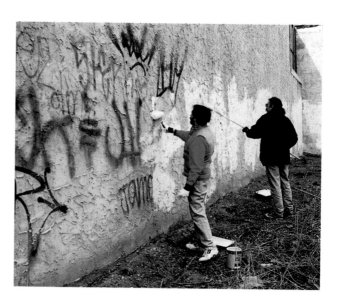

Graffiti is one form youths use to express anger.

family violence. Easy access to illegal drugs and the lure of financial rewards from drug dealing are both powerful attractants for a young person with no money, no education, no job, and no future. For them, gang life is exciting and rewarding.

Gang recruits often have a poor self-image, low self-esteem, and no adult to provide counseling and support. Some gang members are the children of gang members and are following in their parents' footsteps. Gang members often gain recognition from other gang members and from a society that fears them—in this way they gain attention and respect.

Drugs and guns are an integral part of gang acceptance. Often a recruit is not deemed fit until he or she has obtained a gun—and used it, either on a rival gang member or in committing a crime. About half of the juvenile inmates of prisons report that their gang regularly bought and sold guns and that gun theft was an important gang activity. Thus, the ready accessibility of guns in the U.S. directly contributes to gang activities and the destruction of the lives of thousands of young people.

School Violence

The problem of guns in schools became the focus of national attention in 1998. A series of shootings by teenagers in schools across America brought horror and tragedy into the affected families and communities. A partial list of school shootings include:

October 1, 1997, Pearl, Mississippi: A 16-year-old boy shoots and kills his mother, his ex-girlfriend, and a student.

December 1, 1997, West Paducah, Kentucky: A 14-year-old boy shoots and kills three students.

March 24, 1998, Jonesboro, Arkansas: A 13-year-old boy and an 11-year-old boy shoot and kill five students.

April 24, 1998, Edinboro, Pennsylvania: A 14-year-old boy shoots and kills a teacher at a school dance.

May 19, 1998, Fayetteville, Tennessee: An 18-year-old boy shoots and kills a classmate.

May 28, 1998, Springfield, Oregon: A 15-year-old boy shoots and kills his parents and then goes to school and kills two students. Others are critically wounded.

April 20, 1999, Littleton, Colorado: Two Columbine high school boys kill 13 schoolmates and one teacher; 23 are wounded. The two boys kill themselves.

What prompts such senseless violence by teenage boys all across America? Experts of all kinds offer explanations and social theories, but as a friend of the family whose son is accused of the murders in Springfield, Oregon, remarked, "There's no obvious explanation for it.

Managing Stress

Managing the Stress of Adolescence

Adolescence

between thirteen and nineteen they exist
traveling the bridge to adulthood
their parents wishing to be psychiatrists
just to understand, if they could

the journey is long and hard
with many paths to choose
some let down their guard
and turn to drugs or booze

some stay on the yellow brick road
responsible and mature they try to be
increasing the weight on an already heavy load
locking emotions up and throwing away the key

living for the here and now
consequences are seldom thought about

it won't happen to me, they vow
besides the scientists will figure it out

living in a world of violence
desensitized to it all
no longer a time of innocence
roaming around a mini-mall

killing each other with ease
drugs and guns as the source
making violence an age-specific disease
ravaging this population with such force

becoming parents way too fast
dropping out of school to support a child
taking a job and putting fun in the past
no more nights partying and being wild

kids raising kids
violence and gangs and guns and knives
no longer seeing friends because of coffin lids
consuming their everyday lives

being an adolescent is not so simple
too young for this, too old for that
dealing with sex to drugs to violence to pimples
surviving deserves a tip of the hat

thirteen to nineteen, an adolescent
the time flies by, keeping busy
developing an identity and becoming independent
being an adolescent is not so easy

— *Stepanie Vahle*

Printed with permission of author.

Global Wellness

Violence in the U.S. Exceeds That of Any Other Nation

The ultimate measure of violence is homicide, the killing of another person. The U.S. leads all technologically advanced, industrialized nations in the number of homicides per capita (see figure). Compared with Italy, the country with the next highest homicide rate, the U.S. rate is eight times greater. And compared with Japan, it is about 40 times as great. Even compared with Canada, a country that is culturally similar to ours, the U.S. homicide rate is 20 times greater.

If one looks at data on other forms of violence, such as forcible rape, the graph is pretty much the same. In fact, if one looks at the statistical data for any form of interpersonal violence, the U.S. is ahead of every other nation by a factor of 10 or more. A consequence of this violence is that the U.S. also imprisons a higher percentage of its population than any other industrialized nation. Whether a nation can long endure with this level of violence—violence that continues to escalate year after year—is a question that many people ask but are afraid to answer.

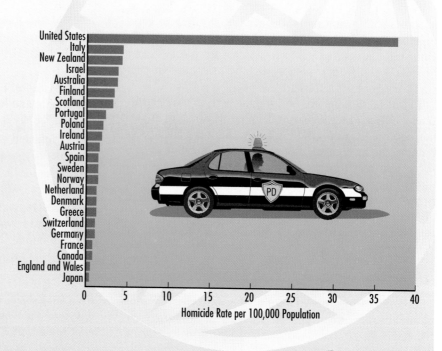

Sources: National Center for Health Statistics, *Vital Statistics*, 1990; World Health Organization, *Statistical Annuals*, 1990, 1991.

Young Kip was just a bad seed" (King and Murr, 1998). These school killings occurred in middle-class American communities and thereby received much more media attention than killings that frequently occur in inner city schools in poor neighborhoods. Today, no parent can feel entirely at ease when a child is at school. All unusual behaviors and threats must be taken seriously.

School killings have rekindled the ongoing controversy about the right of citizens to own firearms in this country, a right that many argue is guaranteed by the U.S. Constitution. The NRA persistently argues that ownership of guns has nothing to do with violence and killings. After the killings in Springfield, Oregon, a spokesman for the NRA stated, "Lawful arms ownership has nothing to do with this tragedy" (Kassirer, 1998). In refuting this, a prominent physician points out that:

"Children and adolescents are by definition immature and may lack judgment. Life's embarrassments, rejections, and torments may send them into fits of temper, even rage, and may prompt a desire for revenge. Impulsively, some children lash out at others and at themselves. Nonetheless, they are only murderous when they have the means, and a loaded gun is the 'perfect' tool" (Kassirer, 1998).

Almost everyone in America has experienced some form of violence in their lives. In many cities and communities, people are afraid to go out at night or to go walking or jogging alone. Now there is fear among students about going to school. Two critical questions must be addressed by American society. First, what are the factors contributing to the continued rise in all forms of violence—child abuse, spousal abuse, bombings, homicide, and sexual abuse of all kinds—and what can be done to reduce violence? Second, will Americans find the will to disarm private citizens and, thereby, reduce the cause of most violent crimes?

Many facts and studies indicate that social and interpersonal violence stems from inequality—inequality in wealth, inequality in education, inequality in medical care, and inequality in job opportunity (Chasin, 1997). Changing these inequalities in American society may prove to be difficult or impossible. If that is so, then violence, and its many negative effects on health and life, is likely to increase in the years ahead.

Many people believe that violence among people and in societies is inevitable, that is, violence is biologically determined and cannot be changed. At best, society can try to limit the amount of violence and punish offenders. This belief is not substantiated by cultural studies of societies around the world that have little or no violence as long as their traditional lifestyle is not disrupted. Examples of nonviolent societies include the Semai Senoi people of Malaysia, Mabuti pygmies of Zaire, the Inuit Eskimos of Canada, the Zuni Pueblo Indians of New Mexico, and the Ladakh people of northwestern India (Adler and Denmark, 1995). The Ladakh, in particular, is a Buddhist culture whose doctrines identify greed, hate, aggression, lust, envy, jealousy, and pride as the ultimate sources of human unhappiness. In American society, we have come to accept these human behaviors.

We believe that the point to remember about violence is that it is a personal decision to be violent or not, just as it is a personal decision to exercise or not. The fact that nonviolent societies do exist and that people may choose to live nonviolent lives should encourage everyone who abhors violence to reduce the level of violence in their lives. In so doing, the violence in society is reduced.

Preventing Unintentional Injuries

Injuries affect the health and well-being of millions of Americans every year. Unintentional injuries and accidents of various kinds are a far greater source of ill health and death than most people realize. Safety warnings and increased public awareness measures have reduced the number of unintentional injuries and deaths in recent years (Figure 13.1). In 1997, the number of unintentional injury deaths from all causes in the United States was 93,800, a

> *God does not play dice.*
> ALBERT EINSTEIN

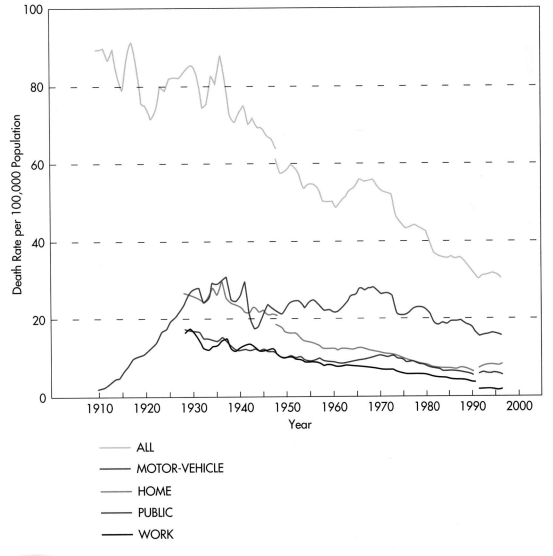

FIGURE 13.1   Trends in Unintentional Injury Deaths Trends in unintentional injury deaths per 100,000 have been reduced 58% between 1912 and 1997 (age-adjusted).

Source: National Safety Council, Accident Facts, 1998 Edition.

decrease of 100 deaths from 1996 (National Safety Council [NSC], 1998). Despite the encouraging reduction in unintentional injury deaths, the adverse health consequences of unintentional injuries are still serious and can be reduced.

In the United States, unintentional injuries are the leading cause of death among all persons aged 1 to 38 and the fifth leading cause of death among all people of all ages (NSC, 1998). Unintentional injuries and accidents are responsible for nearly one-half trillion dollars in medical costs and three-fourths of a trillion dollars in economic costs.

Many people believe accidents are ill-fated occurrences over which people have no control. Whereas it is true that some accidents are the result of bad luck, a vast number of accidents and the injuries resulting from them are caused by social and economic conditions that make the environment hazardous, poor judgment, lapses in attention, recklessness, loss of emotional control, and mental states that are imbalanced by alcohol and drugs. Insofar as the environment can be made safe and individuals made aware and cautious, the degree of unintentional injuries from accidents can be reduced.

Unintentional Injuries and Accidents

What is **safety?** The word "safety" is used in a wide context with various meanings to different individuals. Few individuals or agencies can agree on one universal definition. "Is this a safe part of town to be this late at night?" "He is not a very safe motorcycle driver." "My daughter's safety has been a concern of mine since she obtained her driver's license." "Is that old ladder safe to use?" As you can see, the word "safe" or "safety" may be used in a variety of situations.

One common tie to all these different scenarios is the word **accident.** As defined by the National Safety Council, an accident "is that occurrence in a sequence of events which produces unintended injury, death, or property damage. Accident refers to the event, not the result of the event" (NSC, 1998).

Each year one in four individuals will sustain some type of serious injury that requires medical attention and that is a result of an accident. Injuries are a serious problem, but many individuals lack the necessary knowledge and skills to provide assistance if an emergency does occur. Injuries are the leading cause of disability in young people today and cause more deaths in children than all the infectious diseases combined.

Unintentional injury is a term often used interchangeably with the term "accident," and we also will use both terms. Unintentional injury is the term preferred by public health officials and refers to the *result*

of an accident or the health consequence of an accident (NSC, 1998). Some common examples of unintentional injuries are motor vehicle accidents, home accidents (e.g., falls, poisonings, fires), workplace accidents, unintentional and intentional discharge of firearms, and pedestrian accidents with motor vehicles (Table 13.4).

Unintentional injuries continue to be the fifth leading cause of death overall, exceeded only by heart disease, cancer, stroke, and chronic obstructive pulmonary disease. The five leading causes of death from unintentional injury are motor vehicles; falls; poisoning by solids and liquids; fires and burns; and drowning: these have been the same since 1970. For most of the twentieth century, the rate of death from accidents has steadily dropped because of increased safety and health efforts. However, in the last 4 years, there has been an increase in total deaths from unintentional injury, which should be a warning that greater attention to increased health and safety efforts is needed to reverse this trend.

The causes of death from unintentional injury change with age. Poor diet, sedentary life-style, arthritis, decreased mobility, poverty, chronic diseases, or lack of access to primary medical care may contribute to injuries and accidental death as people get older.

While you are listening to your professor talk for 10 minutes on a personal health topic or are taking a 10-minute walk to class, 2 persons will be killed and approximately 390 will suffer a **disabling injury.** On average, there are 11 deaths from unintentional injury and about 2,200 disabling injuries every hour (Table 13.5).

TABLE 13.4   Leading Causes of Unintentional Deaths in the U.S. in 1995
Cause of death is ascribed to a single category, although many factors contribute to all kinds of unintentional injuries.

Cause of death	Number of deaths, all ages	Number of deaths, 15 to 24 years
Motor vehicle crashes	43,363	10,600
Falls	13,986	245
Poisonings by solids and liquids	8,461	540
Drowning	4,350	790
Fires, burns, and deaths associated with fires	3,761	–
Firearms	–	423
All other unintentional injuries	19,399	1,244
Total	**93,320**	**13,842**

Source: National Safety Council, Accident Facts, 1998 Edition.

TABLE 13.5 **Deaths and Disabling Injuries by Classification, 1997**

Class	Severity	One every . . .	No. per hour	No. per day	No. per week	1997 total
All	Deaths	6 minutes	11	257	1,800	93,800
	Injuries	2 seconds	2,200	52,900	371,200	19,300,000
Motor vehicle	Deaths	12 minutes	5	118	830	43,200
	Injuries	14 seconds	260	6,300	44,200	2,300,000
Work	Deaths	103 minutes	1	14	100	5,100
	Injuries	8 seconds	430	10,400	73,100	3,800,000
Workers off-the-job	Deaths	14 minutes	4	105	730	38,200
	Injuries	5 seconds	660	15,900	111,500	5,800,000
Home	Deaths	19 minutes	3	78	550	28,400
	Injuries	5 seconds	780	18,600	130,800	6,800,000
Public, non–motor vehicle	Deaths	27 minutes	2	53	370	19,400
	Injuries	5 seconds	740	17,800	125,000	6,500,000

Source: National Safety Council, Accident Facts, 1998 Edition.

Reducing the Risk of Accidents

When considering accidents, their prevention, and their consequences, public health professionals focus on **accident mitigation**—methods to reduce damage caused by unplanned events—and **accident prevention**—ways to eliminate the occurrence of unintended injuries. Accident mitigation and prevention can be viewed in two contexts: (1) individual or personal and (2) environmental or community.

Many factors are involved in unintentional injury: knowledge, attitudes, beliefs, and behaviors; economic and social conditions; ability level of the performer of tasks; conditions of the environment; and alcohol and other drug use. Positive changes in these factors will reduce injuries, but more attention should be directed to prevention strategies. Even though unintentional injuries have decreased 57% from 1912 to 1996, the cost is still staggering.

Attitudes and beliefs may be the greatest factor involved in unintentional injuries. Your individual attitude toward safety precautions greatly influences the likelihood of an injury. You may believe that safety precautions are a waste of time, that you have no control over the situation (what will happen, will happen), or you may have a reckless attitude (you like to take risks).

Lack of knowledge and skills also play a role in unintentional injury. In special circumstances, especially when performing a new procedure or task, lacking the proper knowledge or skills could result in unintentional injury (e.g., operating a new power tool before reading the instructions, operating a motorcycle the first time, or using a new kitchen appliance).

Socioeconomic factors also play a role in unintentional injury. Some individuals may lack the necessary funds to replace unsafe or old equipment. Some may even lack the necessary funds to obtain proper training in safety-related matters. Safety training can be received through a local National Safety Council office on such topics as proper storage of household cleaning items, tool safety, and safety tips for the babysitter. Local health departments may also provide educational workshops on safety issues.

Some social settings may lend themselves to accidents. Attitudes and beliefs as well as the social setting can raise or lower the probability of an unintentional injury. For example, alcohol and drug use and abuse definitely affect the frequency of unintentional injuries. Prescribed medications, especially ones with a sedative effect, can increase the likelihood of an accident while operating a motor vehicle, motorcycle, or power tool.

The ability of the individual performing a task or activity may affect the probability of an unintentional injury. The person may be a child who is too young to perform a task competently. At the other end of the spectrum, an elderly individual may not be strong enough or steady enough to perform a simple task like carving Thanksgiving turkey with an electric knife.

Terms

safety: an ever-changing condition in which one attempts to minimize the risk of injury, illness, or property damage from the hazards to which one may be exposed

accident: sequence of events that produces unintended injury, death, or property damage; refers to the event, **not** the result of the event

unintentional injury: preferred term for accidental injury; result of an accident

disabling injury: an injury causing death, permanent disability, or any degree of temporary total disability beyond the day of the injury

accident mitigation: methods to reduce damage caused by unplanned events

accident prevention: ways to eliminate the occurrence of unintended injuries

The environment can be the most unpredictable risk factor in unintentional injuries. Environmental risks include appropriate maintenance of streets, safe power transmission and sewage treatment, and laws that regulate the hazard risk of appliances and tools. Natural disasters such as floods, hurricanes, earthquakes, or tornadoes are also environmental risks. The devastation caused by natural disasters affects every one of us at some point in our lifetime.

Stress and fatigue contribute greatly to higher rates of unintentional injuries. Stress may interfere with your concentration when performing even a simple task or may distract you while you are engaged in an activity. Fatigue causes you to be less alert or have slower reaction times; affects your coordination; and, at worst, can cause you to fall asleep. It is not wise to attempt difficult tasks while you are fatigued or under stress.

Analysis of Unintentional Injury

Scientific study of unintentional injury uncovers why injuries occur, what determinants play a role, and who or what age group is the most susceptible. Analysis of unintentional injury provides us with assessments that are necessary before effective educational, preventive, or enforcement strategies can be implemented.

Injury epidemiology, used to investigate risk factors that cause unintentional injuries, is analogous to the epidemiologic model for disease. For injuries to result, three factors are involved: (1) the agent or source of energy exchange, i.e., mechanical, chemical, electrical, or thermal; (2) the vehicle for the transmission of mechanical energy, i.e., a car, truck, motorcycle, powerline, or poison; and (3) a host or object, i.e., a person, school building, or house (Figure 13.2).

Most unintentional injuries are complex and many factors can be involved. Also, interactions among risk factors affect the likelihood of an accident. For example, cutting trees with a chain saw on a windy or rainy day may increase the risk of accident, whereas choosing a dry, calm day might reduce the chance of an accident.

The Haddon matrix is one of the most famous scientific models used in unintentional injury analysis. Developed by William Haddon, Jr., in the 1960s, this model was used originally to investigate motor vehicle risk factors and to develop and implement programs to prevent or reduce the occurrence of car accidents. The Haddon matrix analyzed accidents in three phases:

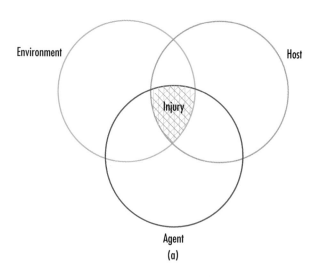

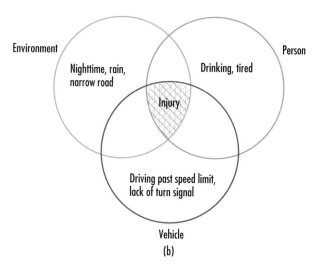

FIGURE 13.2   **Epidemiologic Model for Unintentional Injuries**

- *Phase 1: Pre-event phase.* Includes factors that may determine if an accident will happen; lack of knowledge or skills or alcohol use are the most significant factors.
- *Phase 2: Event phase.* Occurs when the host comes into contact with forces of energy. Many preventive measures, such as the use of helmets, safety belts, or protective goggles, are associated with this phase.
- *Phase 3: Post-event phase.* Includes emergency procedures provided after the injury has occurred. Preventive signaling devices, smoke and carbon monoxide detectors, or fire alarms will increase the speed with which help reaches an injured person. Emergency transportation and care of an injured or sick person occurs in this phase.

All approaches to unintentional injury reduction include: (a) educational and prevention strategies; (b) stricter laws and regulations (e.g., mandates to enforce safety belt and helmet compliance); and (c) better

Terms

injury epidemiology: the study of the occurrence, causes, and prevention of injury

product design and automatic protection devices (e.g., air bags, child-proof car door locks, child-proof safety caps on medicines).

Motor Vehicle Safety

Even though motor vehicle death rates have been declining since 1962, the number of deaths is still a major concern. Motor vehicle travel is the primary means of transportation in the United States, and it provides an unprecedented degree of mobility. Yet, for all its advantages, injuries resulting from motor vehicle crashes are the leading cause of death for every person from age 6 to 27. Traffic fatalities account for more than 90% of transportation-related fatalities. In 1997, 37,280 people were killed in motor vehicle traffic crashes and approximately 2,185,000 people were injured (U.S. Department of Transportation, National Highway Traffic Safety Administration [NHTSA], 1998).

In 1997, there were 16,189 fatalities in alcohol-related automobile crashes. This is a 6% decrease from 1996, and represents an average of one alcohol-related fatality every 32 minutes. However, the 16,189 alcohol-related fatalities in 1997 (38.6% of total traffic fatalities for the year) represent a 32% reduction from the 23,641 alcohol-related fatalities reported in 1987 (51% of the total annual fatalities). The National Highway Traffic Safety Administration estimates that alcohol was involved in 34% of fatal crashes and in 7% of all crashes in 1997 (NHTSA, 1998a). During the year-end holiday season, 50% of all motor vehicle fatalities are alcohol-related. Although all states and the District of Columbia outlaw sale of alcohol to persons under age 21, alcohol-related deaths and injuries among underage persons still occur.

Many accidents involving young persons occur after dark, after parties, and after drinking. Alcohol in the blood and brain impairs a driver's judgment, coordination, and reaction time. The effects of alcohol vary considerably from one person to another, so even small amounts of alcohol may impair driving skills and cause an accident. New laws have been proposed that set a zero tolerance for blood alcohol for persons under age 21.

Many factors other than alcohol use contribute to motor vehicle fatalities and injuries, e.g., road conditions and speed at which the vehicle travels. The interaction between these two factors is particularly risky. In all severe accidents, rural and urban, exceeding the posted speed limit was the most common factor. Speeding while driving kills 13,000 people every year. Defects in a vehicle, such as faulty tires, brakes, headlights, steering system, body, door, and hood, also contribute to the risk of motor vehicle accidents.

> *The best way to avoid something is to cause that which is to be avoided to avoid you of its own accord.*
> SUFI PROVERB

Driving can be difficult even when you are completely concentrating on the road and your surroundings. But driving while you dial a phone or balance it to your ear can be distracting and potentially dangerous. Car phones may be convenient for those who own them, but if not used properly, car phones are a danger to the user and everyone on the road. At 55 miles per hour, a vehicle travels the length of a foot-

---

Wellness Guide

Driving Defensively

Driving defensively means not only taking responsibility for yourself and your actions but also keeping an eye on "the other guy." The National Safety Council offers the following guidelines to help reduce your risks on the road:

- Don't leave the driveway without securing each passenger in the car, including children and pets. Safety belts save thousands of lives each year!

- Remember that driving too fast or too slow can increase the likelihood of collisions.

- Don't kid yourself. If you plan to drink, designate a driver who won't drink. Alcohol is a factor in almost half of all fatal motor vehicle accidents.

- Be alert! If you notice that a car is straddling the center line, weaving, making wide turns, stopping abruptly, or responding slowly to traffic signals, the driver may be impaired.

- Avoid an impaired driver by slowing down, letting the driver pass, pulling onto the shoulder, or turning right at the nearest corner. If it appears that an oncoming car is crossing into your lane, pull over to the roadside, sound the horn, and flash your lights.

- Notify the police immediately after seeing a motorist who is driving suspiciously.

- Follow the rules of the road. Don't contest the "right of way" or try to race another car during a merge. Be respectful of other motorists.

- While driving, be cautious, aware, and responsible.

Source: National Safety Council, Fact Sheet on Driving Defensively, October 20, 1997.

ball field in 3.7 seconds, less time than it takes to dial a phone number. Anything that takes a driver's concentration off the road increases the possibility of an accident. America's growing enchantment with cellular mobile phones in automobiles brings with it the need for renewed emphasis on safe driving practices. Other countries, such as Chile, Panama, and Venezuela, have developed strict traffic laws regarding the use of cellular phones while driving (NSC, October 20, 1997).

Forty-nine states and the District of Columbia have mandatory safety belt use laws in effect. Use rates vary widely from state to state, reflecting factors such as differences in public attitudes, enforcement practices, legal provisions, and public information and education programs. Governmental regulations, and safety belt and child safety seats, which were initially opposed by many individuals, have greatly reduced the number of motor vehicle fatalities and injuries.

In addition to seatbelt use, air bags have also saved many lives in the last decade. Since 1987, there have been about 2.1 million air bag deployments. According to the National Highway Traffic Safety Administration (NHTSA), air bags have saved the lives of more than 2,900 people who otherwise may have died in vehicle crashes. Furthermore, NHTSA estimates that the combination of an air bag plus a lap-shoulder belt reduces the risk of serious head injury by 75% compared with a 38% reduction for seatbelts alone.

The overwhelming majority of Americans and their families can retain the lifesaving benefits of air bags and virtually eliminate the risks by following the **ABCs** of air bag effectiveness (National Safety Council, *Air Bag and Seatbelt Safety Campaign,* April 21, 1998).

- **A**lways slide the seat back as far as possible and sit back.
- **B**uckle everyone up.
- **C**hildren aged 12 and under should ride properly restrained in the back seat.

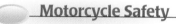

Motorcycle Safety

Motorcycles appeal to many individuals for various reasons: low cost to purchase, repair, and operate; the exciting feeling of open-air riding; and association with fellow motorcycle riders. However, risks include inclement weather, less crash protection than an automo-

---

Managing Stress

Mindfulness Meditation

Ninety percent of all accidents are the result of human error. This fact, cited by the National Safety Council, suggests what those in the field of stress management already know: the mind can focus on only one or two thoughts at a time. When the mind is overwhelmed with thoughts, something always drops. When you are just sitting at your desk studying for an exam and your mind wanders, your life isn't in jeopardy. But when you are engaged in an activity like driving your car, and you have one hand on the cellular phone, the other grabbing your eye liner, electric razor, or radio dial, and your mind is focused on the news broadcast of the latest disaster, an accident is waiting to happen.

Nine times out of ten, accidents occur because your mind is somewhere other than where it is supposed to be. Drifting attention, unfocused thoughts, and mental distractions are normal in the course of a typical day, but the mind *can* be trained to stay focused. Training the mind in this fashion is

called "mindfulness meditation," a type of meditation used to domesticate your thoughts and gain control of your awareness. Athletes, surgeons, and actors practice this technique to improve their performance. It is a technique that everyone should master, in this context specifically to avoid the risk of accidents.

Mindfulness meditation can take many forms and with repeated practice, the effects of one experience (like eating an apple) can transfer to virtually any activity. Mindfulness meditation is a great way to keep focused on whatever task you are engaged in. Try this exercise.

1. Take an apple and hold it in your hand.
2. Sit comfortably with your back straight. You may choose to sit against a wall for support.
3. Hold the apple and feel its weight in your hand. Feel the apple. Feel the texture of the apple's skin. Feel the curves. Feel the stem if there is

one. Notice all the nuances of the apple with your fingers.

4. Look at the apple. What color is it? Look at it carefully. Study it. Know this apple so well, that if it was put back in a barrel of apples, you could easily find it.
5. Now smell the apple. Close your eyes and focus your sense of smell on the apple. What does it smell like?
6. Bite into the apple. Savor its taste, flavor, and texture. Feel your tongue and jaws move as you chew.

Now, sensing and eating an apple may seem far removed from preventing an accident at home, work, or on the road, but the truth is that the skills of concentration and focusing are important in every activity you do. Mindfulness meditation will help you stay focused and attentive to details that require your undivided attention.

Wellness Guide

Protect Your Kids in the Car

The type of child safety seat to buy and how you position it depend on the child's age, weight, and size. Every state and the District of Columbia have child protection laws. The safest place for any child aged 12 and under is in the back seat. Every child should be buckled into a child safety seat or a booster seat or a lap-shoulder belt, if it fits. A few pointers:

Riding with Babies

- Infants up to about 20 pounds and up to age 1 should ride in a rear-facing child seat. The child seat must be in the BACK seat and face the rear of the car, van, or truck.

- Babies riding in a car must never face front. In a crash or sudden stop, the baby's neck can be hurt badly.

- Infants in car seats must never ride in the front seat of a car with air bags. In a crash, the air bag can hit the car seat and hurt or kill the baby.

- Never hold your baby in your lap when you are riding in the car. In a crash or sudden stop, your child can be hurt badly or killed.

Riding with Young Kids

- Kids over 20 pounds and older than 1 year should ride in a car seat that faces the front of the car, van, or truck.

- It is best to keep kids in the foreward-facing car seat for as long as they fit comfortably in it.

- Older kids over 40 pounds should ride in a booster seat until the car's lap and shoulder belts fit them correctly. The lap belt must fit low and

snug on their hips. The shoulder belt must not cross their face or neck.

- Never put a shoulder belt behind a child's back or under a child's arm.

Remember . . .

- All kids are safest in the back seat, in a safety seat or seatbelt.

- Always read the child seat instructions and the car owner's manual. Test the child seat to ensure a snug fit by pulling the base to either side or toward the front of the car.

Source: National Highway Traffic Safety Administration, U.S. Department of Transportation, *Protect Your Kids in the Car,* August 1997.

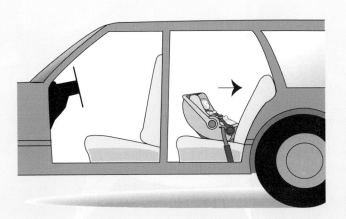

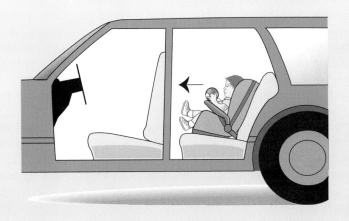

bile, and less visibility by other drivers. Motorcycle operators can ensure a safer ride by securing proper training in operational procedures and by using a helmet and proper protective clothing. Fewer than 1 in 10 motorcycle operators receive any formal training. Wearing a motorcycle helmet may reduce the likelihood of fatal injuries by 29%. Protective clothing, such as long sleeves and pants, jackets, and boots, may lessen the chance for abrasions should an accident occur or protect from the unpredictable elements of weather.

In 1966, Congress mandated that motorcycle riders and passengers use helmets in all states. If states did not enforce this mandate, they would lose federal highway funds, but only three states at first adopted helmet laws. However by 1975, 47 states had helmet laws in force. During this ten-year period (1966–1975), fatal motorcycle accidents declined from 12.8 to 6.5 deaths per 100,000. Nevertheless, the American Motorcycle Association and A Brotherhood Against Totalitarian Enactment (ABATE) have opposed helmet regulations. They argue that riders should not be forced to wear protective equipment, a sentiment also held by many who opposed auto safety belt mandates. Nonetheless, safety belts and helmets *do* reduce motor vehicle injuries and deaths.

All motorcycle helmets sold in the United States are required to meet federal guidelines, which establish the minimum level of protection helmets must afford each user. Currently, 25 states, the District of Columbia, and Puerto Rico require helmet use by all motorcycle operators and passengers. In another 22 states, only persons under a specific age, usually 18, are required to wear helmets. Three states have no laws requiring helmet use.

Pedestrian Safety

Traffic accidents injured 77,000 pedestrians and killed 5,307 pedestrians in the United States in 1997. Nearly 51% of all pedestrian deaths and injuries involve children aged 5 to 9 who are either crossing or entering a street. Among young children, implementation of preventive strategies and educational efforts addressing safety procedures in traffic areas may reduce accidents. Many young children don't know what traffic signals or signs mean. Young children are also unable to judge the distance and speed of vehicles, which puts them in danger when trying to cross a busy intersection. Closer supervision by adults helps. Safety education of childcare workers at school and elsewhere is another preventive strategy.

The elderly are also at risk for pedestrian injuries, as a result of failing eyesight and hearing and mobility problems. Some pedestrian injuries occur when individuals dart into a busy street or are unable to see oncoming traffic because their view is blocked by a parked vehicle. Many pedestrian injuries involve joggers, runners, and walkers. Bright-colored clothes, especially reflective clothes, offer protection for pedestrians during both day and night. Also, just as alcohol impairs the judgment of motor vehicle operators, it also impairs the judgment of pedestrians.

Other preventive strategies help reduce the number of pedestrian injuries and deaths. Underpasses and overpasses in high traffic areas, well-marked crosswalks, and pedestrian guardrails all offer greater protection for the pedestrian. Limiting traffic during peak hours of pedestrian traffic—for instance, before and after school or church—might also be beneficial.

Bicycle Safety

Safety concerns have been increasing as more bicycles are used for exercise and recreation. Bicycling attracts

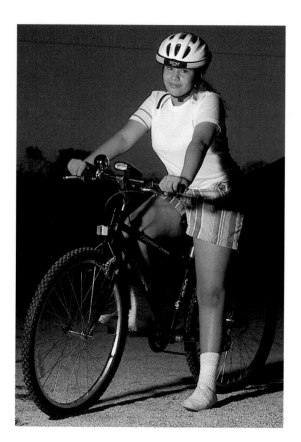

Appropriate helmet and reflector use are crucial to bicycle safety.

more than 67 million riders annually. Very few of these bicyclists wear a protective helmet every time they ride their bike. The estimated annual cost of bicycle-related injuries and deaths for all ages is $8 billion. For every $15 bike helmet purchased and used properly, $30 in direct health care costs and $420 in indirect health care costs could be saved annually. Since 1940, the use of bicycles has increased 15-fold, but the death rate from bicycle accidents is one-fourteenth that of 1940. The single most important factor in reducing bicycle deaths is the use of protective helmets.

A total of 58,000 bicyclists were injured and 813 were killed in traffic crashes in 1997. Bicyclists made up 2% of all the people injured in traffic during the same year. Police reported that for 72% of the bicyclists killed in traffic crashes in 1995, one or more errors in judgment or other factors related to the cyclist's behavior were witnessed. The factor often most noted was "failure to yield right-of-way."

Bicycle riders are required to follow the same rules of the road as automobile operators. But many bicycle riders lack knowledge of these rules, do not use proper hand signals, or ride on the wrong side of the street, contributing to bicycle injuries and fatalities. Also, lack of skill in handling a bicycle increases the risk of an accident. Individuals who purchase a new bicycle should be familiar with all its devices before riding it. Also, many young bicycle riders are unaware of the rules of the road or are too small to see over motor vehicles.

Bicycle riders need to wear bright, reflective clothing, and the bicycle itself should be properly equipped with reflectors and lights. A recent and dangerous phenomenon is wearing headphones while riding. Inability to hear the sounds of traffic, the honk of a horn, or a shout of warning may contribute to an accident. Construction of more bicycle paths, underpasses, overpasses, and guardrails along with defensive riding skills can reduce bicycle injuries and deaths.

Home Safety

Accidental deaths in the home are gradually declining but are still a major source of concern. Accidents in the home take a special toll on both young and elderly persons. As the elderly population continues to grow, accidents in the home will increase. The main categories of home accidents include falls, poisonings, drowning, choking and suffocation, and fires and burns. Although not all falls, drownings, or poisonings occur in the home, they are classified as home accidents.

Between 1912 and 1997, deaths from unintentional home injury per 100,000 population were reduced 61%. One person in 39 in the United States was disabled 1 full day or more by unintentional injuries received in the home in 1997. Disabling injuries are more numerous in the home than they are in the workplace and motor vehicle accidents combined. The National Health Interview Survey indicates that about 19,674,000 episodes of home injuries occurred in 1994. In 1997, there were 28,400 deaths in the home, resulting from numerous causes, including falls, poisonings, drowning, choking and suffocation, and fires (NSC, 1998).

First Aid and Emergencies

First aid and medical emergencies can be handled appropriately if you take a deep breath and tell yourself you can handle the situation until a qualified medical professional arrives to take over. First aid is defined as the immediate care given to an injured or ill person. First aid is temporary assistance given until a person has recovered or until a qualified medical person can provide assistance.

> *The man who is unable to people his solitude is equally unable to be alone in a bustling crowd.*
> CHARLES BAUDELAIRE, poet

Knowledge about first aid and medical emergencies can literally mean the difference between life and death and can help prevent disability or permanent in-

Wellness Guide

Smoke Detectors Give You a Chance

Most deaths and injuries in fires result from inhalation of smoke and toxic gases that reach victims before the flames do. Survival depends on an early warning system that gives you time to vacate the premises at once. The best warning system available is a smoke detector.

According to *Consumer Reports*, installation of a smoke detector in your home cuts your risk of dying in a fire in half. The U.S. Consumer Product Safety Commission offers these suggestions about smoke detectors:

- Many localities require that you have a smoke detector in your home, so buy one—at least one. They're inexpensive and are available at most hardware stores and supermarkets. Check your local codes and regulations; they may require you to purchase a specific kind.

- Read the instructions that come with the detector for advice on where to install it. You should purchase at least one for every floor in your house. Preferably you should place one outside every bedroom.

- Manufacturers know what is best for their products and tell you how to care for them. Follow their instructions. Detectors can save lives, but only if you install and maintain them properly.

- Never disconnect a fire detector. If it goes off at wrong times because of heat from a stove or steam from a bathroom, move it to another location.

- Replace the battery annually (January 1 is an easy day to remember) or when you hear a "chirping" sound. (*Consumer Reports* estimates that one-third of all detectors would not respond to a fire because of dead or missing batteries.) And press the test button regularly to be sure the batteries work.

- Keep your detector clean. Dust, grease, or other materials can interfere with efficient operation. You may want to vacuum the grill work on the detector.

Source: National Safety Council, *Safety and Health,* February 1995.

jury. Knowledge of first aid skills will increase your confidence in dealing with both minor and major emergencies and will be reassuring to an injured person.

Taking Risks and Preventing Accidents

Risks cannot be avoided in life; accidents and unintentional injuries are a consequence of the risks we take. As soon as a child learns to crawl, he or she begins to take risks to explore and understand the environment. At each stage of life we take risks to learn and to expand our capabilities and experiences. We take a risk when we cross the street in traffic, run to catch a bus, or swing from the branch of a tree. When we go hiking or climbing or engage in sports, we are taking risks.

The important question YOU need to ask is: "What risks are necessary and acceptable for me to live the way I want to?" The answer will also, to some extent, determine your risk of unintentional injury. People differ enormously in their need for risk-taking behaviors. Some people thrive on high-risk endeavors, such as playing polo, racing cars, or climbing mountains. However, even people who live more sedate lives may

be at risk for unintentional injuries because of destructive behaviors or unhealthy mental attitudes.

Whatever your personal beliefs, a commitment to safe living can be made at any time. Why not make the commitment now? Eliminating or reducing the use of alcohol can reduce the risk of many kinds of injuries, especially motor vehicle accidents. Lowering your stress level will also contribute significantly to reducing unintentional injuries. Not keeping a loaded firearm in the house can eliminate the risk of an unintentional firearm injury. Reading and following the manufacturer's instructions and warnings before operating a new product will also help to reduce the risk of unintentional injury. Before undertaking any sport activity, climbing a ladder, or riding a bike, take a moment to consider essential safety measures. Observe posted safety rules and warning signs. Keep in good physical condition and have a positive mental attitude when undertaking a potentially dangerous activity.

Although unintentional injuries are usually not a laughing matter, one accident statistic does sound a humorous note. Saturday and Sunday are the two most dangerous days of the week for fatal accidents. Going out on the weekends just to have fun increases the risks of serious injuries. Maybe studying or reading on weekends is a good idea after all.

Critical Thinking About Health

1. Imagine that you are in a debate in school over this question: "Should all Americans over 21 years of age be allowed to own (a) a handgun; (b) a rifle; (c) a semiautomatic weapon; or (d) an automatic weapon?"

   Take a position on this issue with respect to owning or not owning guns in general. If you favor the ownership of guns, give your reasons for owning or not owning each of the four categories of guns. If you do not favor the ownership of guns, explain your reasons. Whatever side of the issue you are on, discuss whether or not you believe that ownership and availability of guns contributes to violence and crime in America.

2. You and Jennifer have been close friends for more than 15 years (since you both were in high school). Jennifer has recently divorced and has a 5-year-old son, Timmy, who is a "handful" in your view. You and Jennifer have shared many thoughts and feelings over the years. One day after work you stop by to see how Jennifer is doing. You notice that Timmy is limping and has several bruises on his legs. When you comment on Timmy's limp, Jennifer looks at the boy sharply and says, "You fell

out of tree. Isn't that right, Timmy?" The boy mumbles, "Yes" and limps from the room. Jennifer seems tense and doesn't want to talk. You soon leave but not before you smell alcohol on her breath.

   Do you think that this might be a case of child abuse? If so, what do you think your actions should be? In your discussion, indicate whether you are a male or female. Do you think a male or female friend of Jennifer's would act differently in this situation?

3. By all statistical measures, the U.S. is the most violent society among all industrialized countries in the world by a large margin. The U.S. has more forcible rapes, more battered women, more homicides, and more suicides than any other nation on a per capita basis. Discuss why you think our society is so violent and what could be done to change its violent nature.

4. Briefly explain a recent injury that occurred to you, a friend, or family member using the epidemiological triad presented in Figure 13.2.

   a. What were the human factors involved in the injury?

b. What were the environmental factors (physical as well as social) involved in the injury?

c. What were the vehicle (or agent) factors involved in the injury?

Which factor(s) could have been modified in such a way that may have prevented the injury from occurring?

5. Alcohol is a contributing factor in about 40% of traffic fatalities. What are your campus and community doing to help prevent people, both young and old, from driving while intoxicated? Some questions to consider:

a. Are there educational programs? If so, what are they and who do they target?

b. How would you design an educational program to keep your peers from drinking and driving?

c. Are there seasonal programs that increase awareness about the dangers of drinking and driving (e.g., high school prom, Fourth of July)?

d. What is the role of local law enforcement, both on and off campus, with regards to decreasing drinking and driving accidents and fatalities?

6. Federal, state, and local governments have written and passed laws and regulations that enforce certain safety behaviors that have an impact on the individual and/or community. Such laws regulate using a seatbelt, restraining your child in a car seat, and wearing a helmet while riding a motorcycle or bicycle. Some people believe that the government (at any level) should not mandate laws regarding individual safety and injury prevention. Others believe that the government has a right to demand certain safe behaviors among its citizens for the public good. What's your opinion? Should the government be allowed to regulate individual safety behaviors? Explain why or why not.

Health in Review

- Domestic violence includes relationship abuse and child abuse. Violence refers to use of force and power.
- Child abuse encompasses physical abuse, emotional abuse, sexual abuse, and neglect.
- Women who have been assaulted may experience anxiety, depression, substance abuse, headaches, and other medical problems. These are symptoms of post-traumatic stress disorder (PTSD). Many long-term consequences of sexual abuse are associated with PTSD.
- Acquaintance rape or date rape occurs when a person known to the victim uses force or power to coerce the victim into having sex. Women of high school and college age are most vulnerable to acquaintance rape.
- Child abuse is a form of domestic violence that reaches across all social, economic, racial, ethnic, geographic, and educational barriers.
- Education is the key to all forms of violence prevention, including firearm violence, relationship abuse, acquaintance rape, and child abuse.
- The United States exceeds all other developed nations in the per capita rate of rapes, homicides and suicides and in the percentage of its population in prisons.
- Violence and the presence of handguns in schools mirror our communities. Violence is generating fear in our schools, not learning.
- Violence is not an essential part of human behavior, and many societies in the world are nonviolent.

- Unintentional injuries and deaths cost Americans billions of dollars in medical costs as well as costs due to loss of work each year. Unintentional injuries and deaths are preventable!
- Many factors contribute to unintentional injuries: knowledge, attitudes, beliefs, and behaviors; economic and social factors; competence; environmental conditions; and use of alcohol and other drugs.
- The Haddon matrix was developed to assess motor vehicle risk factors and is used to develop prevention programs.
- A multidimensional approach to injury prevention includes education, prevention strategies, stricter laws and regulations, and better product design.
- Motor vehicle deaths are decreasing; however, in 1997 about 37,280 people were killed in motor vehicle crashes. Approximately one alcohol-related fatality occurs every 32 minutes.
- Pedestrian and bicycle safety rules and equipment are keys to preventing accidents. Wear reflective clothing and obey the rules of the road.
- Safety in the home includes preventing falls, poisonings, drownings, choking, and fires.
- Accidents and injuries are a consequence of the many risks we take. Although most of what we do has some degree of risk, we can decrease that risk by increasing safety knowledge and taking the necessary precautions.

Health and Wellness Online

The World Wide Web contains a wealth of information about health and wellness. By accessing the Internet using Web browser software, such as Netscape Navigator or Microsoft's Internet Explorer, you can gain a new perspective on many topics presented in *Essentials of Health and Wellness, Second Edition*. Access the Jones and Bartlett Publishers web site at http://www.jbpub.com/hwonline.

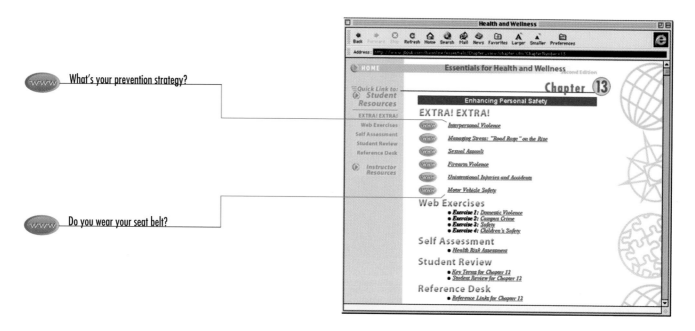

References

Adler, J. (1997, June 2). 'Road rage': We're driven to destruction. *Newsweek, 70.*

Adler, L. L., & Denmark, F. L. (1995). *Violence and the prevention of violence.* Westport, CT: Praeger.

Alexander, L. L., & LaRosa, J. H. (1994). *New dimensions in women's health.* Boston: Jones and Bartlett.

Allen, C. M., & Epperson, D. L. (1993). Perpetrator gender and type of child maltreatment: Overcoming limited conceptualizations and obtaining representative samples. *Child Welfare, 72*(6): 543–554.

Chasin, B. H. (1997). *Inequality and violence in the United States.* New Jersey: Humanities Press.

Dobrin, A., Wiersema, B., Loftin, C., & McDowall, D., (Eds.). (1996). *Statistical handbook on violence in America.* Phoenix, AZ: Oryx Press.

Donat, P. L. N., & D'Emilio, J. (1998). A feminist redefinition of rape and sexual assault: Historical foundations and change. In M. E. Odem & Clay-Warner, J. (Eds.), *Confronting rape and sexual assault* (pp. 35–51). Wilmington, DE: SR Books.

Finkelhor, D., & Dziuba-Leatherman, J. (1994). Victimization of children. *The American Psychologist, 49*(3): 173–184.

Finkelhor, D., & Korbin, J. (1988). Child abuse as an international issue. *Child Abuse and Neglect, 12,* 3–24.

Garbarino, J., & Eckenrode, J. (1997). *Understanding abusive families.* San Francisco: Jossey-Bass, pp. 12–18.

Geles, R. J. (1997). *Intimate violence in families* (3rd ed.). Thousand Oaks, CA: Sage Publications, pp. 3–4.

Gellert, G. A. (1997). *Confronting violence.* Boulder, CO: Westview Press.

Illinois Coalition against Sexual Assault [ICASA] (1993). Springfield, Ill.

Kantor, G. K., & Jasinski, J. L. (1998). Dynamics and risk factors in partner violence. In Jasinski, J. L., & Williams, L. M. (Eds.), *Partner violence* (pp. 1–43).

Kassirer, J. P. (1998). Private arsenals and public peril. *New England Journal of Medicine, 338,* 1375–1376.

Kellerman, A. L. et al. (1992). Suicide in the home in relation to gun ownership. *New England Journal of Medicine, 327*(7): 467.

King, P., & Murr, A. (1998, June 1). A son who spun out of control. *Newsweek,* 32–33.

Koss, M. P., & Harvey, M. R. (1991). *The rape victim: Clinical and community interventions.* Newbury Park, Calif.: Sage Library of Social Research, Sage Publications.

Mitchell, J., Morse, J. (1998). *From victims to survivors.* Washington, DC: Taylor and Francis Group, pp. 25–66.

National Safety Council. (1995, February). *Safety and health.* "Smoke detectors give you a chance." Itasca, IL: Author.

National Safety Council. (1997). *Accident facts, 1997 edition.* Itasca, IL: Author.

National Safety Council. (1997, October 20). *Fact sheet on driving defensively.* Itasca, IL: Author.

National Safety Council. (1997, October 20). *Fact sheet on car phones risk.* Itasca, IL: Author.

National Safety Council. (1998, April 21). *Air bag and seatbelt safety campaign.* Itasca, IL: Author.

Peterson, L., & Gable, S. (1998). Holistic injury prevention. In J. R. Lutzker (Ed.), *Handbook of child abuse: Research and treatment.* New York: Plenum, pp. 291–318.

Quinn, M. J., & Tomita, S. K. (1997). *Elder abuse and neglect.* New York: Springer Publishing, pp. 86–126.

Rapaport, K., Posey, C. D. (1991). Sexually coercive college males. In A. Parrot, ed., *Acquaintance rape: The hidden crime.* New York: John Wiley.

Swenson, C. C., & Hanson, R. F. (1998). Sexual abuse of children. In J. R. Lutzker (Ed.), *Handbook of child abuse research and treatment.* New York: Plenum, pp. 475–500.

U.S. Department of Transportation, National Highway Traffic Safety Administration. (1997, August). *Protect your kids in the car.*

U.S. Department of Transportation, National Highway Traffic Safety Administration. (1998a). *1997 traffic crashes, injuries, and fatalities—Preliminary report, 1998.*

U.S. Department of Transportation, National Highway Traffic Safety Administration. (1998b). *Traffic safety facts—1997.*

Warsaw, R. (1988). *I never called it rape.* New York: Harper and Row.

Suggested Readings

Alexander, L. L., & LaRosa, J. H. (1994). *New dimensions in women's health.* Boston: Jones and Bartlett. The chapter on violence goes into detail about violence issues including rape, relationship abuse, elder abuse, child abuse, and sexual harassment.

Barss, P., Smith, G., Baker, S., & Mohan, D. (1998). *Injury prevention: An international perspective.* Cary, NC: Oxford University Press. Injuries are rapidly assuming epidemic proportions throughout the world. This book provides a worldwide overview of injury problems, including the epidemiology of injury, surveillance, and policy.

Byers, E. S., O'Sullivan, L. F. (1996). *Sexual coercion in dating relationships.* New York: Haworth. Provides a good overview of the growing problem of "date" rape and steps to take to avoid the problem.

Division of Unintentional Injury Prevention. (1999). Motor-vehicle safety: A 20th century public health achievement. *Morbidity and Mortality Weekly Report, 48*(18), 369–374. This report reviews the achievements of motor-vehicle safety during the 20th century, including the passage of the Highway Safety Act and the National Traffic and Motor Vehicle Authorization Act, and the establishment of the National Center for Injury Prevention and Control in 1992.

Elliott, D. S., Hamburg, B. A., & Williams, K. R. (Eds.). (1998). *Violence in American Schools.* Cambridge, MA: Cambridge University Press. This book is written by experts in a variety of disciplines discussing a new strategy for the problem of youth violence. They argue that the most effective interventions use a comprehensive, multidisciplinary approach and take into account stages of development.

Gellert, G. A. (1997). *Confronting violence: Answers to questions about the epidemic destroying America's homes and communities.* Boulder, CO: Westview Press. A thoughtful and comprehensive discussion of all aspects of violence in America. The best source for persons who want to know more about specific kinds of violence and what to do about them. The author was working two miles from the blast that killed 169 people in Oklahoma City on April 19, 1995.

Graham, J. D. (1993). Injuries from traffic crashes: Meeting the challenge. *Annual Review of Public Health, 14,* 515–543. Discusses ways to further reduce traffic fatalities.

Hunnicutt, D. (1996). Using environmental strategies to reduce drinking and driving among college students. *NASPA Journal, 33*(3), 179–91. An excellent review of environmental strategies to reduce drinking and driving among college students.

Injuries in the school environment: A resource guide. (1997). Children's Safety Network, 55 Chapel Street, Newton, MA 02158-1060 (free). The Children's Safety Network designed this packet of information to inform school personnel and other professionals about the extent of the problem of injury and to stimulate discussion.

Munson, L., & Riskin, K. (1995). *In their own words: A sexual abuse workbook for teenage girls.* Washington, DC: Child Welfare League. Two therapists have designed a workbook to help teenage girls work through the pain and emotional damage resulting from sexual abuse.

Shalala, D. E. (1993). Addressing the crisis of violence. *Health Affairs, 12*(4), 30–33. The Secretary of Health and Human Services presents her views on why violence is so prevalent in America and what can be done to reduce and prevent violence.

Turkington, C. (1994). *Poisons and antidotes.* New York: Facts on File. Describes more than 600 toxic substances, symptoms, and treatments for poisoning.

Wissow, L. (1995). Current Concepts: Child Abuse and Neglect. *New England Journal of Medicine, 332*(21): 1425. Defines the various kinds of child abuse and treatment strategies.

Exercises and Activities

WORKBOOK
Intelligent Health Consumer Profile

Health and Wellness Online

 www.jbpub.com/hwonline

Being a Wise Health Care Consumer
Understanding Health Care Financing
Health Care Issues Today

Chapter 14

Making Decisions about Health Care

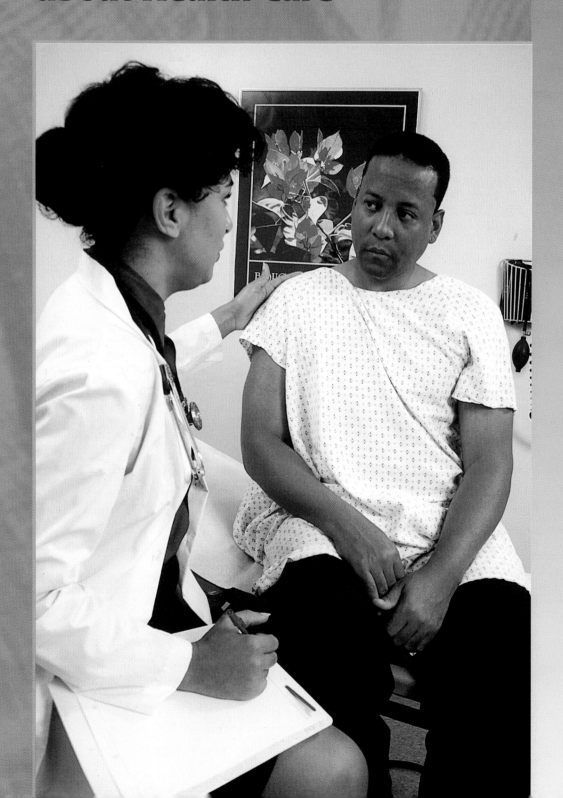

Everyone will need health care at some time. People need to go to health care professionals for vaccinations, physical exams, and diagnostic tests and for assistance when they are not feeling well. Occasionally people need to be hospitalized for serious illness, injury, or surgery. Health care and the cost of medical services are among people's most important concerns. Both state and federal governments have been trying to ensure that all citizens have some form of health insurance and can receive health care when needed, but many people in this country still do not have access to health care services or cannot afford health care.

Modern medicine has become highly technical and expensive. The consumer of health care services must be able to evaluate the risks and benefits of diagnostic tests, treatments, recommended drugs, or surgery if he or she is to maintain control of decisions that affect health. Understanding your rights as a patient and knowing how to communicate your concerns and needs to health professionals will help you stay healthy and help in the healing process when you become sick.

> At one time I had ambitions, but I had them removed by a doctor in Buffalo.
>
> TOM WAITS

Being a Wise Health Care Consumer

Making wise decisions about your health is part of self-care and self-responsibility. As health care consumers, we make important decisions about the health products we purchase, the health services we select, and the information we receive.

Behaviors that can help protect you from health fraud and unnecessary medical procedures include:

- Being well informed and knowing how to make healthy decisions
- Seeking reliable sources of information
- Being skeptical about health information appearing in news media or advertising
- Being wary of unlicensed practitioners and undocumented claims by health practitioners
- Selecting practitioners with great care and asking questions about fees, diagnoses, treatments, and alternative treatments
- Reporting health care fraud and wrongdoing to government regulating agencies

Good health care should be a partnership between you and the health care provider. The quality and cost of health care depend both on you and your doctor. Being a wise health care consumer starts with three basic principles: (1) working in partnership with your health care provider; (2) sharing in health care decision making; and (3) becoming skilled at obtaining health care.

Communication is extremely important in a physician-patient relationship. To work well with your health care provider you need to begin by exercising self-care and self-responsibility (*Consumer Reports*, 1995). As a partner in your own health care, you are responsible for managing minor health problems at home. At the first sign of a health problem, you should observe and record symptoms to share with your health care provider, so that you and your health care provider can better manage problems. When visiting your health care provider, be prepared; you only have a limited time with them. Prepare a checklist of questions you want to ask, as well as a list of your symptoms. During your visit state your concerns, describe the symptoms, and ask questions regarding prescribed drugs, the diagnosis, and treatment recommendations.

The second principle in being a wise health care consumer is shared decision making. In partnership with your health care provider you should actively participate in every medical decision. You have this right except in the emergency room, where informed consent is not necessary. There are numerous ways to share in health care decisions: (1) let your doctor know what you want; (2) do your own research; (3) ask why a test or treatment is recommended; (4) ask about alternatives; (5) consider watchful waiting; (6) state your health care preferences; and (7) accept responsibility.

Being skilled at obtaining health care is the third principle. By communicating and partnering with your health care provider, you can become skilled in purchasing health care services. There are many ways to cut the cost of health care without affecting the quality: (1) exercise self-care and self-responsibility; (2) seek health care from a primary health care provider; (3) reduce unnecessary medical tests; (4) reduce drug use; (5) use specialists only when necessary; (6) use emergency services only for real emergencies; and (7) use hospitals only when required.

Selecting a Health Care Practitioner

The self-care movement became strong in the United States in the 1970s when health care costs began increasing and Americans became more interested in wellness and healthier life-styles. However, self-care is not always appropriate and can be dangerous in some situations. Today's health care system is extremely complex, with numerous medical, dental, and allied health professionals addressing consumers' health care needs. Deciding which health care professional to choose can be confusing. All physicians practice orthodox medicine, sometimes referred to as conventional, Western, or modern medicine. This type of medicine is based on principles of modern science and validated clinical experiments. Practitioners of alternative medicine include chiropractors, homeopaths, and naturopaths, who rely on alternative methods of healing, which may, or may not, be based on science. People often use alternative medicines to complement the treatments they receive from their physicians.

Medical Doctors

Physicians must have at least 3 years of undergraduate work and 4 years of training at an accredited medical or osteopathic school. To be licensed to practice medicine, one must pass a national or state examination. Because the range of medical knowledge is so broad, many medical school graduates choose to become specialists, which requires 3 or more years of specialty training (Table 14.1). Medical specialty boards have high standards of performance and training. Successful specialty training applicants are board certified. Many states and specialty boards require physicians to participate in continuing education programs to maintain their license and specialty license, respectively.

The doctor of medicine (M.D.) and the doctor of osteopathy (D.O.) provide both primary and specialty care. Many states have a single licensing board for doctors of medicine and doctors of osteopathy; others have separate boards for each profession. The training of these two physician groups is similar, except that doctors of osteopathy place greater emphasis on musculoskeletal diagnosis and treatment. The American Medical Association (AMA) estimates that there are over 670,000 physicians practicing in the United States; about 34% of these belong to the AMA.

Dentists

Dentists are licensed in every state and hold either a doctor of dental surgery (D.D.S.) or a doctor of medical dentistry (D.M.D.) degree. Dental schools require at least 2 years of college; however, most entering dental students have a baccalaureate degree. Dental school takes 4 years with at least 2 or more years of training for a dental specialty (Table 14.2). The American Dental Association (ADA) estimates that over 196,000 dentists are practicing in the United States; approximately 71% belong to the ADA.

TABLE 14.1   Selected Medical Specialties

Specialty	Specific focus
Anesthesiology	Administration of drugs to prevent pain or to induce unconsciousness during surgical operations or diagnostic procedures
Cardiology	Diagnosis and treatment of diseases of the heart and blood vessels, including such problems as heart attacks, hypertension, and stroke
Dermatology	Diagnosis and treatment of skin diseases
Endocrinology	Deals with medical problems that result from abnormalities in the endocrine (hormone) system in the body
Family practice	General medical services for patients and their families
Geriatrics/gerontology	Concerned with problems of the elderly
Internal medicine	Diagnosis and nonsurgical treatment of internal organs of the body
Neurology	Diagnosis and nonsurgical treatment of diseases of the brain, spinal cord, and nerves
Obstetrics and gynecology	Care of pregnant women and treatment of disorders of the female reproductive system
Oncology	Diagnosis and treatment of all forms of cancer
Ophthalmology	Medical and surgical care of the eye, including prescription eyeglasses
Orthopedics	Diagnosis and treatment of abnormalities in bone and muscle, especially injuries resulting from sport activities
Pathology	Examination and diagnosis of organs, tissues, body fluids, and excrement
Pediatrics	Medical care of children, usually up to teenage years
Preventive medicine	Prevention of disease through immunization, good health care, and concern with environmental factors
Psychiatry	Treatment of mental and emotional problems
Public health	Subspecialty of preventive medicine that deals with promoting the general health of the community
Radiology	Use of radiation for the diagnosis and treatment of disease
Urology	Treatment of male reproductive system and urinary tract and treatment of female urinary tract

Podiatrists

Doctors of podiatric medicine (D.P.M.) are engaged in the diagnosis, prevention, and treatment of foot problems. Education includes at least 3 years of undergraduate work and 4 years of study at one of seven accredited colleges of podiatric medicine in the United States. The American Podiatric Medical Association (APMA) estimates that there are approximately 13,800 practicing podiatrists in the United States, treating corns, bunions, calluses, and malformations of the foot.

TABLE 14.2   Dental Specialties

Specialty	Specific focus
Endodontics	Prevention and treatment of diseases of the root pulp and related structures
Oral and maxillofacial surgery	Tooth extraction; surgical treatment of diseases, injuries, and defects of the mouth, jaw, and face
Oral pathology	Diagnosis of tumors, other diseases, and injuries of the head and neck
Orthodontics	Diagnosis and correction of tooth irregularities and facial deformities
Pediatric dentistry	Dental care of infants and children
Periodontics	Treatment of diseases of the gums and related structures
Prosthodontics	Treatment of oral dysfunction through the use of prosthetic devices, such as crowns, bridges, and dentures
Public health dentistry	Prevention and control of dental disease and promotion of community dental health

Seeing the Doctor

The majority of people who go to a doctor have minor complaints, have come for a routine follow-up of some chronic problem, or may simply need some kind of reassurance. In general, patients fall into three categories: (1) those who think they are sick and are; (2) those who think they are well but are actually sick; and (3) the "worried well" who come for reassurance that they are not sick. This last group may account for as many as half of all patients who are seen by family practice physicians.

Although some physicians encourage annual checkups, most studies show that frequent medical exams for people who are basically healthy are unnecessary. How often you see a physician depends on your personal needs, but many people go to a physician for minor complaints and illnesses that usually do not require medical attention. Often people are asking more from their doctors than just medicine.

Patient satisfaction with health care usually depends on what occurs in the physician's office. The quality of health care depends to a great degree on the interaction between the physician and the patient. Often, anxiety about what may be wrong, long waits to see the physician, and a seemingly endless number of tests can contribute to patients' stress. You can increase the chance of a successful encounter with your health care provider or hospital if you have a clear understanding of what you want to accomplish in the office visit or hospital stay.

The medical profession recognizes that medical education needs to be about more than biomedical facts. Learning to listen, asking questions, and expressing empathy also need to be part of medical education. A few medical schools have tried to help medical students understand what the patient is going through. Communication skills, like other skills, can

Wellness Guide

How to Have a Successful Interaction with Your Physician

- You should choose a physician you trust and in whose medical skills you have complete confidence. Take the time to find a primary care physician who can satisfy your medical needs. He or she should be someone with whom you can openly express your health concerns.

- Clear and open communication between you and your physician is essential. You should understand the nature of your medical problems and the reasons for any tests that are ordered. You should feel free to ask about different treatment options. You are entitled to all the information pertaining to your condition in language you can understand.

- You should feel confident enough to share with your physician any emotional problems you may have or any stress in your life. This information may be important in arriving at an accurate diagnosis and treatment recommendation. If you are upset in your interaction with a physician, the art of healing is not being practiced.

- Before going to a physician's office, try to relax your mind and body by practicing a meditation or image visualization exercise. This will help calm you when you are discussing your problems with the physician.

- Always remember how suggestible your mind is during a medical consultation. What the physician says about your condition can be as important in the healing process as the treatment. If the physician is positive and encouraging, the likelihood of a cure is increased.

- While negative statements made by the physician cannot be ignored, try not to let your mind be unduly influenced by them. For example, statements regarding complications, adverse effects, chance of permanent disability, and probable duration of the sickness are general comments derived from statistical data collected from thousands of patients. You are not a statistic but an individual and averages need not apply to you. Negative statements that are believed tend to produce negative effects on the body.

be learned. As wise health care consumers you need to select physicians who meet not only your health care needs but your communication needs as well.

Diagnosis is separate and distinct from any agreement you make about treatment. In any illness, there are two important choices: first, admitting that you are sick and finding out what is wrong, which is the process of the **diagnosis;** and second, deciding what is the best course of treatment, based on the diagnosis.

For example, suppose you have had a slight pain in your chest and the diagnostic tests indicate that you have partial blockage of a coronary artery. One physician might recommend dietary changes, exercises, and a drug to control the pain. Another physician might insist on immediate surgery to correct the condition. Only by obtaining as much information as possible can you make a decision that feels right to you.

Hospitals

At some time in your life you will need to use a health care facility, whether a hospital for planned surgery, an emergency room, or as you, your parents, or friends become older, nursing home facilities. To make wise decisions concerning health care facilities, it is important to understand the types of facilities available and whether they meet your needs.

Most Americans will be admitted to a hospital at some time during their lives. For many people the hospital experience is confusing and frightening. To cope with this unpleasant reality, one should understand a hospital patient's rights.

On admission to a hospital, a patient is required to sign a consent form delegating all decisions regarding his or her care to the hospital and physicians. In most instances, physicians obtain informed consent for any invasive procedure, either diagnostic or therapeutic, before proceeding. But the amount of information that is given to the patient and how well a patient understands the proposed treatment usually depend on many factors that affect communication between the patient and the physician. The American Hospital Association publishes a Patient's Bill of Rights covering the situations and questions most often encountered by hospital patients. You are entitled to ask for a list of patients' rights in that hospital.

The most frustrating and anxiety-producing situations for a patient are not understanding what is going to happen and, even worse, not knowing what is happening while being subjected to unfamiliar and uncomfortable procedures. Except in the case of a life-threatening emergency that demands immediate action, you have the right to be fully informed of all medical procedures and the reasons for them. As a pa-

tient, you have the responsibility for deciding what you want done. Once you have made that decision, you should understand how to cooperate fully to gain the most benefit.

Understanding Health Care Financing

In various ways, the United States has attempted to make health care available to Americans. Some employers have provided health care for their employees and dependents; the federal government has provided health care for members of the armed services and their dependents, war veterans, and government employees; and with assistance from local and state governments, the federal government has provided health care for poor families. Nevertheless, a program to ensure universal access and equity in health care services has never materialized. There are three basic types of health insurance plans available: private insurance, health maintenance organizations (HMOs), and preferred provider organizations (PPOs).

> *Some patients, though conscious that their condition is perilous, recover their health simply through their contentment with the goodness of the physician.*
>
> HIPPOCRATES

Private Insurance

Fee-for-service or private health insurance is the traditional type of health care plan in the United States. Fee-for-service plans generally have a deductible the insured person pays before receiving benefits. Most plans pay some physician and hospital expenses; most do not cover preventive health care, such as annual physicals or immunizations. In 1991, there were 670 million visits made to physicians' offices; 36% of these were paid for by private insurance (Green and Ottoson, 1994).

Health Maintenance Organizations

Health maintenance organizations (HMOs) are pre-paid health insurance plans that are an alternative to private insurance. The growth of HMOs has almost tripled

Terms

diagnosis: the cause of a disease or illness as determined by a physician

health maintenance organization (HMO): an organization (either nonprofit or for-profit) of physicians, hospitals, and support staff that provides medical services to members

during the last two decades. HMOs are characterized by four principles defined and described by Congress in the Health Maintenance Organization Assistance Act of 1973: (1) an organized system of health care that accepts the responsibility to provide health care; (2) an agreed-upon set of comprehensive health maintenance and treatment services; (3) a voluntarily enrolled group of people in a specific geographic region; and (4) reimbursement through a prenegotiated and fixed payment schedule on behalf of the enrollee. An example of a large, successful HMO is the Kaiser-Permanente Medical Care Program, in which physicians emphasize early detection and disease prevention.

HMOs and other organizations that deliver medical services of various kinds provide what is known as **managed care.** The simplest definition of managed care is a system that attempts to reduce the cost of health care. The burgeoning cost of health care in the U.S. results from many factors that include excessive use of expensive diagnostic tests, treatments on demand, unnecessary and multiple visits to specialists, high-tech procedures, long stays in hospitals, and unrestricted access to doctors.

In an attempt to control health care costs, President Clinton presented a comprehensive health care plan to Congress in 1993; however, the plan collapsed after intensive lobbying of Congress by medical associations and the insurance industry who argued that the quality of care and freedom of choice would be compromised under the plan. At present, about 50 million Americans are enrolled in HMOs, and this number is expected to increase to 100 million by the year 2000 (Spragins, 1996).

Despite their success, HMOs have also experienced severe criticism. In contracts between physicians and HMOs, physicians are prohibited from recommending certain expensive procedures that are not covered by the HMO and may receive bonuses for not recommending referrals or other services. Physicians are prohibited from disclosing the conditions of their contracts; this so-called "gag rule" has been severely criticized and has generated a backlash against some HMOs (Bodenheimer, 1996). Although managed health care is well established in the U.S., some health care analysts believe that eventually health care will have to evolve into some form of more equitable, universal coverage for all Americans (Ginzberg, 1997).

Choosing the best HMO for your needs is difficult, especially if choices are limited by your place of employment or financial resources. However, some

Wellness Guide

Health Care Insurance Terminology

Terminology to be familiar with when purchasing health insurance

Coinsurance	Arrangements by which the insurer and the insured share, in a specific ratio, payment for losses covered by the policy after the deductible is met
Comprehensive medical expense insurance	Form of health insurance that in one policy provides protection for both basic hospital expenses and major medical expense coverage
Coordination of benefits (COB)	Method of integrating benefits payable under more than one health insurance plan so that the insured's benefits from all sources do not exceed 100% of allowable medical expenses or eliminate appropriate patient incentives to contain costs
Deductible	Amount of covered expenses that must be incurred by the insured before benefits become payable by the insurer
Health insurance	Coverage providing for payment of benefits as a result of sickness or injury; includes insurance for losses from accident, disability, medical expense, or accidental death and dismemberment
Managed care	Those systems that integrate the financing and delivery of appropriate health care services to covered individuals by means of • Arrangements with selected providers to furnish a comprehensive set of health care services to members • Explicit criteria for the selection of health care providers • Formal programs for ongoing quality assurance and utilization review • Significant financial incentives for members to use providers and procedures associated with the plan
Maximum benefit	Highest amount an individual may receive under an insurance contract
Reasonable and customary charges (R&C)	Amounts charged by health care providers that are consistent with charges from similar providers for identical or similar services in a given locale
Utilization	Patterns of usage for a single medical service or type of service (hospital care, prescription drugs, physician visits). Measurement of utilization of all medical services in combination usually is done in terms of dollar expenditures. Use is expressed in rates per unit of population at risk for a given period, such as the number of annual admissions to a hospital per 1000 persons over age 65.
Utilization review	Program designed to reduce unnecessary hospital admissions and to control the length of stay for inpatients through the use of preliminary evaluations, concurrent inpatient evaluations, or discharge planning.

guidelines may help. Some independent organizations attempt to rate the quality of HMOs (*Consumer Reports*, 1996). Check carefully what each HMO offers, especially for emergency care or for chronic conditions. If you are enrolled in an HMO, look until you find a physician that you trust and with whom you can communicate freely. If you are not satisfied with a diagnosis or treatment, consult another doctor or ask for a second opinion.

Preferred Provider Organizations

Preferred provider organizations (PPOs) are a combination of the traditional fee-for-service health care plan and an HMO. Employers or insurance companies negotiate low fee-for-service rates with selected hospitals and health care providers in a specific geographic region. Participants in PPOs must use one of the "preferred" providers for the majority of their medical bills to be paid. If a participant opts for care from a nonprovider, he or she will be charged a substantial fee. Group health insurance costs are reduced for both an HMO and PPO in exchange for a guaranteed pool of patients.

Federal Government Support: Medicare and Medicaid

It was not until the mid-1960s that the federal government played a substantial role in providing health care coverage. Resulting from a concern for the social conditions of the economically disadvantaged and the elderly, Congress passed legislation in 1965 establishing Medicare and Medicaid.

Medicare is a federal health insurance program for Americans over age 65, for certain disabled Americans under age 65, and for people of any age with permanent kidney failure. The basic purpose of Medicare is to provide health care for all eligible persons.

Medicaid provides health insurance for certain poor people in the United States. To be eligible for Medicaid benefits, an individual must be on welfare, have dependent children, or receive supplementary security income for the aged, blind, or disabled. In addition, Medicaid covers nursing home care for many elderly Americans.

 ## Health Care Issues Today

Rising Health Care Costs

Anyone who has been to a physician, filled a prescription, paid a health insurance premium, or been admitted to a hospital realizes how expensive medical care in the United States has become. From the early 1980s to 1994, the costs of medical care more than doubled, exceeding $1 trillion in 1994 (Figure 14.1). These increases have occurred in all areas—physician fees, prescription costs, hospital rooms, emergency services, and health insurance. No single factor explains why our health care costs are increasing.

In 1995, approximately 14% of the U.S. gross domestic product was spent on medical care, more than any other country spends. One reason may be our fascination with medicine, health, and wellness. Every day both print and visual media inform us of new medical technologies, medical science breakthroughs, and promising research in the cures for AIDS and cancer.

To appreciate how much money is spent in the U.S. on health care, consider these statistics from the World Bank (Holden, 1996). In 1990, the average per capita spending on health care in Latin American countries was $105. In really poor countries the average was $16, and in Vietnam, it was only $2. In contrast, U.S. average per capita spending was $2,763. This enormous disparity in government and private support for health care in rich countries in comparison to poor countries will probably increase even further in the future. Whether the U.S. government can continue to increase the amount of money spent on

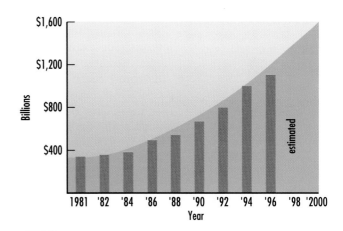

FIGURE 14.1   Skyrocketing Costs of Health Care in the United States
Between 1981 and 1994, spending on health care more than doubled and is now over $1 trillion a year.
Source: U.S. Department of Health and Human Services, 1997.

Terms

managed care: systems of health care in which the primary goal is to reduce costs

preferred provider organization (PPO): physicians who belong to the organization provide medical care at reduced costs that are negotiated by the organization

health care is dubious. This is yet another reason why citizens should do everything that they can to preserve their health and work toward preventing diseases such as cancer and atherosclerosis.

Two issues often surface in analyzing why health care costs are increasing so dramatically: malpractice and health insurance (Robert Wood Johnson Foundation, 1995). Malpractice insurance does cost more for physicians in the United States than for those in other countries, and it is not uncommon for an individual physician in a high-risk specialty (obstetrics, neurology, or anesthesiology) to pay premiums of over $100,000 per year. However, it was estimated that malpractice, including insurance premiums, cost only 3.5% of the projected $1 trillion spent on health care in 1994. Health insurance costs have increased, and Americans are paying more out-of-pocket for their health care than citizens of other countries. Americans pay over 20% of their health care costs, not including health insurance premiums. Another factor affecting health care costs is that more Americans are living longer. As the population ages, so does its risk for chronic and acute illnesses.

Life-style behaviors are another factor contributing to high health care costs. Many health conditions that strain our health care system are preventable. Cancer due to smoking, heart disease due to obesity, automobile accidents due to drinking and driving—all are caused by behaviors that we choose. They cost us billions of dollars each year. Other factors include inefficiency and fraud in health care services. Fraud occurs when an individual files false medical disability claims or dishonest health care providers submit false insurance forms for reimbursement.

Some believe the greatest factor in health care costs is the United States' overdeveloped medical capacity. The medical community has invested heavily in people, facilities, equipment, and drugs. For example, Orange County, California, has more magnetic resonance imaging (MRI) machines for its 2.4 million population than Canada has for 27 million people (Robert Wood Johnson Foundation, 1995). Medical technology in the United States often translates into short waiting times for care, whether urgent or elective, compared to other countries where one is placed on a waiting list for coronary artery surgery or for a computed tomographic (CT) scan.

Overtrained, overspecialized physicians may also be another source of increasing health care costs. It is estimated that the United States may now have an ex-

Where is the wisdom we have lost in knowledge? Where is the knowledge we have lost in information?

T. S. ELIOT
The Rock

cess of 130,000 specialty physicians, almost one-third of the total supply of physicians. This oversupply adds to the cost of health care.

The administrative overhead for health care is enormous. Overhead costs include insurance paperwork as well as internal and external paperwork for hospitals and physicians. Processing all this paperwork requires large numbers of workers. "Many experts estimate that these administrative costs account for at least 10% of the nation's total health bill." (Robert Wood Johnson Foundation, 1995, p. 13).

The health care system in the United States has reached a state of crisis in terms of costs and services. In surveys on consumer satisfaction with health care, a majority of Americans believe our health care system needs a major change. Everyone agrees that change must come, but so far it has been impossible to reach consensus on how to change the health care system and its financing.

Inequities in Health Care

Socioeconomic status plays a crucial role in health (Angell, 1993). Level of education, amount of income, and type of job all contribute to a person's health. A 1993 study showed that people earning less than $9,000 a year died at a rate three to seven times greater than those earning more than $25,000 a year. Black and Hispanic Americans generally have lower incomes than white Americans, experience more health problems, and are less likely to receive medical care. Poor people smoke more cigarettes, drink more alcohol, use more illegal drugs, and are exposed to violence more than people with high incomes and more education; these factors contribute to their increased health risks.

In the past 20 years, the health of economically and educationally disadvantaged Americans has declined steadily. A major challenge facing American society is reversing this trend and increasing the quality of health of its poorest citizens. More health education is necessary, along with universal health insurance that guarantees basic medical services for all.

Quality of Medical Care

Both health care professionals and the general public are worried that the effort to reduce health care costs will result in a lowering of the quality of medical care as well (Blumenthal, 1996). Although medical technology has improved medical care in many areas (notably in neonatal intensive care units and in the care of acute coronary artery disease), overall, many people perceive that the quality of their medical care has been declining.

In recent years, methods have been developed by which the quality of medical care can be measured reliably (Brook et al., 1996). Some of these methods are objective, such as reviewing the medical records of a patient to determine if the tests and treatments were appropriate and were adequate for the condition. But there are also tools for measuring the subjective components of medical care that affect the quality of life.

The term "quality of life" refers to the physical, mental, and social aspects of health that are interrelated with the quality of medical care. Measuring the quality of life of a person can be done with a variety of questionnaires, and the results can be quantified (Testa and Simonson, 1996). Many health professionals believe quality of life should be measured both before and after treatment.

For example, testing for and treating prostate cancer is extremely controversial. Most prostate cancers are very slow-growing and do not cause death. However, a diagnosis of prostate cancer can lead to surgery that severely erodes the patient's quality of life.

Prostate surgery often causes loss of sexual function, incontinence, depression, and other symptoms. For many people confronting serious disease, quality of life is more important that quantity of life, especially among the elderly.

While quality medical care can prevent and cure many forms of illness and prevent suffering, even the best and most costly medical care cannot protect us from health-destroying behaviors. The Centers for Disease Control and Prevention estimate that at least 50% of premature sickness could not be prevented by improved access to medical care (Foster, 1997). Half of the American population becomes sick because of behavioral factors: tobacco use, unsafe sex, poor nutrition, sedentary lifestyle, alcohol and drug abuse, and violent and risk-taking behaviors. We need to accept more responsibility for our behaviors and not expect health to be delivered to us by health care professionals.

Critical Thinking About Health

1. If you are old enough to have had a family physician who ran his or her own office and was not a member of any HMO or PPO, evaluate the health care that you had from them compared with the type of health care that you receive now. Describe what form of health insurance you have now and what form of insurance (if any) you had before.

2. Have you ever been hospitalized for an illness or injury? Describe the condition that caused you to be hospitalized, and discuss the care and tests that you experienced in the hospital. What things were the most positive and healing in the hospital? What things were the most distressing and unhealthy about your hospital experience? Suggest ways (based on your experience) that hospitals might improve the care they provide to patients.

3. The Medicare program, like the Social Security program, will face a fiscal crisis in the near future. The money that is collected by these two federal programs will not cover their costs unless they are restructured. Congress has proposed a new Medicare system for retired persons in which each worker would be required to put away a percentage of earnings during working years to pay for medical needs after retirement. This means that workers would now have to contribute a portion of wages to both Social Security and Medicare. Discuss whether you think this is the proper solution to solve Medicare's financial problems. Can you propose any other alternatives to provide the Medicare program with the money that is needed and that you think would be fair? Or do you think the federal government should not be involved in providing health care for retired persons at all?

4. Joe Windam is in the hospital with liver failure. Joe is only 32 years old but has been a heavy drinker most of his life, just like his father. He also contracted a hepatitis C infection several years ago that has contributed to his liver disease. Joe has been out of work for over a year and does not have any health insurance. The only hope that Joe has is a liver transplant; without a new liver, Joe will probably die in a few months. Do you think Joe should be given a high priority for a liver transplant because of his young age? Who should pay the several hundred thousand dollars in hospital and doctor bills? How should the priority for liver transplants be assigned, since there are not enough livers available for all the patients who need them?

Health in Review

- Everyone needs medical care at some time in his or her life. Knowing what to ask and what to expect from your physician is essential.
- The physician's responsibility is to find the cause of illness. The patient's responsibility is working in partnership with the health care provider, sharing in health care decision making, and becoming skilled at obtaining health care.
- Admission to a hospital is often an unsettling experience. Patients should be aware of their rights and ask questions that will ease their concerns.

- Health care is increasingly provided by large organizations of physicians and hospitals, called preferred provider organizations or health maintenance organizations.
- The costs of medical care in the United States have grown so rapidly that some form of health care reform is needed. Millions of citizens lack health insurance and access to health care.
- "Quality of life" refers to physical, mental, and social aspects of health that may be affected by medical care.

Health and Wellness Online

The World Wide Web contains a wealth of information about health and wellness. By accessing the Internet using Web browser software, such as Netscape Navigator or Microsoft's Internet Explorer, you can gain a new perspective on many topics presented in *Essentials of Health and Wellness, Second Edition.* Access the Jones and Bartlett Publishers web site at http://www.jbpub.com/hwonline.

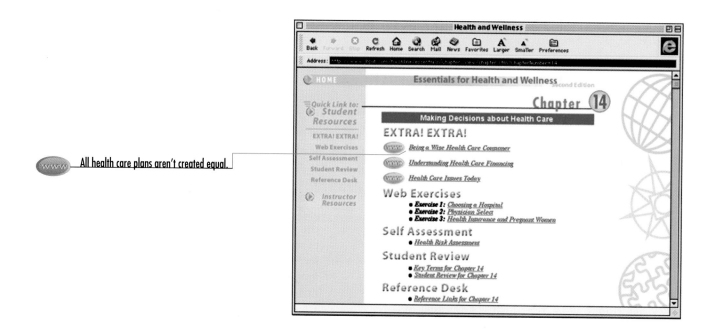

All health care plans aren't created equal.

References

Angell, M. (1993). Privileged and health—What is the connection? *New England Journal of Medicine, 529,* 126–127.

Blumenthal, D. (1996). The origins of the quality of care debate. *New England Journal of Medicine, 335,* 1146–1152.

Bodenheimer, T. (1996). The HMO backlash—Righteous or reactionary? *New England Journal of Medicine, 335,* 1601–1604.

Brook, R. H. et al. (1996). Measuring quality of care. *New England Journal of Medicine, 335,* 966–969.

Fein, R. (1992, November). Health care reform. *Scientific American.*

Foster, H. W. (1997). The enigma of low birth weight and race. *New England Journal of Medicine, 337,* 1232–1233.

Ginzberg, E., & Ostow, M. (1997). Managed care—A look back and a look ahead. *New England Journal of Medicine, 336,* 1018–1020.

Green, L. W., & Ottoson, J. M. (1994). *Community health,* 7th ed. St. Louis: Mosby-Year Book.

Holden, C. (1996). New populations of old add to poor nations' burdens. *Science, 273,* 46–48.

How good is your health plan? (1996). *Consumer Reports, 61,* 28–42.

How is your doctor treating you?" (1995, February). *Consumer Reports,* 81–88.

Robert Wood Johnson Foundation Annual Report, 1994: Cost Containment (1995). Princeton, NJ: Robert Wood Johnson Foundation.

Spragins, E. (1996, June 14). Does your HMO stack up? *Newsweek,* 56–63.

Testa, M. A., & Simonson, D. C. (1996). Assessment of quality of life outcomes. *New England Journal of Medicine, 334,* 835–840.

Suggested Readings

Cundiff, D., & McCarthy, M. E. (1994). *The right medicine.* Totowa, NJ: Humana Press. Discusses the major health care problems in America and how to cure them.

How good is your health plan? (1996, August). *Consumer Reports,* 18–42. Explains and evaluates the country's biggest managed care plans.

Merck manual of medical information—Home edition. (1997). New York: Merck Publishing Group. A very helpful guide to understanding diseases and drugs. This book is based on the book doctors use when they leave the examining room to figure out what is going on.

Miller, M. S. (Ed.). (1997). *Health care choices for today's consumer.* New York: Wiley. A proactive guide to all the the various healthcare options available to consumers.

Russell, L. B. (1994). *Educated guesses: Making policy about medical screening tests.* Berkeley: University of California Press. Documents clearly why many medical screening tests, particularly for cholesterol and some cancers, are unnecessary and a waste of money.

Vickery, D. M., & Fries, J. F. (1993). *Take care of yourself: The complete guide to medical self-care.* New York: Addison-Wesley. A comprehensive guide to physicians and how to obtain good medical care. Also discusses 120 common health problems.

West, S., & Dranov, P. (1995). *The hysterectomy hoax.* New York: Doubleday. Explains why up to 90% of hysterectomies are medically unnecessary and provides other options.

Learning Objectives

1. Describe some of the biological changes that occur with aging.
2. Define aging, maximum life span, average life span, life expectancy, ageism, and gerontology.
3. Discuss some of the health-related and social implications of the average increase in age of the U.S. population.
4. Briefly explain two theories of aging.
5. Explain how undernutrition affects the aging process.
6. Discuss Alzheimer's disease and senile dementia.
7. Describe several ways to prevent osteoporosis.
8. Identify the stages of dying as defined by Elizabeth Kubler-Ross.
9. Explain differences between euthanasia and physician-assisted suicide.
10. Compare palliative care with physician-assisted suicide.
11. Describe factors involved in healthy aging.

Exercises and Activities

WORKBOOK
A Simple Test for Loss of Cognitive Function

Health and Wellness Online

 www.jbpub.com/hwonline

Wellness Guide: Will Hormones Keep You Young?

Theories of Aging

Alzheimer's Disease and Senile Dementia

Wellness Guide: Extracts of Gingko Biloba Slow

Alzheimer's Dementia

Healthy Aging

Chapter 15

Understanding Aging and Dying

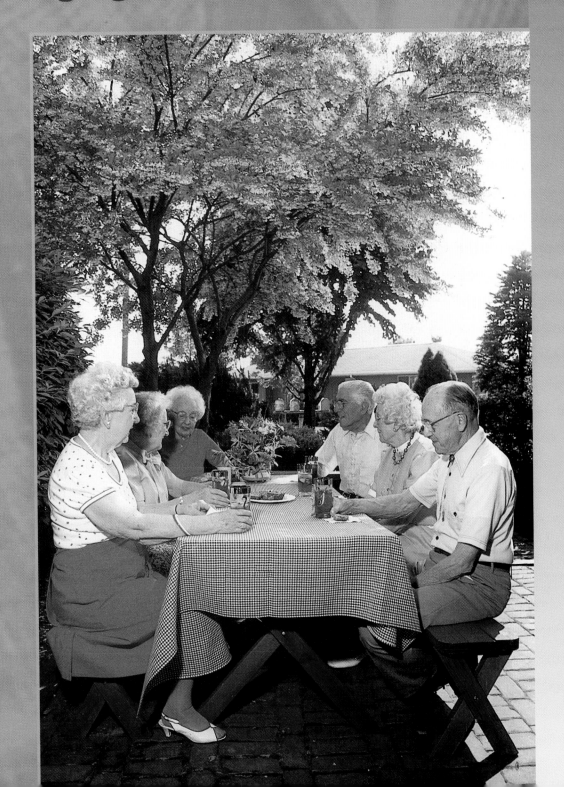

For centuries people have tried to slow down aging and postpone death. Almost everything has been tried, from magic spells to modern drugs. In the sixteenth century, the Spanish explorer Ponce de Leon sought the legendary "fountain of youth," which was supposed to restore the health and youth of anyone who drank its waters. Today, an over-the-counter hormone, DHEA, is being taken by millions of people who hope to rejuvenate their bodies and slow down the aging process. Some people even try to cheat death by having their bodies frozen immediately after dying in the hope that they can be revived and returned to life sometime in the far future, when science has learned to cure all diseases and prevent aging.

> *I don't want to achieve immortality through my work. I want to achieve immortality by not dying.*
> WOODY ALLEN

Many people associate aging with sickness, disability, loneliness, and increased inactivity. However, such negative views of aging are exaggerated; many older persons today are sexually and physically active and continue to work well into their 80s or even 90s. George Burns, comedian and movie star, performed on stage and in movies until he was nearly 100 years old.

In America, negative views about aging are still prominent in movies, television, and, especially, advertising. The ideal American is portrayed as eternally young, active, attractive, and wrinkle-free. Advertisements exhort people to retard the noticeable signs of aging by using face and body creams that restore youth, dyes for graying hair, and special herbs or vitamins that stop aging or by resorting to various kinds of cosmetic surgery.

The normal processes of aging are not caused by disease, so aging cannot be cured. The noticeable effects of aging result from wear and tear on essential functions in the body that change and become less efficient over the years—muscles weaken, immune system functions decrease, and sex drive is reduced. Even the healthiest body wears out slowly. However, by developing healthy habits while young and by understanding aging processes, one can remain vigorous and healthy until the very end of life.

Life expectancy for newborns in the U.S. is close to 80 years. To attain that, however, requires implementing the healthy lifestyles that we have been describing while you are still young.

America's Aging Population

Aging refers to the normal changes in body functions that occur after sexual maturity and continue until death. In an idealized situation, everyone would survive close to the **maximum life span** for the species; for human beings, maximum longevity is about 110 to 115 years (for mice, maximum longevity is only about 2 years). The **average life span** is defined as the age at which half of the members of a population have died.

Wellness Guide

Will Hormones Keep You Young?

Many women use estrogens (called hormone replacement therapy, or HRT) to alleviate the symptoms of menopause, to reduce the risks of osteoporosis and heart disease, and for other health benefits. Now many men are trying hormone therapy to counteract the effects of aging—reduced physical vigor, lowered levels of testosterone and sex drive, difficulty sleeping, and other symptoms that begin to appear after age 50.

An over-the-counter hormone, called dehydroepiandosterone (DHEA), is believed to be used by millions of men in this country to slow down the effects of aging and to increase physical and sexual vigor. DHEA is normally produced in the adrenal glands and is used in the body to manufacture other hormones, such as testosterone. After age 35, the production of DHEA declines and eventually falls to about 20% of the level measured in early adulthood (Eweksler, 1996).

The Food and Drug Administration, which regulates the sales of prescription drugs, does not regulate substances that are marketed as food supplements. Vitamins, herbs, amino acids, and hormones come under this category and, consequently, can be sold without federal regulation.

There is no question that DHEA raises testosterone levels, and many men are convinced that they feel and act younger in many ways after taking it. In fact, at a scientific research meeting on DHEA, about 25% of the investigators acknowledged that they were using it.

Hormones are substances that exert many effects on the body, some of which are not always healthy. Reported side effects of DHEA in men include acne and increased risk of prostate cancer; women who take DHEA may experience increased growth of facial hair and have an increased risk of breast cancer. At present, the official position of the National Institute on Aging and most physicians is that not enough is known about DHEA to justify recommending it as a safe and effective anti-aging medication.

www **www.jbpub.com/hwonline**

Insurance companies use data based on actual populations to determine what insurance premiums are necessary to pay survivor benefits. **Life expectancy** is the average length of time that members of a population can expect to live. The average life expectancy at birth in the U.S. has increased by almost 30 years since 1900 and now averages about 76 years.

Because of disease, accidents, and other factors, populations in the real world do not survive according to the idealized situation but have followed various curves throughout history (Figure 15.1). The average U.S. life span has increased dramatically in the last century. Because of this increase in the average life span, the U.S. population is becoming increasingly older.

Although genes certainly play a significant role in aging and the life span of human beings, studies show that genes account for much less than half of the differences in life span between different persons. If genes were the dominant factor in life span, identical twins should age and die at more or less the same age, but they do not. From identical and fraternal twin studies, genes are estimated to account for no more than 35% of individual differences in life spans (Finch and Tanzi, 1997).

The "graying" of America will create a broad range of social, medical, and economic problems. First and most important is the ability of the federal government to sustain Social Security payments. At the present rate, the government has estimated that the Social Security system will run out of money within 10 to 20 years. To avoid this, Congress has begun to

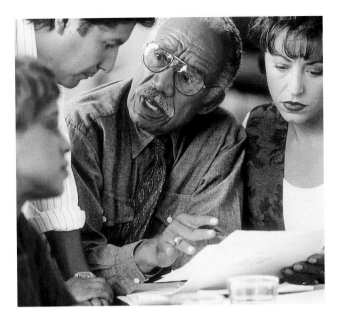

Many elderly people continue to enjoy work long after the "normal" retirement age.

discuss ways to reform Social Security so that future retirees will receive some benefits. Another problem is the extra medical care required by this group of older people. Although many older people are vigorous and healthy, a large number of people over age 65 have chronic illnesses and disabilities that require ongoing medical care and some need expensive, long-term care. The costs of health care for the elderly are going to rise in the years ahead. These rising costs will be a burden to the government and the general public, which is why there is an urgent need for health care reform (see chapter 14).

Age-related prejudice, called **ageism**, is systematic stereotyping and discrimination against people because of age (just as racism and sexism are discrimination based on race and gender). Ageism is based on the misconceptions that older people cannot work efficiently, are sickly, and are mentally less competent than younger people. Older people are asserting themselves more and demanding the same opportunities for work as younger people.

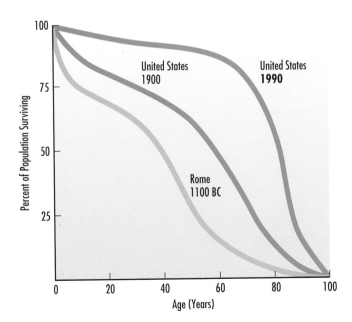

FIGURE 15.1   Approximate Survival Curves for Various Populations The U.S. population is beginning to approximate the idealized curve.

Terms

aging: normal changes in body functions that begin after sexual maturity and continue until death

maximum life span: the theoretical maximum number of years that individuals of a species can live

average life span: the age at which half the members of a population have died

life expectancy: average number of years a person can expect to live

ageism: prejudice against older people

How Long Can Human Beings Live?

Some experts in **gerontology** (the science that studies the causes and mechanisms of aging) believe that populations in many countries are approaching the current maximum average life span, estimated at 85 to 90 years, although a few exceptional individuals may live longer. One bit of evidence for a maximum average life span of 85 to 90 years comes from government estimates that show differences in the life expectancies of people in their countries (Table 15.1). Iceland tops the list with an average life expectancy of 80.5 years. At the bottom of the list are countries where life expectancy is still less than 50 years.

The average life expectancy at birth for Americans is now 75.8 years, but there are significant differences between the sexes and races. White men have a life expectancy of 73.4 years; black men, only 65.4 years. White women have a life expectancy of 79.6 years; black women, only 74.0 years. These differences probably result from socioeconomic factors, education, and access to health care.

Other evidence also suggests that the maximum average life span cannot be increased significantly above 85 to 90 years. Statistical studies can estimate how much average human life expectancy would increase if major diseases were eliminated. For example, if *all* cancers could be cured or prevented, only about 3 years of life would be added to the average baby born today. If *all* heart disease was eliminated, average life expectancy at birth would increase by about 14 years (Hayflick, 1994). Even with remarkable (and unexpected) breakthroughs in medical care, most people still would die in less than 100 years.

A slightly different picture of aging emerges from studies of people between the ages of 85 and 100—a group known as the "oldest old." Statistical studies of oldest old Scandinavians suggest that, in the absence of disease, senescent death (death from old age) could occur as late as 110 years (Barinaga, 1991). However, whether the maximum life expectancy for most people in the absence of disease is 85, 100, or 110 years, no human being is going to live to be as old as Methuselah, the biblical patriarch who is said to have lived for 967 years.

TABLE 15.1 Life Expectancy in Various Countries
Countries at the top of the list have populations that may be approaching the maximum average human life expectancy. Life expectancy in poor, undeveloped countries still is not much more than 50 years. Rank is based on sum of male and female life expectancy.

| Country | Life expectancy at birth | |
	Female	Male
Iceland	83	78
Japan	83	77
Australia	83	76
France	83	75
Italy	82	75
Spain	82	75
United Kingdom	79	74
United States	79	73
Mexico	78	70
China	71	68
Iran	69	66
Brazil	67	57
Bangladesh	56	56
Haiti	51	47
Guinea	48	43
Afghanistan	45	46

Source: *World Almanac*, 1997.

Theories of Aging

Biological Clocks Regulate Aging

Theories of aging fall into two broad categories. One ascribes aging to biological and genetic mechanisms that are specific for each species of animal and determine its maximum life span and rate of aging. The other theories focus on environmental factors that affect aging, such as nutrition, susceptibility to diseases, and exercise. Evidence for a "biological clock" that determines the maximum life span comes from measuring the amount of energy per gram of body weight consumed per day by mammals of different species. This energy consumption per day, called the **specific metabolic rate,** shows a striking correlation with the maximum life span of different species (Figure 15.2). Mammals that have the highest specific metabolic rate have the shortest life span; human beings have the slowest metabolic rate and the longest life span.

Further evidence for a biological clock that governs aging comes from studying the growth of cells in the laboratory. Conditions have been established in which cells from various tissues of different animals can be grown under fixed laboratory conditions. The surprising result of these experiments is that cells grow and divide in a laboratory medium for a fixed number of generations and then die (Hayflick, 1996). The number of generations of growth is related to the

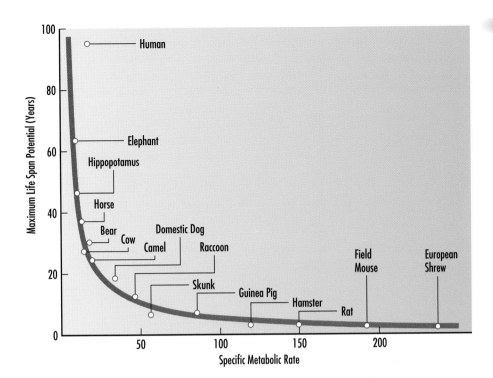

FIGURE 15.2   **Correlation between the Rate of Energy Consumed and Maximum Life Span Potential**   Rate of energy consumption is calculated as energy per gram of body weight per day. Life span of various mammalian species is shown. The correlation suggests that the maximum human life span is a function of human biology and ultimately of human genes.

maximum life span of the animal from which the cells were taken. Mouse cells only divide a few times, but human cells divide many times before dying. The inescapable conclusion from these experiments is that built into the cells of every animal is a genetically controlled clock that determines how many times cells can grow and divide before a signal tells them to stop.

A distinguishing feature of cancer cells is that they are immortal when grown under the same laboratory conditions used for growing normal cells. Cancer cells grow and divide indefinitely; cells taken from human tumors more than 30 years ago are still kept growing in the laboratory. Thus, cancer cells have lost the ability to regulate normal growth and aging.

Environmental Factors Affect Aging

Although genetic factors contribute to aging, environmental factors play an even greater role. The longer we live, the more we are exposed to radiation and chemicals that can damage DNA in cells and, over time, may cause the death of essential cells in the body. For example, most cells possess enzymes that repair damage to their DNA; loss of these cellular repair enzymes with age could lead to widespread cell death. This has been called the "error catastrophe" theory of aging. Accumulated mutations in cells may be responsible for development of cancer and also for aging changes.

It's sad to grow old, but it's nice to ripen.
BRIGITTE BARDOT

Shared activities are healthful at any age.

Terms

gerontology: science that studies the causes and mechanisms of aging

specific metabolic rate: the amount of energy per gram of body weight consumed per day

Another effect of exposure to radiation and chemicals is the production of very reactive molecules in cells, called free radicals (see chapter 10). These substances are normally inactivated in cells, but as we age our cells may be less able to cope with the damaging effects of free radicals. Free radicals also increase the damage to mitochondria, the complex structures in all cells that provide the energy for cellular growth and function. Without enough energy, cells become sick and possibly die; if too many cells die, organs cease functioning and the person dies. In addition, the immune system's functions become less efficient with age so that we become more susceptible to infections and autoimmune diseases. Overall, aging is a complicated process more than likely brought on by a combination of genetic and environmental factors.

Does Undernutrition Slow Aging?

A recurrent idea about aging is that it can be slowed by staying as lean as possible. This notion is not true and may lead to malnutrition. However, there is a large body of evidence from experimental laboratory animals that **undernutrition** does allow them to live longer.

For example, a laboratory rat usually has a maximum life span of about 40 months; rats whose caloric intake is restricted have a maximum life span of about 57 months (Figure 15.3). Moreover, the older rats in the calorie-restricted group are healthier and look younger than old rats in the control group who have been well-fed (Weindruch, 1996).

Undernutrition does not mean malnutrition; the laboratory animals that live longer are not starved or deprived of any essential nutrients. Only the total amount of food that they are allowed to eat each day is

restricted. Calorie restriction studies similar to those performed with rats are now underway with monkeys. Although these studies have been underway for about 10 years, it is still too early to draw any conclusions on changes in the processes of aging or on extension of the normal life span of monkeys in captivity.

One problem with caloric restriction is knowing when to begin restricting the amount of food. Young animals (including young children) require abundant nutrition for physical growth and for brain development. In the rat studies, it was shown that caloric restriction is of no value in prolonging life if it is begun too late in the animal's life. At present not enough is known about undernutrition and life span to make any recommendations to people, except that everyone should consume a varied and healthy diet and not become overweight.

Alzheimer's Disease and Senile Dementia

In the absence of disease, normal mental functions can be maintained to age 100 or longer. However, approximately 20% of people over age 85 have loss of normal cognitive functions that is readily determined by a few simple questions. The medical term for impairment or loss of mental functions in elderly persons is **senile dementia.** Many diseases and conditions can result in senile dementia, but the most common cause is **Alzheimer's disease,** which is characterized by memory loss, reduced ability to use language, losses in perception and problem-solving abilities, and reduced mobility.

More than 4 million Americans suffer from Alzheimer's disease now, and the number will rise dramatically in the next century as the population continues to age (Gambert, 1997). The prevalence of Alzheimer's disease increases linearly with advancing age; more than half of the population at age 90 have symptoms of Alzheimer's disease. Even if Alzheimer's disease cannot be cured, any treatment that delays or prevents symptoms from progressing is of great benefit to society in terms of the number of Alzheimer's patients who need care (Figure 15.4).

The disease is named for Alois Alzheimer, a German physician who, in 1907, described the abnormal brain structures he observed under the microscope in tissues obtained from patients who died from senile dementia. Alzheimer's findings at autopsy revealed what are still the diagnostic criteria for the disease: (a) the presence of bundles of tangled nerve fibrils in certain areas of the brain; and (b) the presence of a specific protein called **amyloid protein,** which is localized in certain areas and blood vessels of the brain (Figure 15.5). How these changes affect the brain to produce loss of cognitive functions is still not understood.

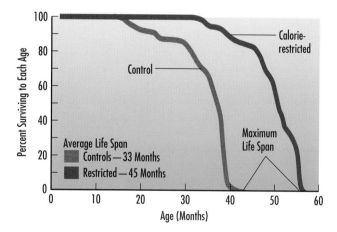

FIGURE 15.3   Survival of Rats Fed Either an Unrestricted Diet or a Calorie-Restricted Diet.   The rats whose diets are restricted in amount live, on average, 45 months compared with 33 months for rats that are allowed to eat as much as they want. The maximum life span of the calorie-restricted rats also is markedly increased.

Source: "Caloric Restriction and Aging," Richard Weindruch. Copyright © 1996 by Scientific American, Inc. All rights reserved.

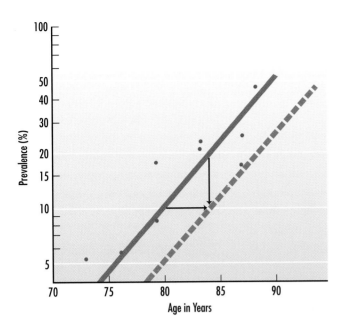

FIGURE 15.4   Benefits of Slowing Onset of Alzheimer's Disease   Approximately 5% of the U.S. population will have Alzheimer's disease by age 75; this increases to 10% by age 80 and to almost 50% by age 90, which shows a linear increase in the disease with increasing age. If the onset of symptoms could be delayed by only 5 years, the prevalence of the disease would be only half as great, about 10% of the population affected at age 85 instead of 20%, which is the current estimate. This marked reduction in the number of persons with symptoms of dementia would be of enormous benefit to society and save a substantial amount of health dollars.

Source: Courtesy Robert Katzman, University of California, San Diego.

No definitive cause for Alzheimer's disease is known, although it seems to develop as a result of both genetic and environmental factors. In some families, Alzheimer's disease occurs over several generations and family members often die at an early age. In these families, inherited genes must contribute to disease susceptibility. However, Alzheimer's disease also occurs in individuals whose families have never had a previous case. Most cases of Alzheimer's disease fall into this category and result from unknown environmental factors.

Researchers have discovered at least four genes that increase a person's susceptibility to Alzheimer's disease (Lendon et al., 1997). Three of these genes *(APP, PS1,* and *PS2)* occur in rare families (only a hundred or so, worldwide), in which many members suffer from Alzheimer's disease, some as young as age 40.

Terms

undernutrition: restricting the daily caloric intake of an animal or person without causing malnutrition

senile dementia: loss of cognitive functions in elderly people

Alzheimer's disease: a common cause of senile dementia and other symptoms, eventually leading to death

amyloid protein: an abnormal protein in the brain of patients with Alzheimer's disease

The presence of one of these genes makes it virtually certain that the carrier will have Alzheimer's disease eventually. The other susceptibility gene (APOE∊4) is associated with increased risk of developing Alzheimer's disease but does not cause it (Roses, 1997). Many people carry this particular gene, which creates a psychological problem for them with respect to genetic testing for their possible increased risk.

The presence of the APOE∊4 gene can be determined by genetic tests, but people need to carefully weigh the benefits and disadvantages of finding out about their Alzheimer's risk status. Although the presence of this gene increases the risk of developing Alzheimer's disease late in life, many people with this gene still will not ever have the disease. Is it useful for people to find out while young that they are at increased risk for Alzheimer's disease many years down the road, even when they may never contract the disease? Genetic testing for susceptibility to Alzheimer's disease raises the same ethical questions as does genetic testing for cancer risks (see chapter 10).

Scientists are on the hunt for other Alzheimer's susceptibility genes. If and when such genes are found and genetic tests become available, people may be able to determine with virtual certainty whether or not they are destined to have Alzheimer's disease. With no cure in sight, knowing that one is doomed to lose mental function eventually may be more than many people can handle, even with counseling.

Despite the current research emphasis on finding defective genes that are linked to Alzheimer's disease, environmental factors are very important. Many epidemiological studies show that people with more education (college graduates) are much less likely to develop Alzheimer's disease than are people with little or no education (Mortimer and Graves, 1993). A study of Catholic nuns who died between ages 76 and 100

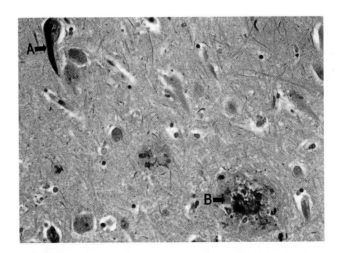

FIGURE 15.5   Photograph of Brain Tissue from a Deceased Alzheimer's Patient   (A) A characteristic tangle of nerves. (B) A characteristic plaque that confirms the diagnosis of Alzheimer's disease.

Wellness Guide

Extracts of Ginkgo Biloba Slow Alzheimer's Dementia

As the population grows increasingly older, the number of persons with dementia, especially of the Alzheimer's type, is increasing rapidly. Although an intensive effort is under way to find drugs that will prevent or slow the symptoms of Alzheimer's disease, no available drugs are very effective. But careful, placebo-controlled, double-blind studies in both the U.S. and Europe indicate that an extract of the herb *Ginkgo biloba* (Egb 761) is effective in

stabilizing and, in some cases, reversing the symptoms of dementia (LeBars et al., 1997).

Ginkgo biloba is one of the most popular herbs used in Europe to alleviate cognitive disorders of various kinds. Recently it has been approved in Germany for the treatment of dementia. Although the mechanism of action of ginkgo biloba extract is not well understood, it does act as an antioxidant and can scavenge free radicals that destroy cells. The

Egb 761 extract of the herb contains many compounds that probably act synergistically to protect cell membranes and neurotransmitter functions. This is an excellent example of an herb being much better than a single drug. The extract is made by a standardized procedure developed in Germany that uses dried *Gingko biloba* leaves.

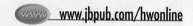 **www.jbpub.com/hwonline**

has confirmed the importance of education. All of these Catholic nuns were college-educated and had a much lower prevalence of Alzheimer's disease than the general population. And among the few who did develop the disease, it could be shown by studying their brains after death that stroke was a primary trigger of the clinical symptoms of Alzheimer's disease (Snowden et al., 1997).

It is not simply the level of education that helps to prevent the development of Alzheimer's disease. The key is to use the brain throughout life. Keep learning new things, explore new ventures—even doing crossword puzzles may help. It is now clear that brain cells continue to grow and establish new connections throughout life and that brain growth and health is dependent on mental stimulation. Just as exercise is necessary to maintain the body's fitness at all ages, exercising the brain is necessary to maintain mental functions.

If you were thinking of dropping out of school, remember how education is helping to protect your brain's health. Take more challenging courses. Take night classes if you have a job all day. And remember that watching TV is *not* a useful form of physical or mental exercise!

Osteoporosis

The bone density that we build up during our growing years is important in later life to prevent life-threatening fractures. **Osteoporosis** is a condition in older persons, particularly women, that results from loss of bone material, causing bones to become thin, porous, and brittle. The brittleness of bones make them extremely vulnerable to fractures with even a minimal amount of stress. Fracture of the hip is the most frequent result of osteoporosis and can lead to death.

Osteoporosis affects 25 million women in the United States and is responsible for 250,000 hip frac-

tures each year (Barzel 1996). Medical costs of caring for people with bone fractures from osteoporosis are $10 billion each year and will rise sharply as the American population ages.

Osteoporosis occurs because the rate of bone breakdown exceeds the rate of bone renewal; many factors contribute to this. In older women, estrogen loss following menopause contributes to loss of bone material. In both older men and women, aging results in bone loss and increases the risk of fracture, depending on how much bone mass is reduced (Figure 15.6). Generally, the bone loss in women caused by low estrogen levels is significantly greater than the bone loss caused by normal aging processes.

The risk of osteoporosis in older women can be lessened by replacing the lost estrogen with **hormone replacement therapy (HRT).** For most women HRT is beneficial because it reduces the risk of osteoporosis (and heart disease, to some degree) but for other women HRT may increase the risk of breast and uterine cancer.

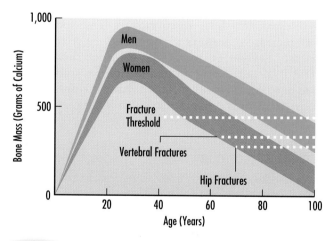

FIGURE 15.6   Changes in Bone Mass in Aging Men and Women   The risk of bone fracture from osteoporosis occurs when bone mass falls below a theoretical threshold and even a slight strain can cause a fracture.

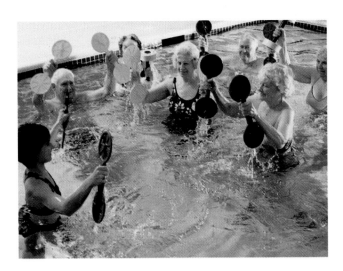

Regular exercise is important for reducing the risk of osteoporosis.

Another benefit of HRT is that women who take estrogen for even a limited time during menopause have about half the risk of developing Alzheimer's disease compared with women who do not take the hormone. Thus, the use of HRT must be carefully weighed by each postmenopausal woman. Women whose families have a history of breast cancer or blood clotting problems are not good risks for estrogen supplementation.

The best way to avoid osteoporosis is to build up as much bone mass as possible while young through calcium consumption and exercise. After maturity, calcium and vitamin D are still needed to maintain bone density (Dawson-Hughes et al., 1997). Nearly half of all Americans do not consume enough calcium to maintain bone mass. Consuming at least a gram of calcium a day throughout life can reduce the risk of osteoporosis and bone fractures later in life. In addition, adequate vitamin D in the diet is essential in the assimilation of calcium. The best sources of calcium are dairy products and green vegetables. Calcium also can be obtained in supplements such as calcium lactate or calcium citrate.

Exercise, especially weightlifting, running, hiking, and walking briskly, reduces the risk of osteoporosis because bone is renewed with exercise. A sedentary lifestyle contributes to the risk of osteoporosis. Regular exercise throughout life will help keep bones strong and prevent fractures later. Not smoking and not consuming alcohol excessively also help prevent osteoporosis.

Some people are genetically more susceptible to osteoporosis than others because they inherited a gene that produces a variant of the vitamin D receptor protein. Regardless of one's vitamin D receptor gene, adequate calcium in the diet and regular exercise are the keys to preventing osteoporosis.

Fear of Aging and Dying

Nobody wants to grow old or die. When we are young, we never think about becoming old nor can we imagine what it is like not to be strong, vigorous, and ac-

Terms

osteoporosis: a condition in older people, particularly women, in which bones lose density and become porous and brittle

hormone replacement therapy (HRT): administration of estrogen to menopausal and postmenopausal women to help prevent symptoms of menopause, osteoporosis, and heart disease

Global Wellness

Can Beliefs Influence Life Span?

Just how powerful are thoughts and feelings in influencing health? Can beliefs affect the duration of a person's life? A recent survey of the causes and ages of death among Chinese-Americans shows that strongly held beliefs can affect the cause of death and how long a person lives (Phillips et al., 1993).

In Chinese astrology, a particular phase — metal, water, wood, fire, or earth — is associated with the year of a person's birth. Also associated with each phase is susceptibility to particular diseases (see table). According to Chinese astrology and medicine, being born in a particular year makes a person more likely than usual to succumb to diseases associated with the phase of their birth year. An analysis of almost 30,000 death certificates of Chinese-Americans showed that people with the predicted combination of birth year and disease susceptibility died 2 to 5 years before white Americans with the same diseases and phases.

The more traditional the Chinese life-style of the person, the shorter their life was once they contracted the disease associated with their birth year. The most plausible explanation of the findings is that Chinese-Americans who believe in the predictions of Chinese astrology are the most likely

Birth year ends in	Phase	Susceptibility to
0 or 1	Metal	Pulmonary diseases
2 or 3	Water	Kidney disease
4 or 5	Wood	Cirrhosis of liver
6 or 7	Fire	Heart attack
8 or 9	Earth	Cancer, diabetes, ulcers

to succumb to the disease that they expect will kill them. It appears that beliefs not only affect health through the onset of disease but also affect life span.

tive. With few exceptions, the media portray aging as a time of life beset with sickness, inactivity, and slow deterioration of physical and mental functions. These negative views of aging are used to sell products and do not truthfully portray the experiences of most older Americans.

Fear of aging and death may lead to anxiety and stress that may hasten aging processes. A few of the many fears that people associate with aging are illness, poverty, being attacked or victimized, falling and being injured while alone, loss of responsibility for one's life, memory loss, and sexual inadequacy. Most of these fears are unfounded, but they may turn out to be self-fulfilling prophesies. However, chronological age often does not correlate with biological age. Some people feel and act young even in old age.

Death with Dignity

Death can strike without warning in the form of an accident or an unexpected heart attack. However, for most people, thoughts of death do not occupy their daily lives until old age. People in their 20s are too busy living to think about dying. But people in their 70s and 80s realize the inevitability of death and may modify their lives and affairs accordingly. Younger people who acquire a life-threatening disease such as cancer also are forced to face the reality of death.

Most people would prefer to die peacefully in their sleep after living a full, satisfying life. Some may be fortunate to die like this, but others may have to endure considerable pain and suffering for years. In addition to wondering how they are going to die, people usually wonder what will happen to them after death. Christianity provides a heaven where one's "soul" can exist in the grace of God for all eternity. Buddhism embraces a belief in reincarnation; after a series of deaths and rebirths a person can attain "Buddhahood," a perpetual state of enlightenment.

Of all human fears none is greater than the fear of death. When we are young, thoughts of death and dying are rare. Instead we are occupied with living, learning, and daily activities. We can't imagine that someday we will die. As we grow older and see parents, relatives, and friends die, we become more aware of our own mortality. We may begin to ponder our own death.

Terms

euthanasia: helping someone who is on the verge of death or in a coma to die without suffering

physician-assisted suicide: a form of active euthanasia in which a physician helps a patient who no longer desires to live because of pain or an incurable illness to commit suicide

In our society, death is not discussed openly, although this is beginning to change. (In 1997, public radio ran a series of programs on death and dying that included interviews with people who had been diagnosed with a terminal illness and were facing death within weeks or months.) Dying people are often isolated in hospitals and their care is left to physicians who may perform unwanted or unnecessary treatments. Sterile, impersonal death in a hospital or nursing home has increased many people's fears of death and the process of dying.

Fear is a crippling emotion; it paralyzes thoughts and actions and stifles spiritual growth. Here are some suggestions to help you overcome fears associated with death.

- Become a volunteer with the American Cancer Society or American Hospice Centers. Spend time with cancer or AIDS patients who are dying and who may be willing to share their thoughts with you.

- Write down your feelings about death and dying. Record any experiences you have had at funerals or with someone who was dying. Write down how you felt and how you coped with your feelings and fears.

- A powerful technique for dealing with fear is humor. Humor associated with death and dying is called "black humor" because it deals with the dark side of thoughts and feelings. Black humor was used to cope with issues of death in the long-running TV show M*A*S*H. Many movies also portray death in a humorous way in order to make audiences comfortable. Many cartoons by Gary Larson (*The Far Side*) and John Callahan (who has quadriplegia) portray death and dying in humorous ways. Confront your fears by drawing cartoons or writing a humorous story about dying.

Stages of Dying

People have different attitudes toward death and dying. In conversations with many persons who were facing death, Elisabeth Kubler-Ross (1975) identified five distinct stages in the process of dying. Not all persons experienced all stages, but most experienced some of them. These stages of dying are: 1) denial and isolation, 2) anger, 3) bargaining, 4) depression, and 5) acceptance.

The work of Kubler-Ross has found widespread acceptance, especially among counselors and those who help dying patients, but it has also received much criticism (Fulton and Metress, 1995). The leading criticism is the fact that the studies were not conducted scientifically but were based on personal observation and interpretation. Another criticism is that because the stages of dying that Kubler-Ross proposed have been widely accepted and publicized, some dying patients may feel obliged to follow the stages she described.

More and more it is recognized that dying, like living, is an individual, personal matter. People can do as poet Dylan Thomas recommended and "Rage, rage against the dying of the light." Or they can quickly come to a place of inner peace and accept the idea that the soul will soon be free of its body.

Euthanasia

Almost everyone would like to live a full, active, satisfying life right up to the moment of death. But some people will experience illnesses that bring on a prolonged period of disability, suffering, and pain that cannot be relieved by medical care. Modern medical technology often has the means to prolong life beyond the point where the dying person wishes to live. Given the choice, some terminally ill patients would elect **euthanasia,** which is defined as the act of helping a person experience a peaceful, painless death. In recent years **physician-assisted suicide** has become an alternative to active euthanasia.

In physician-assisted suicide, a terminally ill patient who is mentally competent must express a desire to die on a number of occasions. Then a second physician would be consulted. Finally, if both physicians agree that the patient is mentally competent and has an incurable, painful disease, one physician would supply the patient with the drugs needed to commit suicide or otherwise help the patient end his or her life.

Thousands of people in the United States are kept alive in hospitals in a permanent vegetative state. They are fed artificially and maintained by machines and medical technology. There is no hope of recovery for these persons and most would die if they were un-hooked from the machines that keep them

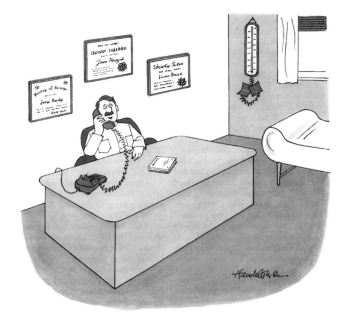

"Before we try assisted suicide, Mrs. Rose, let's give the aspirin a chance."

J. B. Handelsman © 1997 from The New Yorker collection. All rights reserved.

alive. There is intense legal and ethical controversy about proper choices regarding these individuals and about those who want the option of physician-assisted suicide.

Physicians are trained to prolong human life as long as possible and it is illegal in most instances to help a person die or to remove life support systems even from a person in a vegetative state. However, support for physician-assisted suicide has been growing; in public surveys, a majority of Americans now favor some form of physician-assisted suicide (Orentlicher, 1996). Surveys of physicians also show that a majority

Global Wellness

Physician-Assisted Suicide Is Practiced in the Netherlands

Even though active euthanasia is technically illegal in the Netherlands, it is estimated that physicians assist in over 3,000 deaths of terminally ill persons each year. Many advocates of active euthanasia believe that most countries, including the United States, will adopt some form of physician-assisted suicide in the near future.

In the Netherlands, the practice of euthanasia must conform to the following rules.

- The patient must repeatedly and explicitly express the desire to die.

- The patient's decision must be well informed, free, and enduring.

- The patient must be suffering from severe physical or mental pain with no prospect of relief.

- All other options for care must have been exhausted or refused by the patient.

- Euthanasia must be carried out by a qualified physician.

- The physician must consult at least one other physician.

- The physician must inform the local coroner that euthanasia has occurred.

of them favor being able to help terminally ill patients voluntarily end their lives.

Public referendums on physician-assisted suicide were passed in Oregon and narrowly defeated in California and Washington State in recent years. In response to the controversy over physician-assisted suicide, New York State and Washington State passed laws banning any form of physician-assisted suicide. Two Federal Appeals courts struck down the laws as being unconstitutional; however, on June 26, 1997, the U. S. Supreme Court reversed the lower courts' decisions and upheld the right of New York State and Washington State to ban physician-assisted suicide. However, pressure is mounting to permit physicians to help terminally ill patients die. In 1997, the executive editor of the *New England Journal of Medicine*, one of the country's most prestigious medical journals, argued in favor of physician-assisted suicide (Angell, 1997).

Physician-assisted suicide has been practiced in the Netherlands for more than 20 years, although it is officially illegal. However, the practice has strong public support, and the government has monitored the extent of physician-assisted suicide with several large studies in the 1990s. About 2% of all deaths in the Netherlands in 1990 were the result of active euthanasia or physician-assisted suicide. Studies of deaths in the Netherlands over the years do not show any significant increase in the use of physician-assisted suicide. Because aging populations will increase dramatically in most countries in the next century, it is likely that eventually most of them, including the United States, will adopt some form of physician-assisted suicide in response to public pressure and the need for compassion.

Palliative Care

Palliative care is a newly recognized branch of medicine that focuses on noncurative treatments for the dying (Goodlin, 1997). The World Health Organization (WHO) defines palliative care as follows:

- Affirms life and regards dying as a normal process
- Neither hastens nor postpones death
- Provides relief from pain and other distressing symptoms
- Integrates the psychological and spiritual aspects of patient care
- Offers a support system to help patients live as actively as possible until death
- Offers a support system to help families cope with the patient's illness and death

When a person elects palliative care, the emphasis of treatment shifts from prolonging life to enhancing the quality of life that remains, preserving a person's dignity, and relieving suffering. Usually a team of health professionals, in consultation with the patient and family, will decide if palliative care is appropriate.

Many opponents of physician-assisted suicide embrace the concept of palliative care and believe that it is more in accord with the ethics of medical practice. Now that palliative care is seen as a reimbursable form of therapy by many health insurance programs, eventually all terminally ill patients may have access to such care and no longer have to fear prolonged pain and suffering.

The Hospice

The term **hospice** originally applied to medieval Christian hospitals caring for the poor, the aged, and

Managing Stress

The Need for Palliative Care

As the population ages, the need to care for persons with terminal illnesses also is going to increase. In many instances of cancer and other diseases that cannot be cured, the primary goal of medicine should be to relieve suffering and to improve the quality of life in the final weeks or days. Unfortunately, aggressive, high-tech medicine has largely ignored this aspect of patient care. Hospitals can only keep patients as long as they are being treated for a disease; when nothing more can be done in the form of treatments, patients must be

released to a nursing home or a hospice or sent home.

Because many older people do not wish to be treated for ailments that are incurable, attempts are being made to change the care of seriously ill older people. In 1996, a new hospital code was approved for palliative care, which allows hospitals to provide palliative (as opposed to curative) care to patients who are approaching death. Efforts can be made simply to relieve suffering, to provide support, and to make the patient as comfortable as possible until death.

Physicians are finally acknowledging that "dignity, choice, comfort, and the involvement of family members and other loved ones are the basic principles that should govern care at the end of life. . . . The role of medicine is sometimes to cure, but always to comfort. It is ironic that the concept of comfort care has been in eclipse in this high-technology era" (Cassel and Vladeck, 1996). Knowing that palliative care is available can relieve a great deal of stress and suffering that normally would be the fate of terminally ill patients and their families.

the sick. Hospices also provided refuge for people on religious pilgrimages. Providing physical necessities, medical care, and spiritual comfort was the primary purpose of the early religious hospices. In the United States today there are over 2,000 hospices offering comprehensive care for terminally ill patients. The goal of a hospice is to meet the total health needs—physical, psychological, and spiritual—of patients who have weeks or months to live. Medications are given to ease pain, but heroic treatments are not attempted. Family and friends are free to visit with the patient in a comfortable setting, whether it is in a patient's home or a hospital with a hospice attached.

The hospice philosophy is that dying is part of living and should not be resisted with every weapon in the modern medical arsenal. Hospice care is designed to control pain and make patients comfortable, but staff also are trained to discuss emotional and spiritual issues relevant to death. Counseling and social services are available in hospices and close family members are encouraged to participate in daily activities. About two-thirds of hospices in the United States are certified for Medicare reimbursement.

More than 200,000 patients each year in the United States elect to spend their final weeks or months in hospice care. As the population in this country becomes older, more and more families and individuals will have to face the issues raised by terminal illness and death. Although hospices do everything possible to make patients comfortable, they do not permit active euthanasia.

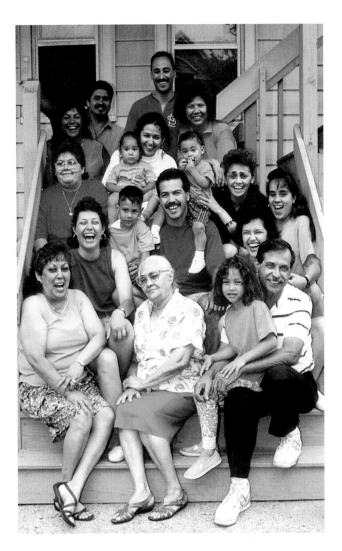

Strong family ties are healthy for young and old alike.

Healthy Aging

With the dramatic upward shift in average life expectancy in the U.S. and other countries, finding ways to improve health in elderly people has become a major challenge. Generally, increasing age is associated with increasing disability and functional impairments, such as loss of mobility, sight, or hearing. One goal of gerontology is to find ways to minimize or postpone the disabilities that accompany aging so that quality of life extends to, or close to, the end of life (Khaw, 1997).

The scientific evidence is now quite overwhelming that most of the disability and long-term medical care in elderly persons results from major chronic diseases that were already present in mid-life (Reed et al., 1998). The most significant predictors of a healthy old age are low blood pressure and low serum glucose levels, not being obese, and not smoking cigarettes while young. These factors are also important in predicting such diseases as cardiovascular disease, cancer, and diabetes. Thus, the evidence points to the importance of developing healthy habits while young if the "golden years"

are going to be enjoyed with ones' physical and mental abilities intact.

Persons surviving to age 55 today can expect to live, on average, another 25 years; those surviving to age 75 can expect to live another 10 to 12 years. Many of these older people are relatively healthy and the length of time that they will be disabled before death is short. In general, people who live to the oldest ages without disabilities are those who have practiced good

Dying is only bad when it takes a long time and hurts so much that it humiliates you.

ERNEST HEMINGWAY
For Whom the Bell Tolls

Terms

hospice: a place for terminally ill patients to spend the time before death in an environment that attends to their physical, emotional, and spiritual needs but no further treatments are administered; hospice care also can be given in a patient's home

nutrition, were physically and mentally active, and did not use tobacco or drink alcohol excessively.

More and more attention is being paid to the role of nutrition in healthy aging. Increased consumption of fresh fruits and vegetables are thought to slow the aging processes; those containing antioxidant chemicals are regarded as particularly potent anti-aging foods. These include avocado, berries, broccoli, cabbage, carrots, citrus, grapes, onions, tomatoes, and spinach. But according to believers in the antioxidant theory of aging, supplements still are needed to ensure that you are getting sufficient amounts of antioxidant vitamins and minerals (Table 15.2). Taking vitamin and mineral supplements from early adulthood on may contribute to a healthier old age (Carper, 1995).

There is no way of knowing how or when we are going to die or what we will do or think when confronted with death. Most of us only think about death when someone close to us dies or if we ourselves become seriously sick or injured. However, if thoughts of death do arise often, or if you feel that you are unreasonably afraid of death, then it is advisable to seek help to overcome fears.

Every age of life provides opportunities for growth and satisfaction. Even though we have no way of knowing when serious illness or death will confront us, we do have control of how we live each day and the satisfactions we find in life. The way we choose to live when we are young will greatly affect our health later. For example, smoking while young increases the

TABLE 15.2   Anti-Aging Supplements and Recommended Maximum Daily Doses

If you take a multivitamin and mineral supplement, you may want to reduce the recommended amounts shown below.

Supplement	Recommended amount
Vitamin E	400 IU
Vitamin C	1,000 milligrams (1 gram)
Beta carotene (vitamin A)	10 milligrams*
Chromium	200 micrograms
Selenium	200 micrograms
Calcium	1,000–1,500 milligrams (1 to 1.5 grams)
Zinc	15 milligrams
Magnesium	200–300 milligrams
Coenzyme Q	30 milligrams (probably not worth the money)

*may increase risk of lung cancer in smokers

likelihood of developing cancer and heart disease later. Drinking alcohol to excess and taking unnecessary chances invite accidents that can cause death or permanent disability. While each person's life span is partly determined by genes, environmental factors, such as nutrition, exercise, and life-style, are also important not only in determining how long we live, but how well we live.

Critical Thinking About Health

1. Since the breakup of the former Soviet Union, the life expectancy of people in Russia has been declining dramatically. Make a list of all the factors you can think of that would contribute to a shorter life expectancy in Russia now compared with previously. Discuss each factor and how important you think it is in contributing to the decline. Also indicate if any of the factors you have discussed for the decline of life expectancy in Russia are important in explaining the difference in life expectancy between black and white Americans discussed in this chapter.

2. Imagine that you have just learned that your mother is suffering from terminal cancer that cannot be treated. The physician estimates that death can occur at any time within a few months and that your mother's pain will be considerable. While drugs can alleviate some of the pain, the doctor honestly does not know how effective the pain relief will be. Your mother is 75 years old and is aware of her condition. When you and she dis-

cuss her condition, she expresses a strong desire not to suffer in order to survive a few weeks or months. She asks you to help her obtain drugs that she can use to end her life peacefully whenever she chooses.

Describe how you would feel in such a situation and what actions you would take. Would you discuss the problem with her physician, with a religious counselor, or with someone else? Would you be concerned about legal problems if you did obtain the lethal drugs and give them to your mother? Would you tell your mother that you want to keep her alive at all costs and you will do all that you can to reduce her suffering? Make a list of all the steps you would take in this situation, and explain your reasons for each action.

3. Make a list of all the health-related factors in your life that you think might play a role in how healthy you will be at age 70 (e.g., you smoke cigarettes, you are significantly overweight). After thinking about the list you have made, ask your-

self if some behaviors or life-style factors are worth changing to help ensure that you will enjoy a healthy old age. Or perhaps you feel that it is not worth worrying about old age now and that the important thing is how to enjoy life at the present time. Discuss these different views and try to develop a personal philosophy of aging that is right for you.

4. Because both of your grandmothers have Alzheimer's disease, the other members of your family are very concerned over their own future mental health, even though both of your parents are only in their 50s. Having read that a particular gene contributes to the risk of Alzheimer's disease and that doctors can test for the presence of this gene, your mother and father have been discussing the advisability of getting the test. They also have asked if you would like to be tested for the Alzheimer's gene. What advice would you give them? Would you want to be tested for the Alzheimer's susceptibility gene? Discuss in detail the reasons for your advice to them and the decision you would make for yourself.

Health in Review

- Aging and dying are natural stages of life. People should strive to remain physically, emotionally, mentally, and spiritually active at all stages of life regardless of chronological age.
- The maximum human life span is approximately 115 years; the average life span in many countries is 80+ years, which means that a majority of people in those countries will live to be 80 years of age or older.
- The average age of the population in the United States is increasing, causing increasing health care costs and financing problems for the Social Security system.
- Aging is partly determined by genes and partly by environmental factors that cause cellular changes with age. Undernutrition slows aging in laboratory animals and may slow down aging processes in people.

- Loss of cognitive mental functions in older people is called senile dementia; the most common cause of this is Alzheimer's disease. Bone loss with age is called osteoporosis and occurs most often in postmenopausal women.
- Active euthanasia refers to helping someone die without pain or suffering. Physician-assisted suicide is a form of active euthanasia that is presently illegal in the United States, although some states have attempted to enact laws legalizing it.
- Palliative care is treatment that does not cure but relieves pain and suffering of dying patients and deals with the distress of family members.
- Hospice care provides terminally ill patients with medical, emotional, and spiritual support during the final weeks or months of their lives.

Health and Wellness Online

The World Wide Web contains a wealth of information about health and wellness. By accessing the Internet using Web browser software, such as Netscape Navigator or Microsoft's Internet Explorer, you can gain a new

perspective on many topics presented in *Essentials of Health and Wellness, Second Edition.* Access the Jones and Bartlett Publishers web site at http://www.jbpub.com/hwonline.

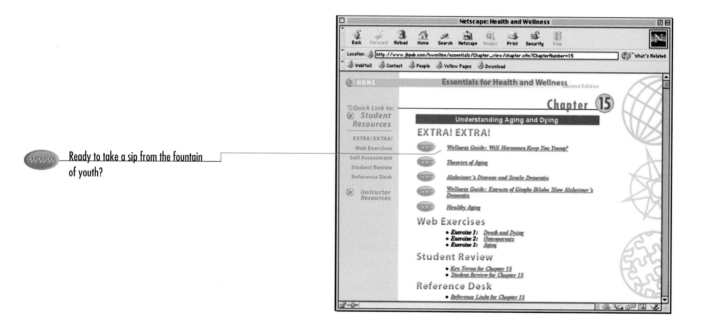

Ready to take a sip from the fountain of youth?

References

Angell, M. (1997). The supreme court and physician-assisted suicide—The ultimate right. *New England Journal of Medicine, 336,* 50–53.

Barzel, U. S. (1996, May 15). Osteoporosis: Taking a fresh look. *Hospital Practice,* 59–68.

Carper, J. (1995). *Stop aging now!* New York: Harper Collins.

Cassel C. K., & Vladeck, B. C. (1996). ICD-9 code for palliative or terminal care. *New England Journal of Medicine, 335,* 1232–1233.

Dawson-Hughes, B., Harris, S. S., Krall, E. A., & Dallal, G. E. (1997). Effect of calcium and vitamin D supplementation on bone density in men and women 65 years of age or older. *New England Journal of Medicine, 337,* 670–676.

Eweksler, M. (1996). Hormone replacement for men. *British Medical Journal, 312,* 859–860.

Finch, C. E., & Tanzi, R. E. (1997). Genetics of aging. *Science, 278,* 407–411.

Gambert, S. R. (1997). Is it Alzheimer's disease? *Postgraduate Medicine, 101,* 42–90.

Goodlin, S. J. (1997, February 15). What is palliative care? *Hospital Practice,* 13–16.

Hayflick, L. (1996). *How and why we age.* New York: Ballantine.

Khaw, K-T. Healthy aging. *British Medical Journal, 315,* 1090–1095.

Lendon, C. L., Ashall, F., & Goate, A. M. (1997). Exploring the etiology of Alzheimer's disease using molecular genetics. *Journal of the American Medical Association, 277,* 825–830.

Le Bars, P. L., et al. (1997). A placebo-controlled, double-blind, randomized trial of an extract of ginkgo biloba for dementia. *Journal of the American Medical Association, 278,* 1327–1332.

Mortimer, J. A., & Graves, A. B. (1993). Education and other socioeconomic determinants of dementia and Alzheimer's disease. *Neurology, 43* (Suppl 4), S39–S44.

Orentlicher, D. (1996). The legalization of physician-assisted suicide. *New England Journal of Medicine, 335,* 663–667.

Phillips, D. P., Ruth, T. E., & Wagner, L. M. (1993, November 6). Psychology and survival. *The Lancet, 342,* 142–145.

Reed, D. M., et al. (1998). Predictors of healthy aging in men with long lives. *American Journal of Public Health, 88,* 1463–1468.

Roses, A. D. (1997, July 15). Alzheimer's disease: The genetic risk. *Hospital Practice,* 51–69.

Snowden, D. A., et al. (1997). Brain infarction and the clinical expression of Alzheimer's disease—The nun study. *Journal of the American Medical Association, 277,* 813–817.

Weindruch, R. (1996, January). Caloric restriction and aging. *Scientific American,* 46–52.

Suggested Readings

Fulton, G. B., & Metress, E. K. (1995). *Perspectives on death and dying.* Boston: Jones and Bartlett. A textbook covering dying and death in detail.

Hayflick, L. (1996). *How and why we age.* New York: Ballantine Books. Excellent discussion of all aspects of aging by an eminent researcher.

Horgan, J. (1997, May). Seeking a better way to die. *Scientific American,* 100–105. Explores the pros and cons of physician-assisted suicide and alternatives to relieving pain and suffering in dying patients.

Humphrey, D. (1991). *Final exit: The practicalities of self-deliverance and assisted suicide for the dying.* Eugene, Ore.: The Hemlock Society. A controversial book that explains euthanasia and how it can be done with or without assistance.

The Merck manual of geriatrics. (1995). New York: Merck and Company. A comprehensive guide to all aspects of aging and geriatric medical care.

Rowe, J. W., & Kahn, R. L. (1998). *Successful aging.* New York: Pantheon. Stresses the importance of life-style, diet, exercise, and mental stimulation to maintain strength and mental acuity in old age.

Weindruch, R. (1996, January). Caloric restriction and aging. *Scientific American,* 46–52. Discusses how restriction of food intake in rats prolongs their lives by almost one-third. Speculates on the usefulness of caloric restriction in human beings to prolong life.

Learning Objectives

1. Discuss the relationship between environment and health.
2. Describe the health effects of air pollution, including smog and the hole in the ozone layer.
3. Explain the greenhouse effect and the predicted consequences of global warming.
4. Describe the effects of lead on children's health and intelligence.
5. Describe substances that pollute water in the United States.
6. Discuss the impact of land pollution on food production and health.
7. Describe sources of pesticide contamination and their effects on health.
8. Identify the potential health problems associated with noise pollution and EMFs.
9. Discuss how human population growth will affect global health and environmental issues.

Exercises and Activities

WORKBOOK
How Do You Score on Environmental Awareness?

Health and Wellness Online

 www.jbpub.com/hwonline

Outdoor Pollution

Indoor Pollution

Land Pollution

Pesticides

Noise Pollution

Chapter 16

Working Toward a Healthy Environment

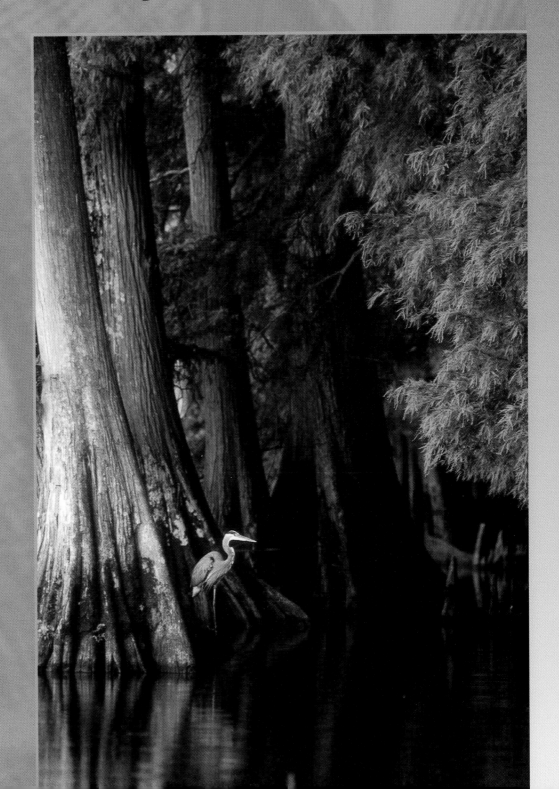

The term **environment** refers to all external physical factors that affect us. In order to survive, all animals, including human beings, require a certain amount of high quality air, water, food, and shelter. If people are deprived of any essential environmental factors, or if the environment is polluted with toxic substances, health is adversely affected. Anyone who has experienced difficulty breathing smoggy, dusty, or smoke-filled air realizes the unhealthy effects of polluted air.

More than any other time in history, mankind faces a crossroads. One path leads to despair and utter hopelessness. The other, to total destruction. Let us pray we have the wisdom to choose correctly.
WOODY ALLEN

To achieve optimal health, we must live in a high quality environment. Unfortunately, the quality of many aspects of the environment is deteriorating from pollution, degradation, and depletion of environmental resources. Environmental health hazards stem from many different causes, which is why environmental problems are not easily solved. However, underlying all environmental problems is human overpopulation and the consequent overuse of natural resources. The United States is making progress in reducing environmental pollution and in preserving natural resources, but the government can only do so much. All of us need to pay more attention to protecting the environment if future generations are to have a safe and healthy environment. As the comic strip character Pogo declared years ago, *"We have met the enemy and he is us."* People's activities are at the root of almost *all* environmental pollution.

 ## Outdoor Pollution

Smog

Each of us breathes about 35 pounds of air per day—more than 6 tons over the course of a year. Fresh, clean air consists of about 21% oxygen, 78% nitrogen, and trace amounts of seven other gases. It is the oxygen in air that is essential for life. If the oxygen content of air drops below 16%, body and brain functions are affected. If breathing stops for even a few minutes, a person becomes unconscious and will die unless breathing is restored.

Everybody has heard of **smog,** a term first used in England to describe a hazardous combination of smoke and fog. Smog causes breathing problems, coughs, bronchitis, asthma, and can even result in death among people with lung diseases. In most U.S. cities, smog is not associated with fog but results from the action of sunlight on various chemicals and particles in the air that come from automobiles, oil refineries, electricity generating plants, and other industrial sources (Table 16.1).

Smoggy, polluted air not only irritates eyes and lungs, but also contributes to health problems, such as allergies, lung infections, and heart disease. Carbon

Managing Stress

Honoring Mother Earth

"All things connect. Man did not weave the web of life. He is merely a strand in it. Whatever he does to the web, he does to himself."

These prophetic words were written by Chief Seattle over a century ago and still ring true today. The neglect and abuse that human beings have inflicted on the planet, primarily in the last few centuries, are beginning to take their toll. Water and air pollution, nuclear and chemical wastes, depletion of the ozone layer, deforestation, and the increased rate of extinction of plant and animal life are all signs of a sick planet.

It may seem hard to believe that the earth is a living entity. Western thought, heavily grounded in science and technology, tends to regard such an idea as foolish or more suitable to myths. But if you

really pay attention to the words of Native Americans and tribal elders around the world, you begin to see the wisdom of viewing the earth as a living entity. But human beings have grown distant and separate from nature and these attitudes have caused major harm to the planet that nourishes all of us.

Whether we realize it or not, we are all connected to the earth like threads of a web. Despite all the advances of technology, we still depend on Mother Earth for the air, water, and food that keeps us alive. Wellness means living in an environment that is healthy, not one that is sick. We can begin to interact with the environment in less harmful ways; even small actions are important, as the slogan "Think globally, act locally" points out.

Here are some questions you can reflect on to become more environmentally aware and proactive.

1. How would you best describe your relationship with the earth?

2. Do you see the earth as a rock spinning in space or as a living entity that provides sustenance in one form or another to all her species of flora and fauna?

3. Getting back to nature can take many forms, from gardening to exotic vacations. What do you do to get back to nature when the urge strikes?

4. Any good relationship takes work. What steps do you feel you can take to enhance your relationship with the earth?

TABLE 16.1   Major Air Pollutants and Their Health Effects

These pollutants affect breathing, damage lungs, and cause a wide range of health problems. The primary sources of these air pollutants are industrial emissions, automobiles and trucks, and coal and oil burning in industry and homes.

Pollutant	Health effects and symptoms
Carbon monoxide gas	Low levels cause dizziness, headache, and fatigue. High levels lead to coma and death. Especially dangerous for persons with asthma and heart disease.
Nitrogen oxide gas	Causes a smelly brown haze that irritates the eyes, nose, and lungs.
Sulfur oxide gas	Sulfur dioxide gas is poisonous. Irritates the eyes, nose, throat, and lungs. Kills plants and rusts metals.
Particulate matter (Particles from dust and smoke that are less than 10 microns in diameter)	Causes throat irritation and permanent lung damage. Some industrial soot particulates may cause cancer.
Ozone (O_3)	In the stratosphere ozone protects us from UV light. Can be formed at ground level from nitrous oxides and organic compounds. Causes eye irritation, cough, and breathlessness.
Photochemical oxidants	A mixture of gases and particles oxidized by the sun from gasoline and other fuels. Cause eye, nose, and throat irritation and make breathing difficult.
Volatile organic compounds	Smog-forming chemicals, such as benzene, toluene, methylene chloride, and methyl chloroform. All VOCs can cause serious health problems.

monoxide, one of the most common pollutants in urban air, interferes with oxygen use in the body. If the air contains 80 parts per million (ppm) of carbon monoxide, the oxygen supplied to the body is reduced by 15%. In heavy freeway traffic, the levels of carbon monoxide may reach levels of 400 ppm. It is no surprise that many commuters in large cities who get stuck in traffic jams arrive home with headaches.

The world's automobile "population" is exploding along with its human population. In 1950, there were about 50 million cars worldwide; by 1990, the number had increased to at least 400 million. As nations such as India and China, which together comprise 38% of the world's population, continue to progress economically, the car population in these and other less developed countries also will increase. Car manufacturers will rejoice, but the effects on air and land pollution will be devastating.

A modern U.S. car with a catalytic converter to reduce emissions still produces about 20 pounds of carbon dioxide for every gallon of gas that is burned; this is a significant factor in global warming. Over an average 10-year life, each American car spews 50 tons of carbon dioxide into the atmosphere. If mileage standards were increased and cars were made more fuel efficient, CO_2 emissions could be reduced significantly.

One major victory in the battle against air pollution was the elimination of lead in gasoline in the United States. There is evidence that the phaseout of leaded gasoline, which began in 1984, has markedly reduced the blood levels of lead in the U.S. population Figure 16.1).

Sulfur oxides are produced when coal or oil, both of which contain sulfur, is burned in industrial or home furnaces and by active volcanos. If the air is damp, sulfuric acid is formed, which is a corrosive substance either as a gas or a liquid. Air containing sulfur oxides can erode stone, pit metal, and harm lungs. Sulfur oxides can also combine with water vapor in the air to form acid rain, a phenomenon responsible for widespread damage to aquatic ecosystems and forests in many parts of the world.

Nitrogen oxides, which come primarily from automobile exhausts, also interfere with the body's use of oxygen. Photochemical smog, common over Los Angeles and other cities, is caused by nitrogen gases produced by sunlight acting on pollutants from automobiles.

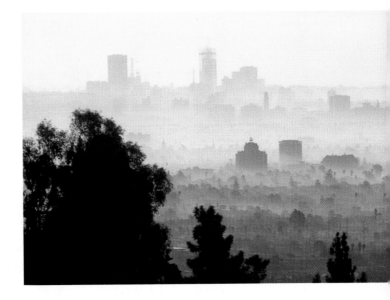

Polluted, "smoggy" air over many large cities contributes to respiratory problems and other diseases.

T e r m s

environment: all external physical factors that affect us

smog: air polluted by chemicals, smoke, particles, and dust

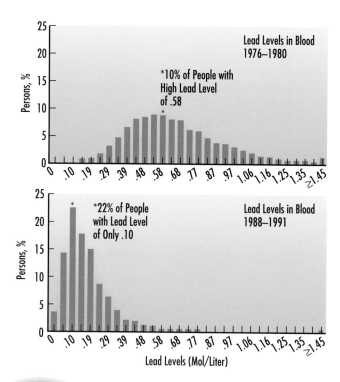

FIGURE 16.1   **Reduction in Blood Lead Levels in the U.S. Population as a Result of the Elimination of Leaded Gasoline**

Source: Data from the National Health and Nutrition Examination Survey, 1990.

Cities that have many smoggy days have higher-than-expected death rates and admissions to hospitals for emergency lung conditions (Dockery et al., 1993).

The battle over clean air pits the Environmental Protection Agency (EPA), which is responsible for air quality and pollution standards, against much of U.S. industry, which finds flaws in the scientific research on the causes and effects of air pollution. Most industries balk at making changes that will cut into profits and make them less competitive with foreign companies that do not have to be concerned about pollution (Kaiser, 1997).

The evidence that particulate matter is a health hazard is quite strong, but industries argue that other air pollutants underlie the health problems and that particulates are not responsible. It required more than 10 years of heated debate and legal wrangling to prove that lead from gasoline was damaging the brains of young children. Many years of effort and research were devoted to showing that chlorofluorocarbons (CFCs) were destroying the ozone layer that protects the earth's surface from harmful UV irradiation. Eventually, both lead in gasoline and CFCs were banned. These two examples show that improving air quality is a long and tedious process.

Acid Rain

Acid rain is rainwater containing large amounts of sulfur dioxide and other gases that have been released into the atmosphere. When these gases combine with water, they produce sulfuric acid and nitric acid, which are dispersed in the rain. Acid rain harms forests, and raises the acidity of lakes and rivers to levels that kill fish and vegetation. Acid rain is a global problem.

Solutions to the acid rain problem involve difficult economic and political decisions. Acid rain can fall hundreds of miles from the source of the sulfur dioxide emission, making it difficult to determine the exact source and responsibility. Acid rain does not observe national boundaries, so countries must cooperate if the problem is to be solved. Like other atmospheric pollution problems, acid rain is likely to fall far into the future.

The Greenhouse Effect

Greenhouses came into widespread use in seventeenth-century Europe to prevent plants from freezing in winter. The glass roofs over a greenhouse allow heat to build up inside because the sun's rays penetrate the glass and warm the air. However, heat does not radiate back through the glass very efficiently. Carbon dioxide (CO_2) in the earth's atmosphere acts much like the glass in a greenhouse, hence the term **greenhouse effect** (Figure 16.2).

The greenhouse effect was first described in 1861 by an English scientist who pointed out that carbon dioxide is a good absorber of infrared (heat) radiation. As the sun's rays warm the earth, heat is radiated back

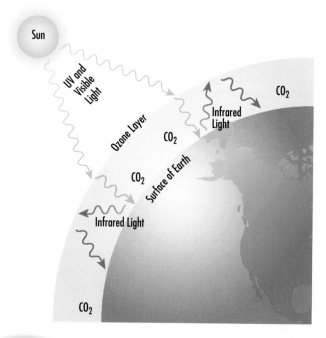

FIGURE 16.2   Greenhouse Effect Carbon dioxide (CO_2) in the earth's atmosphere acts like the glass roof in a greenhouse. Carbon dioxide is transparent to the radiation from the sun and lets it pass to the ground, which warms up.

into the atmosphere. But some of the radiated heat is absorbed by carbon dioxide in the atmosphere and radiated back to earth. As the amount of carbon dioxide in the atmosphere increases, the temperature of the earth tends to rise slightly because more of the sun's heat is absorbed by the atmosphere.

Until the recent widespread industrialization, the carbon dioxide content of the atmosphere was relatively constant because plants and trees use the carbon dioxide in the atmosphere and give off oxygen. Carbon dioxide also is washed from the air by rain and is absorbed into the oceans and used in the formation of carbonate-containing rocks. However, with the great increase in the burning of wood, coal, and oil for transportation, cooking, heating, and industrial uses, the carbon dioxide in the atmosphere has been rising steadily.

Global Warming

Global warming is becoming a major threat to the planet in the coming century. Despite years of acrimonious debate on whether carbon dioxide (CO_2)

emissions are causing global warming, there is now a strong concensus among scientists that the projected increase in global surface temperatures in the next century are real (Figure 16.3). No one can say for sure what the increase will be, but the world's leaders have finally realized that something must be done to reduce the global emissions of carbon dioxide that are responsible for global warming. At present, the countries that emit the most CO_2 are the United States, China, Russia, Japan, Germany, India, Ukraine, and the United Kingdom. As many underdeveloped countries industrialize in the next century, their CO_2 emissions will also increase dramatically.

Life is what happens while you're making other plans.
TOM SMOTHERS

The effects of global warming are far reaching but all are destructive in one way or another (Moore, 1997). Some of the predicted serious effects of global warming include:

- Sea levels will rise. During the past century, global sea levels have risen between 4 to 10 inches. A further rise in sea levels will wipe out islands and flood many low-lying coastal areas. The number of refugees fleeing flooded areas could exceed all existing refugee problems.

- Ice shelves in Antarctica should begin to break up, causing chunks of ice as large as Rhode Island to begin to float away. Ice breakups of this magnitude have already been observed and will lead to major changes in the Antarctic continent.

- Mountaintop glaciers will shrink. Plants that live in warm weather should move up mountains, pushing cold weather varieties into shrinking ranges.

- Animals on land and fish in the oceans will shift their populations northward. Warm water fish will be found in previously cold ocean waters. As the climate changes, many species of plants and animals will become extinct.

- Many diseases, particularly insect-borne diseases, will spread to new regions. Dengue fever, previously unknown in South America, is now prevalent and has spread as far north as Texas. Malaria will spread widely to warmer areas (Patz et al., 1996).

- The number and intensity of violent storms—hurricanes, cyclones, drought, blizzards, and wildfires—

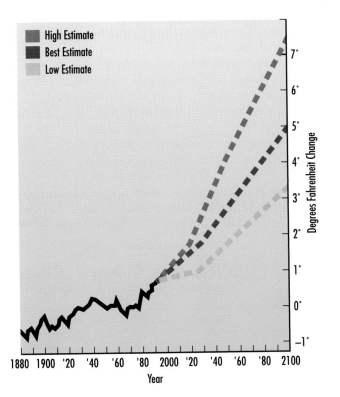

FIGURE 16.3   Measured and Projected Increase in Average Global Temperature as a Result of CO_2 Emissions   Although the phenomenon of global warming has just begun, the average temperature of the planet is expected to increase several degrees in the next century as a result of CO_2 emissions and the greenhouse effect. An increase in global temperatures will have catastrophic effects on climate, oceans, and plant and animal life.
Source: San Francisco Chronicle, Monday, April 17, 1995, A6.

Terms

acid rain: rain, snow, fog, mist, etc., with a pH lower than 5.6

greenhouse effect: the ability of atmospheric carbon dioxide to reflect heat radiated from the earth back to the earth and to thereby raise the earth's temperature globally

will increase globally. Since 1992, record-setting storms have struck countries around the world and produced weather changes including record rainfall, drought, hurricanes, and tornados in regions of the United States.

At an international conference on global warming in Kyoto, Japan, in December 1997, a historic treaty was signed that will dramatically reduce the global emissions of CO_2 by all of the industrialized nations. The U.S., which produces about 25% of the world's CO_2 emissions, agreed to reduce levels to 7% below the 1990 levels by the year 2012. Accomplishing this reduction in the U.S. will be enormously difficult. At the present rate, the CO_2 emissions in the U.S. are predicted to rise by 35% over the next decade. This commitment to drastically curtail CO_2 emissions will require a complete revamping of the coal, petroleum, automotive, electricity-generating, and other major industries in the United States.

The Ozone Layer

The **ozone layer** consists of ozone molecules (i.e., 3 atoms of oxygen bonded together: O_3) that form a layer in the outermost region of the earth's atmosphere. The ozone layer absorbs much of the dangerous ultraviolet (UV) light that is radiated from the sun, and protects us from excessive exposure to UV radiation that can increase the risk of skin cancer and cataracts in the lens of the eye.

A class of chemicals called **chlorofluorocarbons (CFCs)** have been widely used as refrigerant gases and as propellant gases in cans during the past 30 years. These CFCs escape into the atmosphere and rise to the ozone layer where they destroy ozone molecules. In the 1970s it was discovered that the ozone layer was thinning; over the Antarctic an **ozone hole** appears during the Antarctic spring (September to October) and ozone disappears completely in that region. The ozone hole has now spread over populated areas of Asia and northern Europe (Figure 16.4).

When the seriousness of the thinning of the ozone layer was realized, 31 industrialized countries agreed in 1987 to phase out the use of CFCs. Even though CFC use has now dropped significantly, the large amounts of these chemicals already in the atmosphere will cause the ozone layer to continue to thin well into the next century and will cause health problems for millions of people.

Evaluating the Risks of Air Pollution

In evaluating the health hazards of toxic air pollutants, two important factors must be evaluated separately. **Emission** refers to the amount of a substance that is released into the atmosphere from an automobile or other source of air pollution. **Exposure** refers to

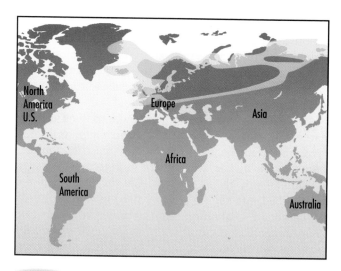

FIGURE 16.4   The "Ozone Hole"   Since its discovery in 1985, the ozone hole has spread dramatically. Lighter color shows the area of most damage to the ozone layer; the darker color shows somewhat less damage.
Source: NASA.

the amount of the substance to which people are exposed. Frequently, emission can be high, while exposure is low. Alternatively, emission can be low, while exposure is high.

For many air pollutants, such as carbon monoxide, benzene, and chloroform, the major sources of emissions are automobiles, industry, and sewage treatment plants, respectively. However, the major health risks from these substances are *not* from the sources of highest emission, but from gas stoves, cigarettes, and chloroform in shower water, respectively (Table 16.2).

To regulate all of the possible pollutants of the air is impossible, so it is important to identify both the sources of greatest emission and the sources of greatest exposure. For example, benzene is an important chemical used in many industrial processes; it also can cause leukemia in people who are exposed to it. Of all the benzene released into the air, 50% comes from automobiles. However, although cigarettes emit

TABLE 16.2   Major Sources of Emission of a Pollutant versus Major Sources of Exposure to It*

Pollutant	Major emission sources	Major exposure sources
Benzene	Industry; automobiles	Smoking
Tetrachloroethylene	Dry-cleaning shops	Dry-cleaned clothes
Chloroform	Sewage treatment plants	Showers
p-Dichlorobenzene	Chemical manufacturing	Air deodorizers
Particulates	Industry; automobiles; home heating	Smoker at home
Carbon monoxide	Automobiles	Driving; gas stoves
Nitrogen dioxide	Industry; automobiles	Gas stoves

*For many hazardous airborne pollutants, the health risk is not related significantly to the major source of emission (as shown in Figure 16.5).

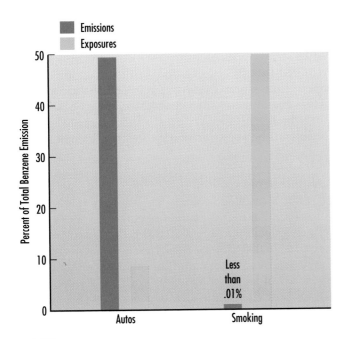

FIGURE 16.5   Benzene Emissions Automobiles emit the greatest amount of benzene into the air—about 50% of the total. However, in terms of the amount of benzene that people inhale, most exposure comes from cigarette smoking.

only a tiny amount of benzene compared with automobiles, at least half of the total population's exposure to benzene comes from smoking cigarettes (Figure 16.5). Even nonsmokers get most of their exposure to benzene from second-hand cigarette smoke as opposed to benzene from automobile exhausts. The most serious indoor air pollutant is cigarette smoke.

Indoor Pollution

Cigarette smoke is not only harmful to the person who smokes, but the "second-hand smoke" that is produced is harmful to others who breathe it (see

chapter 12). The carbon monoxide levels in smoke-filled rooms can rise to hazardous levels. For example, in bars and conference rooms where many people are smoking, the air may contain levels of carbon monoxide as high as 50 ppm. This level is sufficient to produce headache, nausea, impaired judgment, and other symptoms (Table 16.3).

Radon

Another form of indoor air pollution is **radon,** a radioactive gas that is invisible and odorless. Radon is naturally produced in the ground in areas that contain uranium ore. In New Jersey, for example, some homes built on top of rocks that contain uranium ore have over one hundred times the safe level of radon in air inside the house. Homes also may be constructed from bricks or building materials that contain radioactive minerals, one of the decay products of which is radon gas. The radon is slowly released into the house over many years.

Long-term exposure to radon increases the risk of lung cancer. Uranium miners exposed to radon for

Terms

ozone layer: a layer of ozone molecules located in the stratosphere in a diffuse band extending from 10 to 30 miles above the earth's surface

chlorofluorocarbons (CFCs): chemicals formerly used as coolants that are released into the atmosphere and are responsible for destroying stratospheric ozone

ozone hole: an ozone-deficient portion of the atmosphere above Antarctica that has been steadily growing since the problem was first reported in 1985

emission: amount of substance that is released into the atmosphere

exposure: actual amount of the substance people are exposed to

radon: a radioactive gas found in some homes that can increase the risk of cancer

TABLE 16.3   Symptoms of Carbon Monoxide (CO) Poisoning

CO blood level (%)	Symptoms
0–2	No symptoms.
2–5	No symptoms in most people, but sensitive tests reveal slight impairment of arithmetic and other cognitive abilities. Levels of 2–5% are found in light or moderate smokers.
5–10	Slight breathlessness on severe exertion. Levels of 5–10% are found in smokers who inhale one or more packs of cigarettes per day.
10–20	Mild headache, breathlessness on moderate exertion. These levels are sometimes seen in smokers who are exposed to additional CO from other sources.
20–30	Throbbing headache, irritability, impaired judgment, defective memory, rapid fatigue.
30–40	Severe headache, weakness, nausea, dimness of vision, confusion.
40–50	Confusion, hallucinations, ataxia, hyperventilation, and collapse.
50–60	Deep coma with possible convulsions.
Above 60	Usually results in death.

years have a much higher risk of lung cancer than average people not occupationally exposed to the gas. Cigarette smoking seems to act synergistically with radon; smokers who also are exposed to radon get lung cancer at rates much higher than individuals whose exposure is limited solely to cigarette smoke or solely to radon (Peto & Darby, 1994).

Lead Pollution

Lead is a heavy metal that is a serious threat to the health of millions of Americans, especially children. Lead contaminates air, land, water, and houses that still contain lead-based paints. Early symptoms of **plumbism** (lead poisoning) are loss of appetite, weakness, and anemia. Lead poisoning also causes brain damage and is responsible for an enormous number of learning disabilities among children.

Federal studies show that a level of 10 μg/dl of lead in blood puts children under age 6 at risk of learning and behavioral disorders (CDC report, 1997). At least 1.7 million children have this blood level. Another 200,000 children under age 6 have blood lead levels above 20 μg/dl. Even though blood lead levels have declined by more than 80% over the past 20 years because of removal of lead from gasoline, paint, and canned foods, lead toxicity in young children and in fetuses is still of great concern. Even at the current low levels, lead is capable of causing neurological damage to developing brains (Goyer, 1996).

One recent study has documented that attention-deficit disorders, aggression, and delinquency are associated with low levels of lead toxicity and that the higher the blood lead levels are, the greater the symptoms of aberrant behaviors among affected children (Needleman et al., 1996). Despite the progress society has made in reducing lead contamination of the environment, the neurological development of millions of children is still at risk from lead toxicity.

A source of lead poisoning among children, especially those living in old, decrepit inner-city housing, is ingestion of lead paints. In old houses, paint flakes off, and as children crawl around they are apt to pick up and eat paint flakes. A main source of childhood lead poisoning is now believed to be ingestion of lead-containing house dust. The lead ingested is often sufficient to hinder brain development, causing mental deficits later on.

Lead is important to many industries, particularly the battery industry, so it is still an uphill battle to reduce the amount of lead released into the environment and to clean up all sources of lead poisoning. Most of the children who suffer from lead poisoning come from poor families with little political power, so the government has not conducted an all-out effort to further reduce the lead in the environment.

Water Pollution

After air, water is probably the body's most essential requirement. We can survive without air for only a few minutes and without water perhaps for several days. The human body is composed of about 60% water, which is essential to every function carried out by organs in the body, including digestion, blood circulation, and excretion.

Agriculture, cities, and industry in this country are enormous consumers of water. For example, producing a gallon of gasoline requires five gallons of water; brewing a barrel of beer consumes a thousand gallons; a ton of newspaper takes about 50,000 gallons; a ton of steel requires 25,000 gallons; and irrigating an acre of orange trees requires almost a million gallons of water a year. A family of four uses about 600 gallons of water daily. Water is as vital to the maintenance of our life-style as it is to the body's continued health.

Water is continuously recycled in the environment by evaporation and rain. However, as more and more water becomes polluted from pesticides, chemicals, oil spills, and sewage, less and less water is suitable for human consumption and agricultural use. Of special concern is the chemical contamination of rivers, lakes, and underground water supplies, which provide most of our water needs.

Waterborne diseases, such as cholera, typhoid fever, and dysentery, have been virtually eliminated in North America through sanitation and water treatment methods. In many communities, the water supplied to homes is purified by sedimentation, filtration, or chlorination. The addition of chlorine to water kills dangerous bacteria; however, it may create other health hazards. Interaction of chlorine with other chemicals in the water produces toxic substances, such as chloroform and chloramines, which are cancer-causing agents. The widespread use of detergents, herbicides, pesticides, fertilizers, and other chemicals also has contributed to increased water pollution.

In the early 1970s, the Environmental Protection Agency found that the water supplies of many towns and cities were dangerously contaminated with pathogenic organisms and toxic chemicals. As a result of these findings, Congress passed the Safe Drinking Water Act of 1974, which covers 58,000 community water supply systems and another 160,000 private systems. The Act requires that these systems meet federal drinking water safety standards; but it is one thing to pass such a law and another thing to enforce it.

In 1996, Congress renewed the Safe Drinking Water Act of 1974. Under the new act, consumers must be notified whenever contaminants are found in drinking water and not merely when the water does not meet federal standards for contamination and safety. Because millions of Americans still are supplied with water that does not meet federal standards for health and

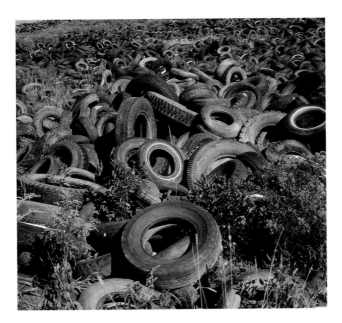

Do you ever think about what happens to your old tires? It's not a pretty picture, but it's a problem we have to solve.

safety, people are purchasing bottled water and water purifying equipment in ever-increasing amounts.

Land Pollution

Until relatively recently, little attention was paid to the disposal of garbage and solid wastes in landfills around the country. Now, however, we are beginning to run out of space to dump the stuff we want to get rid of. Each year in the U.S., we junk about 8 million cars and trucks; 100 billion cans, bottles, and jars; and more than 200 million tons of garbage. The average American generates more than twice as much garbage as citizens of other industrialized countries. The United States produces 1,584 pounds of trash per person annually; Japan, 902 pounds; and the European Union, only 660 pounds.

Many old, abandoned solid waste disposal sites are dangerous to health because they contain hazardous materials that may be corrosive, flammable, or contain toxic chemicals (Table 16.4). In 1980, Congress passed the Superfund Act, which was supposed to pro-

vide for the clean-up of the most dangerous waste sites. Despite spending many billions of dollars, the Superfund Act has only made a small dent in cleaning up hazardous waste sites. By 1993, only 217 of almost 1,300 hazardous sites on the Superfund list had been cleaned up (Stix, 1993). The average cost to clean up a site has been $27 million. These high costs prompt many people to believe we should be looking for more environmentally safe ways of manufacturing what we need and of recycling what we discard.

For example, discarded automobile tires are a major problem for landfills. Americans throw away about 250 million tires a year. Experts have suggested that the government should investigate environmentally safe ways to use the scrapped tires to generate electricity. Each automobile tire is the equivalent of about 2.5 gallons of oil. Stacked up in landfills around the country are tires that add up to about 178 million barrels of oil. But political and economic pressures force the U.S. to import foreign oil, rather than explore new ways to clean up the environment and produce energy.

Pesticides

Soil, water, and some foods have become increasingly contaminated with chemicals used to control weeds, insects, and plant diseases in the environment. Any chemical capable of killing unwanted organisms is called a **pesticide.** Specific kinds of chemicals that destroy certain kinds of organisms are **insecticides** (kills insects), **fungicides** (kills molds and fungi), **herbicides** (kills weeds), and **rodenticides** (kills rats and mice). Pesticides are important to the agriculture industry,

Terms

plumbism: disease caused by lead poisoning
pesticide: a chemical that kills unwanted organisms
insecticide: a pesticide that kills insects
fungicide: a chemical that kills fungi
herbicide: a chemical that kills weeds
rodenticide: a chemical that kills mice and rats

TABLE 16.4   Hazardous Wastes That Escape into the Environment Cause Many Health Problems
Millions of tons of these substances are discarded every year in the U.S.

Substance	Source	Health effects
Mercury	Sludge from chloralkali plants; electrical equipment, fluorescent lights	Tremors, mental retardation, loss of teeth, kidney damage, neurological damage
Arsenic	Arsenic trioxide from coal combustion and from metal smelters	Diarrhea, vomiting, paralysis, skin cancers
Cadmium	Waste from electroplating industry; paint containers, nickel-cadmium batteries	Lung diseases
Cyanide	Electroplating industry waste	Poisoning, interferes with cellular energy metabolism
Pesticides	Solid wastes and wastes in solutions	Multiple effects including rashes, respiratory and gastrointestinal symptoms, neurological disorders, hemorrhages

which has claimed over the years that the abundance and quality of food grown in the United States depend on the use of chemicals to destroy crop pests. While pesticides may contribute to agricultural productivity (although this is contested by people who practice organic farming), widespread dissemination of pesticides in the environment has created health and pollution problems.

The evidence over the safety of pesticide use is both confusing and controversial. Pesticide manufacturers claim that their products are safe when used as directed. Monitoring of pesticide residues on food shows that the levels are not dangerous. However, consumer groups and many scientists argue that pesticides cause much more harm than good both to people and to the environment and are responsible for many serious health problems.

Many pesticides have been found to be so dangerous that their use has been banned by the EPA, the federal agency that regulates pesticide use. One of the most widely used pesticides, DDT, was found to be carcinogenic and was banned by the EPA more than 20 years ago.

The use of other pesticides such as heptachlor, kepone, dieldrin, mirex, and toxophene has been banned and these chemicals have been off the market in the United States for a number of years. The quandary faced by the EPA is balancing the necessary use of chemicals by agriculture and other industries while safeguarding the public's health.

For example, millions of homes in the United States have been treated for termite control. Until recently, the two most commonly used chemicals for killing termites were chlordane and heptachlor, both related in chemical structure to DDT. These chemicals do not break down; they persist in houses and the environment for at least 25 years. Exposure to these pesticides is claimed by some to cause headaches, breathing problems, fatigue, nervous system disorders, liver and kidney damage, and possibly cancer. Some people have had to abandon their homes because of health problems resulting from the pesticides used to kill termites.

Generally, the health effects of pesticides on people and other animals are subtle. For the most part, pesticides do not cause sudden, severe sickness or death unless the amount of exposure is extremely high. The amount of pesticide capable of causing death varies widely depending on the specific chemical in question as well as on individual susceptibility to these poisons. For some insecticides and rodenticides, a very small amount can kill a full-grown person. However, there is growing concern over pesticide residues in the environment that may be responsible for the increase in breast and uterine cancer (Davis et al., 1993).

Year after year, thousands of tons of various pesticides are released into the environment. Most of these chemicals do not degrade easily, and they accumulate in soil, lakes, and rivers. Plants and animals in the environment absorb chemicals, which become more and more concentrated as they move up the food chain.

Many large animals, birds, and fish now have high levels of pesticides in their tissues. For example, in a lake in Florida, 80% to 95% of alligator eggs have failed to hatch in recent years, a mortality rate of 10 times normal. The alligator eggs contain abnormal levels of estrogen and testosterone, which are essential reproductive hormones in all animals. The few male and female alligators that do survive are reproductively abnormal, and males have abnormally small penises. A pesticide called **dicofol**, similar to DDT in structure, is present in the lake as a result of dumping by a chemical company that used to operate on its shore. Dicofol mimics the action of estrogen and causes abnormalities in reproduction and in sexual development (Raloff, 1995).

As a society, we are not ready to abandon the use of pesticides. However, as individuals we should restrict our use of pesticides as much as possible to protect ourselves and the environment. To achieve this goal, many people now grow their own vegetables without the use of pesticides. Others shop at stores that sell fruits and vegetables grown without the use of pesticides and herbicides.

Polychlorinated Biphenyls (PCBs)

Polychlorinated biphenyls (PCBs) belong to a family of more than 200 structurally related chemicals that were widely used from 1930 until the late 1970s as industrial coolants, especially in power transformers. PCBs were found to cause cancer in laboratory animals and have been banned for more than 20 years in the United States. However, they persist in the envi-

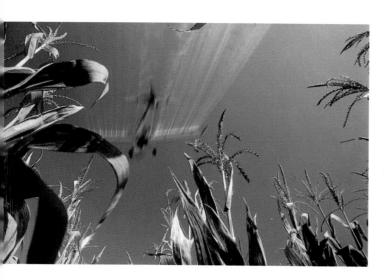

Many people would like to see the use of pesticides on our food supply reduced.

Wellness Guide

Precautions for Pesticide Use

- Before you buy a pesticide product, read the instructions for use and any health and safety warnings. When mixing, do not increase the concentration of the pesticide above the label-recommended amount. Do not purchase the product if you can't use the pesticide properly (you may not have the right equipment). If you don't understand or feel completely comfortable with the health and safety information provided, get more information before you buy the product. Also, consider whether you have adequate storage space for the pesticide. A

bigger bottle may be cheaper, but can you store it safely?

- Use the least toxic pesticide available for your pest control problem. Try to strike a balance between effective pest control and the safety of people, pets, and other nontarget organisms. Minimize skin and respiratory contact with pesticides. Wear rubber gloves. When you select gloves, consider both the solvent used in the pesticide formulation and the possibility that the pesticide itself can penetrate skin. You may want to use a respirator to guard against inhaling pesticide spray or dust.

- Use pesticides only for the uses for which they are intended. For instance, some wood preservatives are meant for outside use only, so don't use them inside the house!

- Don't leave seemingly empty pesticide containers where children can get them. Children have been poisoned by drinking from "empty" containers that actually contained leftover pesticide.

- Never smoke, eat, or drink while using pesticides.

---

ronment and may have contributed to the death of seals and other animals in water contaminated with PCBs. Now scientists have found that PCBs mimic the action of **thyroxin,** a hormone produced by the thyroid gland that in excess causes abnormal development of the thyroid (Stone, 1995).

Thyroxin controls many essential functions in the body and is involved in regulating sperm production. Based on studies of laboratory rats exposed to PCBs, scientists speculate that PCBs may be contributing to the decline in sperm production in men that has been observed in many countries. PCBs and some pesticides share similar chemical structures and may affect human hormones in ways that are just beginning to be discovered.

Even though use of PCBs has been banned for years, they persist in the environment and in the bodies of people who were exposed. The World Wildlife Fund estimates that at least a billion pounds have been dispersed into the environment worldwide.

Studies of children born in the 1980s in Michigan indicate that prenatal exposure to PCBs caused developmental delays, learning impairment, and lower IQ

scores. While most of these middle-class children are still within the normal range of IQ, they are at the lower end of normal (Jacobson & Jacobson, 1996).

Electromagnetic Fields (EMFs)

Electric power lines, appliances, motors, TV sets, microwave ovens, and power tools all emit very low frequency **electromagnetic fields (EMFs).** Except for the earth's electromagnetic field, all EMFs come from electricity that is generated by electrical devices of all kinds (Table 16.5).

Terms

dicofol: a pesticide that mimics the action of estrogen and causes reproductive abnormalities

polychlorinated biphenyls (PCBs): a family of banned synthetic, organic chemicals that affect the human thyroid gland and reproductive systems of animals

thyroxin: a hormone produced by the thyroid gland

electromagnetic fields (EMFs): a form of radiation produced by electrical power lines and appliances that may increase the risk of cancer

TABLE 16.5   Strength of Electromagnetic Fields from Household Sources

Many electrical appliances, especially ones with motors, produce very strong magnetic fields, but the strength of the field falls rapidly with increasing distance from the appliance.

Source	Intensity (milligauss) at distance from source	
	At 4 cm	At 20 cm
100-watt bulb	2.5	—
Refrigerator (back)	11	5
200-watt stereo	27	5
80-watt fluorescent bulb	34	18
Coffeemaker	90	7
Electric drill	600	6
Hair dryer	1,000	0.1

Some studies have found an association between the incidence of childhood leukemia and brain tumors and exposure to EMFs. Families that live close to high voltage power lines or electrical distribution boxes tend to experience more sickness and more cancers. However, a very careful study of the risks of childhood leukemia and exposure to EMFs showed that the risk of cancer was not increased (Linet et al., 1997). While some medical experts believe that this study should put the issue of health and EMFs to rest, it has not. Many experts still believe that further research is required and that caution in exposure to EMFs is still advisable (correspondence, 1997).

All of us are exposed to EMFs every day. An electric shaver or hair dryer puts out a strong EMF, although users are exposed for only a few minutes a day (Figure 16.6). If a person lives near a high voltage transmission line, exposure to EMFs may be considerable depending on the distance between the house and the wires. And the exposure goes on day and night.

Based on current research, the risk to health from exposure to EMFs must be regarded as small compared with the risks of chemical pollutants in air, soil, water, and food. Moreover, our lives are so dependent on electricity and the gadgets that make life more comfortable that major changes in electrical use are not anticipated. Despite ongoing uncertainty about the health effects of EMFs, certain precautions can be taken that will reduce exposure (Salvatore, 1996).

Noise Pollution

Have you ever been kept awake at night by a dripping faucet or a neighbor's party? Does the sound of sirens and horns put you on edge? Have you ever found yourself thinking, "If that noise doesn't stop, I'm going to scream." Everyone is sensitive to noise, and excessive noise produces stress and can cause health problems. Noise interferes with sleep and over periods of time can cause fatigue, irritability, tension, and anxiety.

Sound activates the nervous system, thereby affecting functions of the endocrine, cardiovascular,

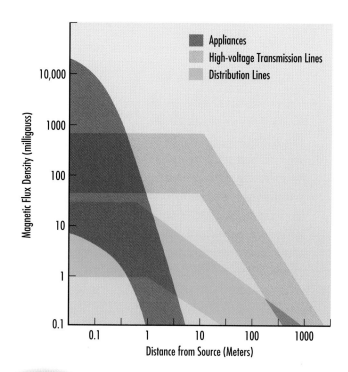

FIGURE 16.6   **Strength of Magnetic Fields from Sources of Electromagnetic Fields (EMFs)**   Small appliances produce strong fields, but the strength disappears within a few feet. High voltage lines produce less dense magnetic fields but they cover a large area.
Source: Adapted from Keith Florig.

and reproductive systems. Noise is a "stressor" and can increase blood pressure, alter hormone levels, constrict blood vessels, and cause intense pain at high levels.

Sound levels are measured in **decibels** (dB). The danger zone for hearing loss begins at about 85 dB, a level present on schoolbuses crowded with kids or driving in freeway traffic with the window open (Table 16.6). Many daily activities expose us to sound levels that can permanently damage hearing. An estimated 20 million men, women, and children in the United States are exposed to dangerous levels of sound every day that can cause hearing loss (Flodin, 1992).

Rock musicians and people who listen to loud rock music are particularly at risk for hearing loss. Members of many famous rock bands suffer from **tinnitus**, a per-

Wellness Guide

Ways to Reduce Your Exposure to EMFs

- Don't use an electric blanket or water bed heater unless it is a newer model with reduced EMFs.

- Use battery-operated shavers and hair dryers. Battery-operated appliances and toys do not put out EMFs.

- Don't sit too close to computers, TVs, fans, or light fixtures.

- If your work requires long exposure to EMFs, look for ways to reduce it. Do not sit too close to computer screens for long periods.

- If you rent or buy a house, choose one that is not near a high voltage line or distribution transformer.

TABLE 16.6   **Noise Levels Produced by Daily Activities and Machines**
A noise level above 85 dB can damage hearing and cause hearing loss over time.

Source of noise	Sound level (dB)
Firearms	140 to 170
Jet engines	140
Rock concerts	90 to 130
Amplified car stereos	140 (at full volume)
Portable stereos (e.g., Sony Walkman)	115 (at full volume)
Power mowers	105
Jackhammers	100
Subway trains	100
Video arcades	100
Freeway driving in a convertible	95
Power saws	95
Electric razors	85
Crowded school buses	85
School recesses or assemblies	85

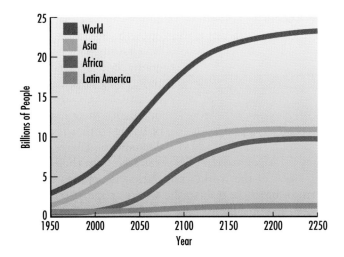

FIGURE 16.7   **Estimated Population Increases**   A global population of more than 20 billion is predicted before growth levels off.

sistent ringing in the ears, or have lost a significant amount of their hearing. Children are especially prone to turning up the volume and to listening to music with earphones at dangerously high sound levels.

Many people live and work amidst the din of urban life, and have forgotten the rest and peacefulness that come with silence. If you have the good fortune to spend time at isolated spots in the woods or at the ocean, you become aware of the beneficial effects of quiet. The human need for stillness was expressed eloquently in 1854 by Chief Seattle, after whom the modern city in Washington is named:

> There is no quiet place in the white man's cities. No place to hear the unfurling of leaves in spring or the rustle of insects' wings. But perhaps it is because I am a savage and do not understand. The clatter only seems to insult the ears. And what is there to life if a man cannot hear the lonely cry of the whippoorwill or the arguments of the frogs around a pond at night?

How Human Population Growth Affects Us

In 1995, the world's population was estimated at 5.7 billion people. By 2050, the world's population is expected to increase to 11.5 billion, assuming fertility continues to fall and that the average family produces just 2.6 children (Figure 16.7). However, the average global fertility rate is still 3.6 children per woman (Calne, 1995).

What do these numbers mean with respect to environmental degradation and human health? One unresolved question of a rapidly growing population is whether the world can produce enough food to feed its people (Bongaarts, 1994). In addition, crowding and poverty lead to disease epidemics and increased crime, conditions that are already appearing in some areas of this country and around the world.

All of the world's environmental problems stem, in one way or another, from human activities and human overpopulation (Vitousek, 1997). Deforestation; loss of native species of plants and animals; depletion of natural resources; and air, water, and land pollution are all related to too many people needing too many scarce resources. The demand for modern life-styles and products adds to the destruction and pollution of the environment. Indeed, as one close observer of nature has observed, we already may be witnessing the "end of nature," a process that progressed for billions of years before the emergence of human beings a few million years ago (McKibben, 1989).

The actions, needs, and goals of people are at the root of all environmental problems and the ongoing destruction of nature. As the economies of nations become stronger and aspirations of people around the globe increase, so does the rate of environmental destruction. Political and economic solutions to the population problem are discussed, but many nations

Terms

decibel: a measure of noise level

tinnitus: persistent ringing in the ears often caused by repeated or sudden exposure to loud noises

are unable or unwilling to undertake the measures that might curb population growth. Some countries have family planning programs, but the success of these programs depends on educating people and in raising their standard of living so that they understand that large families are not in their interest. Most of the world's population is opposed to any form of birth control, so the world's population is expected to continue to increase for at least the next 50 years.

> *The greatest problem of communication is the illusion that it has been accomplished.*
> GEORGE BERNARD SHAW

The United States has made progress in reducing environmental pollution and in slowing population growth (the goal of most industrialized nations is zero population growth). Thanks to legislation, environmental lawsuits, and improved technology, air quality has improved, many waterways are cleaner than they were 20 years ago, and disposal of hazardous wastes has declined dramatically. While all this is good news, we have a long way to go in solving environmental and population problems. Most observers of the world's population growth are pessimistic about the future. As one physician observed: "*Homo sapiens* is destined to become *Homo extinctus* if the population increase continues without constraint and the resources of the planet are exhausted" (Wall, 1995).

> What we call the beginning is the end
> And to make an end is to make a beginning.
> The end is where we start from.
>
> —*T.S. Eliot*
> *Four Quartets*

Critical Thinking About Health

1. Check around your house or apartment, and make a list of all pesticides or herbicides that are stored anywhere. Decide which ones you really need to keep and which ones can be discarded. (Check with your local waste management authorities for proper disposal of pesticides and herbicides.) Make a list of how and when you use pesticides and what precautions you take when you use them. After doing this, write a report on how you can reduce your use and exposure to pesticides and herbicides.

2. The United States has made a committment to lower carbon dioxide (CO_2) emissions dramatically in the next few years. To accomplish this, society must make major readjustments in the use of energy and transportation and in industrial output. Everyone will have to contribute to this effort. Begin by making a list of how you can:
   a. Reduce your electricity use by 30%. What appliances use the most electrical energy and what changes can you make to reduce their use?
   b. Reduce the use of your automobile by 30% or more. What changes in your life-style can you make that will reduce your dependence on car transportation?
   c. Find out what industries release the most CO_2 in manufacturing their products. Are these products essential to your life, or would you be able to live without some of them?

3. The major global threats to the environment are (a) nuclear, chemical, and biological warfare; (b) depletion of the ozone layer; (c) global warming; (d) land and ocean degradation; and (e) extinction of species of plants and animals. Indicate which of these global environmental problems is of the most concern to you personally. What can you personally do about the problem? What do you think governments should do about the problem? Discuss any effects that you think this problem will have on your life now and in the future.

4. If you had the option of living anywhere in the world, where would you choose to live? Is your choice largely determined by job opportunities, environmental concerns, access to a favorite sport (e.g., swimming), or by some other variable? Discuss your choice in detail, and explain the things that are most important to you in making your selection. Do you think your choice will be the same 10 years from now? Why might it change?

Health in Review

- To maintain good health, people require adequate unpolluted air, water, food, and shelter.
- The air we breathe is often polluted with ozone, carbon monoxide, hydrocarbons, nitrogen and sulfur oxides, lead, cigarette smoke, and other contaminants.
- Drinking water may be contaminated with particulates or microorganisms that can cause disease.

Pesticides in land, water, and food that have hormone-like properties may be damaging human endocrine and reproductive systems.

- The greenhouse effect and the ozone hole are examples of global environmental problems caused by human activities.
- Pollution of air, land, and water from heavy metals, such as lead, is particularly hazardous to health. Children with even small amounts of lead

or PCBs in their bodies may suffer from learning deficits.

- Global warming is expected to cause serious environmental disruptions in the next century.
- Noise pollution can cause a wide range of health problems, including stress, tinnitus, and hearing loss.
- World population is expected to double in the next 50 years, severely taxing an already depleted environment and creating more health and environmental problems.

Health and Wellness Online

The World Wide Web contains a wealth of information about health and wellness. By accessing the Internet using Web browser software, such as Netscape Navigator or Microsoft's Internet Explorer, you can gain a new

perspective on many topics presented in *Essentials of Health and Wellness, Second Edition.* Access the Jones and Bartlett Publishers web site at http://www.jbpub.com/hwonline.

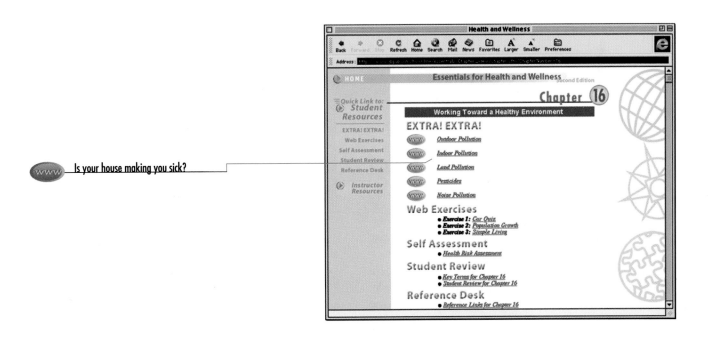

References

Bongaarts, J. (1994, March). Can the growing human population feed itself? *Scientific American*, 36–42.

Calne, R. (1995). *Too many people*. New York: Riverrun Press.

Centers for Disease Control and Prevention. (1997). Children with elevated blood lead levels attributed to home renovation and remodeling activities—New York, 1993–1994. *Journal of the American Medical Association, 277*, 1030–1031.

Davis, D. L., et al. (1993). Medical hypothesis: Xenoestrogens as preventable causes of breast cancer. *Environmental Health Perspectives, 101*(5), 372–377.

Dockery, D. W., et al. (1993). An association between air pollution and mortality in six U.S. cities. *New England Journal of Medicine, 329*(24), 1753–1759.

Flodin, K. C. (1992, January/February). Now hear this. *American Health*, 59–62.

Goyer, R. A. (1996). Results of lead research: Prenatal exposure and neurological consequences. *Environmental Health Perspectives, 104,* 1050–1053.

Jacobson, J. L., & Jacobson, S. W. (1996). Intellectual impairment in children exposed to polychlorinated biphenyls in utero. *New England Journal of Medicine, 335,* 783–789.

Kaiser, J. (1997). Showdown over clean air science. *Science, 277,* 466–469.

Linet, M. S., et al. (1997). Residential exposure to magnetic fields and acute lymphoblastic leukemia in children. *New England Journal of Medicine, 337,* 1–7.

McKibben, B. (1989). *The end of nature.* New York: Random House.

Moore, C. A. (1997, January/February). Warming up to hot new evidence. *International Wildlife,* 21–25.

Needleman, H. L. (1996). Bone lead levels and delinquent behavior. *Journal of the American Medical Association, 275,* 363–369.

Patz, J. A., et al. (1996). Global climate change and emerging infectious diseases. *Journal of the American Medical Association, 275,* 217–223.

Peto, J., & Darby, S. (1994). Radon risk assessment. *Nature, 368,* 97–98.

Postel, S. L., et al. (1996). Human appropriation of renewable fresh water. *Science, 271,* 785–788.

Raloff, J. (1995). Beyond estrogens. *Science News, 148,* 44–46.

Salvatore, J. R. (1996). Low-frequency magnetic fields and cancer. *Postgraduate Medicine, 100,* 183–190.

Stix, G. (1993, December). Clean definitions: The nation contemplates what to do with Superfund. *Scientific American,* 26–27.

Vitousek, P. M., et al. (1997). Human domination of Earth's ecosystems. *Science, 277,* 494–499.

Wall, W. J. (1995). Too many people. *New England Journal of Medicine, 333,* 464.

Wartenberg, D. (1997). Leukemia and exposure to magnetic fields. *New England Journal of Medicine, 337,* 1471–1474.

Suggested Readings

Brodeur, P. (1993). *The great power line coverup.* Boston: Little, Brown.

Calne, R. (1995). *Too many people.* New York: Riverrun Press. An excellent, authoritative explanation of what overpopulation means to the future of the planet and to the people of the next century.

50 simple things you can do to save the earth. (1989). Berkeley, CA: The Earthworks Group. Simple, practical things each person can do to help heal the environment.

Gelbspan, R. (1997). *The heat is on: The high stakes battle over earth's threatened climate.* New York: Addison-Wesley. A candid portrayal of the brutal politics behind the battle over global warming. The author believes that scientists will have to become more proactive and aggressive if significant reduction in global warming is to be accomplished.

McKibben, B. (1989). *The end of nature.* New York: Random House. Discusses why we may have gone too far in conquering nature.

Meyer, W. B. (1996). *Human impact on the earth.* New York: Cambridge University Press. Describes in detail the environmental changes that have occurred over the past 300 years as a result of human activities.

Needleman, H. L., & Landrigan, P. J. (1994). *Raising children: Toxic free.* New York: Farrar, Straus, and Giroux. Two physicians concerned with environmental hazards to health explain how to protect children from the most dangerous ones.

Ott, W. R., & Roberts, J. W. (1998, February). Everyday exposure to toxic pollutants. *Scientific American,* 86–91. Describes the toxic substances we are exposed to in our daily routines. An excellent article if you want to learn how to avoid pollutants in the environment.

Making Healthy Changes

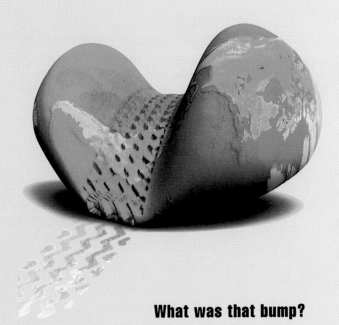

What was that bump?

Although we may do everything that is reasonably possible to live a healthy life—eat a healthy diet and not become overweight, exercise regularly, practice stress reduction techniques, leave time for fun and relaxation—we will still require medical care when we become sick. Also, we live on a planet that is becoming increasingly polluted and whose resources, oceans, forests, and species are being depleted at a faster rate than at any time in earth's history. The feverish consumerism that has engulfed the entire world also has an important impact on our lives, work, behaviors, and health. High technology and environmental changes on a global level affect our ability to live healthy lives, especially if we strive to live simply in a technologically complex world.

More than 30 years ago, one of the most important (and often quoted) scientific articles of the century was published, entitled "Tragedy of the Commons" (*Science, 162,* 1243, 1968). It contained no data, described no unusual experiments, nor offered a radical new theory. The article pointed out clearly and graphically that the growing human population problem has no "technical solution" and can only eventually result in a worsening state of living and health for all of us on the planet.

The "Tragedy of the Commons" is illustrated by a simple example. A group of herdsmen have access to a finite amount of land on which to graze their sheep. As long as the number of herdsmen and sheep are small,

the land will support them all. However, eventually a herdsman discovers that by increasing the number of sheep he grazes on the pasture, the more he will earn and the better his life will become. Of course, eventually all herdsmen realize this and add more and more sheep to the pasture. The end result is that all suffer when the pasture dies and the sheep have nothing to eat. This is the "Tragedy of the Commons."

Earth is our pasture and its resources are finite. As more and more people consume more and more goods that use up the planet's resources faster and faster, the "Tragedy of the Commons" seems less like a fable and more like reality. Since our overall health, the health of our children, and of their children depend on the health of the planet we all live on, consideration of environmental issues, consumerism, and advertising also become essential health concerns. As one mother put it, "One day I would like to show my daughter how to see the forest for the trees."

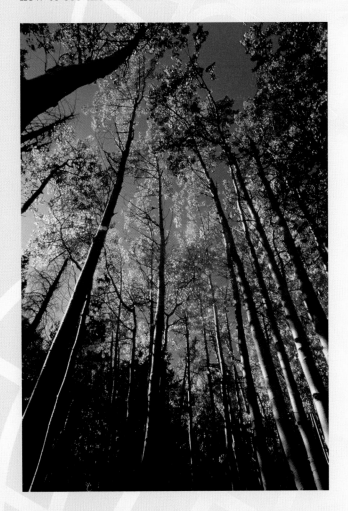

Emotional Wellness: Avoiding Neurotoxins in the Environment

The daily news reminds us of the widespread increase in depression, anxiety, and anger in the United States and elsewhere. These unhealthy emotional states also are increasingly associated with violence—both against oneself (suicide) and against others (homicide). Many environmental toxins that are inhaled daily are neurotoxins, chemicals that affect the brain and alter emotional responses. A partial list of inhaled substances that may act as neurotoxins in susceptible individuals includes household cleaners, copy machine toners, nail polish and remover, hair sprays, ink markers, paint and solvents, air fresheners, pesticide sprays, and glues.

List in your journal all the potential neurotoxic substances that you are exposed to at home, school, or work. Circle ones that you are exposed to most often. For the next week or two monitor your moods, especially if you become angry or depressed. Keep a record in your journal of any substances that you were exposed to that may have accounted for the emotional changes, especially if there was no other obvious cause.

Think of ways to eliminate potentially unhealthy chemical substances from your environment. Consider using face masks that protect against vapors if you have to spray pesticides or use volatile solvents. Make a list of chemicals that you can eliminate completely from your environment and ones for which a safe substitute is available.

Improving Your Diet: Fasting for Health

Fasting means not eating for a period of time, ranging from a day to weeks, depending on the goal of the fast. Lengthy fasts are usually used for spiritual journeys, since restricting food intake over a long period changes body chemistry and frequently induces altered states of consciousness. However, even letting your digestive system clean out for a day or two is healthy. Anyone can safely try a clear juice and water fast for a day or two to help eliminate solid wastes and toxins from the body. Also, a liquid fast can help you to relearn the signals of "hunger" and help you not to eat simply because it's dinner time or because you can't think of anything else to do. In today's world we often eat by the clock and not by the dictates of our body. And we also ignore the signals from our body to stop eating.

If you think a fast might be beneficial for you, pick a day when you have no pressing obligations. You can drink as much water as you want and you can have several servings of clear fruit juices such as cranberry or apple juice. The goal is to not take in solid food for 24 hours or longer. When you break your fast, do so slowly. Eat small amounts of food. Do *not* eat a large amount of food all at once.

Describe in your journal your reasons for fasting and what you experienced during and after the fast. Has fasting changed your eating habits in any way?

Emotional Wellness: Trying a News Fast

Just as a "food fast" is good for the body, a "news fast" is good for the mind and even easier to try. Just decide that for one day (or one week) you are not going to watch, listen to, or read any news. This means giving up TV news, newspapers, weekly news magazines, radio news, computer news. If someone asks you what you think about such and such, you can answer: "I'm on a news fast for my health."

Describe in your journal what it felt like to try a "news fast." Did you notice any change in your thoughts or emotions? Were you able to complete your daily activities with less stress? Did you feel less anxious because you did not have to think about the latest disaster?

Stress Management: Writing to Reduce Stress

Everyone has experienced the relief from talking with a close friend or counselor about a personal tragedy or stressful experience. The old advice to "get it off your chest" is still valid. However, telling someone what you are feeling is not always easy and often an appropriate someone is unavailable, unaffordable, or both. There is an easier way to relate what you are thinking and feeling, and that is to write it down.

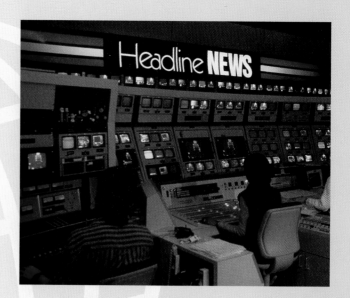

A growing scientific literature demonstrates that writing about stressful experiences can not only relieve mental stress, but can improve physical health as well. Writing about stressful experiences appears to bolster the immune system, relieve symptoms of asthma and rheumatoid arthritis, and reduce visits to doctors. Given the positive health effects that derive from writing about stressful experiences, it should be one of the first things a person should do after any stressful experience, such as the death of a family member, being physically attacked, or having witnessed something very upsetting. Even a breakup with a partner, failure to get a job, or not getting acceptable grades in school may cause stress that should be explored in writing.

If you have had some stressful experiences in the last year or even many years ago, or if there are unhappy or unpleasant things that you think about more or less daily, take time to write about them. You can use your journal or you can write about them separately so that you do not worry about someone reading what you have written. The point is for you to write about what you experienced and how you feel. You do not even have to save the written material unless you want to read it again or add to it. The important health benefits come from the writing and expressing what was, until now, bottled up inside.

Wise Consumer: Freezing Your Credit

Money management (i.e., not having enough) often produces stress for many people and can destroy relationships. By causing stress and damaging relationships, overspending and debt contribute significantly to loss of wellness and even to illness. At every turn we are urged to buy and consume more—more food, sportier cars, new computers, bigger houses. For most people, the credit card is the means to having everything they desire. But paying off the bills when they arrive is often impossible, so a new credit card is used to pay off the old one, until credit runs out. As a nation, we spend more and save less than people in any other industrialized country.

One creative solution for people who cannot control the urge to use their credit card to make purchases, often for things that are not essential, is to freeze your credit. Literally. When you find your credit card balances getting out of hand, place all your credit cards in a large plastic tub of water and put the tub in the freezer. The inaccessibility of the cards is a reminder to curb your purchases. If you really need a credit card, you must take time to thaw them out, which forces you to think about whether you need to make the purchase on credit or not. For many people

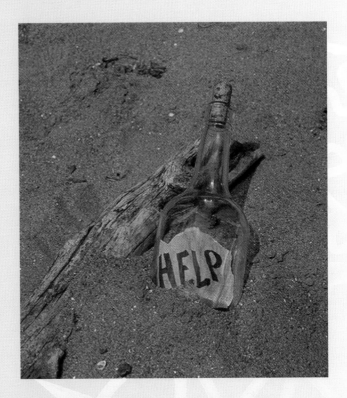

who cannot control their spending, "freezing" their credit has proved helpful.

Describe in your journal whether you get into financial trouble from overspending or buying things you really do not need. Do you think your money troubles ever affect your health? Does "freezing" your credit seem like a good idea?

Wise Consumer: Evaluating Alternative Medicines

More and more people are turning to alternative medicines and therapies, not only to relieve their aches and pains, but for treating serious diseases such as cancer, arthritis, depression, and many others. One problem is that very few doctors can (or are willing to) provide information or advice on the usefulness and safety of alternative medicines. Doctors are not trained to evaluate herbal remedies, massage, acupuncture, dietary interventions, magnetic healing, and hundreds of other alternative medicines. However, millions of people use these alternative medicines and many say they feel some benefit.

If you have used or are thinking of using an alternative medicine, describe in your journal how you arrived at your decision. Did you do any research on the efficacy and safety of the treatment? Was it recommended by a friend? Did you discuss the usefulness of the alternative medicine with a doctor? What do you think is the best way to evaluate whether an alternative medicine works or not?

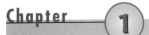

Chapter 1

Explore your own health by completing the following self-assessment as honestly and completely as possible.

Exploring Your Health

How Well Are You?

Complete the following health and wellness inventory to gauge your present degree of wellness. For each of the questions, circle the number

5 if the statement is ALWAYS true
4 if the statement is FREQUENTLY true
3 if the statement is OCCASIONALLY true
2 if the statement is SELDOM true
1 if the statement is NEVER true

1. I am able to identify the situations and factors that overstress me.   5 4 3 2 1
2. I eat only when I am hungry.   5 4 3 2 1
3. I don't take tranquilizers or other drugs to relax.   5 4 3 2 1
4. I support efforts in my community to reduce environmental pollution.   5 4 3 2 1
5. I avoid buying foods with artificial colorings.   5 4 3 2 1
6. I rarely have problems concentrating on what I'm doing because of worrying about other things.   5 4 3 2 1
7. My employer (school) takes measures to ensure that my work (study) place is safe.   5 4 3 2 1
8. I try not to use medications when I feel unwell.   5 4 3 2 1
9. I am able to identify certain bodily responses and illnesses as my reactions to stress.   5 4 3 2 1
10. I question the use of diagnostic X-rays.   5 4 3 2 1
11. I try to change personal habits that are risk factors for heart disease, cancer, and other life-style diseases.   5 4 3 2 1
12. I avoid taking sleeping pills to help me sleep.   5 4 3 2 1
13. I try not to eat foods with refined sugar or corn sugar as ingredients.   5 4 3 2 1
14. I accomplish goals I set for myself.   5 4 3 2 1
15. I stretch or bend for several minutes each day to keep my body flexible.   5 4 3 2 1
16. I support immunization of all children for common childhood diseases.   5 4 3 2 1
17. I try to prevent friends from driving after they drink alcohol.   5 4 3 2 1
18. I minimize my salt intake.   5 4 3 2 1
19. I don't mind when other people and situations make me wait or lose time.   5 4 3 2 1
20. I climb four or fewer flights of stairs rather than take the elevator.   5 4 3 2 1
21. I eat fresh fruits and vegetables.   5 4 3 2 1
22. I use dental floss at least once a day.   5 4 3 2 1
23. I read product labels on foods to determine their ingredients.   5 4 3 2 1
24. I try to maintain a normal body weight.   5 4 3 2 1
25. I record my feelings and thoughts in a journal or diary.   5 4 3 2 1
26. I have no difficulty falling asleep.   5 4 3 2 1
27. I engage in some form of vigorous physical activity at least three times a week.   5 4 3 2 1
28. I take time each day to quiet my mind and relax.   5 4 3 2 1
29. I want to make and sustain close friendships and intimate relationships.   5 4 3 2 1
30. I obtain an adequate daily supply of vitamins from my food or vitamin supplements.   5 4 3 2 1
31. I rarely have tension or migraine headaches or pain in the neck or shoulders.   5 4 3 2 1
32. I wear a safety belt when driving.   5 4 3 2 1
33. I am aware of the emotional and situational factors that lead me to overeat.   5 4 3 2 1
34. I avoid driving my car after drinking any alcohol.   5 4 3 2 1
35. I am aware of the side effects of the medicines I take.   5 4 3 2 1
36. I am able to accept feelings of sadness, depression, and anxiety, realizing that they are almost always transient.   5 4 3 2 1
37. I would seek several additional professional opinions if my doctor recommended surgery for me.   5 4 3 2 1
38. I agree that nonsmokers should not have to breathe the smoke from cigarettes in public places.   5 4 3 2 1
39. I agree that pregnant women who smoke harm their babies.   5 4 3 2 1
40. I feel I get enough sleep.   5 4 3 2 1
41. I ask my doctor why a certain medication is being prescribed and inquire about alternatives.   5 4 3 2 1
42. I am aware of the calories expended in my activities.   5 4 3 2 1
43. I am willing to give priority to my own needs for time and psychological space by saying "no" to others' requests of me.   5 4 3 2 1
44. I walk instead of drive whenever feasible.   5 4 3 2 1
45. I eat a breakfast that contains about one-third of my daily need for calories, proteins, and vitamins.   5 4 3 2 1
46. I prohibit smoking in my home.   5 4 3 2 1
47. I remember and think about my dreams.   5 4 3 2 1
48. I seek medical attention only when I have symptoms or feel that some (potential) condition needs checking, rather than have routine yearly checkups.   5 4 3 2 1

Self-Assessment

Self-Assessment

49. I endeavor to make my home accident-free.   5 4 3 2 1
50. I ask my doctor to explain the diagnosis of my problem until I understand all that I care to.   5 4 3 2 1
51. I try to include fiber or roughage (whole grains, fresh fruits, vegetables, or bran) in my daily diet.   5 4 3 2 1
52. I can deal with my emotional problems without alcohol or other mood-altering drugs.   5 4 3 2 1
53. I am satisfied with my school or job.   5 4 3 2 1
54. I require children riding in my car to be in infant seats or in shoulder harnesses.   5 4 3 2 1
55. I try to associate with people who have a positive attitude about life.   5 4 3 2 1
56. I try not to eat snacks of candy, pastries, and other "junk" foods.   5 4 3 2 1

57. I avoid people who are "down" all the time and who bring down those around them.   5 4 3 2 1
58. I am aware of the calorie content of the foods I eat.   5 4 3 2 1
59. I brush my teeth after meals.   5 4 3 2 1
60. (for women only) I routinely examine my breasts.   5 4 3 2 1
    (for men only) I am aware of the signs of testicular cancer.   5 4 3 2 1

How to Score

Enter the numbers you've circled above next to the question number in the columns below and total your score for each category. Then use the wellness status key to determine your degree of wellness for each category.

Emotional health	Fitness and body care	Environmental health	Stress	Nutrition	Medical self-responsibility
6 ____	15 ____	4 ____	1 ____	2 ____	8 ____
12 ____	20 ____	7 ____	3 ____	5 ____	10 ____
25 ____	22 ____	17 ____	9 ____	13 ____	11 ____
26 ____	24 ____	32 ____	14 ____	18 ____	16 ____
36 ____	27 ____	34 ____	19 ____	21 ____	35 ____
40 ____	33 ____	38 ____	28 ____	23 ____	37 ____
47 ____	42 ____	39 ____	29 ____	30 ____	41 ____
52 ____	44 ____	46 ____	31 ____	45 ____	48 ____
55 ____	58 ____	49 ____	43 ____	51 ____	50 ____
57 ____	59 ____	54 ____	53 ____	56 ____	60 ____
Total ____	Total ____	Total ____	Total ____	Total ____	Total ____

Wellness Status

To assess your status in each of the six categories, compare your total score in each column to the following key: **0–34,** need improvement; **35–44,** good; **45–50,** excellent.

Contracting with Yourself

Based on your wellness status results, make appropriate changes in categories you would like to improve. List the changes you wish to make, set a time to begin making them, and decide when you want the change to be fully integrated into your life.

For example:

Change Desired

- quit smoking
- take up meditation
- record dreams

Begin Change

- in 1 week
- immediately
- after quitting smoking

Time Allotted

- 1 month
- 2 weeks
- 1 week

Do not try to make all the changes on your list at the same time. Begin with either the one or two most important or the one or two you know you can accomplish. Then make one or two changes at a time after that.

Chapter ⑵

Explore your own health by completing the following self-assessment as honestly and completely as possible.

Exploring Your Health

What Are Your Stress Reactions?

Many people experience particular physical reactions to excessive stress. Here's a list of some common stress reactions. Which ones do you frequently experience? Can you add some reactions that are not on the list?

Reaction	Once a day	Once every 2–3 days	Once a week	Once a month	Not in the last 2 months
Headaches	____	____	____	____	____
Nervous tics and twitches	____	____	____	____	____
Blurred vision	____	____	____	____	____
Dizziness	____	____	____	____	____
Fatigue	____	____	____	____	____
Coughing	____	____	____	____	____
Wheezing	____	____	____	____	____
Backache	____	____	____	____	____
Muscle spasms	____	____	____	____	____
Itching	____	____	____	____	____
Excessive sweating	____	____	____	____	____
Palpitations	____	____	____	____	____
Constipation	____	____	____	____	____
Jaw tightening	____	____	____	____	____
Rapid heart rate	____	____	____	____	____
Impotence	____	____	____	____	____
Pelvic pain	____	____	____	____	____
Stomachache	____	____	____	____	____
Diarrhea	____	____	____	____	____
Frequent urination	____	____	____	____	____
Dermatitis (rash)	____	____	____	____	____
Hyperventilation	____	____	____	____	____
Irregular heart rhythm	____	____	____	____	____
High blood pressure	____	____	____	____	____
Delayed menstruation	____	____	____	____	____
Vaginal discharge	____	____	____	____	____
Nail biting	____	____	____	____	____
Heartburn	____	____	____	____	____

Self-Assessment

Self-Assessment

How Susceptible Are You to Stress?

Some persons are more susceptible to the harmful effects of stress than others. The following inventory can give you an indication of your susceptibility. Score each item from 1 (almost always) to 5 (never) as it applies to you. A total score lower than 50 indicates you are not particularly vulnerable to stress. A score of 50 to 80 indicates moderate vulnerability, and a score of more than 80, high vulnerability—time to make some changes.

_____ 1. I eat at least one hot, nutritious meal a day.
_____ 2. I get 7 to 8 hours sleep at least 4 nights a week.
_____ 3. I am affectionate with others regularly.
_____ 4. I have at least one relative within 50 miles on whom I can rely.
_____ 5. I exercise to the point of sweating at least twice a week.
_____ 6. I smoke fewer than 10 cigarettes a day.
_____ 7. I drink fewer than five alcoholic drinks a week.
_____ 8. I am about the proper weight for my height and age.
_____ 9. I have enough money to meet basic expenses and needs.
_____ 10. I feel strengthened by my religious beliefs.
_____ 11. I attend club or social activities on a regular basis.
_____ 12. I have several close friends and acquaintances.
_____ 13. I have one or more friends to confide in about personal matters.
_____ 14. I am basically in good health.
_____ 15. I am able to speak openly about my feelings when angry or worried.
_____ 16. I discuss problems about chores, money, and daily living issues with the people I live with.
_____ 17. I do something just for fun at least once a week.
_____ 18. I am able to organize my time and do not feel pressured.
_____ 19. I drink fewer than three cups of coffee (or tea or cola drinks) a day.
_____ 20. I allow myself quiet time at least once during each day.

TOTAL
SCORE _____

Source: Adapted from a test developed by L. H. Miller and A. D. Smith.

Do You Have "Hurry Sickness"?

Behavior	Almost always	Only sometimes	Almost never
1. Do you interrupt other people before they have finished speaking?	___	___	___
2. Are you irritated when you have to wait in line?	___	___	___
3. Do you eat fast?	___	___	___
4. Do you try to do more than one thing at a time?	___	___	___
5. Are you annoyed if you lose at sports or games?	___	___	___
6. How often do you forget what you were going to say?	___	___	___
7. Do you tap your fingers or bounce your feet while sitting?	___	___	___
8. Do you speed up and drive through yellow caution lights at intersections?	___	___	___
9. Do you race the car engine while waiting for the signal to change?	___	___	___
10. Do you fall behind in the things you need to accomplish?	___	___	___

Here's how to determine your score: If you checked _Almost always,_ give yourself 3 points; if you checked _Only sometimes,_ 2 points; and if _Almost never,_ 1 point. Add up all the points. If you scored 25 to 30, you probably have hurry sickness (don't worry, it's not fatal) and need to work on slowing down or relaxing more. If you scored 16 to 24, you have a potential for hurry syndrome. If you scored less than 16, you are probably pretty laid back.

Chapter ③

Explore your own health by completing the following self-assessment as honestly and completely as possible.

Exploring Your Health

Identify Your Fears or Phobias

Frightening situations or objects	No fear	Mild fear	Strong fear
Airplanes	____	____	____
Birds	____	____	____
Bats	____	____	____
Blood	____	____	____
Cemeteries	____	____	____
Dead animals	____	____	____
Insects	____	____	____
Crowds of people	____	____	____
Dark places	____	____	____
Dentists or doctors	____	____	____
Hospitals	____	____	____
Dirt or germs	____	____	____
Lakes or oceans	____	____	____
Dogs or cats	____	____	____
Other animals	____	____	____
Guns	____	____	____
Closets or elevators	____	____	____
Heights	____	____	____
Public presentations	____	____	____
Loud noises	____	____	____
Driving in a car	____	____	____
Being shouted at	____	____	____
Being rejected	____	____	____
Walking alone at night	____	____	____
Other fears	____	____	____

Self-Assessment

Keep a Sleep and Dream Record

Each morning for 1 week, assess your sleep behavior with the aid of a chart like the one below; also record the details of your dreams in your journal or notebook. Hints for dream recording:

Sleep Assessment Chart

1. Keep a pen or a pencil and a pad of paper near your bed.
2. Remind yourself before going to sleep that you want to remember your dreams.
3. Write down your dreams immediately upon awakening.

	Sun	Mon	Tues	Wed	Thurs	Fri	Sat
Time to bed							
Time fell asleep (estimate on waking)							
Feelings before falling asleep							
Trouble falling asleep? (yes or no)							
Take sleeping aid? (e.g., milk or pills)							
Number of times awake in the night							
Time woke up							
Time arose							
Feelings on awakening							
Dreams? (yes or no)							
Total sleep time							

Chapter 4

Explore your own health by completing the following self-assessment as honestly and completely as possible.

Exploring Your Health

Food Diary

Data Collection

For 2 days, keep a list of *everything* you eat. You should choose days that are representative of your usual food consumption patterns. You should also record the quantity of each food item, the time of day it was consumed, whether consumption was part of meal or a snack, whether you ate because of hunger or for other reasons, your feelings at the time you ate, and the social circumstances surrounding eating (e.g., alone, with friends, family).

Food	Quantity	Time of day	Meal or snack	Hungry? Other?	Feelings?	Social?
cereal	bowlful	6:30 AM	meal	hungry	sleepy	alone
banana	one	"	"	"	"	"
milk, skim	cup	"	"	"	"	"

Data Analysis

Analyze the nutrient content of a representative meal from your food diary.

1. Choose a representative meal.
2. Log on to the Nutritional Analysis Calculator at the University of Illinois and submit your meal for a nutrition analysis. You can find the link to the calculator on the Health and Wellness website.
3. Print out the analysis.
4. Write a one-page paper in which you compare your food intake (the number of servings in each category) with the guidelines offered by the "Food Guide Pyramid" (see pages 63–64).

My Eating Habits: Some Clues to Calories

Calories come from food—all kinds of food. Do you get enough? Or more than you need? Think about your eating patterns—and why you eat what you eat. Check all the answers that describe your eating patterns.

What Do I Usually Eat?

_____ A varied and balanced diet.
_____ A diet with only moderate amounts of fats and sugars.
_____ Deep-fat-fried and breaded foods.
_____ "Extras," such as salad dressings, potato toppings, spreads, sauces, and gravies.
_____ Sweets and rich desserts, such as candies, cakes, and pies.
_____ Snack foods high in fat and sodium, such as chips and other "munchies."
_____ Soft drinks.

When Do I Usually Eat?

_____ At mealtime.
_____ While studying.
_____ While preparing meals or clearing the table.
_____ When spending time with friends.
_____ While watching TV or participating in other activities.
_____ Anytime.

Where Do I Usually Eat?

_____ At home at the kitchen or dining room table.
_____ In the school cafeteria.
_____ In fast-food places.
_____ In front of the TV or while studying.
_____ Wherever I happen to be when I'm hungry.

Why Do I Usually Eat?

_____ It's time to eat.
_____ I'm hungry.
_____ Foods look tempting.
_____ Everyone else is eating.
_____ Food will get thrown away if I don't eat it.
_____ I'm bored or frustrated.

Changes I Want to Make

1. _____

2. _____

3. _____

Source: U.S. Department of Agriculture, *Dietary Guidelines and Your Health: Health Educator's Guide to Nutrition and Fitness* (Washington, D.C.: U.S. Government Printing Office, 1992).

Eat for Good Nutrition

Are you "in action"? Are you ready to stay in shape—for a lifetime? From these statements, check seven sense guidelines for smart eating that can help you stay healthy.

_____ Use salt and sodium only in moderation.
_____ Choose a diet low in fat, saturated fat, and cholesterol.
_____ Avoid snacking.
_____ Eat an apple a day for good health.
_____ Use sugars only in moderation.
_____ Avoid desserts.
_____ Maintain a healthy weight.
_____ Avoid alcoholic beverages.
_____ Eat green vegetables every day.
_____ Avoid candy, chips, and soft drinks.
_____ Choose a diet with plenty of vegetables, fruits, and grain products.
_____ Eat a variety of foods.
_____ Avoid fast foods.

I want to follow the dietary guidelines so I stay healthy. Here's how I'll eat smart:

_____

_____

_____

_____

_____

_____

SIGNED _____

DATE _____

Source: U.S. Department of Agriculture, Dietary Guidelines and Your Health: Health Educator's Guide to Nutrition and Fitness (Washington, D.C.: U.S. Government Printing Office, 1992).

How Does Your Diet Rate for Variety?

A varied diet is a healthful diet. How would you describe the variety in your food choices?

How often do you eat:	Seldom or never	1 or 2 times a week	3 to 4 times a week	Almost daily
1. At least six servings of breads, cereals, rice, crackers, pasta, or other foods made from grains (a serving is one slice of bread or a half cup cereal or rice) per day?	□	□	□	□
2. Foods made from whole grains?	□	□	□	□
3. Three different kinds of vegetables per day?	□	□	□	□
4. Cooked dry beans or peas?	□	□	□	□
5. A dark-green vegetable, such as spinach or broccoli?	□	□	□	□
6. Two kinds of fruit or fruit juice per day?	□	□	□	□
7. Three servings of milk, yogurt, or cheese per day?	□	□	□	□
8. Two servings of lean meat, poultry, or fish, or eggs, dry beans, or nuts per day?	□	□	□	□

Count the number of check marks in each column.   TOTAL   _____   _____   _____   _____

To eat a varied diet, I will _____

_____

Chapter (5)

Explore your own health by completing the following self-assessment as honestly and completely as possible.

Exploring Your Health

What Are Your Weight Statistics?

Fill in the blanks below.

Your height in inches
(without shoes) _____ inches (multiply by .0254 = _____ meters)

Your weight (with
clothes) _____ pounds (divide by 2.2 = _____ kilograms)

Highest adult weight _____ pounds, when age_____

Lowest adult weight _____ pounds, when age_____

Recommended weight for height (see page 89) _____

Body mass index (see page 89) _____ Divide your weight (in kilograms)
by your height (in meters, squared)

Body Image

How do you feel about the appearance of these regions of your body?

	Quite satisfied	Somewhat satisfied	Somewhat dissatisfied	Very dissatisfied
Hair	☐	☐	☐	☐
Arms	☐	☐	☐	☐
Hands	☐	☐	☐	☐
Feet	☐	☐	☐	☐
Waist	☐	☐	☐	☐
Buttocks	☐	☐	☐	☐
Hips	☐	☐	☐	☐
Legs and ankles	☐	☐	☐	☐
Thighs	☐	☐	☐	☐
Chest or breasts	☐	☐	☐	☐
Posture	☐	☐	☐	☐
General attractiveness	☐	☐	☐	☐

1. Which of your thoughts and actions enhance your body image?

_____

2. Which of your thoughts and actions are detrimental to your body image?

_____

3. What societal forces (expectations of friends and parents, advertising, celebrities and professional athletes, etc.) influence your body image most strongly?

_____

4. What could you do to become more satisfied with your body image?

_____

Self-Assessment

Chapter **6**

Explore your own health by completing the following self-assessment as honestly and completely as possible.

Self-Assessment

Exploring Your Health

Determine Your Fitness Index

The Harvard Step Test is a standardized measure of cardiorespiratory fitness. To carry out the Harvard Step Test, you need to be comfortably dressed (athletic clothes are best); and you need a chair, stool, or bench 12 to 18 inches high, a stopwatch or clock with a second hand, a pencil and paper, and a metronome or some other method to produce a rhythmic 100 to 120 beats per minute, such as a recording of a march or some disco music. Once all this is assembled, you can begin.

1. Make a 15-second recording of your resting pulse and multiply by 4 to obtain your heartbeat rate per minute.

2. Start the metronome or music at 120 beats per minute.

3. Step completely up on the bench with the left leg first, followed by your right leg, then step back down with the left leg first, followed by the right. The stepping should be done on a four-count: up-up-down-down; up-up-down-down . . .

4. Continue the exercise for 3 minutes unless you are over 30 years old and have been rather inactive for more than 6 months. In that case, do the test for only a minute or two, whichever you think you can do. If you are sure you cannot do the test for even a few seconds, don't.

5. When the 3 minutes of exercise are through, immediately take your pulse. Record the number of heartbeats between 15 and 30 seconds after exercising. Make additional heart rate measurements between 60 and 75 seconds, 120 and 135 seconds, 180 and 195 seconds, 240 and 255 seconds, and a final measurement between 300 and 315 seconds.

6. Multiply each of the 15-second heart rates by 4 to give the beats per minute. Record your data on a graph below.

7. Compute your fitness index: Add the per-minute heart rates for the first 3 minutes after exercise. Then divide that number into 30,000.

Fitness index	Rating
Above 90	Excellent
80–89	Good
65–79	Average
55–64	Low Average
Below 55	Poor

Determine Your Flexibility Index

Body flexibility is a fundamental aspect of feeling good and keeping your body young. Use this simple YMCA test to determine your degree of body flexibility, and continue to use it to determine your progress in becoming more limber. You can consult exercise and yoga books to find exercises that will help you improve your flexibility.

1. Warm up with some stretching before the test.

2. Sit on the floor with your legs extended and feet a few inches apart.

3. With a piece of adhesive tape, mark the place where your heels touch the floor. Your heels should touch the near edge of the tape.

4. Place a yardstick on the floor between your legs and parallel to them. The beginning of the yardstick should be closest to you and the 15-inch mark should align with the near edge of the tape.

5. Slowly reach with both hands as far forward as possible. Touch your fingers to the yardstick to determine the distance reached. Do not jerk to increase your distance—this may cause damage to your leg muscles.

6. Repeat the exercise two or three times and record your best score.

Inches reached		Rating
Men	Women	
22–23	24–27	Excellent
20–21	21–23	Good
14–19	16–20	Average
12–13	13–15	Fair
0–11	0–12	Poor

Harvard Step Test data record			
Time	Heartbeats per 15 seconds		Heartbeats per minute
At rest	_____	× 4 =	_____
15–30 sec	_____	× 4 =	_____
60–75 sec	_____	× 4 =	_____
120–135 sec	_____	× 4 =	_____
180–195 sec	_____	× 4 =	_____
240–255 sec	_____	× 4 =	_____
300–315 sec	_____	× 4 =	_____

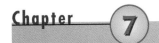

Chapter 7

Explore your own health by completing the following self-assessment as honestly and completely as possible.

Exploring Your Health

An Assessment of Sexual Communication

Communication skills contribute to rewarding relationships in many ways. Many of the problems couples experience could be avoided or easily resolved with more effective communication skills. How are your communication skills? For each statement, circle the appropriate number of points.

	Usually	Sometimes	Seldom
1. I find it easy to express my nonsexual needs and feelings to others.	2	1	0
2. I find it easy to express my sexual needs and feelings to others.	2	1	0
3. I am sensitive to the needs and feelings expressed by others, and especially their nonverbal expressions.	2	1	0
4. My relationships with other people are pleasant and rewarding.	2	1	0
5. When a conflict arises in one of my relationships, it is resolved with ease.	2	1	0
6. I find it easy to communicate with people of both genders.	2	1	0
7. I can communicate effectively with people of various ethnic groups.	2	1	0
8. I can find the right words to express the ideas I want to convey.	2	1	0
9. I am good at interpreting nonverbal messages from other people.	2	1	0
10. I try very hard not to interrupt someone who is speaking to me.	2	1	0
11. I try very hard to be nonjudgmental in my responses when people share their ideas and feelings with me.	2	1	0
12. When a discussion is causing me to feel uncomfortable, I try hard not to withdraw from the discussion or change the subject.	2	1	0
13. I try to help people open up by asking open-ended, rather than yes-or-no questions.	2	1	0
14. When I want to express my feelings, I try to phrase them as "I" statements, rather than "you" statements.	2	1	0
15. I feel that I am adequately assertive.	2	1	0
16. I let someone know when they are not respecting my rights or feelings.	2	1	0
17. I find it easy to say no to pressure for unwanted sexual activity.	2	1	0
18. I find it easy to talk to a potential sexual partner about prevention of sexually transmitted diseases.	2	1	0
19. When conflicts arise in my relationships, I am, if necessary, willing and able to make a compromise to resolve the conflict.	2	1	0
20. When conflicts arise in my relationships, I try to find a resolution that satisfies the needs of both persons involved.	2	1	0

TOTAL POINTS: _____

Interpretation:

36 to 40 points: You have developed highly effective patterns of communication and assertiveness.

32 to 35 points: You have above-average communication and assertiveness skills.

28 to 31 points: You have about average communication and assertiveness skills. Sharpening these skills will improve your relationships and need fulfillment.

27 points or less: It would be very rewarding for you to improve your communication skills. Your relationships would function much better, and you would experience much greater need fulfillment.

Source: Byer, C. O., Shainberg, L. W. & Galliano, G. (1999). *Dimensions of Human Sexuality.* Boston, MA: McGraw-Hill College, p. 68. Reproduced with permission of The McGraw-Hill Companies.

Self-Assessment

Gender Roles and Society

Purpose: This inventory will aid you in becoming aware of your attitudes toward stereotypical masculine and feminine roles in society. The views of many people in regard to these traditional roles are changing but not necessarily in the same way. Therefore, it is important that you understand your own values as well as the values of those with whom you interact.

Directions: Read each statement carefully and respond by using the scale given below. Use the first column of blanks for your own responses. Then use a sheet of paper to cover your responses and have your partner or friend use the second column of blanks to respond to the statements.

You	Friend	Strongly agree 1	Agree 2	Disagree 3	Strongly disagree 4

____ ____ 1. Men should feel comfortable receiving flowers from a woman.

____ ____ 2. Women should take the steps necessary to prevent pregnancy, as contraception is the woman's responsibility.

____ ____ 3. The woman's role is to stay home, take care of the children, and support her husband in his work; the man's role is to support the family financially.

____ ____ 4. A man should be open to relocating because of his wife's job, regardless of whose salary is higher.

____ ____ 5. Men should be expected to stand when a woman enters the room and to open doors for women.

____ ____ 6. Men and women should share equally in the role of decision maker in the home.

____ ____ 7. Women should pay their half of the expenses on dates.

____ ____ 8. Women should be able to ask men for dates.

____ ____ 9. A woman who pursues a career cannot be a good mother.

____ ____ 10. Men should be free to express their emotions as openly as women do.

____ ____ 11. Women should be free to initiate the sex act.

____ ____ 12. Education is equally important for husband and wife.

____ ____ 13. Only men should be drafted into the army.

____ ____ 14. Society discriminates against women in certain occupations.

____ ____ 15. Society discriminates against men in certain occupations.

____ ____ 16. Parents should allow their sons to play with dolls.

____ ____ 17. A woman should be free to pursue whatever interest or career she would like, as long as it does not inconvenience her husband.

____ ____ 18. Girls should be raised feeling proud to say that their vocation is wife and mother.

____ ____ 19. The movement toward desexualization in clothes, jobs, recreation, and education is dangerous.

____ ____ 20. Maternal and nurturing feelings are instinctive only to women.

____ ____ 21. Men are sexual, women are productive.

____ ____ 22. Boys play at love when what they desire is sex, and girls play at sex when they desire love.

____ ____ 23. Married women should feel comfortable keeping their maiden names.

____ ____ 24. Men stand to gain just as much from the women's movement as women do.

____ ____ 25. The ideal couple should go everywhere together.

____ ____ 26. Women should be allowed to serve in combat in the armed forces.

Reactions: Use the space provided to respond to the following questions.

1. For which statements were your responses different from those of your partner?

2. After discussing the differences in your responses, decide if these are potential problem areas. Explain why or why not.

3. Discuss whether you feel your beliefs regarding these statements are the same as most people your age.

Source: Valois, R.F. & Kammerman, S. (1992). *Your Sexuality* (2nd ed.). New York, NY: McGraw-Hill, 4–6. Reproduced with permission of The McGraw-Hill Companies.

Chapter

8

Explore your own health by completing the following self-assessment as honestly and completely as possible.

Exploring Your Health

Contraceptive Comfort and Confidence Scale

In assessing your answers to these questions, you will be helping yourself decide whether the method of control you are using or considering is a realistic choice. (Members of a couple should answer these questions separately.)

Method of birth control you are considering using: _____
Length of time you used this method in the past: _____

Check **Yes** or **No** for each of the following questions:	Yes	No
1. Have I had problems using this method before?	____	____
2. Have I or my partner ever become pregnant while using this method?	____	____
3. Am I afraid of using this method?	____	____
4. Would I really rather not use this method?	____	____
5. Will I or my partner have trouble remembering to use this method?	____	____
6. Will I or my partner have trouble using this method correctly?	____	____
7. Do I still have unanswered questions about this method?	____	____
8. Does this method make menstrual periods longer or more painful?	____	____
9. Does this method cost more than I can afford?	____	____
10. Could this method cause me or my partner to have serious complications?	____	____
11. Am I opposed to this method because of my religious or moral beliefs?	____	____
12. Is my partner opposed to this method?	____	____
13. Am I using this method without my partner's knowledge?	____	____
14. Will using this method embarrass my partner?	____	____
15. Will using this method embarrass me?	____	____
16. Will I or my partner enjoy intercourse less because of this method?	____	____
17. If this method interrupts lovemaking, will I avoid it?	____	____
18. Has a nurse or physician ever told me or my partner NOT to use this method?	____	____
19. Is there anything about my or my partner's personality that could lead me or my partner to use this method incorrectly?	____	____
20. Am I or is my partner at risk of being exposed to HIV or another STD if I use or my partner uses this method?	____	____

Most persons will have a few "yes" answers. "Yes" answers mean that problems might arise. If you have more than a few "yes" responses, you may want to talk with a physician, counselor, partner, or friend to help you decide whether to use this method or how to use it so that it will really be effective for you. In general, the more "yes" answers you have, the less likely you are to use this method consistently and correctly at every act of intercourse.

Source: Byer, C. O., Shainberg, L. W., & Galliano, G. (1999). *Dimensions of Human Sexuality.* Boston, MA: McGraw-Hill College, p. 455. Reproduced with permission of The McGraw-Hill Companies.

Self-Assessment

Self-Assessment

Exploring Your Health

Knowledge of STIs

In response to each infectious disease/concept, circle the number that best represents your current knowledge.

Key:
1. I have never heard of this.
2. I have heard of it, but don't really know what it means.
3. I have some idea of what this means, but it's vague.
4. I have a clear idea what this is and can explain it.

Infectious disease/concept	Never heard of it	Don't really know	Vague idea	Clear idea
Ways that HIV can be transmitted	1	2	3	4
Indicator or opportunistic diseases related to AIDS	1	2	3	4
Testing for HIV	1	2	3	4
Treatment for AIDS	1	2	3	4
AIDS Antibody Test	1	2	3	4
Preventing transmission of HIV	1	2	3	4
Syphilis	1	2	3	4
Chlamydia	1	2	3	4
Gonorrhea	1	2	3	4
Genital warts	1	2	3	4
Herpes infections	1	2	3	4
Trichomoniasis	1	2	3	4
Yeast infection	1	2	3	4
Prevention of other sexually transmitted infections	1	2	3	4

Chapter **9**

Explore your own health by completing the following self-assessment as honestly and completely as possible.

Self-Assessment

Exploring Your Health

Are You Current on All Your Vaccines?

Adult Vaccination Schedules

Vaccine	Indication	Precautions and contraindications
Bacille Calmette-Guérin	Debatable benefits for adults at high risk of multiple drug-resistant tuberculosis	Immunocompromised
Hæmophilus influanzae type B	Patients with splenic dysfunction, other at-risk conditions	Safety in pregnancy unknown
Hepatitis A	Adults at increased risk, e.g., travelers to endemic areas, gay men, injecting drug users, day care workers	Pregnancy risk not fully evaluated
Hepatitis B	Healthcare workers in contact with blood, persons residing for ≥ 6 months in areas of high endemicity, others at high risk	Safety to fetus unknown, pregnancy not a contraindication in high-risk persons
Influenza	Adults with high-risk conditions, healthy persons ≥ 65 years, health care personnel	Anaphylaxis in response to eggs, first trimester of pregnancy (relative contraindication)
Measles	Adults born after 1956 without measles (diagnosed by a physician or immunologic test) or live-virus immunization, for revaccination of persons given killed measles vaccine (1963–1967)	Pregnancy, immunocompromised, history of anaphylaxis to eggs or neomycin
Meningococcal polysaccharide	Travel to areas with epidemic meningococcal disease	Safety in pregnancy unknown
Mumps	Susceptible adults	Pregnancy, immunocompromised, history of anaphylaxis in response to eggs or neomycin
Pneumococcal polysaccharide	Persons at increased risk of pneumococcal disease and its complications, healthy adults ≥ 65 years	Safety in pregnancy unknown
Polio (inactivated)	Preferred for ≥ 18-year-olds for primary immunization; one-time booster dose for travelers	Safety to fetus unknown, anaphylactic reactions to streptomycin or neomycin
Polio (oral)	One-time booster for previously immunized persons, completion of the series in partially immunized adults, alternative to inactivated polio vaccine when there is < 1 month before travel, not used for primary immunization in persons ≥ 18 years	Immunocompromised host or contact
Rubella	Susceptible adults, particularly women of childbearing age	Pregnancy, immunocompromised, history of anaphylactic reaction to neomycin
Tetanus-diphtheria	Adults	First trimester of pregnancy, hypersensitivity or neurologic reaction to previous doses, severe local reaction
Varicella	Susceptible adolescents and adults, especially health care workers and others likely to be exposed	Pregnancy, immunocompromised

Source: Adapted in part from data of the Centers for Disease Control and Prevention.

Chapter 10

Explore your own health by completing the following self-assessment as honestly and completely as possible.

Self-Assessment

Exploring Your Health

Testing For Risk of Heart Disease

Total the Points for All Your Risk Factors from the Tables Below

Age	
HDL Cholesterol	+
Total Cholesterol	+
Syst. Blood Press.	+
Cigarette Smoker	+
Diabetes	+
LVH	+
POINT TOTAL	+

Note: Add plus points and subtract minus points

Age Risk

Find the Points that Correspond to Your Age			
Men		Women	
Age	Points	Age	Points
30	−2	≤30	−12
31	−1	31	−11
32–33	0	32	−9
34	1	33	−8
35–36	2	34	−6
37–38	3	35	−5
39	4	36	−4
40–41	5	37	−3
42–43	6	38	−2
44–45	7	39	−1
46–47	8	40	0
48–49	9	41	1
50–51	10	42–43	2
52–54	11	44	3
55–56	12	45–46	4
57–59	13	47–48	5
60–61	14	49–50	6
62–64	15	51–52	7
65–67	16	53–55	8
68–70	17	56–60	9
71–73	18	61–67	10
74	19	68–74	11

Blood Lipid Risks

HDL Cholesterol		Total Cholesterol	
HDL	Points	Total	Points
25–26	7	139–151	−3
27–29	6	152–166	−2
30–32	5	167–182	−1
33–35	4	183–199	0
36–38	3	200–219	1
39–42	2	220–239	2
43–46	1	240–262	3
47–50	0	263–288	4
51–55	−1	289–315	5
56–60	−2	316–330	6
61–66	−3		
67–73	−4		
74–80	−5		
81–87	−6		
88–96	−7		

Blood Pressure Risks

Systolic Blood Pressure	
SBP	Points
98–104	−2
105–112	−1
113–120	0
121–129	1
130–139	2
140–149	3
150–160	4
161–172	5
173–185	8

Other Risks

Factor	Points
Cigarette smoker	4
Diabetic male	3
Diabetic female	6
Left ventricular hypertrophy (LVH)	9

Measure the Risk Corresponding to Your Point Total

	Probability of developing heart disease	
Points	5-Yr. Risk	10-Yr. Risk
1 or less	Less than 1%	Less than 2%
2	1%	2%
3	1%	2%
4	1%	2%
5	1%	3%
6	1%	3%
7	1%	4%
8	2%	4%
9	2%	5%
10	2%	6%
11	3%	6%
12	3%	7%
13	3%	8%
14	4%	9%
15	5%	10%
16	5%	12%
17	6%	13%
18	7%	14%
19	8%	16%
20	8%	18%
21	9%	19%
22	11%	21%
23	12%	23%
24	13%	25%
25	14%	27%
26	16%	29%
27	17%	31%
28	19%	33%
29	20%	36%
30	22%	38%
31	24%	40%
32	25%	42%

Compare Your Risk to 10-Year Average Risks for U.S. Population

	Average 10-year risks	
Age	Women	Men
30–34	less than 1%	3%
35–39	less than 1%	5%
40–44	2%	6%
45–49	5%	10%
50–54	8%	14%
55–59	12%	16%
60–64	13%	21%
65–69	9%	30%
70–74	12%	24%

Copyright 1998 CSPI. Reprinted/Adapted from *Nutrition Action Healthletter* (1875 Connecticut Ave., N.W., Suite 300, Washington DC 20009-5728. $24.00 for 10 issues.).

Self-Assessment

Chapter 11

Explore your own health by completing the following self-assessment as honestly and completely as possible.

Exploring Your Health

The Drugs You Take

Keep a list of all the nonessential drugs that you ingest for a week. Be sure to include coffee, tea, and cola drinks (which contain caffeine); alcohol; nicotine; and pain relievers. After the first week, look at your list. Are you surprised by how many of these nonessential drugs you use? Now, keep the list for another week, but eliminate just one of the nonessential drugs that you ingest and make notes about how you feel.

Week 1	Sun	Mon	Tues	Wed	Thurs	Fri	Sat
Caffeine (How many cups of coffee or 12-oz. servings of cola drinks per day?)							
Alcohol (How many 12-oz. beers, glasses of wine, or mixed drinks per day?)							
Nicotine (How many cigarettes, cigars, pipes, or dips of snuff or chewing tobacco per day?)							
Pain relievers (How many tablets per day?)							
Other:							
Other:							

Week 2	Sun	Mon	Tues	Wed	Thurs	Fri	Sat
Caffeine (How many cups of coffee or 12-oz. servings of cola drinks per day?)							
Alcohol (How many 12-oz. beers, glasses of wine, or mixed drinks per day?)							
Nicotine (How many cigarettes, cigars, pipes, or dips of snuff or chewing tobacco per day?)							
Pain relievers (How many tablets per day?)							
Other:							
Other:							

Self-Assessment

Be a Knowledgeable Consumer

If you are taking a prescribed drug, consult the library or your pharmacist or physician to find out any side effects and contraindications of the drug.

Drug	Side Effects	Contraindications

1. Evaluate the risks of taking the drug in relationship to its therapeutic benefits.

2. Discuss with your physician ways to deal with your medical needs without the use of drugs.

Self-Assessment

Chapter 12

Explore your own health by completing the following self-assessment as honestly and completely as possible.

Exploring Your Health

Why Do You Smoke?

Here are some statements made by people to describe what they get out of smoking cigarettes. How often do you feel this way when smoking? Circle one number for each statement.

Important: Answer every question.

	Always	Frequently	Occasionally	Seldom	Never
A. I smoke cigarettes in order to keep myself from slowing down.	5	4	3	2	1
B. Handling a cigarette is part of the enjoyment of smoking it.	5	4	3	2	1
C. Smoking cigarettes is pleasant and relaxing.	5	4	3	2	1
D. I light up a cigarette when I feel angry about something.	5	4	3	2	1
E. When I have run out of cigarettes I find it almost unbearable until I can get them.	5	4	3	2	1
F. I smoke cigarettes automatically without even being aware of it.	5	4	3	2	1
G. I smoke cigarettes to stimulate me, to perk myself up.	5	4	3	2	1
H. Part of the enjoyment of smoking a cigarette comes from the steps I take to light up.	5	4	3	2	1
I. I find cigarettes pleasurable.	5	4	3	2	1
J. When I feel uncomfortable or upset about something, I light up a cigarette.	5	4	3	2	1
K. I am very much aware of the fact when I am not smoking a cigarette.	5	4	3	2	1
L. I light up a cigarette without realizing I still have one burning in the ashtray.	5	4	3	2	1
M. I smoke cigarettes to give me a "lift."	5	4	3	2	1
N. When I smoke a cigarette, part of the enjoyment is watching the smoke as I exhale it.	5	4	3	2	1
O. I want a cigarette most when I am comfortable and relaxed.	5	4	3	2	1
P. When I feel "blue" or want to take my mind off cares and worries, I smoke cigarettes.	5	4	3	2	1
Q. I get a real gnawing hunger for a cigarette when I haven't smoked for a while.	5	4	3	2	1
R. I've found a cigarette in my mouth and didn't remember putting it there.	5	4	3	2	1

How to Score

1. Enter the numbers you have circled in the spaces below, putting the number you have circled to Question A over line A, to Question B over line B, etc.

2. Add the three scores on each line to get your totals. For example, the sum of your scores over lines A, G, and M gives you your score on *Stimulation*, lines B, H, and N give the score on *Handling*, and so on.

			Totals
A + G + M =			Stimulation
B + H + N =			Handling
C + I + O =			Pleasurable relaxation
D + J + P =			Crutch; tension reduction
E + K + Q =			Craving: psychological addiction
F + L + R =			Habit

Scores of 11 or above indicate that this factor is an important source of satisfaction for the smoker. Scores of 7 or less are low and probably indicate that this factor does not apply to you. Scores in between are marginal.

Source: Smoker's Self-Testing Kit developed by Daniel Horn, Ph.D. Originally published by National Clearinghouse for Smoking and Health, Department of Health, Education, and Welfare.

Do You Have a Drinking Problem?

This questionnaire is designed to help you determine whether you have a problem with alcohol. Answer each question yes or no and record your choice in the right-hand column.

		Yes	No
1.	Do you feel you are a normal drinker?	___	___
2.	Have you ever awakened the morning after drinking the night before and found that you could not remember a part of the evening before?	___	___
3.	Does your wife, husband, a parent, or other near relative ever worry or complain about your drinking?	___	___
4.	Can you stop drinking without a struggle after one or two drinks?	___	___
5.	Do you ever feel bad about your drinking?	___	___
6.	Do friends or relatives think you are a normal drinker?	___	___
7.	Do you ever try to limit your drinking to certain times of the day or to certain places?	___	___
8.	Are you always able to stop drinking when you want to?	___	___
9.	Have you ever attended a meeting of Alcoholics Anonymous?	___	___
10.	Have you gotten into fights when drinking?	___	___
11.	Has drinking ever created problems between you and your wife, husband, boyfriend, girlfriend, a parent, or other near relative?	___	___
12.	Has your wife, husband, boyfriend, girlfriend, a parent, or other near relative ever gone to anyone for help about your drinking?	___	___
13.	Have you ever lost friends because of drinking?	___	___
14.	Have you ever gotten into trouble at work because of drinking?	___	___
15.	Have you ever lost a job because of drinking?	___	___
16.	Have you ever neglected your obligations, your family, or your work for two or more days in a row because you were drinking?	___	___
17.	Do you drink before noon fairly often?	___	___
18.	Have you ever been told you have liver trouble? Cirrhosis?	___	___
19.	After heavy drinking have you ever had delirium tremens (DT's) or severe shaking?	___	___
20.	After heavy drinking have you ever heard voices or seen things that weren't really there?	___	___
21.	Have you ever gone to anyone for help about your drinking?	___	___
22.	Have you ever been in a hospital because of drinking?	___	___
23.	Have you ever been a patient in a psychiatric hospital or in a psychiatric ward of a general hospital?	___	___
24.	Have you ever been in a hospital to be "dried out" (detoxified) because of drinking?	___	___
25.	Have you ever been in jail, even for a few hours, because of drunk behavior?	___	___

Scoring: Item keying for alcoholic responses are 1. N; 2. Y; 3. Y; 4. N; 5. Y; 6. N; 7. Y; 8. N; 9–25, Y.

To score, add one point for each alcoholic response. The total score is the number of alcoholic responses.

No. of Alcoholic Responses	*Interpretation*
0–2	No problem with alcohol
3–5	Early warning signs that drinking is becoming problematic
6 or more	Problem drinker/alcoholic

If you think you have a drinking problem, seek professional help.

Chapter ⬤13

Explore your own health by completing the following self-assessment as honestly and completely as possible.

Self-Assessment

Exploring Your Health

Crime Prevention Tips

Be street wise and safe:

- Stand tall and walk confidently. Watch where you're going and what's happening around you.
- Stick to well-lit and busy streets. Walk with friends. Avoid shortcuts through a dark alley or deserted street.
- If harassed from a car, walk quickly or run in the opposite direction to safety. If you are really scared, scream.
- Never hitchhike. Accept rides only from people you know and trust.
- Don't flash your cash. Always have *emergency* change for a telephone call.
- Know your neighborhood. What hours are stores and restaurants open? Where are the police and fire stations, libraries, and schools? You might need them in an emergency.
- If you go out for a late night snack or a midnight movie, take a friend. Don't go alone. Most assaults happen to a lone victim.
- Let someone know where you are going and when you will come back. Call if you're going to be late.
- If you are driving, park your car in well-lit places and lock it when you leave. Check for uninvited passengers in the back seat or on the floor before you get in.
- Have your keys in hand when approaching your car. Don't wait until you get to the car to look for your keys.
- Alter your routine. Change daily patterns and, if possible, take different routes to work or to school. Park in different locations.

When jogging or bicycling:

- Go with a friend and take familiar and well-traveled routes.
- Don't jog or bike at night.
- Try it without your stereo headphones. It's safer to remain alert to what's around and behind you.

If you are the victim of a crime:

- If someone attacks you, try not to panic. Look at the attacker carefully so you can give a good description to the police. Try to remember key things like age, race, complexion, body build, clothing, height and weight, hair, eyes, or unusual features.
- Report all crimes to your local police. For life-threatening emergencies, call 911.
- If the attacker has a weapon and only wants your money or possessions, don't fight. Your life and safety are more important.
- If you're harassed by a gang, go to an open store, gas station, firehouse, or anywhere there are people present.

Source: Courtesy of the Columbus, Ohio, Police Department, 1998.

Prevention of Intentional Injury

Answer yes or no to the following questions.

1. I have guns in my home.	Y	N
If yes, are they stored safely?	Y	N
When used, are they always used safely?	Y	N
2. I am involved in an abusive relationship.	Y	N
3. I live in a heavy-crime area.	Y	N
4. I abuse alcohol or other drugs.	Y	N
5. I work in a high-risk job.	Y	N
6. I clearly communicate my intentions and boundaries in a dating situation.	Y	N
7. I know, and have immediate access to, emergency phone numbers.	Y	N
8. I have sources of personal support.	Y	N
9. I know the warning signs of suicide.	Y	N
10. I know resources for mental health counseling in my community.	Y	N

Based on your responses to the questions above, are there behaviors or situations in your life that need to be addressed? If so, what are they?

_____

_____

_____

_____

_____

What concerns do you have, both as an individual and a member of your community, related to intentional injury and death?

_____

_____

_____

_____

_____

Source: Birch and Creary, *Managing Your Health: Assessment and Action,* © 1996 by Jones and Bartlett Publishers, Inc.

Chapter 14

Explore your own health by completing the following self-assessment as honestly and completely as possible.

Self-Assessment

Exploring Your Health

Intelligent Health Consumer Profile

This exercise can help determine the extent to which consumers act intelligently when exposed to misleading and inaccurate information, health fraud, and health quackery. Place an X in the column to the right that best represents your answer:

	VM	M	S	L	N
Are you sufficiently informed to be able to make sound decisions?					
Where do you go for information when needed?					
Professional health organizations or individuals					
Health books, magazines, newsletters					
Government health agencies					
Advertisements					
Newspapers or magazines					
Radio or television					
People you know					
To what extent do you accept statements appearing in news reports or advertisements at face value?					
To what extent can you identify quacks, quackery, fraudulent schemes, and hucksters?					
When selecting health practitioners to what extent do you:					
Talk with or visit before first appointment					
Check or inquire regarding qualifications or credentials					
Ask friend or neighbor about reputation					
Inquire about fees and payment procedures					
When you have been exposed to a fraudulent practice, quack, quackery, or a poor product or service, to what extent do you report your experience?					

Key: VM = very much; *M* = much; *S* = some; *L* = little; *N* = none.

Source: H. J. Cornacchia and S. Barrett, *Consumer Health: A Guide to Intelligent Decisions*, 5th ed. (St. Louis, MO: Mosby, 1993), p. 11.

Alternative Therapies Checklist

The decision to use alternative treatments is an important one. The following topics should be considered before selecting an alternative therapy—the safety and effectiveness of the therapy or treatment, the expertise and qualifications of the health care practitioner, and the quality of the service delivery. Consider these when selecting any practitioner or therapy.

Assess the Safety and Effectiveness of the Therapy

Generally, *safety* means that the benefits outweigh the risks of a treatment or therapy. A safe product or practice is one that does no harm when used under defined conditions and as intended.

Effectiveness is the likelihood of benefit from a practice, treatment, or technology applied under typical conditions by the average practitioner for the average patient.

Examine the Practitioner's Expertise

Health consumers may want to take a close look into the background, qualifications, and competence of any potential health care practitioner, whether a physician or a practitioner of alternative health care.

This can be accomplished by contacting a state or local regulatory agency with authority over practitioners who practice the therapy or treatment you want. However, the practice of alternative medicine is usually not as regulated as the practice of conventional medicine. So, it may be helpful to talk both with other health practitioners and with patients who have had experience with the practitioner you are considering. Find out whether there have ever been any complaints from patients. Finally, talk to the practitioner in person. Find out how open the practitioner is to communicating with patients about technical aspects of methods, possible side effects, and potential problems.

Consider the Service Delivery

The quality of the service delivery, or how the treatment or therapy is given and under what conditions, is an important issue. However, quality of service is not necessarily related to the effectiveness or safety of a treatment or practice.

Visit the practitioner's office, clinic, or hospital. Ask the practitioner how many patients are typically seen in a day or week and how much time is spent with each patient. Look at the conditions in the office or clinic. Consider whether the service delivery adheres to regulated standards for medical safety and care.

Consider the Costs

Costs are an important factor to consider, because many alternative treatments are not currently reimbursed by health insurance. Many patients pay directly for these services. Ask your practitioner and your health insurer which treatments or therapies are reimbursable. Also, find out what several practitioners charge for the same treatment to assess the appropriateness of costs.

Consult your Health Care Provider

Most importantly, discuss all issues concerning treatments and therapies with your health care provider, whether a physician or practitioner of alternative medicine. A complete picture of your treatment plan requires knowledge of both conventional and alternative therapies you are undergoing.

Chapter (15)

Explore your own health by completing the following self-assessment as honestly and completely as possible.

Exploring Your Health

A Simple Test for Loss of Cognitive Function

Forgetting a person's name or an appointment is not a sign that you are "losing your mind." Loss of cognitive function as a result of disease or injury can prevent a person from answering even simple questions. Following is a simple test to determine loss of some cognitive functions Score 1 point for each correct answer. Most older persons score at least 17 points out of a possible 19 points.

- Name the season, year, date, month, and day.   (5 answers)
- Name three objects that you see.   (3 answers)
- Name the last five letters of the alphabet backwards.   (5 answers)
- Repeat the sentence: "No ifs, ands, or buts."   (3 answers)
- Repeat the three objects that you mentioned before.   (3 answers)

Chapter 16

Explore your own health by completing the following self-assessment as honestly and completely as possible.

Self-Assessment

Exploring Your Health

How Do You Score on Environmental Awareness?

Circle the number that is your most appropriate response to each question.

Do you use pesticides in the house to kill insects, such as ants, roaches, or flies?

1. Frequently
2. Occasionally
3. Almost never

Do you use pesticides or herbicides around the garden and yard to kill insects and weeds?

1. Frequently
2. Occasionally
3. Almost never

Do you recycle newspapers or other kinds of paper?

1. Almost never
2. Sometimes
3. Regularly

Do you recycle bottles, cans, or plastics?

1. Hardly ever recycle these items
2. Some of these items sometimes
3. Most of the items regularly

When you go on a picnic or hike do you pack out and dispose of all trash in proper trash receptacles?

1. Very infrequently
2. Sometimes
3. All of the time

If you need to run an errand that is less than a half mile away, do you walk or bike instead of drive?

1. Almost never
2. Occasionally
3. Most of the time

Do you conserve electricity by turning off unneeded lights and by not running appliances when you don't really need to (like the air conditioner)?

1. Hardly ever
2. Some of the time
3. Almost always

Do you make an effort to conserve water when showering, flushing, washing the car, etc.?

1. Almost never
2. Sometimes
3. Almost always

Do you pour dangerous chemicals like gasoline or paint solvents down the drain or into sewer systems instead of arranging for proper disposal?

1. Often
2. Sometimes
3. Almost never

Have you thrown an empty can or bottle into the environment?

1. Within the past week
2. Within the past month
3. Not within the past year that you can remember

If you smoke, do you throw your butts into the environment when smoking outside?

1. Usually
2. Occasionally
3. Never

What kind of mileage does your automobile average?

1. Less than 20 miles per gallon
2. 20 to 30 miles per gallon
3. More than 30 miles per gallon

If you play a radio outdoors, how loud do you play it?

1. About as loud as it will go
2. Just loud enough for me to hear
3. Never play a radio outdoors where it might disturb others

When shopping for needed products, do you look for environmentally safe ones?

1. Never, just look for the cheapest and best product
2. Sometimes, depends on what is needed
3. Almost always, if I can find one.

How many motor vehicles do you own, including cars, motorcycles, motorboats, jet skis, and others.

1. More than four
2. Two to four
3. Only one

A perfect score on these specific environmental questions is 45, but remember that no one is perfect. Perhaps by reviewing your answers you can find ways to improve your environmental awareness—and also contribute to your own health.

Chapter   **1**

Use these study questions to test your knowledge of the chapter material. The answer key is located at the end of the study guide.

Multiple Choice

Choose the best answer from the available options:

1. Though health can be defined many ways, a common theme in all definitions is:
   a. nutrition and weight control
   b. exercise and fitness
   c. self-responsibility for life-style
   d. self-esteem and stress reduction

2. The model that measures health by the prevalence and incidence of disease is the:
   a. environmental model   c. holistic model
   b. medical model   d. life-style

3. Susan has a mind that is open to new ideas and concepts. This characteristic is best described as:
   a. physical wellness   c. social wellness
   b. intellectual wellness   d. spiritual wellness

4. The concept of holistic health emphasizes:
   a. self-healing   c. maintenance of health
   b. prevention of disease   d. all of the above

5. The Surgeon General's Report on Health Promotion and Disease Prevention stressed:
   a. finding a cure for chronic diseases
   b. increased research on HIV immunization
   c. increasing personal responsibility for health
   d. increased funding for medical schools

6. AIDS is a leading cause of death for:
   a. young people between 15–24
   b. men between 30–50
   c. women between 25–40
   d. all ages, all races, and both genders

7. Sexual health issues affecting college students include:
   a. STIs   c. sexual assault
   b. unplanned pregnancies   d. all of the above

8. College students concerned with failure to achieve, academic stress, and lack of social support are dealing with issues related to:
   a. sexual health   c. spiritual health
   b. mental health   d. environmental health

9. *Healthy People 2000* goals were to:
   a. increase the life span of health life for Americans
   b. reduce differences in health status among Americans
   c. give access to preventive health services for all Americans
   d. all of the above

10. Which of the following statements about health is correct?
    a. the characteristics of health change throughout life
    b. if you eat a nutritious diet, you always will be healthy
    c. not taking risks is one characteristic of people who are healthy
    d. being able to endure pain is a sign of health

11. Which of the behavioral changes listed below would reduce the annual death rate in the United States by the greatest amount?
    a. stop drinking alcohol   c. always using a seatbelt
    b. stop using illegal drugs   d. stop smoking cigarettes

12. The mind can produce disease in the body by:
    a. exposure to intense sunlight c. smoking cigarettes
    b. sexual promiscuity   d. somatization

13. Mortality is a measure of:
    a. the number of people with AIDS in the U.S.
    b. the number of people in the U.S. that become sick each year
    c. the number of deaths in a population
    d. the number of people who are buried each year in the U.S.

14. Which of the following is part of the holistic model of health but absent from the medical model of health?
    a. exercise   c. spirituality
    b. death and dying   d. herbal remedies

15. Using the mind to improve physical health and to change behaviors is called:
    a. meditation   c. somatization
    b. image visualization   d. all of the above

True/False

Determine whether each of the following statements is true or false:

1. Wellness is a state of complete physical well-being.
2. The environmental model of health focuses on disease and mortality.
3. Wellness is a dynamic and continuous process.
4. Emotional wellness requires an ability to understand your feelings and cope with daily problems.
5. Heart disease is the leading cause of death for 15- to 24-year-olds.
6. Infectious diseases were the leading cause of death in 1900.
7. Currently the leading causes of death are related to life-style factors.
8. Mental health is a major health issue for college students.
9. Diabetes can be caused by modern life-styles.
10. Physical wellness involves good nutrition, regular exercise, and responsible decision making.

Study Guide

Use these study questions to test your knowledge of the chapter material. The answer key is located at the end of the study guide.

Study Guide

Multiple Choice

Choose the best answer from the available options:

1. A condition that produces a disruption in mind-body harmony is referred to as a (an):
   a. stressor
   b. virus
   c. ulcer
   d. accident

2. How does stress contribute to illness?
   a. it suppresses immunity
   b. it increases susceptibility to disease
   c. it induces the use of unhealthy behaviors (smoking, drinking, etc.) as coping strategies
   d. all of the above

3. Effects of a reaction to stress, such as use of tranquilizers, drugs, or cigarettes, are called:
   a. activators
   b. stressors
   c. consequences
   d. headaches

4. During what phase of the General Adaptation Syndrome does the body adapt to a stressor with physiological changes like elevated blood pressure and increased alertness?
   a. alarm
   b. resistance
   c. exhaustion
   d. homeostasis

5. The best way to manage stress is to:
   a. use anti-depressant drug therapy
   b. find a good counselor
   c. use tranquilizers to cope with stressful events
   d. replace stressful ways of living with attitudes and behaviors that promote mind-body harmony

6. Confidence that you can master or deal with many situations that you encounter is called:
   a. self-control
   b. avoidance
   c. self-efficacy
   d. self-appraisal

7. Stress can lead to changes in the:
   a. nervous system
   b. endocrine system
   c. immune system
   d. all of the above

8. Life changes, such as the death of parent, can produce stress because they act as:
   a. activators of stress
   b. consequences of stress
   c. reactions to stress
   d. frustrating experiences

9. The expectation that we behave in a certain way is called:
   a. frustration
   b. a desire to please
   c. reaction
   d. pressure

10. The fight-or-flight response activates:
    a. the nervous system
    b. the endocrine system
    c. the digestive system
    d. all of the above

11. The relaxation response can be induced by:
    a. yoga exercises
    b. taking tranquilizer drugs
    c. posttraumatic stress disorders
    d. the general adaptation syndrome

12. The belief that you can master the stressful situations that you encounter in life is called:
    a. the relaxation response
    b. self-efficacy
    c. meditation
    d. a harm-and-loss situation

13. Both recently divorced couples and recently married couples may experience:
    a. posttraumatic stress disorders
    b. one thousand life change units
    c. reduced immune system functions
    d. image visualizations

14. When a person says that he or she is "stressed out," it means that the person is:
    a. looking for drugs to help with anxious feelings
    b. experiencing a disruption of mind-body harmony
    c. about to become sick
    d. going to perform a violent act in the near future

True/False

Determine whether each of the following statements is true or false:

1. Activators are occurrences, situations, or events that are potential stressors.
2. Coping refers to one's success at solving a problem.
3. Knowing that a stressful situation will occur produces less stress than being in a state of uncertainty.
4. In modern society, a physical reaction to stress is usually the most appropriate response.
5. Activation of the GAS can cause dramatic changes in body organs.
6. Stress can suppress the effectiveness of the immune system.
7. Failing to pass an exam may lead to a posttraumatic stress disorder.
8. Approach-avoidance situations usually result in inaction.
9. Unresolved problems that cause stress may increase a person's risk of infection.
10. Stress at school or work contributes to smoking and alcohol abuse.

Chapter

Multiple Choice

Choose the best answer from the available options:

1. Needs involving self-esteem as well as mental and psychological stimulation are:
   a. growth needs
   b. maintenance needs
   c. basic needs
   d. social needs

2. When basic, urgent needs are met and a person has achieved a high level of growth and achievement potential, this state is called:
   a. nirvana
   b. cognition
   c. self-actualization
   d. maintenance

3. Thoughts, beliefs, and attitudes that we are not clearly aware of are called:
   a. conscious
   b. subterranean
   c. unconscious
   d. subliminal

4. Perception, learning, and problem solving are part of the mental process called:
   a. self-actualization
   b. homeostasis
   c. cognition
   d. awareness

5. There are various ways of dealing with emotional distress when needs are not met. These are called:
   a. coping strategies
   b. created needs
   c. self-actualization
   d. cognitions

6. The strategy of denial is commonly used as a form of:
   a. humor therapy
   b. defense mechanism
   c. self-actualization
   d. counseling therapy

7. Which of the following might help reduce emotional distress?
   a. exercise
   b. meditation
   c. viewing distress as temporary
   d. all of the above

8. An intense fear of an object or situation is called a:
   a. panic attack
   b. denial
   c. phobia
   d. defense mechanism

9. The human brain is capable of the process of cognition. This means that every person is capable of:
   a. interpreting data gathered by the five senses
   b. learning new things and storing them in memory
   c. reasoning and problem solving
   d. all of the above

10. It is appropriate to express anger when:
    a. someone knowingly abuses you
    b. someone you care for abuses himself or herself
    c. someone breaks a promise
    d. people do not support you in your actions

11. Mental disorders can be caused by:
    a. ingesting a toxic substance
    b. an injury to the brain
    c. a genetic disorder
    d. all of the above

12. Some people become depressed during winter months because:
    a. they cannot go skiing
    b. they suffer from cold weather
    c. they do not get enough sunlight
    d. they suffer from a bipolar disorder

13. One of the most worrisome aspects of depression is the risk of:
    a. becoming addicted to antidepressive drugs
    b. suicide
    c. psychosis
    d. becoming violent

14. Which of the following is true about suicide?
    a. it is the leading cause of death among teenagers
    b. the number of reported suicides represents only about 10% to 15% of all suicide attempts
    c. suicide is a disease
    d. suicide is an inherited disorder that runs in families

True/False

Determine whether each of the following statements is true or false:

1. Maintenance needs involve physical safety and survival.

2. Physical requirements for satisfying hunger and thirst are at the lowest level of the Hierarchy of Needs.

3. Exercise can be an effective strategy for coping with emotional distress.

4. Defense mechanisms help people distort perception in order to avoid unpleasant situations.

5. Loss of appetite, sleep disturbances, and social withdrawal may signal depression.

6. A person's emotional state can produce physical symptoms of a disease through a process called somatization.

7. Few people have difficulty dealing with anger because it is such a common emotion.

8. If depression is not addressed, it can intensify and create a depressive cycle.

9. Schizophrenia is a mental disorder characterized by multiple personalities.

10. To be emotionally healthy means that a person almost never experiences anger or becomes depressed.

Study Guide

Use these study questions to test your knowledge of the chapter material. The answer key is located at the end of the study guide.

Study Guide

Multiple Choice

Choose the best answer from the available options:

1. In the food guide pyramid, complex carbohydrates like bread, rice, and pasta are located:
   - a. at the top
   - b. at the bottom
   - c. on the side
   - d. in the middle

2. If a food label reads: honey, brown sugar, corn syrup solids, oat flour, corn meal, hydrogenated vegetable oil, and sodium, the product contains more _____ than anything else.
   - a. fat
   - b. flour
   - c. sugar
   - d. salt

3. Food energy is measured in units of energy called:
   - a. nutrients
   - b. proteins
   - c. amino acids
   - d. calories

4. Countries with the highest per capita meat consumption also have the highest rates of:
   - a. mad cow disease
   - b. rabies
   - c. colon cancer
   - d. lung cancer

5. The preferred source of energy for the body is:
   - a. protein
   - b. carbohydrate
   - c. fat
   - d. vitamins

6. The classes of complex carbohydrates are:
   - a. liver and onions
   - b. fructose and sucrose
   - c. fruits and leaves
   - d. starch and fiber

7. Carbohydrate is stored in the liver and muscles in the form of:
   - a. glucose
   - b. cellulose
   - c. glycogen
   - d. fiber

8. Antioxidant vitamins are associated with a lower risk of:
   - a. cancer
   - b. cataracts
   - c. heart disease
   - d. all of the above

9. Many Americans consume too much of this mineral, which may contribute to high blood pressure:
   - a. calcium
   - b. iron
   - c. sodium
   - d. potassium

10. Which of the following is true of vegetarians?
   - a. they consume poultry and fish, but no beef or pork
   - b. all vegetarians must take dietary supplements
   - c. they are at reduced risk for coronary heart disease and some cancers
   - d. they are often anemic and in poorer health than nonvegetarians

11. Proteins are made up of smaller chemical units called:
   - a. calories
   - b. triglycerides
   - c. amino acids
   - d. vitamins

12. Lactose intolerance means that people:
   - a. do not like a person of another skin color
   - b. get indigestion if they eat candy
   - c. have a vitamin deficiency
   - d. cannot drink milk

13. The organ in the body that is responsible for removing toxic chemicals is the:
   - a. pancreas
   - b. gallbladder
   - c. liver
   - d. all of the above

14. The function of food is:
   - a. to provide chemicals that the body needs
   - b. to provide energy
   - c. to satisfy hunger and provide pleasure
   - d. all of the above

15. Basal metabolism is defined as:
   - a. the minimum amount of energy needed to keep the body alive
   - b. the energy expended when you are sleeping
   - c. the energy needed for growth and physical activity
   - d. all of the above

16. People choose to become vegetarians because:
   - a. they object to killing animals for food
   - b. they believe it helps to conserve the world's food supply
   - c. they believe they will live longer and be healthier
   - d. all of the above

True/False

Determine whether each of the following statements is true or false:

1. A product marked "light" should have one third the calories or one half the fat of the original product.

2. Essential nutrients are those produced by the body.

3. All of the essential amino acids can be found in chicken.

4. Simple carbohydrates are primarily found in whole grain products.

5. Fiber may be instrumental in preventing heart disease and cancer.

6. The fats in animal products such as meat and milk are saturated.

7. Vegetable shortenings and margarine contain high levels of cholesterol and saturated fat.

8. All major artificial sweeteners have been associated with health risks.

9. A fish sandwich is the healthiest option at a fast-food restaurant.

10. Phytochemicals from plants can help eliminate toxins in humans.

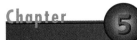

Use these study questions to test your knowledge of the chapter material. The answer key is located at the end of the study guide.

Multiple Choice

Choose the best answer from the available options:

1. The term obesity refers specifically to:
   a. having an ideal height to weight ratio
   b. having excess muscle tissue on the body
   c. an increased risk of disease associated with fat
   d. having an excess of body fat

2. The most important issue regarding excess weight is:
   a. the amount of excess weight
   b. the location of extra weight
   c. the percentage of body fat
   d. the percentage of lean body mass

3. Fat necessary for normal physiological functioning is:
   a. essential fat   c. brown fat
   b. storage fat   d. body fat

4. The body stores carbohydrate in the form of:
   a. adipose tissue   c. insulin
   b. glycogen   d. connective tissue

5. The theory that each person has an internal "mechanism" designed to regulate the amount of body fat within a narrow range is called:
   a. The Dietary Fat Theory   c. The Fat-Cell Theory
   b. The Set-Point Theory   d. The Yo-Yo Theory

6. Which of the following statements about obesity is (are) correct?
   a. there is a definite connection between weight fluctuation and increased risk of illness or death
   b. weight cycling increases risk for heart disease and hurts future attempts at weight loss
   c. data are inconclusive regarding long-term effects of weight cycling
   d. all of the above

7. Which is (are) true of diet programs?
   a. lost weight is usually regained in a short time
   b. they seldom include provisions for life-style changes to prevent future weight gain
   c. they are often expensive, difficult to maintain, or both
   d. all of the above

8. Anorexia athletica is a condition which:
   a. can result from excessive training and food restriction by those obsessed with athletic performance
   b. can affect both males and females
   c. can be fueled by high expectations of coaches and parents
   d. can be described by all of the above

9. Characteristics of those afflicted with anorexia nervosa include:
   a. high self-esteem and self-efficacy
   b. families that encourage independence and honest expression of emotions
   c. strong personal identity and goal-oriented attitude
   d. a sense of powerlessness and lack of control over most aspects of life

10. The primary reason that people are overfat is:
    a. they eat too many carbohydrates
    b. they consume too much saturated fat
    c. they consume most of their daily calories late in the evening
    d. their physical activity is insufficient to use up the calories they ingest

11. Managing body weight not only involves nutritional choices but also includes issues such as:
    a. living a sedentary lifestyle
    b. being confused by nutrition advice
    c. being "stressed out" most of the time
    d. all of the above

12. A young woman wants to lose 10 pounds in 10 weeks. She needs 2,000 calories a day to maintain her present weight. To lose the desired weight in this time frame, how many calories a day should she consume?
    a. 500   c. 2,000
    b. 1,600   d. 2,500

13. Which sport burns the most calories per minute?
    a. golf   c. roller skating
    b. tennis   d. skiing

True/False

Determine whether each of the following statements is true or false:

1. Cells, bone, muscle, and water are elements of lean body mass.
2. Life-style changes have resulted in a decreased incidence of obesity among children during the last few decades.
3. Adipose tissue serves to store carbohydrate energy in the body.
4. Yo-yo dieting refers to repeated cycles of weight loss and gain.
5. Increased activity of lipoprotein lipase reduces the efficiency of fat storage.
6. Adipsin is a protein that signals the brain when fat cells are "full."
7. Body wraps reduce body size and result in permanent weight loss.
8. Though eating disorders are serious conditions, they are never fatal.
9. Bulimia is characterized by binge eating followed by self-induced vomiting.
10. As a group, bulimics are characterized by high self-esteem.

Use these study questions to test your knowledge of the chapter material. The answer key is located at the end of the study guide.

Study Guide

Multiple Choice

Choose the best answer from the available options:

1. With respect to the physiological benefits of physical activity:
   a. regular exercise can reduce the risk of chronic disease
   b. regular exercise can reduce the risk of heart attack
   c. regular exercise promotes psychological well-being
   d. all of the above are true

2. Which is a psychological outcome of regular exercise?
   a. increased self-consciousness
   b. reduced self-awareness
   c. irregular breathing rhythms
   d. reduced psychic tension and stress

3. During exercise, the hormone that stimulates the heart, releases fat from fat cells, and makes carbohydrates available from the liver and muscles is:
   a. enkephalin   c. epinephrine
   b. insulin   d. adipsin

4. _____ are substances secreted by the brain during exercise. These mitigate pain and produce a feeling of well-being.
   a. endorphins   c. sex hormones
   b. enzymes   d. amino acids

5. Components of fitness include:
   a. gain strength and endurance   c. cardiovascular efficiency
   b. joint flexibility   d. all of the above

6. The most effective exercise for increasing heart capacity is:
   a. aerobic exercise   c. isometric exercise
   b. strength training   d. endurance training

7. Aerobic exercise can produce collective changes in physiology known as:
   a. the fitness effect   c. the collective effect
   b. the training effect   d. the toning principle

8. The ability of a joint to move through its range of motion is called:
   a. endurance   c. flexibility
   b. efficiency   d. toning

9. Calisthenics and yoga are good exercises for:
   a. endurance   c. flexibility
   b. strength   d. aerobic fitness

10. The most common form of exercise abuse is:
    a. being "addicted" to exercise
    b. exercising beyond biological limits to the point of injury
    c. athletic amenorrhea
    d. diarrhea

11. Which of the following are reasons to begin an exercise program?
    a. to reduce stress
    b. to strengthen the cardiovascular system
    c. to lose weight
    d. all of the above

12. Athletes take steroid supplements to:
    a. help maintain body weight
    b. increase sexual prowess
    c. build muscle mass and stamina
    d. increase flexibility

13. Training effect refers to the:
    a. physiological changes needed to compete in sports
    b. beneficial changes in physiology resulting from exercise
    c. psychological effects of exercise
    d. ability to stay in shape

14. Regular physical activity increases:
    a. the risk of a heart attack
    b. basal metabolic rate
    c. blood flow through the heart and arteries
    d. the amount of fat in the body

True/False

Determine whether each of the following statements is true or false:

1. Regular physical activity helps increase blood pressure in people with hypertension.

2. Exercising regularly can lower cholesterol levels.

3. The Centers for Disease Control and Prevention recommends 30 minutes of exercise at least twice a week.

4. Isometric training is another term for strength training.

5. Synthetic male hormones used to increase muscle size and strength are called anabolic steroids.

6. Strength training produces little improvement in cardiovascular fitness.

7. Athletic amenorrhea refers to painful menstruation due to excessive participation in athletics.

8. Excessive exercising and poor equipment are common causes of overuse injuries.

9. Physical stress of exercise helps counteract the negative effects of daily psychological stressors.

10. To produce aerobic benefits, walking must be done for longer periods than more strenuous exercises.

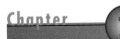

Chapter

7

Use these study questions to test your knowledge of the chapter material. The answer key is located at the end of the study guide.

Multiple Choice

Choose the best answer from the available options:

1. A little girl who is encouraged to wear frilly dresses, avoid competitive games, and be be submissive in social situations is having her _____ influenced by her caregivers.
   a. sexual orientation   c. gender role
   b. gender   d. hormones

2. Secondary sex characteristics include:
   a. fallopian tubes   c. testicles
   b. pubic hair   d. eye color

3. The discharge during menstruation consists of:
   a. the endometrium   c. gonadotropins
   b. birth products   d. endorphins

4. Together, the testes, seminal vesicles, prostate gland, and Cowper's gland produce a fluid called:
   a. urine   c. sperm
   b. smegma   d. semen

5. Sharing private information about goals, weaknesses, desires, and fears is:
   a. intimacy   c. self-disclosure
   b. commitment   d. foreplay

6. The feeling of being emotionally obligated or compelled to be with someone is part of:
   a. commitment   c. self-disclosure
   b. a metamessage   d. excitement

7. The most effective strategy for expressing anger constructively is to:
   a. try to agree on a time, place and content for arguments or fights
   b. use you-statements to criticize the other's personal qualities
   c. wait until anger has built to a sufficient point before you address it
   d. stick to your guns and avoid compromise

8. Sperm are produced in the:
   a. seminal vesicles   c. seminiferous tubules
   b. prostate gland   d. ovaries

9. Pregnancy is detected by the presence of _____ in the women.
   a. estrogen   c. progesterone
   b. testosterone   d. Human Chorionic Gonadotropin

10. When a fertilized egg implants anywhere other than the uterus, it is called:
    a. ectopic pregnancy   c. endorphic pregnancy
    b. placental pregnancy   d. chorionic pregnancy

11. The organ that supplies nutrients to the fetus, eliminates fetal waste, and consequently supports growth and development of the fetus is the:
    a. amnion   c. chorion
    b. placenta   d. gestation

12. Discomfort during labor can often be controlled by:
    a. breathing exercises   c. relaxation strategies
    b. massage techniques   d. all of the above

13. Which of the following is NOT recommended during pregnancy?
    a. supplementing the diet with iron and folic acid
    b. a weight gain of up to 30 pounds
    c. abstaining from alcohol and tobacco use
    d. use of appetite suppressants to control weight

14. Artificial insemination involves:
    a. inserting semen directly into the cervix with a syringe
    b. inserting a fertilized egg into the uterus
    c. using sound waves to produce images of internal structures
    d. use of an egg from a donor

15. In vitro fertilization (IVF) involves:
    a. placing fertilized eggs into a woman's uterus
    b. placing equal numbers of eggs into each fallopian tube and introducing semen (GIFT)
    c. placing an embryo into the fallopian tube
    d. all of the above

True/False

Determine whether each of the following statements is true or false:

1. Feeling sexually attracted to members of a particular gender is part of the physical dimension of sexuality.

2. A woman attracted to two men at the same time is a bisexual.

3. Menopause signals physical deterioration and emotional instability in women.

4. Circumcision is a surgical procedure to remove the foreskin of the penis.

5. The release of sexual tension, usually accompanied by rhythmic contractions in pelvic muscles and feelings of pleasure, is called orgasm.

6. When fertilization takes place, the resulting cell is called an embryo.

7. Unless special problems exist, sexual intercourse can continue throughout pregnancy.

8. High blood pressure during pregnancy may indicate toxemia.

9. Sexually transmitted infections can cause infertility.

10. A stillbirth is the abortion of an embryo or fetus too young to live outside the uterus.

Study Guide

Use these study questions to test your knowledge of the chapter material. The answer key is located at the end of the study guide.

Multiple Choice

Choose the best answer from the available options:

1. The likelihood of becoming pregnant when using a particular contraceptive method for one year is called the:
   a. fertility rate
   b. success rate
   c. failure rate
   d. experimental rate

2. The most common oral contraceptives contain:
   a. estrogen only
   b. estrogen and progesterone
   c. progesterone only
   d. prostaglandins

3. The diaphragm is highly effective if used correctly. Another advantage is:
   a. absence of side effects (other than allergic reactions to latex)
   b. once inserted, it is effective for 24 hours
   c. it is available without a prescription
   d. one size diaphragm will fit most women

4. The calendar method, temperature method, and mucus method are all:
   a. hormonal methods of contraception
   b. barrier methods of contraception
   c. fertility awareness methods of contraception
   d. methods of sterilization

5. When a man has a vasectomy, he should be aware that:
   a. a vasectomy is considered a reversible form of contraception
   b. the vas deferens will be removed so sperm cannot be transported
   c. he will continue to ejaculate semen, but it will contain no sperm
   d. the semen will contain sperm, but they will not be viable (able to fertilize an egg)

6. The principal sterilization procedure for women:
   a. is called a tubal ligation
   b. involves blocking the fallopian tubes in some way
   c. can be performed in a clinic or doctor's office
   d. all of the above

7. An epidemic of sexually transmitted infections persists in the United States partly because:
   a. most of the STIs are incurable
   b. negative attitudes toward STIs keep people from getting checkups and from communicating with partners about possible exposure to these diseases
   c. almost all STIs are caused by viruses that cannot be killed by antibiotics
   d. most STIs are not detectable during a medical examination

8. Which of the following STIs is caused by a virus?
   a. gonorrhea
   b. chlamydia
   c. syphilis
   d. hepatitis B

9. Scabies is caused by:
   a. mites
   b. HIV
   c. *Treponema pallidum*
   d. pubic lice

10. When individuals first become infected with HIV, within a few weeks they usually experience:
    a. flu-like symptoms
    b. pneumonia
    c. Kaposi's sarcoma
    d. there are no symptoms early in HIV infection

11. Before HIV screening was available, thousands of _____ were infected through blood transfusions.
    a. homosexuals
    b. heterosexuals
    c. hemophiliacs
    d. IV drug users

12. Vaginal infections that can be transmitted by sexual contact include:
    a. trichomonas and gardnerella
    b. chlamydia and herpes
    c. gonorrhea and syphilis
    d. treponema and papilloma

13. The human papilloma virus (HPV) causes:
    a. AIDS
    b. scabies
    c. venereal warts
    d. cold sores

True/False

Determine whether each of the following statements is true or false:

1. Oral contraceptive use is the most effective method of birth control.

2. Withdrawing the penis prior to ejaculation will prevent sperm from entering the vagina.

3. About 50 percent of women taking birth control pills experience unwanted side effects.

4. Fertility awareness involves monitoring ovulation, body temperature, and mucus changes.

5. Once inserted, the cervical cap is theoretically effective for 24 hours.

6. Most abortions are performed on married women who feel they have had enough children.

7. People with oral herpes infections can transmit the infection to their sexual partners via oral sex.

8. Antiviral drugs can cure a genital herpes infection.

9. Gonorrhea can be contracted from contaminated bedsheets, clothing, towels, or toilet seats.

10. The most prevalent STI in the United States each year is chlamydia infections.

Chapter 9

Use these study questions to test your knowledge of the chapter material. The answer key is located at the end of the study guide.

Multiple Choice

Choose the best answer from the available options:

1. The factor having the most adverse effect on the development of the immune system is:
   a. poor nutrition   c. alcohol
   b. stress   d. tobacco

2. The body's first line of defense against infectious disease is (are):
   a. cilia   c. skin
   b. microphages   d. enzymes

3. Histamine is released by the body in response to:
   a. invasion of bacteria
   b. a viral infection
   c. the presence of an allergen
   d. the presence of an antibody

4. Which of the following is true with respect to food allergies?
   a. over 50 percent of the population reports some type of food allergies
   b. fewer than 10 percent of foods account for 90 percent of food allergies
   c. food allergies only occur in children
   d. most people who report food intolerance are found to have actual food allergies

5. What do lupus, multiple sclerosis, and rheumatoid arthritis have in common?
   a. they are triggered by viral infections
   b. they are autoimmune diseases
   c. they are more common in cold climates
   d. they can be cured with appropriate diagnosis and therapy

6. People with Type O blood are called:
   a. universal donors   c. universal recipients
   b. perfect matches   d. Rh positive

7. Recent research on ulcers indicates that:
   a. stress and anxiety are primary causes of ulcers
   b. specific bacteria must be present for an ulcer to develop
   c. the best treatment for ulcers is a "bland" diet without spices
   d. ulcers can be removed by surgery

8. Infectious diseases are fought by:
   a. antibiotic treatment   c. good sanitation and hygiene
   b. vaccination   d. all of the above

9. Immune system cells are transported to all parts of the body through the:
   a. lymphatic system   c. endocrine system
   b. nervous system   d. all of the above

10. The main source of nosocomial infections is:
    a. bacteria
    b. viruses
    c. hospitals
    d. oral–genital sex with an infected person

11. The organ most often transplanted is the:
    a. heart   c. lung
    b. kidney   d. none of the above

12. Allergies:
    a. can be caused by a person's emotional and mental state
    b. are usually imaginary diseases
    c. can be cured with allergy shots
    d. are usually the result of eating contaminated food

13. Vaccines prevent infections by eliciting the production of
    _____ in the body.
    a. antigens   c. fever
    b. antibodies   d. all of the above

14. Which of the following has a major influence on the functioning of the immune system?
    a. nutrition   c. antihistamines
    b. viruses and bacteria   d. sexual activity

True/False

Determine whether each of the following statements is true or false:

1. Antigens are foreign proteins found on infectious organisms.
2. Extreme stress may make asthma attacks more frequent or more severe.
3. Anaphylactic shock is a common allergic reaction but is not serious.
4. If food allergies are imagined, they do not need to be treated.
5. An autoimmune disease causes antibodies to attack the body's own cells.
6. People with Type AB blood can safely donate blood to anyone.
7. Malaria is an infectious disease transmitted by a vector.
8. Antibiotics are extremely effective against diseases caused by viruses.
9. Colds and flu are caused by bacteria.
10. Throughout the world, public health measures have largely eliminated infectious diseases.

Study Guide

Chapter 10

Multiple Choice

Choose the best answer from the available options:

1. If blood supply to the heart is blocked and cells die, the condition is called:
   a. ischemia
   b. stroke
   c. infarction
   d. edema

2. Fibrous, fatty deposits on the walls of arteries are called:
   a. lipoproteins
   b. plaques
   c. cholesterol
   d. cardiolytes

3. Chest pain resulting from blocked arteries is called:
   a. angina pectoris
   b. atherosclerosis
   c. an angiogram
   d. a plaque attack

4. In a procedure called _____, a balloon-tipped catheter is used to push plaques back against arterial walls.
   a. coronary bypass
   b. angina pectoris
   c. angioplasty
   d. angiography

5. Cerebral thrombosis and cerebral embolism are caused by:
   a. plaques on arterial walls
   b. ruptured blood vessels
   c. clots that plug an artery to the brain
   d. HDL cholesterol

6. The cholesterol that is deposited in plaques and blocks arteries comes from:
   a. low-density lipoproteins (LDLs)
   b. triglycerides
   c. hi-density lipoproteins (HDLs)
   d. lipoprotein lipase

7. Major risk factors for hypertension include:
   a. obesity
   b. stress
   c. smoking
   d. all of the above

8. Which of the following is (are) true?
   a. smokers are twice as likely to have a heart attack as non-smokers
   b. smoking is a major contributor to both heart disease and cancer
   c. stopping smoking can reverse many of tobacco's harmful effects
   d. all of the above

9. The type of cancer that is increasing dramatically in both men and women is:
   a. colon
   b. lung
   c. breast
   d. stomach

10. The unregulated or uncontrolled growth of certain body cells is called:
   a. oncology
   b. osmosis
   c. metastasis
   d. cancer

11. When an abnormal mass of cells grows rapidly and invades other areas of the body it is said to be:
   a. malignant
   b. benign
   c. lymphatic
   d. narcotic

12. When cancerous cells enter the lymph system and spread to other organs, the process is called:
   a. osmosis
   b. pathology
   c. metastasis
   d. oncology

13. Investigating the causes and frequencies of certain diseases is called:
   a. pathology
   b. scientology
   c. epidemiology
   d. psychology

14. Risk factors for breast cancer include:
   a. a high fat diet
   b. high exposure to radiation
   c. late menopause
   d. all of the above

15. The substance having the most carcinogenic potential with respect to the number of cancers caused is:
   a. nitrosamine
   b. tobacco
   c. asbestos
   d. lead

16. Which dietary choices may help to prevent cancer?
   a. foods containing B-vitamins
   b. foods containing vitamin C
   c. foods with folic acid
   d. all of the above

17. _____ is considered the best treatment for tumors that have not spread.
   a. radiation therapy
   b. chemotherapy
   c. surgical removal
   d. biopsy

True/False

Determine whether each of the following statements is true or false:

1. A stroke occurs when blood supply to the heart is blocked.

2. During recent decades the rate of cardiovascular diseases in the United States has declined steadily.

3. Recent research indicates that certain life-style changes may help reduce arterial blockage.

4. Physical inactivity and stress are major risk factors for stroke.

5. Hypertension means high blood pressure.

6. Antioxidant vitamins can help reduce the risk of heart disease and cancer.

7. Tumors that do not spread and are not a threat to life are malignant.

8. Life-style factors contribute relatively little to cancer risk.

9. Though incidence of melanoma is increasing, this condition is seldom dangerous.

10. Emotional support and group therapy have a positive effect on cancer survival rates.

Study Guide

Use these study questions to test your knowledge of the chapter material. The answer key is located

at the end of the study guide.

Multiple Choice

Choose the best answer from the available options:

1. A substance that alters the structure or function of a biological process is:
   - a. a receptor
   - b. a drug
   - c. a teratogen
   - d. a dose

2. An unintended drug action is called:
   - a. a side effect
   - b. an allergy
   - c. a teratogen
   - b. all of the above

3. Body size, food consumption, and digestion can all influence effectiveness of:
   - a. a placebo
   - b. a receptor
   - c. a drug dose
   - d. all of the above

4. In a _____ study, neither patients nor researchers know who is receiving a placebo.
   - a. therapeutic
   - b. double blind
   - c. volunteer
   - d. clinical

5. When progressively larger doses of a drug are needed to produce the same effect, the condition is called:
   - a. habituation
   - b. withdrawal
   - c. tolerance
   - d. dependance

6. Drugs that affect thoughts, perceptions, and moods are called _____ drugs.
   - a. hypnotic
   - b. psychedelic
   - c. teratogenic
   - d. psychoactive

7. Those most likely to abuse _____ to fight fatigue and enhance performance are drivers, students, and athletes.
   - a. depressants
   - b. opiates
   - c. amphetamines
   - d. hallucinogens

8. Morphine, codeine, and heroin are all classified as:
   - a. stimulants
   - b. opiates
   - c. amphetamines
   - d. hallucinogens

9. Phencyclidine (PCP) is classified as:
   - a. a stimulant
   - b. a depressant
   - c. an hallucinogen
   - d. all of the above, depending on the route of administration

10. Which of the following is true of inhalants?
    - a. they produce physical dependence
    - b. they produce tolerance
    - c. withdrawal symptoms occur when use is stopped
    - d. they are dangerous substances that can cause kidney, liver, and lung damage

11. Repeated use of a drug to the point where a person is consumed with drug-seeking behavior is called:
    - a. habituation
    - b. tolerance
    - c. addiction
    - d. physiological dependence

12. A drug found in many cold remedies and analgesics is:
    - a. codeine
    - b. caffeine
    - c. nicotine
    - d. thorazine

13. Once in the body, drugs are degraded or inactivated by the _____ and the _____.
    - a. kidneys; brain
    - b. liver; blood
    - c. liver; lungs
    - d. kidney; urine

14. The most widely used and abused stimulant drug is:
    - a. smoked cocaine
    - b. smoked methamphetamine
    - c. inhaled cocaine
    - d. injected heroin

15. Risk factors for drug addiction include:
    - a. tendency to develop tolerance to the drug
    - b. posttraumatic stress disorder
    - c. availability of drugs
    - d. all of the above

16. Drugs cause chemical changes in the body by binding to:
    - a. neurotransmitters
    - b. antibodies
    - c. receptors
    - d. all of the above

True/False

Determine whether each of the following statements is true or false:

1. A contraindication is a reason for prescribing a drug.

2. A person's expectations or attitude can influence drug effectiveness.

3. Habituation refers to psychological dependence on a drug.

4. Withdrawal symptoms from depressants are the same as withdrawal symptoms from stimulants.

5. Amphetamines are commonly prescribed as therapeutic drugs.

6. All depressants have potential for physical and psychological dependency.

7. Use of hallucinogens results in physical addiction and withdrawal symptoms.

8. The National Academy of Science has concluded that long-term marijuana use is extremely harmful.

9. Hashish and marijuana are derived from the same plant.

10. Cycling and stacking are patterns of anabolic steroid use.

Chapter

Use these study questions to test your knowledge of the chapter material. The answer key is located at the end of the study guide.

Multiple Choice

Choose the best answer from the available options:

1. Cigarette advertising is now aggressively targeting:
   a. women and teens
   b. young professionals
   c. middle-aged men
   d. young urban males

2. The smoker's "rush" and non-smoker's nausea when inhaling tobacco are due to:
   a. the effects of burning tar in the cigarette
   b. the effects of radon gas in tobacco smoke
   c. the effects of carbon monoxide on the body
   d. the effects of nicotine on the body

3. The most hazardous form of smokeless tobacco is:
   a. chewing tobacco
   b. dry snuff
   c. moist snuff
   d. twist/rope tobacco

4. Smokeless tobacco has been linked to:
   a. tooth decay
   b. receding gums
   c. oral cancer
   d. all of the above

5. The constituent of cigarettes that is a documented cause of lung cancer is:
   a. burning paper
   b. tar
   c. nicotine
   d. carbon monoxide

6. The strongest predictor of alcohol consumption, especially among young people, is:
   a. parental attitudes
   b. exposure to media advertising
   c. peer influence
   d. number of liquor stores in an area

7. Alcohol is metabolized by the:
   a. spleen
   b. pancreas
   c. liver
   d. kidneys

8. What is the relationship between alcohol and sexual behavior among college students?
   a. impaired judgment may result in unintended pregnancies and sexually transmitted diseases
   b. intoxication may cause sexual dysfunction (problems) and frustration
   c. alcohol consumption is linked to sexual assault
   d. all of the above

9. Paul has found that his tolerance for alcohol has increased. He has started to focus on opportunities for drinking, and has concealed drinks at work several times. Paul is most likely in the:
   a. warning phase of alcoholism
   b. crucial phase of alcoholism
   c. chronic phase of alcoholism
   d. controlled phase of alcoholism

10. If Mary calls in sick for her alcoholic husband, or assumes his responsibilities when he cannot, she is a (an):
    a. rescuer
    b. enabler
    c. counselor
    d. codependent

11. One cigar may contain as much tobacco as:
    a. a pinch of snuff
    b. a pack of cigarettes
    c. two cigarettes
    d. a pouch of pipe tobacco

12. Which of the following questions should someone ask if he or she wants to quit smoking?
    a. How much do I smoke?
    b. Why do I smoke?
    c. What will be the hardest part of quitting?
    d. all of the above

13. Smoking decreases the average person's life expectancy by:
    a. several months
    b. 1 or 2 years
    c. 7 years
    d. more than 10 years

14. The liver detoxifies alcohol at a rate of:
    a. 1 ounce an hour
    b. 1 ounce every 6 hours
    c. 1 ounce every 12 hours
    d. 6 ounces an hour

15. Approximately what percentage of all highway fatalities each year involve people who have been drinking alcohol?
    a. 1 percent
    b. 10 percent
    c. 25 percent
    d. 40 percent

True/False

Determine whether each of the following statements is true or false:

1. Smoking is the most prevalent cause of death in the United States.
2. Bronchitis is reversible, but emphysema is not reversible.
3. It has been determined that nicotine is as addictive as heroine.
4. Chewing tobacco and snuff are safe alternatives to smoking.
5. Switching to low tar and nicotine cigarettes will significantly reduce the cancer risks for smokers.
6. The United States government supports the tobacco industry as well as anti-smoking educational programs.
7. Alcohol is not a nutrient or food and contains no calories.
8. Alcohol is capable of promoting disease in nearly all body organs.
9. Alcohol abuse is the principal drug problem in the United States.
10. Codependency involves believing you are responsible for the moods and emotions of others.

Chapter 13

Use these study questions to test your knowledge of the chapter material. The answer key is located at the end of the study guide.

Multiple Choice

Choose the best answer from the available options:

1. What types of violence are occurring in today's society?
   a. firearm violence
   b. domestic and child abuse
   c. interpersonal violence
   d. all of the above

2. A factor that contributes to domestic violence is:
   a. high level of conflict and stress in the family
   b. female dominance
   c. cultural norms that prohibit family violence
   d. lack of alcohol or drugs in the household

3. Forced sexual activity can occur between:
   a. women and men
   b. men and men
   c. women and women
   d. all of the above

4. Views that may contribute to acquaintance rape include:
   a. sexual assault can only occur between strangers
   b. blaming themselves for allowing it to happen
   c. women really don't mean "no" when they say "no"
   d. all of the above

5. Ways to prevent violence include all of the following EXCEPT:
   a. confronting the abuser with a taste of his own medicine
   b. providing shelters
   c. training law enforcement in mediation techniques
   d. reducing the amount of violent imagery on television

6. The idea that "people get what they deserve" is an example of:
   a. male dominance
   b. victim blaming
   c. PTSD
   d. denial

7. Neglect is:
   a. a form of childhood sexual abuse
   b. probably the most common form of maltreatment of children
   c. intentional force that results in injury
   d. psychological abuse

8. Programs that have been implemented to help reduce the incidence of child abuse include:
   a. stress management
   b. conflict resolution
   c. parenting skills
   d. all of the above

9. The physical, sexual, or emotional maltreatment of an adult, age 60 or over, is:
   a. ageism
   b. elder abuse
   c. self-neglect
   d. aggravated battery

10. Which of the following is true about youth gangs?
    a. youth gangs are primarily an urban phenomenon restricted to large cities.
    b. gang recruits usually have a strong sense of self-esteem
    c. most gang members are pacifists
    d. gang members attempt to gain respect by making society fear them

11. Which of the following might lead to an increased risk of unintentional injury?
    a. decreased mobility
    b. chronic disease
    c. poverty
    d. all of the above

12. Ways to eliminate the occurrence of unintended injuries are called:
    a. epidemiology
    b. accident prevention
    c. accident mitigation
    d. accident investigation

13. According to the National Highway Traffic Safety Administration:
    a. seatbelts alone are adequate and airbags contribute little to passenger safety
    b. airbags have caused more injuries than they have prevented
    c. the combination of an airbag and a seatbelt can reduce the risk of serious head injury by 75 percent
    d. airbags should be banned from all vehicles

14. Which of the following is a factor that can potentially lead to a motor vehicle fatality?
    a. road construction
    b. poor weather conditions
    c. exceeding the posted speed limit
    d. all of the above

True/False

Determine whether each of the following statements is true or false:

1. Violence refers to the use of force or power that results in injury or death.

2. The National Rifle Association supports legislation to limit the sale of guns.

3. Violence is often glamorized in TV shows and movies.

4. The FBI estimates that a woman is beaten every 15 seconds either by her husband or a male friend.

5. Unemployment, racism, and poverty are factors that contribute to domestic violence.

6. Sexual assault is an act of power and humiliation rather than a sexual act.

7. There is no relationship between being abused as a child and abusing one's own children.

8. In about 80 percent of all sexual assaults, the victim knows the assailant.

9. Injuries are the leading cause of disability among young people today.

10. Fewer than 10 percent of all motorcycle operators receive any formal training.

Study Guide

Chapter 14

Use these study questions to test your knowledge of the chapter material. The answer key is located at the end of the study guide.

Multiple Choice

Choose the best answer from the available options:

1. In order to be an effective partner in health care, it is important to:
   a. maintain effective communication with health care providers
   b. be an active participant in making medical decisions
   c. be informed about available alternatives and options
   d. all of the above

2. Conventional, "scientific" medicine and procedures are offered by:
   a. doctors (M.D.s) and dentists
   b. homeopaths
   c. naturopaths
   d. herbalists

3. With respect to health insurance, "managed care" means:
   a. patients receive only one bill for all medical procedures
   b. support staff see patients more frequently than doctors
   c. alternative therapies are used whenever possible
   d. companies attempt to control costs of health care by a variety of strategies

4. _____ can be classified as alternative medicine.
   a. meditation and faith healing
   b. nutritional supplements and fasting
   c. acupuncture, massage, and yoga
   d. all of the above

5. The discipline of chiropractic medicine:
   a. relies primarily on surgery and nutrition therapy
   b. focuses on realigning subluxation of vertebrae
   c. licenses practitioners to prescribe drugs
   d. all of the above

6. Acupuncture is most effective when used to:
   a. treat chronic disease
   b. treat acute, infectious diseases
   c. provide relief from chronic pain and reduce stress
   d. treat mental illness

7. Jason is insured by a medical plan that only pays for certain doctors in a specific region. If Jason sees other physicians or providers, he pays most or all of the fees himself. This insurance plan is best described as using:
   a. a conventional fee-for-service plan
   b. a preferred provider organization
   c. a part of Medicaid
   d. a traditional, private insurance policy

8. The insurance plan providing care to those below a certain income level is:
   a. a health maintenance organization
   b. a preferred provider organization
   c. Medicaid
   d. Medicare

9. A number of reasons have been given to explain the rise in health care costs. One of the following is not a primary reason. Choose the INCORRECT statement from the following options.
   a. Population increases, unemployment, and single-income families have caused health care costs to rise dramatically.
   b. Increased costs for malpractice insurance have driven insurance costs up.
   c. Overspecialization of physicians, facilities and equipment has increased costs of health care.
   d. Rising costs for administration and processing "paperwork" are passed on to the consumer in the form of higher health care costs.

10. How does socioeconomic status play a role in health care?
    a. those with lower incomes have less education on appropriate self-care
    b. those with lower incomes have poorer access to medical care and resources
    c. health risks like smoking, excessive drinking, and exposure to violence are more prevalent among lower income groups
    d. all of the above

True/False

Determine whether each of the following statements is true or false:

1. Questioning diagnoses and treatments is part of being a wise health care consumer.

2. Using emergency rooms instead of your family doctor will help cut medical costs.

3. The quality of health care can be influenced by the interaction between patient and physician.

4. The Patient's Bill of Rights provides information on common situations and questions encountered by hospital patients.

5. All citizens of the United States have universal access to health care.

6. Homeopathy advocates giving tiny doses of drugs to produce disease symptoms and stimulate the body's natural defenses.

7. Because their training is similar, osteopathic physicians and medical doctors can both prescribe drugs and perform surgery.

8. Scientific validation of acupuncture has made it a fairly common, medically reimbursable procedure in the United States.

9. The United States spends more on medical care than any other country.

10. People's health can be influenced by their education, income, and employment.

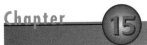

Chapter 15

Use these study questions to test your knowledge of the chapter material. The answer key is located at the end of the study guide.

Multiple Choice

Choose the best answer from the available options:

1. The average life expectancy at birth in the United States has _____ over the past several decades.
   a. increased
   b. decreased
   c. stayed the same
   d. increased, then decreased sharply

2. What are consequences of the "graying of America"?
   a. extra medical care will be required by a larger group of older people
   b. social security reform will be necessary to ensure retirement benefits
   c. there will be more people with chronic illnesses and disabilities
   d. all of the above

3. The discipline of gerontology focuses on:
   a. the causes and mechanisms of aging
   b. disease processes in the specific body organs
   c. dying with dignity
   d. ethical issues related to terminal illness

4. Evidence for a "biological clock" focuses on studies of:
   a. the amount of protein consumed by laboratory animals
   b. elderly populations in Japan and Iceland
   c. the energy consumption, or specific metabolic rate, in animals
   d. animals that live longest in the wild

5. Choose the true statement(s).
   a. Osteoporosis occurs when the rate of bone breakdown exceeds the rate of bone renewal.
   b. Regular exercise reduces the risk of osteoporosis.
   c. Risk of osteoporosis increases for women after menopause.
   d. all of the above

6. When people are incapacitated, a previously prepared _____ can communicate their wishes about medical treatment to relatives and medical personnel.
   a. hospice
   b. living will
   c. informed consent
   d. statement of intent

7. _____ can be defined as assisting someone to experience a peaceful death.
   a. suicide
   b. anesthesia
   c. euthanasia
   d. homicide

8. Which of the following statements is NOT true?
   a. Hospices offer comprehensive care for the terminally ill.
   b. Hospice care involves medication to control pain.
   c. Hospices use innovative treatments to extend life as long as possible.
   d. Hospice care may be given in a patient's home, hospital, or clinic.

9. People with Alzheimer's disease have an accumulation of _____ in certain parts of the brain.
   a. aluminum
   b. low density lipoprotein
   c. amyloid protein
   d. cholesterol

10. Most people in the United States view old age as a time:
    a. of sickness, disability, loneliness, and inactivity
    b. to enjoy the fruits of a life of work
    c. for further growth and development
    d. in the life cycle that is to be expected and even welcomed

11. According to the "error catastrophe" hypothesis of aging:
    a. the thymus gland produces a hormone that causes aging
    b. cellular repair mechanisms become increasingly damaged
    c. the cells of each species of animal have a specific, biologically determined life span
    d. immune system functions decline, causing aging

12. When told that they are going to die soon, people tend to respond with:
    a. denial first, followed eventually by acceptance
    b. anger first, then denial to the end of life
    c. depression that often lasts until death
    d. fear first, followed by anger and denial

True/False

Determine whether each of the following statements is true or false:

1. Ageism is a social movement working to ensure the rights of older citizens.
2. The United States has the longest life expectancy of any nation.
3. For most people, midlife transition occurs in their early 30s.
4. Research indicates that certain genes contribute to the development of Alzheimer's disease.
5. Evidence strongly indicates that undernourished lab animals live longer than those on unrestricted diets.
6. Alzheimer's disease can be treated effectively with drug therapy.
7. The more education you have, the less likely you are to develop Alzheimer's disease.
8. Estrogen replacement therapy can reduce the risk of osteoporosis in older women.
9. Heart disease is the leading killer of adults over 65.
10. Physician-assisted suicide is a form of euthanasia.

Study Guide

Chapter **16**

Multiple Choice

Choose the best answer from the available options:

1. Species extinction and habitat destruction are issues most closely related to the environmental concern of:
   a. global warming
   b. ozone depletion
   c. the greenhouse effect
   d. loss of biodiversity

2. One of the most common pollutants in urban air is _____, which causes health problems by interfering with oxygen use in the body.
   a. carbon dioxide
   b. nitrous oxide
   c. carbon monoxide
   d. sulfur oxide

3. The greenhouse effect occurs because _____ in the atmosphere act (s) like the glass in a greenhouse, letting the sun's rays in and "trapping" the warmth.
   a. ozone
   b. chlorofluorocarbons
   c. carbon dioxide
   d. carbon monoxide

4. Plants and trees:
   a. absorb carbon dioxide
   b. give off oxygen
   c. are critical to global temperature stability
   d. all of the above

5. The most serious indoor air pollutant is:
   a. wood smoke
   b. radon gas
   c. lead residue
   d. cigarette smoke

6. People using wood stoves and fireplaces should be aware that:
   a. prolonged exposure to wood smoke may increase susceptibility to lung infections
   b. heating with wood is a healthier alternative to gas or electric heat
   c. wood stoves should be open, not airtight, to allow heat circulation
   d. rooms should be airtight to maintain heat and conserve energy

7. What do producing gasoline, brewing beer, and making steel have in common?
   a. they use large amounts of water
   b. they require fossil fuels
   c. they contribute to acid rain
   d. they hasten the process of species extinction

8. Which of the following statements is true?
   a. Pesticides are monitored by the EPA and are seldom dangerous.
   b. Pesticides do not affect large animals like alligators.
   c. When pesticides are discontinued, residues rapidly wash out of the soil.
   d. Soil and water are becoming increasingly contaminated by pesticides and many have been banned by the EPA.

9. Polychlorinated biphenyls (PCBs):
   a. have been banned in the United States for decades
   b. were found to cause cancer in laboratory animals
   c. may cause abnormal activity in the thyroid gland
   d. all of the above

10. The world's population is expected to _____ during the first part of the 21st century.
    a. increase
    b. decrease
    c. stay the same
    d. stabilize and then decrease

11. Which of the following is NOT a major air pollutant?
    a. carbon monoxide
    b. carbon dioxide
    c. nitrogen dioxide
    d. sulfur dioxide

12. At least half of people's exposure to benzene, a cancer-causing chemical, comes from:
    a. automobile exhausts
    b. fumes that leak out when people fill their gas tanks
    c. manufacturing of chemicals and plastics
    d. cigarette smoke

13. Plumbism is a term for:
    a. chemical pollution of the environment
    b. lead poisoning
    c. toxic exposure to pesticides
    d. poisoning by mercury and cadmium

True/False

Determine whether each of the following statements is true or false:

1. Overpopulation is the single most significant environmental problem.

2. Taking lead out of gasoline has little effect on air pollution.

3. Photochemical smog is produced when gases from sunlight mix with auto pollutants.

4. The ozone layer protects the earth from dangerous ultraviolet radiation.

5. Exposure refers to the amount of a substance released into the atmosphere from a source of pollution.

6. Radon is a gas found in ultraviolet radiation.

7. The best solution to the problem of contaminated water is to add chlorine to the water supply.

8. Congressional legislation such as the Superfund Act has succeeded in having most hazardous waste sites "cleaned up."

9. Research has found a strong association between electromagnetic fields and cancer.

10. All environmental problems can be related to human activities.

Answers to Study Guide Questions

Chapter 1: Answers to Multiple Choice

1. c	2. b	3. b	4. d	5. c
6. d	7. d	8. b	9. d	10. a
11. d	12. d	13. c	14. c	15. b

Chapter 1: Answers to True/False

1. false	2. false	3. true	4. true	5. false
6. true	7. true	8. true	9. true	10. true

Chapter 2: Answers to Multiple Choice

1. a	2. d	3. c	4. b	5. d
6. c	7. d	8. a	9. d	10. d
11. a	12. b	13. c	14. b	

Chapter 2: Answers to True/False

1. true	2. false	3. true	4. false	5. true
6. true	7. false	8. true	9. true	10. true

Chapter 3: Answers to Multiple Choice

1. a	2. c	3. c	4. c	5. a
6. b	7. d	8. c	9. d	10. b
11. d	12. c	13. b	14. b	

Chapter 3: Answers to True/False

1. true	2. true	3. true	4. true	5. true
6. true	7. false	8. true	9. false	10. false

Chapter 4: Answers to Multiple Choice

1. b	2. c	3. d	4. c	5. b
6. d	7. c	8. d	9. c	10. c
11. c	12. d	13. c	14. d	15. a
16. d				

Chapter 4: Answers to True/False

1. true	2. false	3. true	4. false	5. true
6. true	7. false	8. true	9. false	10. true

Chapter 5: Answers to Multiple Choice

1. d	2. b	3. a	4. b	5. b
6. c	7. d	8. d	9. d	10. d
11. d	12. b	13. d		

Chapter 5: Answers to True/False

1. true	2. false	3. false	4. true	5. false
6. true	7. false	8. false	9. true	10. false

Chapter 6: Answers to Multiple Choice

1. d	2. d	3. c	4. a	5. d
6. a	7. b	8. c	9. c	10. b
11. d	12. c	13. b	14. c	

Chapter 6: Answers to True/False

1. false	2. true	3. false	4. true	5. true
6. true	7. false	8. true	9. true	10. true

Chapter 7: Answers to Multiple Choice

1. c	2. b	3. a	4. d	5. c
6. a	7. a	8. c	9. d	10. a
11. b	12. d	13. d	14. a	15. d

Chapter 7: Answers to True/False

1. false	2. false	3. false	4. true	5. true
6. fasle	7. true	8. true	9. true	10. false

Chapter 8: Answers to Multiple Choice

1. b	2. b	3. a	4. c	5. c
6. d	7. b	8. d	9. d	10. a
11. c	12. a	13. c		

Chapter 8: Answers to True/False

1. false	2. false	3. true	4. true	5. true
6. false	7. true	8. false	9. false	10. true

Chapter 9: Answers to Multiple Choice

1. a	2. c	3. c	4. b	5. b
6. a	7. b	8. d	9. a	10. c
11. b	12. a	13. b	14. a	

Chapter 9: Answers to True/False

1. true	2. true	3. false	4. false	5. true
6. false	7. true	8. false	9. false	10. false

Chapter 10: Answers to Multiple Choice

1. b	2. b	3. a	4. c	5. c
6. a	7. d	8. d	9. b	10. d
11. a	12. c	13. c	14. d	15. b
16. d	17. c			

Chapter 10: Answers to True/False

1. false	2. true	3. true	4. false	5. true
6. true	7. false	8. false	9. false	10. true

Chapter 11: Answers to Multiple Choice

1. b	2. a	3. c	4. b	5. c
6. d	7. c	8. b	9. d	10. d
11. a	12. b	13. c	14. b	15. d
16. c				

Chapter 11: Answers to True/False

1. false	2. true	3. true	4. false	5. false
6. true	7. false	8. false	9. true	10. true

Study Guide

Chapter 12: Answers to Multiple Choice

1. a	2. d	3. c	4. a	5. b
6. c	7. c	8. d	9. a	10. b
11. b	12. d	13. c	14. a	15. d

Chapter 12: Answers to True/False

1. true	2. true	3. true	4. false	5. false
6. true	7. false	8. true	9. true	10. true

Chapter 13: Answers to Multiple Choice

1. d	2. a	3. d	4. d	5. a
6. b	7. b	8. d	9. b	10. d
11. d	12. b	13. c	14. d	

Chapter 13: Answers to True/False

1. true	2. false	3. true	4. true	5. true
6. true	7. false	8. true	9. true	10. true

Chapter 14: Answers to Multiple Choice

1. d	2. a	3. d	4. d	5. b
6. c	7. b	8. c	9. a	10. d

Chapter 14: Answers to True/False

1. true	2. false	3. true	4. true	5. false
6. true	7. true	8. false	9. true	10. true

Chapter 15: Answers to Multiple Choice

1. a	2. d	3. a	4. c	5. d
6. b	7. c	8. c	9. c	10. a
11. b	12. a			

Chapter 15: Answers to True/False

1. false	2. false	3. false	4. true	5. true
6. false	7. true	8. true	9. true	10. true

Chapter 16: Answers to Multiple Choice

1. d	2. c	3. c	4. d	5. d
6. a	7. a	8. d	9. d	10. a
11. b	12. d	13. b		

Chapter 16: Answers to True/False

1. true	2. false	3. true	4. true	5. false
6. false	7. false	8. false	9. false	10. true

Index

Photo Credits